Management of Periprosthetic Joint Infection

Klaus-Dieter Kühn (Ed.)

Management of Periprosthetic Joint Infection

A global perspective on diagnosis, treatment options, prevention strategies and their economic impact

With 196 figures

Springer

Editor
Klaus-Dieter Kühn
Department of Orthopaedic Surgery
Medical University Graz
Austria

Library of Congress Control Number: 2017946542

ISBN 978-3-662-54468-6 978-3-662-54469-3 (eBook)
https://doi.org/10.1007/978-3-662-54469-3

Springer

Cover Design: deblik Berlin
Cover illustration: © Kindly licensed by Heraeus Medical GmbH

Printed on acid-free paper

This Springer imprint is published by Springer Nature
The registered company is Springer-Verlag GmbH, DE
The registered company address is: Heidelberger Platz 3, 14197 Berlin, Germany

Medical University of Graz

The Roman encyclopaedist Aulus Cornelius Celsus (ca. 25 BC–ca. 50 AD) described the diagnosis and therapy of fistulae caused by infectious disease, followed by the Andalusian physician and surgeon Abulcasis (Abu al-Qasim al-Zahrawi; 936 AD–1013 AD), who had already developed sophisticated surgical instruments to probe and excise these fistulae (see ◘ Fig. 1). At a time when electronically downloadable open-access articles are en vogue, the present volume stands in the tradition of good old-fashioned books with the great advantage of giving the readers a concise overview of the different topics. Professor Kühn has successfully managed to motivate a large number of internationally renowned experts in the diagnosis and treatment of periprosthetic joint infection to put their compressed experience, ideas, and recommendations into this volume. I sincerely thank him for this effort and hope you, the reader, gain new ideas from this book that will contribute towards the successful treatment of your patients.

A. Leithner

Albucasis

Forma experientis ex plumbo medij.

Forma experientis ex plumbo parui.

Forma vncinorum ⁊ sunt multarũ spẽruz: qm̃ ex eis sunt simplices. s. quibus est curuitas vna: ⁊ sunt trium speciez sicut vides: magni medij ⁊ parui: ⁊ ex eis sunt vncini ceci: ⁊ sunt trium specierũ: ⁊ ex eis sunt vncini habentes duas curuaturas: ⁊ sunt triũ specierũ: ⁊ ex eis sunt vncini hñtes tres curuaturas: ⁊ sunt triũ spẽz: ⁊ oẽs isti sũt necẽij in loco suo. Forma vncini simplicis magni.

Forma vncini simplicis medij.

Forma vncini simplicis parui.

Forma vncini ceci magni.

Forma vncini ceci medij.

Forma vncini ceci parui.

Forma vncini magni hñtis duas curuaturas.

Forma vncini medij hñtis duas curuaturas.

Forma vncini parui hñtis duas curuaturas.

Forma vncini magni hñtis tres curuaturas.

Forma vncini medij hñtis tres curuaturas.

Forma vncini parui hñtis tres curuaturas.

Et iste sunt forme scalpellorum quibus secantur ⁊ excoriantur nodi: ⁊ apostemata ⁊ sunt trium specieruz: quoniã ex eis est magnum medium ⁊ paruum. Eorum extremitates quibus fit sectio sunt acute: extremitates alie sunt nõ acute: ⁊ non ponuntur taliter nisi vt cum eis fiat iuuamẽtum in excoriatione nodorũ apud timorem incisionis vene aut nerui: Et vt sanetur per ea infirmus: ⁊ inueniat trãquillitatem parumper ex adustione quã inuenit apud excoriationem apostematis.

Forma scarpelli magni.

Forma scarpelli medij.

Forma scalpelli parui.

Iste sunt forme amagdea ⁊ sunt specierum trium.

Forma magda magni.

Forma magda medij.

Forma magda parui.

Forma vẽtose magne.

Forma vẽtose medie.

Forma vẽtose parue.

Forma spatumilis magni.

Forma spatumilis medij.

Forma spatumilis parui.

Fiunt ex ere ⁊ sunt similia radio: cum quo fit alcobol: ⁊ in extremitate lata est puncta spatumilis occultata: ⁊ in ea currit ad interiora: ⁊ ad exteriora quando vis sicut vides. Forma spatumiliũ que absconduntur inter digitos apud perforationẽ apostematũ: ⁊ non pcipiunt ea ĩfirmi: ⁊ sunt trium spẽrum magnũ medium ⁊ paruũ. Forma spatumili magni medij ⁊ parui rotundi cum extremitate puncte nunc dixi eos. Forma ventosarum cum quibus abscinditur fluxus sanguinis ⁊ sunt trium specierũ magne medie ⁊ parue. Fiant ex ere aut citrino rotunde ad longitudinez parũper sicut vides: ⁊ sint ad subtilitatẽ ⁊ oportet vt sint

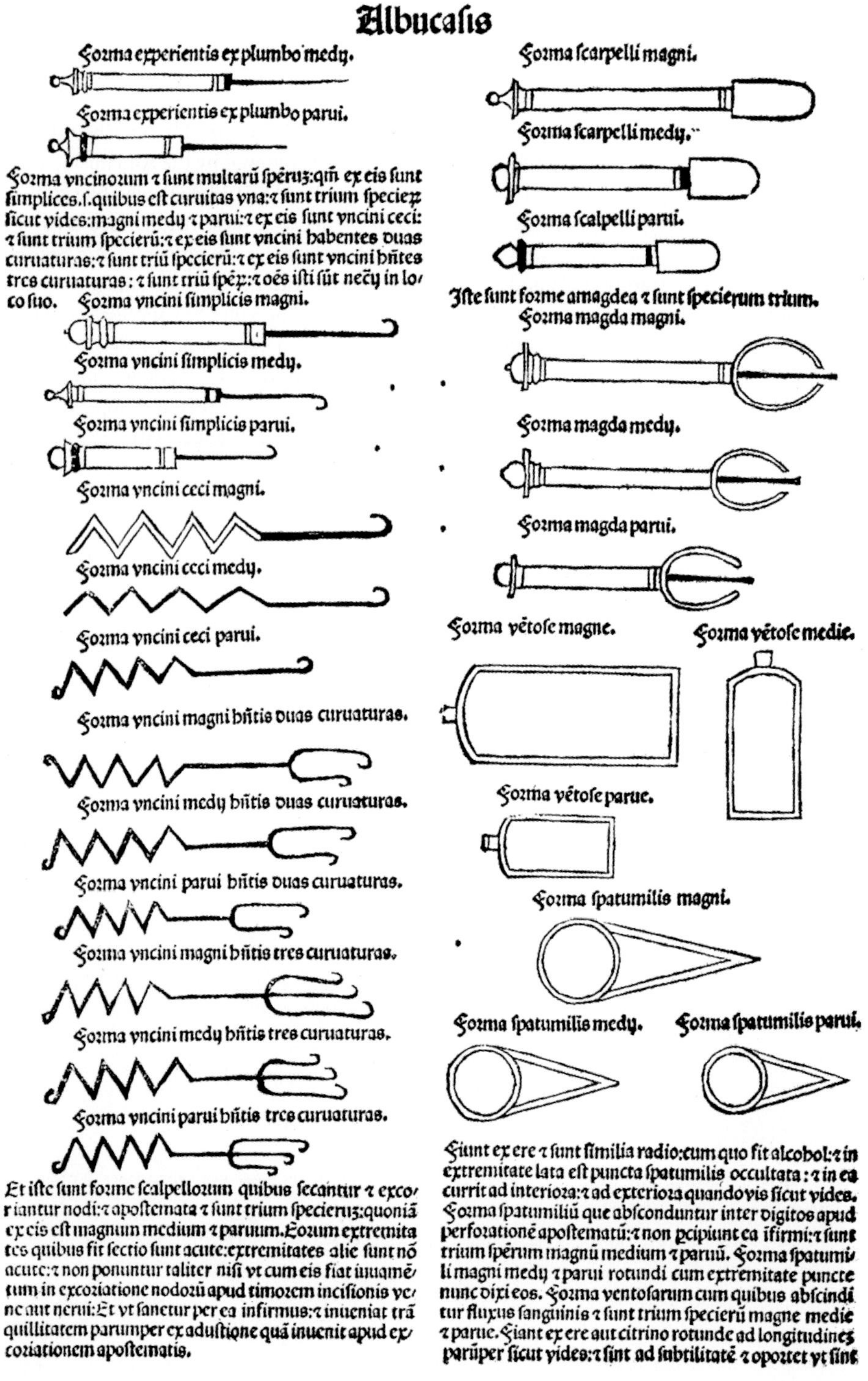

Fig. 1 Surgical instruments; anon, after designs originally drawn by Abulcasis (ca. 1000); Woodcut circa 1500; Chauliac, Guy de, Chirurgia parva. (Wellcome Library, London; https://wellcomeimages.org/indexplus/image/L0002051.html)

Foreword

The editor of this book, Klaus-Dieter Kühn, has succeeded in motivating many well-known experts to present their knowledge in the field of periprosthetic joint infections (PJI). Amongst these authors you will find different specialists – orthopaedic surgeons, infectious disease specialists and microbiologists. The chapters focus on a range of issues related to PJI, including economic factors, clinical aspects, diagnosis, prevention, microbiologic analyses, treatment algorithms, antibiotic-loaded bone cement, spacers and the potential of implants with anti-infective coating.

The strength of this book lies in the generously illustrated chapters that present a great variety of PJI cases. In presenting these cases, the authors explain the basis of their decisions for an adequate treatment. The careful study of this illustrative material allows the reader to choose the most appropriate algorithm for their practice. However, there is not much discussion on the results achieved with these algorithms.

This volume can be recommended to anyone dealing with PJI as a treasure trove of ideas. It is of special interest for orthopaedic surgeons or infectious disease specialists who are confronted with clinical infections. It will be the duty of each individual reader to gather their own clinical experience on the basis of the new ideas presented in this book.

The treatment of musculoskeletal infections has changed a great deal in the past few decades. One of the most important achievements is that treatment of musculoskeletal infections is decided in a team. This should be composed of at least an orthopaedic surgeon and an infectious disease specialist, supported on a case-by-case basis by a microbiologist, a pathologist and a plastic surgeon. In countries that do not have the speciality of infectious diseases, internists should be motivated to acquire special knowledge in this field.

As a young resident in the 1970s, I was shocked by the fate of patients affected by PJI. I often saw them suffering from large open wounds after incomplete removal of the implants and the bone cement. Frequently, they remained handicapped for the rest of their life. Fortunately, step by step, we learnt how to improve this situation. After realizing that debridement means the complete removal of all foreign bodies – including any gentamicin beads left behind – healing of the wounds could be achieved. New ideas such as loading bone cement with gentamicin, re-implantation of a prosthesis after a successful Girdlestone situation and the method of Buchholz, daring to carry out a one-step exchange in PJI, came into the picture.

At the orthopaedic department in Liestal Hospital near Basel we were faced with a growing number of patients who were referred to us with bone infections. Progressively, we learnt about the key elements necessary for a better handling of these cases. A thorough debridement included not only the removal of all foreign bodies, but also an adequate resection of necrotic bone. We tested the quality of debridement by analysing the resected bone in our own laboratory for non-decalcified histology so as to be sure not to resect neither too much nor too little. After debridement we proceeded to immediate closure of all wounds, if necessary with the help of the plastic surgeon instead of allowing for a delay by application of negative pressure dressing. Any imminent leaking of a postoperative wound was prevented by an immediate re-intervention completed with new drainage.

Re-implantation of a total joint after a Girdlestone hip was successfully changed to a two-step replacement with an interval of only 2–3 weeks. Following the idea of Buchholz, in cases of PJI proven by arthrocentesis presenting with uneventful tissues we favoured a one-step exchange. Finally, revision with retention of the prosthesis was chosen for early infections of up to 3 weeks. By introducing this Liestal algorithm the number of recurrences gradually decreased, as proved in the repeated scientific follow-ups of all our cases.

Using the following additional diagnostic measures, the number of PJI without known micro-organisms dropped below 4%: discontinuation of the antibiotic therapy for 2 weeks, harvesting of three to five tissue samples instead of swabs, sonication of the removed foreign bodies and leucocyte count in the synovial fluid.

Feeling that I was not sufficiently trained to manage the antibiotic therapy, I looked for help, which I found with the infectious disease specialist Werner Zimmerli, who worked at the University of Basel. He later changed to Liestal where he became the head of the internal medicine department. To treat early biofilms without exchange of the prosthesis represented a significant challenge. We could achieve much better results treating early staphylococcal infections by adding rifampicin to the conventional antibiotic. This was proven with a randomized study.

A number of micro-organisms were resistant to our two-step exchange with a short interval. Infections by so-called difficult-to-treat bacteria – such as small colony variants of common bacteria, enterococci, rifampicin-resistant staphylococci, fungi and some others – could be treated by another type of two-stage procedure that included a long interval of 8–10 weeks without a spacer. During this period, a curative antibiotic treatment of the infection without foreign material can be achieved.

The main secrets for a successful treatment of PJI are:

- Clear definition of the different elements of the treatment and their application without compromise.
- Rigorous application of an algorithm once it has been selected as a basis for a scientific control
- Collaboration of the orthopaedic surgeon and the infectious disease specialist with access to specialized partners in microbiology, histology and plastic surgery
- Long-term follow-up of all the patients treated, including a scientific analysis of the results in order to prove the quality of the chosen algorithm

To promote better treatment, »Swiss orthopaedics« in 2006 created an expert group on »infections of the musculoskeletal system« comprising a representative number of orthopaedic surgeons and infectious disease specialists. This group edited a pocketbook including an e-book version on the treatment of these infections, which can be ordered for free on www.swissorthopaedics.ch or www.ebjis.org.

If this present book on PJI motivates the reader to do a better job in the therapy of these unfortunate patients by following strict algorithms and practising an interdisciplinary treatment, then it has achieved an important goal.

Peter E. Ochsner
Emeritus Extraordinarius Professor in Orthopaedics at the University of Basel

Preface

Periprosthetic joint infection (PJI) is among the most serious complications in the field of endoprosthetics. The number of PJIs is increasing worldwide and poses a real interdisciplinary challenge for everyone involved. Beside its immense impact on patients and the health-care system, the diagnosis and management of PJI are very difficult, since there is no »gold standard«.

This book provides basic and advanced knowledge of the diverse aspects of periprosthetic joint infections and a comprehensive overview on a global scale, which was possible only because of the close collaboration of international experts. Various issues such as diagnosis, treatment options, prevention strategies and their economic impact are addressed in order to exchange versatile experience and know-how. Furthermore, attention was given to antibiotic-loaded bone cements (ALBC), spacer management and anti-infective implant coatings.

This compilation offers an ample summary to a multidisciplinary audience. Not only for the microbiologist, who is responsible for identifying the causative germs, the infectious disease specialist, who can recommend the appropriate antibiotic therapy, the clinical pharmacist, who is consulted regularly throughout the therapy to discuss the risk of potential drug interactions, or the surgeon, who will proceed with the revision surgery, following defined algorithms, but also for any other interested reader. Moreover, it may also help affected patients to understand the clinical procedure.

This book aims to contribute to a fruitful international debate concerning the ideal management of PJI. In addition, the reader can use this book as a solid platform for comparing their own approach to PJI treatment with the specialists' recommendations.

Prof. Dr. Klaus-Dieter Kühn
Department of Orthopaedic Surgery
Medical University of Graz
Austria

Acknowledgements

My sincere thanks to all the authors for agreeing to provide a scientific contribution to this book. Despite having many other obligations, they took the time to share their clinical experience and offer valuable information for the reader. Based on this essential support, it was possible to give a comprehensive overview of the topic of periprosthetic joint infections on a global scale.

Because of the abundant clinical data, it would have been impossible to produce a successful compilation of all the multifaceted contributions without additional scientific support. Thus, I would like to express a special thanks to S. Vogt and C. Berberich for our great scientific discussions, as well as E. Lieb, L. Schell, M. Schulze, J. Schmiedel, O. Vornkahl, D. Müller, and A. Klotz for their support during the review procedure. In particular, I thank A. Roggeman, who was always willing to offer assistance in the international correspondence and networking.

Since the book includes various contributions from many different countries it was often necessary to contact the authors directly. This would have been impossible without S. Buitendag and A. Peyper (SA), M. Zaaijer (B, NL), T. Smith (UK), S. Tye and C. Berberich (AUS), L. Kiontke (UK, AUS, USA), E. Lieb (F), and T. Kluge (USA), whom I want to thank for their commitment.

Furthermore, I would like to thank M. Zimni for the creation of the book cover and other graphics, U. Dächert of Springer for managing the publication of the book, I. Athanassiou for professional editing, and S. Janka for the initial compilation of the submitted contributions.

Special thanks to A. Holl for her competent assistance in creating figures as well as in viewing and editing the contributions all the way to the printing stage.

My thanks to Prof. Dr. A. Leithner, Medical University of Graz, Department of Orthopaedic Surgery, for the opportunity and freedom to create the present book.

Last, but not least, I would like to thank Prof. P. Ochsner for the friendly and professional foreword.

Table of Contents

List of Contributors

Florian Ludwig Amerstorfer
Department of Orthopaedics and Trauma Surgery, Medical University of Graz
Auenbruggerplatz 5
8036 Graz
Styria, Austria
FlorianLudwig.Amerstorfer@klinikum-graz.at

Frédéric Auburn
Department of Anesthesia, Hôpital de la Croix-Rousse, Hospices Civils de Lyon; CRIOAc Lyon
Université Claude Bernard Lyon 1
Quai des Célestins 3
69002 Lyon
Auvergne-Rhône-Alpes, France
frederic.auburn@chu-lyon.fr

Christoph Berberich
Heraeus Medical GmbH
Philipp-Reis-Straße 8–13
61273 Wehrheim
Hesse, Germany
christof.berberich@heraeus.com

James Robert Berstock
Musculoskeletal Research Unit, Department of Orthopaedics, Avon Orthopaedic Centre, Southmead Hospital
Dorian Way
BS10 5NB Bristol
South West England, UK
James.Berstock@gmail.com

Isabelle Bobineau
Department of Anesthesia, Hôpital de la Croix-Rousse, Hospices Civils de Lyon; CRIOAc Lyon
Université Claude Bernard Lyon 1
Quai des Célestins 3
69002 Lyon
Auvergne-Rhône-Alpes, France
isabelle.bobineau@chu-lyon.fr

Willemijn Boot
Department of Orthopaedics, University Medical Center Utrecht
Heidelberglaan 100
3584 CX Utrecht
Utrecht, The Netherlands
W.Boot@umcutrecht.nl

Olivier Borens
Service d'Orthopédie et de Traumatologie, Centre Hospitalier Universitaire Vaudois (CHUV)
Rue de Bugnon 46
1011 Lausanne
Canton of Vaud, Switzerland
Olivier.Borens@chuv.ch

David G. Campbell
Wakefield Orthopaedic Clinic
University of Adelaide
Wakefield Street 270
5000 Adelaide
South Australia, Australia
hipknee@tpg.com.au

Jason H. H. Chan
Royal National Orthopaedic Hospital (RNOH) NHS Trust
Brockley Hil
HA7 4LP, Stanmore
Greater London, UK
jhhchan@doctors.org.uk

Yuhan Chang
Division of Joint Reconstruction, Department of Orthopaedic Surgery, Chang Gung Memorial Hospital, Linko
Fuxing Street 5
333 Taoyuan City
Guishan District, Taiwan
yhchang@cloud.cgmh.org.tw

Ben Clark
Fremantle Hospital
Alma Street
6160 Fremantle
Western Australia, Australia
ben.clark@health.wa.gov.au

Elena De Vecchi
Laboratory of Clinical Chemistry and Microbiology,
IRCCS Galeazzi Orthopaedic Institute
Via Festa del Perdono 7
20122 Milan
Lombardy, Italy
elena.devecchi@grupposandonato.it

Lorenzo Drago
Laboratory of Clinical Chemistry and Microbiology,
IRCCS Galeazzi Orthopaedic Institute
Laboratory of Clinical Microbiology, Department of
Biomedical Sciences for Health, University of Milan
Via R. Galeazzi 4
20161 Milan
Lombardy, Italy
lorenzo.drago@unimi.it

Tristan Ferry
Infectious Disease Unit, Hôpital de la Croix-Rousse,
Hospices Civils de Lyon; CRIOAc Lyon
Université Claude Bernard Lyon 1
Quai des Célestins 3
69002 Lyon
Auvergne-Rhône-Alpes, France
tristan.ferry@chu-lyon.fr

Bernd Fink
Clinic of Joint Replacement, General and
Rheumatic Orthopaedics, Orthopaedic Clinic
Markgröningen gGmbH
Kurt-Lindemann-Weg 10
71706 Markgröningen
Baden-Württemberg, Germany
Bernd.Fink@okm.de

Lars Frommelt
Helios Endo-Klinik Hamburg
Holstenstraße 2
22767 Hamburg
Hamburg, Germany
lars.frommelt@me.com

Enrico Gallazzi
Department of Reconstructive Surgery and
Osteo-articular Infections C.R.I.O. Unit - I.R.C.C.S.
Galeazzi Orthopaedic Institute
University of Milan
Via R. Galeazzi 4
20161 Milan
Lombardy, Italy
enrico.gallazzi@gmail.com

Thorsten Gehrke
Helios Endo-Klinik Hamburg
Holstenstraße 2
22767 Hamburg
Hamburg, Germany
Thorsten.Gehrke@helios-kliniken.de

Mathias Glehr
Department of Orthopaedics and Trauma Surgery,
Medical University of Graz
Auenbruggerplatz 5
8036 Graz
Styria, Austria
Mathias.Glehr@klinikum-graz.at

Sascha Gravius
Clinic for Orthopaedics and Trauma Surgery, Bonn
University Hospital
Sigmund-Freud-Straße 25
53105 Bonn
North Rhine-Westphalia, Germany
sascha.gravius@ukb.uni-bonn.de

Tim Hanstein
Heraeus Medical GmbH
Philipp-Reis-Straße 8–13
61273 Wehrheim
Hesse, Germany
tim.hanstein@heraeus.com

Hans J.G.E. Hendriks
Máxima Medisch Centrum (MMC)
Ds Theodor Fliednerstraat 1
5631 BM, Eindhoven
Noord-Brabant, The Netherlands
jge_hendriks@hotmail.com

Yannick Herry
Department of Anesthesia, Hôpital de la Croix-Rousse, Hospices Civils de Lyon; CRIOAc Lyon
Université Claude Bernard Lyon 1
Quai des Célestins 3
69002 Lyon
Auvergne-Rhône-Alpes, France
yannick.herry@chu-lyon.fr

Christopher W. Jones
Fremantle Hospital
University of Sydney
Alma Street
6160 Fremantle
Western Australia, Australia
cjon0040@gmail.com

Tamon Kabata
Department of Orthopaedic Surgery,
Graduate School of Medicine, Kanazawa University
Takara machi 13-1
920-8641 Kanazawa shi
Ishikawa Prefecture, Japan
tamonkabata@yahoo.co.jp

Susann Klimas
Heraeus Medical GmbH
Philipp-Reis-Straße 8–13
61273 Wehrheim
Hesse, Germany
susann.klimas@hotmail.de

Thomas Kluge
Heraeus Medical GmbH
Philipp-Reis-Straße 8–13
61273 Wehrheim
Hesse, Germany
thomas.kluge@heraeus.com

Hendrik Kohlhof
Clinic for Orthopaedics and Trauma Surgery, Bonn University Hospital
Sigmund-Freud-Straße 25
53105 Bonn
North Rhine-Westphalia, Germany
Hendrik.Kohlhof@ukb.uni-bonn.de

Andreas Kolb
Heraeus Medical GmbH
Philipp-Reis-Straße 8–13
61273 Wehrheim
Hesse, Germany
andreas.kolb@heraeus.com

Klaus-Dieter Kühn
Department of Orthopaedics and Trauma Surgery,
Medical University of Graz
Auenbruggerplatz 5
8036 Graz
Styria, Austria
klaus.kuehn@medunigraz.at

Frederic Laurent
Microbiology Laboratory, Hôpital de la Croix-Rousse, Hospices Civils de Lyon; CRIOAc Lyon
Université Claude Bernard Lyon 1
Quai des Célestins 3
69002 Lyon
Auvergne-Rhône-Alpes, France
frederic.laurent@univ-lyon1.fr

Andreas Leithner
Department of Orthopaedics and Trauma Surgery,
Medical University of Graz
Auenbruggerplatz 5
8036 Graz
Styria, Austria
andreas.leithner@medunigraz.at

Elke Lieb
Heraeus Medical GmbH
Philipp-Reis-Straße 8-13
61273 Wehrheim
Hesse, Germany
elke.lieb@heraeus.com

Sébastien Lustig
Orthopaedic Surgery Unit, Hôpital de la Croix-Rousse, Hospices Civils de Lyon; CRIOAc Lyon
Université Claude Bernard Lyon 1
Quai des Célestins 3
69002 Lyon
Auvergne-Rhône-Alpes, France
sebastien.lustig@chu-lyon.fr

Ashutosh Malhotra
Heraeus Medical GmbH
Philipp-Reis-Straße 8–13
61273 Wehrheim
Hesse, Germany
ashutosh.malhotra@heraeus.com

John McManus
Service d'Orthopédie et de Traumatologie, Centre Hospitalier Universitaire Vaudois (CHUV)
Rue du Bugnon 46
CH-1011 Lausanne
Canton of Vaud, Switzerland
John.McManus@chuv.ch

Ilaria Morelli
Department of Reconstructive Surgery and Osteo-articular Infections C.R.I.O. Unit - I.R.C.C.S. Galeazzi Orthopaedic Institute
University of Milan
Via R. Galeazzi 4
20161 Milan
Lombardy, Italy
ilaria.morelli90@gmail.com

Vincent M. Moretti
Rothman Institute at Thomas Jefferson University
9th Street 125 S
PA 19107 Philadelphia
Pennsylvania, USA
vincent.moretti@gmail.com

Jeroen G.V. Neyt
University Hospitals Leuven - Campus Pellenberg
Weligerveld 1
3212 Lubbeek
Flanders, Belgium
jeroen.neyt@uzleuven.be

Peter E. Ochsner
University of Basel
Petersplatz 1
4003 Basel
Canton Basel City, Switzerland
peter.ochsner@hin.ch

Dean F.M. Pakvis
OCON Orthopedic Clinic Hengelo
Geerdinksweg 141
7555 DL Hengelo
Overijssel, The Netherlands
d.pakvis@ocon.nl

Paul F. Partington
Spire Washington Hospital
Northumbria Healthcare NHS Foundation Trust
Picktree Lane
NE38 9JZ Washington
Tyne & Wear, UK
paul.partington@btopenworld.com

Javad Parvizi
Rothman Institute, Thomas Jefferson University
9th Street 125 S
PA 19107 Philadelphia
Pennsylvania, USA
javadparvizi@gmail.com

Carlo Luca Romanò
Department of Reconstructive Surgery and Osteo-articular Infections C.R.I.O. Unit – I.R.C.C.S. Galeazzi Orthopaedic Institute
University of Milan
Via R. Galeazzi 4
20161 Milan
Lombardy, Italy
carlo.romano@grupposandonato.it

Vincent Ronin
Prevention and Infection Control Unit, Hôpital de la Croix-Rousse, Hospices Civils de Lyon; CRIOAc Lyon
Université Claude Bernard Lyon 1
Quai des Célestins 3
69002 Lyon
Auvergne-Rhône-Alpes, France
vincent.ronin@ars.sante.fr

Pablo Sanz-Ruiz
Orthopedic and Trauma Service, Gregorio Marañon General University Hospital
Complutense University
Calle del Dr. Esquerdo 46
28007 Madrid
Madrid, Spain
pablo.sanzruiz@gmail.com

Sara Scarponi
Department of Reconstructive Surgery and Osteo-articular Infections C.R.I.O. Unit – I.R.C.C.S. Galeazzi Orthopaedic Institute
University of Milan
Via R. Galeazzi 4
20161 Milan
Lombardy, Italy
scarponi1981@libero.it

John Segreti
University Infectious Diseases, Rush University Medical Center
Paulina St. 600 S.
IL 60612 Chicago
Illinois, USA
john_segreti@rush.edu

Kiran Singisetti
Sheffield Teaching Hospitals NHS Foundation Trust, Royal Hallamshire Hospital
Glossop Rd
S10 2JF Sheffield
South Yorkshire, UK
kiransingisetti@gmail.com

Ralf Skripitz
Zentrum für Endoprothetik, Fußchirurgie, Kinder - und Allgemeine Orthopädie, Roland-Klinik
Niedersachsendamm 72/74
28201 Bremen
Bremen, Germany
rskripitz@roland-klink.de

Ian Stockley
Sheffield Teaching Hospitals NHS Foundation Trust, Royal Hallamshire Hospital
Glossop Rd
S10 2JF Sheffield
South Yorkshire, UK
ianstockley56@gmail.com

René H.M. ten Broeke
Department of Orthopaedic Surgery, Maastricht University Medical Centre
P. Debyelaan 25
6229 HX Maastricht
Limburg, The Netherlands
r.tenbroeke@compaqnet.nl

Hiroyuki Tsuchiya
Department of Orthopaedic Surgery, Graduate School of Medicine, Kanazawa University
Takara machi 13-1
920-8641 Kanazawa shi
Ishikawa Prefecture, Japan
tsuchi@med.kanazawa-u.ac.jp

Florent Valour
Infectious Disease Unit, Hôpital de la Croix-Rousse, Hospices Civils de Lyon; CRIOAc Lyon
Université Claude Bernard Lyon 1
Quai des Célestins 3
69002 Lyon
Auvergne-Rhône-Alpes, France
florent.valour@chu-lyon.fr

Laura van Dommelen
Máxima Medisch Centrum (MMC)
Ds Theodor Fliednerstraat 1
5631 BM Eindhoven
Noord-Brabant, The Netherlands
L.vanDommelen@pamm.nl

Robin W.T.M. van Kempen
Máxima Medisch Centrum (MMC)
Ds Theodor Fliednerstraat 1
5631 BM Eindhoven
Noord-Brabant, The Netherlands
robin.v.kempen@catharinaziekenhuis.nl

Manuel Villanueva-Martinez
Avanfi - Instituto Avanzado en Medicina Deportiva, Traumatología, Podología y Fisioterapia
Orense 32
28020 Madrid
Madrid, Spain
mvillanuevam@gmail.com

Anthony Viste
Orthopaedic Trauma and Surgery Unit, Centre Hospitalier Lyon-Sud, Hospices Civils de Lyon; CRIOAc Lyon
Université Claude Bernard Lyon 1
Quai des Célestins 3
69002 Lyon
Auvergne-Rhône-Alpes, France
viste.anthony@gmail.com

H. Charles Vogely
University Medical Center Utrecht, Department of Orthopaedics
Heidelberglaan 100
3584 CX Utrecht
Utrecht, The Netherlands
h.ch.vogely@umcutrecht.nl

Götz von Foerster
Helios Endo-Klinik Hamburg
Holstenstraße 2
22767 Hamburg
Hamburg, Germany
goetz.vonfoerster@helios-kliniken.de

Frank-Christiaan B.M. Wagenaar
OCON Orthopedic Clinic Hengelo
Geerdinksweg 141
7555 DL Hengelo
Overijssel, The Netherlands
f.wagenaar@ocon.nl

Jason C.J. Webb
Avon Orthopaedic Centre, Southmead Hospital
Dorian Way
BS10 5NB Bristol
South West England, UK
jcjwebb@doctors.org.uk

Piers Yates
Department of Orthopaedics and Trauma
Fremantle Hospital
Alma Street
6160 Fremantle
Western Australia, Australia
piers.yates@uwa.edu.au

Introduction

K.-D. Kühn (Ed.), *Management of Periprosthetic Joint Infection*
DOI 10.1007/978-3-662-54469-3_1

1.1 Interview

Javad Parvizi and Thorsten Gehrke

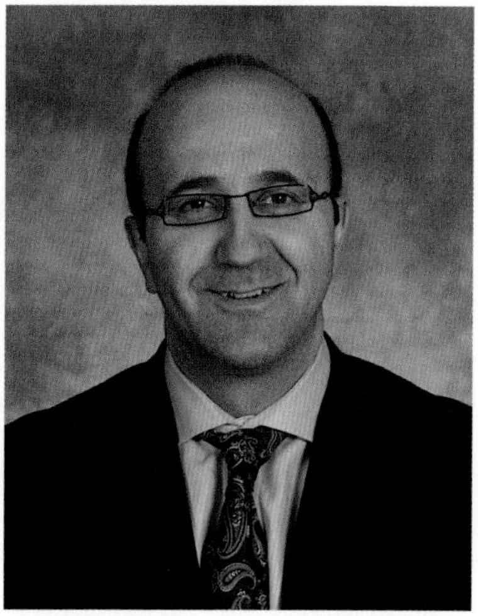

Fig. 1.1 Javad Parvizi

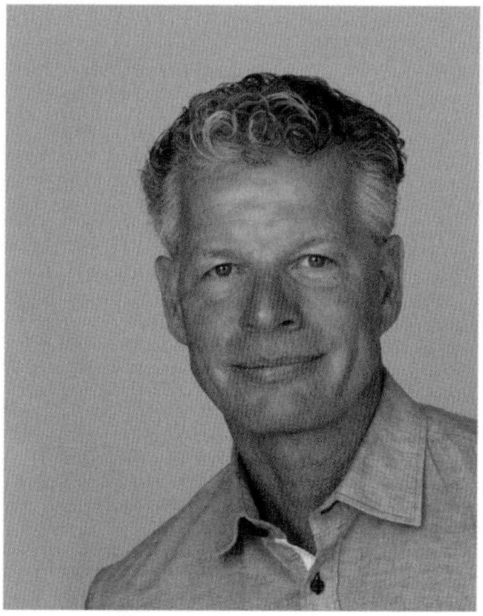

Fig. 1.2 Thorsten Gehrke

- **How important is it to know the pathogen profile before surgery? What if you do not have complete confidence in the pathogen profile before surgery?**

Isolation of the pathogen causing periprosthetic joint infection (PJI) allows the clinicians to refine the treatment to cover the infecting organism. By this, we mean the type of antibiotic added to cement or administered to the patient is based on the nature and sensitivity of the infecting organism. If the culture has been negative and we have not been able to isolate the infecting organism, then we attempt to gain information about the pathogen using molecular techniques.

- **How confident do you feel with poly-microbial infections?**

We believe that majority of PJIs are poly-microbial in nature. The inability of the traditional culture to isolate more than one organism is partly because one of the organisms is more dominant than the others and hence only the dominant pathogen, or a pathogen that appears to grow better in a given culture, is isolated. This raises the issue that moving forward we need to seek better technologies that will identify *all* the infecting organisms and not only the dominant organism that happens to grow in the given culture conditions. The poly-microbial nature of the PJI may explain why some treatments of patients with surgical infection fail at a later date with a new organism. This is not, in our opinion, a re-infection but rather a persistence of an infection that was not covered by the initially administered antibiotics. Acknowledging the poly-microbial nature of PJI then allows us to implement a wider scope of treatment that covers all organisms. Moving forward there is a need for molecular techniques that isolate the pathogen DNA and do not rely on the growth of organisms on a traditional culture plate.

- **How appropriate is your approach for patients with additional host-related risk factors?**

It is a known fact that patients who are immunocompromised or those with severe comorbidities are at a higher risk for failure following treatment for PJI. Therefore, it is extremely important to prepare and optimize patients properly prior to surgical intervention in an attempt to reduce the failure rate. This may include halting immunosuppressive drugs, optimization of nutritional status, better diabetes control, and so on.

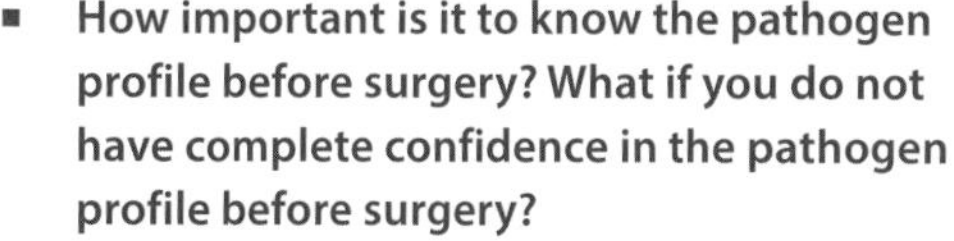

- **How appropriate is your approach for re-revisions?**

Re-revisions are complex cases. These require investment of much more time and effort to optimize the patient prior to surgical intervention. The aforementioned strategies in dealing with the issue of hyperglycaemia, malnutrition, anaemia, and other conditions becomes much more of a critical step in the management of these patients.

- **Are there any preferences with regard to cemented or uncemented fixation of revision implants in your approach?**

For management of patients with PJI who are undergoing one-stage exchange arthroplasty, the Endo-Klinik philosophy is that these patients should receive cemented fixation of the implant with the cement carrying the antibiotic directed towards the pathogen. In other circumstances, the treatment needs to be individualized and attention to the use of uncemented components should also be given, especially in cases of massive bone loss and other patients with challenging conditions.

- **What role do antibiotics play in bone cements in your approach?**

The use of antibiotic X (ABX)-loaded bone cement for management of PJI is, in our opinion, mandatory. The delivery of high doses of antibiotics at the site of infection contributes to improving outcome and infection control. In circumstances when cement fixation is being used for patients with prior PJI, careful attention should be given to the use of ABX-loaded cement.

- **How excessive should the debridement be in your approach?**

It has been our philosophy that management of PJI is much like treating cancer. The late George Cierney touted on numerous occasions the fact that surgical debridement should aim to obtain a »clear margin« in order to enhance the success of surgical intervention. Surgical debridement and the effort to reduce bio-burden are critical in optimizing the chances of surgical intervention. Basically we need to consider that surgical debridement is the most important step in the management of patients with PJI.

- **How experienced must the surgeon be to choose your pathway?**

The experience of the surgeon is important in dealing with patients with PJI. The experienced surgeon is likely to get better visualization of the surgical field and perform a more thorough debridement, which leads to a better outcome.

- **What about hospitalization and patient satisfaction in recovery?**

Every effort should be invested to minimize the hospital stay for patients with PJI. The rationale for this strategy is to reduce the risk of additional nosocomial infections. In addition, the patients who are discharged from the hospital are more likely to engage in activities of daily living earlier and clear functional milestones earlier. This in turn leads to higher satisfaction.

- **If you compare your approach with others regarding medicolegal aspects, where are the risks and the benefits?**

Management of patients with PJI is very complex and the outcome in many patients is unfortunately suboptimal. Management of PJI suffers from the lack of a standardized treatment regimen that compels surgeons to resort to the use of unconventional methods for treatment, sometimes with the devices being used on an off-label basis. The latter occurs despite the fact that patients may have to endure numerous operations.

- **Is there an algorithm you would propose before choosing the one- or two-stage procedure in a patient-adapted way?**

There is an algorithm that was designed by the international consensus on PJI. There are clear contraindications for the implementation of one-stage exchange arthroplasty. These contraindications have been clearly spelled out in the ICM document, such as the lack of inability to close the soft tissues, or culture-negative cases of PJI etc. In the rest of the circumstances we believe one-stage exchange arthroplasty offers an acceptable outcome and has a lower economic burden. This also allows patients to return to a functional status earlier. The outcome of one-stage exchange arthroplasty appears to parallel that of two-stage exchange in centres that perform high-volume surgical procedures for management of PJI.

- **Do you see a trend towards one or the other approach in the future?**

There is an increase in the popularity of one-stage exchange arthroplasty thanks to the emergence of data from centres like the Endo-Klinik and others. We feel that one-stage exchange arthroplasty is a great option for many patients with PJI and is currently underutilized in North America.

- **Prof. Javad Parvizi (Fig. 1) and Prof. Thorsten Gehrke (Fig. 2), thank you very much for this interview.**

Economic Aspects

K.-D. Kühn (Ed.), *Management of Periprosthetic Joint Infection*
DOI 10.1007/978-3-662-54469-3_2

2.1 Economic Aspects of Periprosthetic Joint Infections

Tim Hanstein and Ralf Skripitz

2.1.1 Economization of Health Care

With the introduction of lump sum reimbursements in the European health-care systems, economic pressure on hospitals has risen. Inpatient care is increasingly influenced by economic considerations and forces physicians to take – beside medical aspects – economic aspects into account. Contribution margins of elective procedures are calculated by hospital controllers and the cost for the operation, care, diagnostics, consumables, and stay should remain within the imputed average costs. If the treatment costs of a patient are below the average calculated costs, the hospital can gain an increased contribution margin with the least possible efforts, while a patient with treatment costs above the average costs leads to an economic burden for the hospital (Hanstein et al. 2015).

Similarly, economic pressure also exists in countries without a lump sum reimbursement system: In these countries, hospitals usually agree annually with their superordinate health authority on global budgets and on a certain number of patients or procedures to treat within this budget and period (Stargardt 2008; Geissler et al. 2011).

With each unplanned severe case or any additional case, the hospital's budget pressure grows. Lump sums have replaced single-cost reimbursement, although in some countries certain cost components of the treatment, such as the implant, are still reimbursed additionally. However, focussing on the total procedure costs is of utmost importance for the hospital for an effective and profitable treatment.

2.1.2 Orthopaedic Treatments

Total hip replacement (THR) and total knee replacement (TKR) are one of the most frequent elective operations in Europe and they have undergone steady improvements in the past few decades. Owing to process improvements in hospitals, which led to remarkably shortened lengths of stay for THR and TKR patients compared with previous decades, and the competition among hospitals for patients, there is great pressure to optimize the treatment from an economic and time perspective (Hanstein et al. 2015). Primary procedures are considered as cost-covering treatments from the hospital's perspective (Stargardt 2008; Haenle 2012a).

With infection rates below 2% of all total joint replacements (TJR) and a rate of approximately 10–20% for revisions (Bozic et al. 2009, 2010), periprosthetic joint infection (PJI) does not seem to be a major epidemiological issue. However, PJI can have a huge economic impact on the hospital and a personal impact for the affected patient (Alijanipour and Parvizi 2014).

Furthermore, PJIs are not only a challenge for the medical team and the patients alike, but the treatment costs are also expected to be high. While primary joint replacement procedures are said to be cost-covering and cost-effective, any adverse event such as a PJI poses a threat to the hospital's budget. But even with optimized surgical techniques, improved theatre conditions and prophylaxis measures, PJIs still occur. Therefore, it is essential to be aware of the economic consequences of PJIs for a hospital.

2.1.3 Reimbursement

The idea behind diagnosis-related groups (DRGs) is to combine a group of similar treatments in one reimbursement code; even within these groups it is possible to sub-classify the severity of a treatment with sub-groups (Kobel et al. 2011). For the calculation of a DRG, similar treatments are combined as a group and average costs are calculated. For most treatments, the concept of DRGs is well established and is working well. On the other hand, complex and costly treatments in the field of PJI might not fit into this rigid system of groups. The main problem is the method of grouping with average cost consideration (Lieb et al. 2015). Both aseptic revisions as well as septic revisions are included in the same DRG. Aseptic procedures often include comparatively simple treatments – such as the exchange of prosthesis parts only. While the serious procedures of septic treatment – with often difficult and complex surgical measures and more expensive materials – are most likely above the average costs of this heterogeneous DRG.

However, both the number of PJIs and the awareness among surgeons are increasing (Bozic et al. 2009, 2010). From a payer perspective, the treatment of PJI plays only a minor role in the field of revisions. Unless a systemic sepsis needs to be treated, no specific reimbursement for a PJI is usually granted. And even in the case of sepsis, the reimbursement is focused on the sepsis treatment in an intensive care unit and not on an orthopaedic treatment. Hence the treatment of PJI is reimbursed with the same amount as an aseptic revision. This applies to most European countries with DRG payment systems. Although within the group of revisions there might be different levels – depending on the severity of a procedure – of reimbursement, complex aseptic procedures and septic revisions are usually put in the highest group without further distinction.

2.1.4 Cost of PJI Treatment

From a hospital perspective, the main cost factors for inpatient procedures are the cost centre operating theatre, consumables, medical and non-medical services, and the general ward. Usually the implant costs, the duration of the operation and the length of stay are the main costs within these cost areas (Maradit Kremers et al. 2013). The amount of these costs is strongly influenced by the severity of the condition and the efforts required for treatment (Fisman et al. 2001).

Detailed cost data for the treatment of PJI in France, Germany and the UK have been published (Klouche et al. 2010; Haenle et al 2012a, 2012b; Vanhegan et al. 2012). If applicable, these data are compared with the costs of an aseptic revision and compared with the reimbursement afterwards to check whether PJIs are cost-covering procedures or not.

France: Cost of PJI Treatment After Total Hip Replacement

In France the average cost for the treatment of a PJI after total hip arthroplasty is €23,757 and for an aseptic revision procedure it is €12,049. Both procedures can gain a maximum reimbursement (based on the severity) of €14,062 (aseptic) or €15,081 (septic; Klouche et al. 2010). While the cost for septic treatment increases by 97.1%, the reimbursement – which is only granted for national revision centres – increases by 7.2% only. Aseptic revisions seem to be a cost-covering procedure, while septic revisions lead to a loss for the hospital (▣ Tab. 2.1).

The biggest cost factor in the treatment of PJI in France is the cost for personnel, which is directly linked to the length of stay (Klouche et al. 2010). For septic revisions this adds up to €9,948 on average. Further relevant cost aspects are the costs for the operation (€2,900), medical consumables (€2,742) and general expenses for non-medical services (€3,594). It is remarkable that the costs for the prosthesis and operation are lower for septic revision procedures than for aseptic revisions, while all other cost areas significantly increase with PJI treatment (▣ Tab. 2.2).

Germany: Cost of PJI Treatment After Total Hip Replacement

In Germany three studies including costs for septic or aseptic revisions have been identified: Assmann et al. found average costs of US $14,379 for septic revisions and US $5,487 for aseptic revisions, which is an increase by 262% (Assmann et al. 2014). The average costs for the treatment of a PJI after total hip arthroplasty published by Haenle et al. is €29,322. No data for aseptic revisions have been published

▣ **Tab. 2.1** Costs for aseptic and septic revisions in France (modified from Klouche et al. 2010)

	Aseptic revision	Septic revision	Difference in costs
Average costs for treatment	€12,049	€23,757	+97.1%
Maximum reimbursement	€14,062	€15,081	+7.2%
Cost coverage	116.7%	63.4%	–

Tab. 2.2 Cost factors in aseptic and septic revisions in France (from Klouche et al. 2010)

Cost area	Aseptic revision	Septic revision	Difference in costs, %
Human resources	€2,210	€9,948	+450.1%
Medical prescriptions besides prostheses	€146	€2,742	+1,878.1%
Prosthesis	€2,047	€1,862	-9.0%
General expenses, amortization and financial expenses	€23	€39	+169.6%
Surgical unit + anaesthesia	€3,079	€2,900	-5.8%
Physiotherapy	€244	€388	+159.0%
Diagnostics (radiology, laboratory)	€404	€1,019	+252.2%
Pharmacy	€245	€706	+288.2%
General expenses	€850	€3,594	+422.8%

(Haenle et al 2012a). Lieb et al. (2015) found average costs for septic hip revisions of €20,166 (Tab. 2.3).

However, each cost analysis approach differs regarding the methods of cost collection from the other studies: Assmann and colleagues worked with the fixed and variable costs approach as used in business administration. While the other studies used a bottom–up cost analysis (Haenle et al.) or the matrix calculation as used in the »Institut für das Entgeltsystem im Krankenhaus« (Institute for the Hospital Remuneration System; Lieb et al. 2015).

The findings regarding coverage of the costs with the reimbursement are inconsistent. While Haenle et al. found a huge deficit, Lieb et al. found the procedure to be cost covering (Tab. 2.3). The reason for this difference might be the different approaches used to collect and analyse the costs.

From aseptic to septic revisions, the cost increased in all areas. The additional costs for the intensive care unit were the highest with a 507% increase (Tab. 2.4). Similar to the findings in France, an extended stay in the hospital increases the total costs (Assmann et al. 2014). According to Haenle et al. (2012a), the main cost factors in the treatment of PJI are implant (€5,133) and medical supplies (€6,254) and the cost for the general ward (€7,134) and intensive care unit (€5,395). Lieb et al. have not published detailed cost areas.

Tab. 2.3 Costs for aseptic and septic hip revisions in Germany (from Assmann et al. 2014, Haenle et al. 2012a, 2012b; Lieb et al. 2015)

	Aseptic hip revision (Assmann et al. 2014)	Septic knee revision (Assmann et al. 2014)	Difference in costs	Septic hip revision (Haenle et al 2012a)	Septic hip revision (Lieb et al. 2015)
Average costs for treatment	US $5,487 (€7,286[a])	US $14,379 (€19,095[a])	+262%	€29,322	€20.166
Average reimbursement	–	–		€16,645	€21,580
Cost coverage	–	–		56.7%	107.0%

[a] Converted with original exchange rate from authors (€1 = US $1.3280)

Tab. 2.4 Cost factors in aseptic and septic revisions in Germany (from Assmann et al. 2014)

Cost area	Aseptic revision	Septic revision	Difference in costs
Operation theatre	US $3,394	US $6,737	198.5%
Intensive care unit	US $403	US $2,046	507.7%
General ward (nursing costs)	US $934	US $3,015	322.8%
Diagnostic procedures	US $104	US $258	248.1%
Radiology, laboratory	US $650	US $2,321	357.1%

Tab. 2.5 Costs for septic knee revisions in Germany (from Haenle et al. 2012b; Lieb et al. 2015)

	Septic (Haenle et al. 2012b)	Septic knee revision (Lieb et al. 2015)
Average costs for treatment	€25,195	€19,946
Average reimbursement	€18,838	€19,010
Cost coverage	74.7%	104.9%

Germany: Cost of PJI Treatment After Total Knee Replacement

Another study by Haenle et al. investigated the costs of the treatment of an infected total knee replacement. Average costs for the treatment of a PJI after total knee replacement were €25,195, while the reimbursement covers €18,838 only, leading to a deficit of €6,357 or 25.3% of the total treatment costs (Tab. 2.5). The main cost areas were implant (€5,892), medical supplies (€4,520) and general ward (€6,760). Again the extended length of stay was identified as one of the main cost drivers beside higher costs for medical supplies (Haenle et al. 2012b). In the cost analysis of Lieb et al., an average cost of €19,946 for septic knee revisions was reported, with a cost coverage of 104.9%.

UK: Cost of PJI Treatment After Total Hip Replacement

Vanhegan et al. (2012) investigated the cost of treatment for PJI in the UK after total hip replacement. They found average costs of GBP 21,937 for the treatment, while an aseptic revision procedure generated mean costs of GBP 11,897. This represents a cost increase of 184.4% (Tab. 2.6). The calculation of cost coverage is more difficult for the UK, as beside a basic reimbursement additional funds for specialization are paid to the hospital. The procedure reimbursement is GBP 8,152, both for aseptic and septic procedures, which means both procedures are, without surcharge, not cost covering. In the cost analysis of Vanhegan and co-workers, septic procedures were found to have a loss of GBP 860 per

Tab. 2.6 Costs for septic and aseptic hip revisions in the UK (from Vanhegan et al. 2012)

	Aseptic revision	Septic revision	Difference in costs
Average costs for treatment	GBP 11,897	GBP 21,937	+184.4%
Maximum reimbursement	GBP 8,152	GBP 8,152	+0%
Cost coverage	68.5%	37.1%	–

Tab. 2.7 Cost factors in aseptic and septic revisions in the UK (from Vanhegan et al. 2012)

Cost centre	Aseptic revision	Septic revision	Difference in costs
Inpatient stay	GBP 3,688	GBP 6,800	184.4%
Investigation costs	GBP 342	GBP 988	288.9%
Drug costs	GBP 200	GBP 854	427.0%
Implant costs	GBP 2,298	GBP 3,345	145.6%
Theatre costs	GBP 1,216	GBP 1,744	143.4%
Other costs	GBP 4,153	GBP 8,206	197.6%

case after taking additional payments for the hospital into account (Vanhegan et al. 2012).

Spending for drugs accounted for the highest relative increase in costs at 427%. This was followed by the costs for inpatient stay (GBP 6,800), other costs (GBP 8,206) and implant costs (GBP 3,345) (Tab. 2.7).

2.1.5 Major Factors Increasing the Costs

All studies reported on the drug or antibiotic costs, and showed that treatment of PJI increases the costs for antibiotics disproportionately compared with the total cost increase (Haenle et al. 2012a, 2012b; Klouche et al. 2010). In clinical practice this can result in further worsening of the cost and cost coverage situation: Antibiotic costs can vary widely depending on which pathogens were identified by the laboratory tests as the cause of the PJI. Klouche et al. (2010) reported a range of €77–336 for the cost of antibiotic therapy in their patients. In the case of difficult-to-treat or resistant pathogens, these costs can be even higher. According to Haenle et al. (2012a), the cost of antibiotics has increased from €5 for primary hip procedures to €600 per PJI, which represents an increase of more than 14,000%. The costs for other drugs have increased, too, but the increase from €114 to €404 (355%) is less significant than for the antibiotics (Fig. 2.1).

Our own calculation with drug prices according to the *Rote Liste* from Germany has shown a wide range of costs: from €184 in the case of an Enterobacteriaceae (quinolone-susceptible) infection with a ciprofloxacin therapy only, up to €13,167 for the antibiotic regimen in the treatment of penicillin-resistant *Enterococcus* spp. with daptomycin. However, the total duration of antibiotic therapy was used for this calculation, which does not necessarily take place in the hospital for the full therapy period and thus is not at the expense of hospital budgets (Fig. 2.2).

Appropriate diagnostic procedures are necessary for an adequate antibiotic therapy, which is also reflected in the increased costs for diagnostic or laboratory tests. Thus, all authors, as far as reported, determined a significant increase in the costs for laboratory, radiology, and other diagnostic services (Vanhegan et al. 2012; Klouche et al. 2012; Haenle et al 2012a, 2012b).

The severity of a treatment is reflected in the need to use the intensive care unit (ICU). With daily costs of up to €2,000, use of the ICU is a major cost factor in the treatment of PJI (Kasch et al. 2016). In their analysis, Haenle et al. found ICU costs of €5,395 for hip and €3,081 for knee procedures. These costs contribute to a large part of the additional costs in treating PJI (Haenle et al. 2012a, 2012b). On the other hand, even the regular ward care for patients with PJI is labour-intensive. Increased costs for personnel by up to 36% (Kasch et al. 2016) or 40% (Klouche et al. 2010) reflect this. At the same time, the length of stay for PJI patients is prolonged. In the various analyses, mean treatment duration of up to 52 days was determined. On average, 4.5 operations per patients were performed (Haenle et al. 2012a). The duration of surgery is

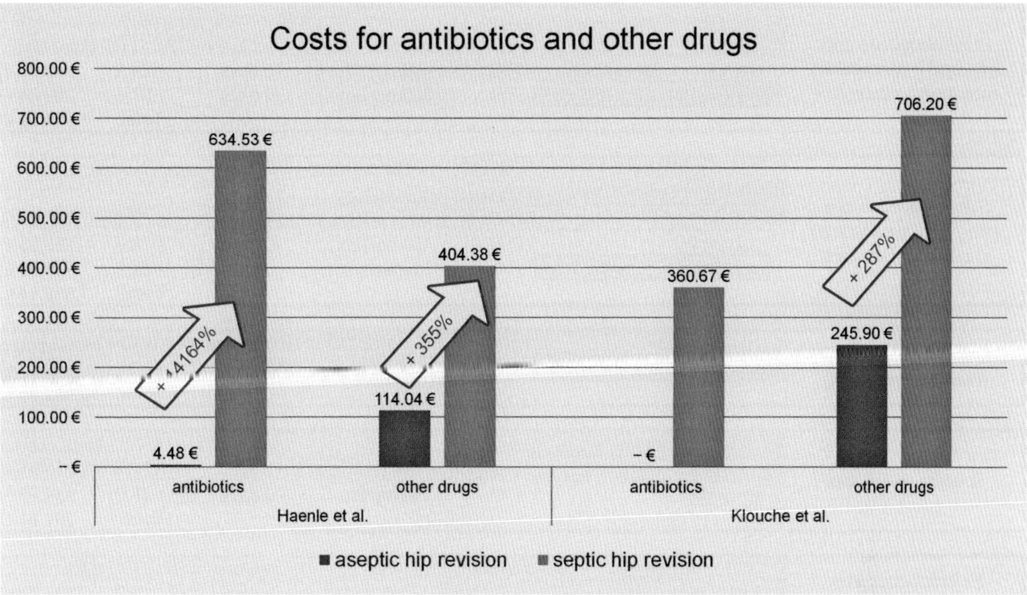

Fig. 2.1 Cost increase for primary versus septic revision cases (own calculation; from Haenle et al. 2012a; Klouche et al. 2010)

another cost factor. The duration of these operations is extended compared with aseptic procedures. Simultaneously, intraoperative complications, such as the loss of blood and thus the need for costly blood products, also increase significantly with the length of operation (Vanhegan et al. 2012). In total, the materials needed for the treatment account for up to one third of the treatment costs of a PJI (Kasch et al. 2016; Haenle et al. 2012a).

2.1.6 Consequences for Hospital Management and the Health-Care System

Compared with aseptic revisions, PJIs are associated with significantly increased treatment costs. This is valid for several countries and for both PJI of the knee and the hip. The cost analyses, however, differ considerably in terms of cost areas and the methodology of the investigation, and therefore no direct comparison between the results can be made. Except for one study, all studies have shown that reimbursement for PJI treatment does not cover the hospital's expenses. And even if the lower costs reported by Assmann et al. may lead to the conclusion that the procedure can be cost covering with the reimbursement, we should avoid drawing this conclusion: Owing to a completely different calculation approach, in which only the costs of the orthopaedic department for the treatment are taken into account, a large share of the costs that were identified in the other cost surveys were not included in the cost analysis of Assmann et al. – a positive contribution margin is still no evidence of a genuine profit from the hospital perspective. For this purpose, imputed daily hospital costs per patient should be compared. And especially since the analysis was made in a university hospital it is expected that the imputed day costs are quite high because of the high fixed costs. The surplus coverage for aseptic revisions should not be considered as profit. Almost no hospital meets the calculated average costs, and it needs to provide special equipment and is hence confronted with fixed costs. Furthermore, the average costs for the calculation of the DRG are retrospectively collected (Dittmann 2015), and retrospective calculation does not necessarily represent the current costs.

It is evident that PJIs are highly complex cases that require interdisciplinary collaboration in hospital. Therefore, in addition to the surgical manage-

	antibiotic	route	dose	duration	cost DDD	total costs
Staphylococcus spp. (rifampin - susceptible) methilicin - susceptible	rifampicin + flucoxacillin	iV	450mg/12h + 2g/6h	14 days	87.11 €	1,219.54 €
	rifampicin + flucoxacillin	P O	450mg/12h	70 days	4.28 €	299.25 €
	+ levofloxacin	P O	500mg/12h	70 days	2.97 €	208.04 €
					Total:	**1,726.83 €**

	antibiotic	route	dose	duration	cost DDD	total costs
Staphylococcus spp. (rifampin - susceptible) methilicin - resistant	rifampicin	iV	450mg/12h	14 days	49.95 €	699.30 €
	+ vancomycin	iV	1g/12h	14 days	53.79 €	753.00 €
	rifampicin	P O	450mg/12h	70 days	4.28 €	299.25 €
	+ ciprofloxacin	P O	750mg/12h	70 days	2.64 €	184.59 €
					Total:	**1,936.14 €**

	antibiotic	route	dose	duration	cost DDD	total costs
Staphylococcus spp. (rifampin - resistant)	daptomycin	i.V	10mg/kg/24h	42 days	261.00 €	10,962.00 €
					Total:	**10,962.00 €**

	antibiotic	route	dose	duration	cost DDD	total costs
Streptococcus spp.	ceftriaxon	i.V	2g/24h	14 days	18.71 €	261.94 €
	amoxicillin	P O	750mg/8h	70 days	1.98 €	138.25 €
					Total:	**261.94 €**

	antibiotic	route	dose	duration	cost DDD	total costs
Enterococcus spp. (penicillin - susceptible)	amoxicillin	i.V	2g/6h	42 days	5.26 €	220.92 €
					Total:	**220.92 €**

	antibiotic	route	dose	duration	cost DDD	total costs
Enterococcus spp. (penicillin - resistant)	daptomycin	i.V	12mg/kg/24h	42 days	313.50 €	13,167.00 €
					Total:	**13,167.00 €**

	antibiotic	route	dose	duration	cost DDD	total costs
Enterobacteriaceae (quinolone-susceptible)	ciprofloxacin	P O	750mg/12h	70 days	2.64 €	184.59 €
					Total:	**184.59 €**

	antibiotic	route	dose	duration	cost DDD	total costs
Nonfermentative bacilli (quinolone - susceptible)	cefepime	iV	2g/8h	14 days	137.96 €	1,931.41 €
	ciprofloxacin	P O	750mg/12h	84 days	2.64 €	221.51 €
					Total:	**2,152.92 €**

	antibiotic	route	dose	duration	cost DDD	total costs
Gram-positive anaerobes	penicillin G	iV	5 Mio U/6h	14 days	17.42 €	243.82 €
	amoxicillin	P O	750mg/8h	70 days	1.98 €	138.25 €
					Total:	**382.07 €**

	antibiotic	route	dose	duration	cost DDD	total costs
Gram-negative anaerobes	amoxicillin/clavulanic acid	iV	2.2g/8h	14 days	8.27 €	115.78 €
	clindamycin	P O	600mg/8h	70 days	2.89 €	202.30 €
					Total:	**318.08 €**

Fig. 2.2 Therapy costs for selected pathogens and antibiotics (own calculation, list prices according to the *Rote Liste*)

ment, a case management is necessary to ensure the costs are controlled. In this case, the lengths of stay should be kept as short as possible, within a feasible medical perspective, and the same applies to material and other costs. However, the optimization potential is limited: The investigated cost analyses have all demonstrated that a majority of the costs arise at the beginning of treatment by surgery and possibly by the necessary ICU stays.

Lieb et al. describe innovative approaches to optimize the treatment duration in German hospitals, which are associated with a reduction in treatment costs. However, the reimbursement system does not reward approaches like this and in fact »penalizes«

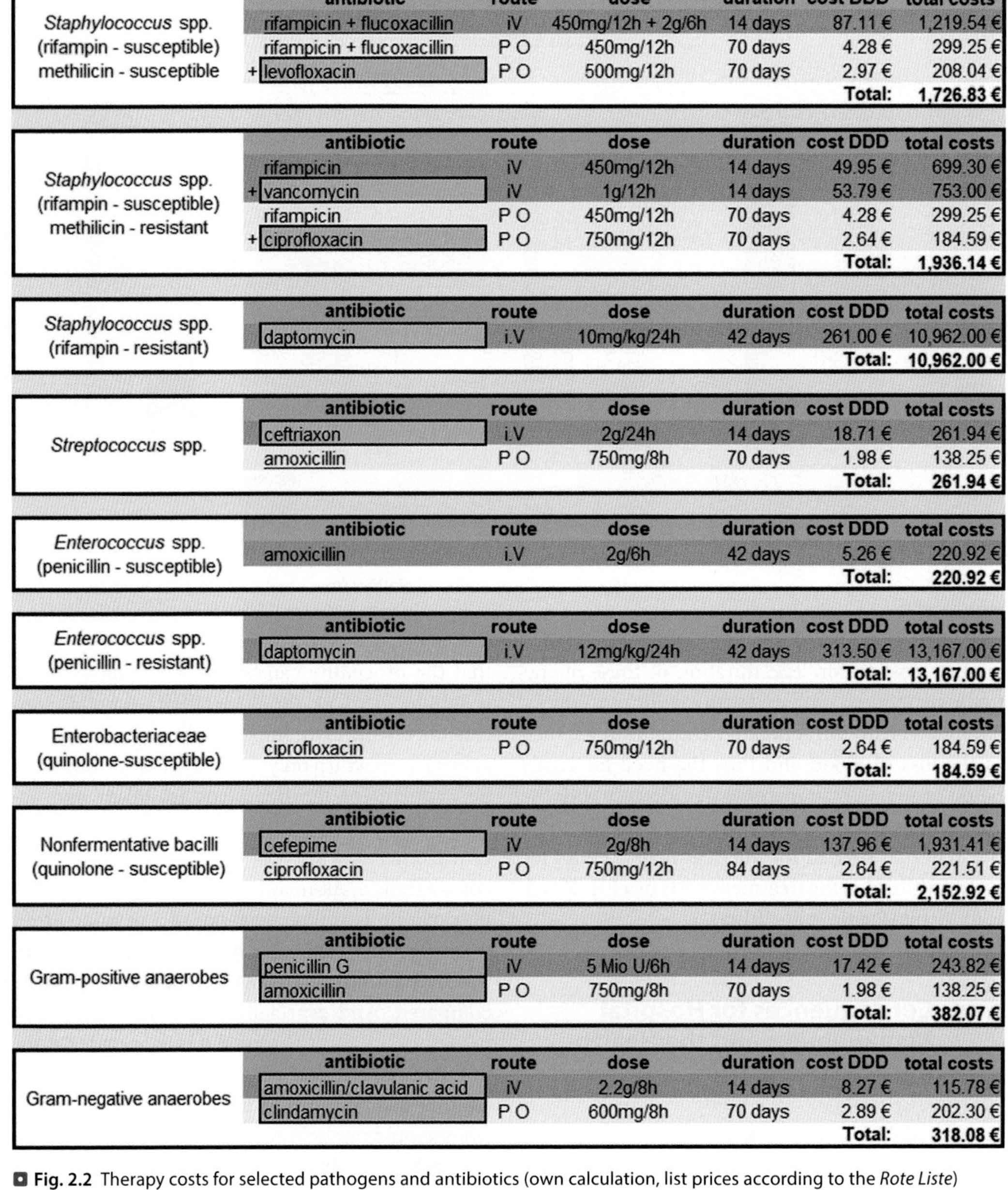

Take-Home Message

- PJI can have a huge economic impact for the hospital and personal impact for the affected patient and his or her surroundings; it is also a challenging situation.
- The number of PJIs and the awareness among surgeons are increasing; however, from a payer perspective, the treatment of PJI plays only a minor role in the field of revisions.
- Compared with aseptic revisions, PJIs are associated with significantly increased treatment costs while they are reimbursed with the same amount as an aseptic revision. This applies to most European countries with a DRG system.
- It is evident that PJIs are highly complex cases that require interdisciplinary collaboration in hospital. Therefore, in addition to the surgical management, a case management is necessary to maintain control of the costs.
- Specific coding is essential for specific reimbursement.

them with a significant reduction in the reimbursement (Lieb et al. 2015). Hospitals should have better opportunities to decide to focus on procedures such as PJI but be able to get alternative or additional payment options. A similar approach exists in The Netherlands, France or the United Kingdom. Here, focal centres for the treatment of PJI are appointed by the health authorities, which have better equipment and/or special refunds.

A specific code for the operations performed and the therapeutic measures is still missing; only with a more specific coding of PJI treatment, can a DRG split end the merging of septic and aseptic revisions into one reimbursement.

From the health-care system perspective, it should be better recognized that hospitals select these patients only in the rarest cases. And that these procedures are not elective procedures, but are also associated with a sense of urgency, so that a prospective calculation of the number of procedures is impossible. The hospitals instead have to fulfil their duties, as often highly specialized, maximum-care centres. Therefore, both the ability and the willingness to treat these cases should be honoured, at least through cost-covering reimbursement for the treatment.

References

Alijanipour P, Parvizi J (2014) Infection post-total knee replacement: current concepts. Curr Rev Musculoskelet Med 7(2):96-102

Assmann G, Kasch R, Maher CG, Hofer A, Barz T, Merk H, Flessa S (2014) Comparison of health care costs between aseptic and two stage septic hip revision. J Arthroplasty 29(10):1925-1931

Bozic KJ, Kurtz SM, Lau E, Ong K, Chiu V, Vail TP, Rubash HE, Berry DJ (2010) The epidemiology of revision total knee arthroplasty in the United States. Clin Orthop Relat Res 468(1):45-51

Bozic KJ, Kurtz SM, Lau E, Ong K, Vail TP, Berry DJ (2009) The epidemiology of revision total hip arthroplasty in the united states. J Bone Joint Surg Am 91(1):128-33

Dittmann H (2015) [Analysis of the conceptual structure of the DRG payments from a cost-accounting point of view]. Gesundheitswesen 77(9):880

Fisman DN, Reilly DT, Karchmer AW, Goldie SJ (2001) Clinical effectiveness and cost-effectiveness of 2 management strategies for infected total hip arthroplasty in the elderly. Clin Infect Dis 32(3):419-430

Geissler A, Quentin W, Scheller-Kreinsen D, Busse R (2011) Introduction to DRGs in Europe: Common objectives across different hospital systems. In: Quentin W, Busse R, Geissler A (eds) Diagnosis-related Groups in Europe: Moving towards transparency, efficiency and quality in hospitals (European Observatory on Health Systems and Policies Series). McGraw-Hill

Haenle M, Skripitz C, Mittelmeier W, Skripitz R (2012a) [Economic impact of infected total hip arthroplasty in the German diagnosis-related groups system]. Orthopäde 41(6):467-476

Haenle M, Skripitz C, Mittelmeier W, Skripitz R (2012b) Economic impact of infected total knee arthroplasty. Scientific World Journal 196:515

Hanstein T, Kumpe O, Mittelmeier W, Skripitz R (2015) [Hybrid and uncemented hip arthroplasty: Contribution margin in the German lump sum reimbursement system]. Orthopäde 44(8):617-622

Kasch R, Assmann G, Merk S, Barz T, Melloh M, Hofer A, Merk H, Flessa S (2016) Economic analysis of two-stage septic revision after total hip arthroplasty: What are the relevant costs for the hospital's orthopedic department? BMC Musculoskelet Disord 17:112

Klouche S, Sariali E, Mamoudy P (2010) Total hip arthroplasty revision due to infection: a cost analysis approach. Orthop Traumatol Surg Res 96(2):124-132

Kobel C, Thuillez J, Bellanger MM, Aavikso A, Pfeiffer K (2011) Diagnosis related group (DRG) systems and similar Patient Classification Systems in Europe. In: Busse R, Geissler

A, Quentin W, Wiley MM (eds) Diagnosis related groups in Europe: moving towards transparency, efficiency and quality in hospitals? Open University Press, Maidenhead
Lieb E, Hanstein T, Schuerings M, Trampuz A, Perka C (2015) [Reduction of Treatment duration in periprosthetic infection with a fast-track concept is economically not feasible]. Z Orthop Unfall 153(6):618-623
Maradit Kremers H, Visscher SL, Moriarty JP, Reinalda MS, Kremers WK, Naessens JM, Lewallen DG (2013) Determinants of direct medical costs in primary and revision total knee arthroplasty. Clin Orthop Relat Res 471(1):206-214
Stargardt T (2008) Health service costs in Europe: cost and reimbursement of primary hip replacement in nine countries. Health Econ 17[1 Suppl]:S9-20
Vanhegan IS, Malik AK, Jayakumar P, Ul Islam S, Haddad FS (2012) A financial analysis of revision hip arthroplasty: the economic burden in relation to the national tariff. J Bone Joint Surg Br 94(5):619-623

2.2 Periprosthetic Joint Infections in the Spectrum of the German Diagnosis-Related Groups System

Sascha Gravius and Hendrik Kohlhof

2.2.1 Introduction

Periprosthetic joint infection (PJI) is among the most devastating complications following artificial joint replacement, affecting 0.4–2% of patients following primary implantation (Peersman et al. 2001) and 5–15% following revision surgery (Marculescu et al. 2006; Pulido et al. 2008; Trampuz and Zimmerli 2008). Owing to the high number of implants, the steadily increasing number of primary implantations, and the aging of the population, the number of PJIs can be expected to rise. Estimates of the anticipated increase in the PJI rate are as high as 600% (Kurtz et al. 2007). Treatment of infected prostheses is very costly in resources and time, with each infected prosthesis costing €40,000–50,000 (Lavernia et al. 2006). In addition to the serious adverse psychosocial effects on patients, PJI treatment places a medico-economic burden on the care provider and on the health-care system –especially because of the inadequate representation of treatment costs in the diagnosis-related groups (G-DRG) system of the German health-care system (Haenle et al. 2012).

In the present chapter we attempt to clarify the depiction of costs for treatment of PJI in the G-DRG system according to specific therapeutic procedures. A retrospective analysis was made of the treatment costs at an endoprosthetics centre providing the maximum level of care to determine whether the application of current operation and procedure codes (OPS codes) allows for the recovery of real costs from the G-DRG system and whether there are any over- or underpayments for certain procedures. In addition, an assessment was made as to which cost categories within the DRG matrix represent the major generators of cost.

2.2.2 The DRG System

The DRG system is a medico-economic patient classification system that reproduces the services provided by hospitals via a fee-for-service payment system. The goal of the DRG system is to ensure fair payment based on the true cost of treatment incurred by care providers (resource use and associated costs).

The DRG system was introduced in Germany on an obligatory basis as the German DRG (G-DRG) in January 2004 and is based on the Australian Refined (AR) DRG system.

The G-DRG system groups patients with similar medical conditions incurring similar treatment costs into »diagnosis-related groups« (DRG). The legal basis is § 17b of the German hospital financing act (KHG). Patients are assigned to a specific DRG group (lump sum) based on patient and case data routinely documented during hospital stays. Diagnoses and procedures are coded according to the German modification of the ICD-10 (ICD-10GM) and the operation and procedure codes (OPS codes).

Complications, comorbidities, and demonstration of causative pathogens can complicate and increase the treatment costs of PJI and are accounted for in the G-DRG system by an increase in the patient clinical complexity level (PCCL) as an expression of the severity of a disease.

DRG are defined by a four-digit alpha numerical code (e.g. I03A). The first letter indicates the major diagnostic category (MDC), the two-figure number designates the MDC subcategory, and the second letter differentiates DRGs based on how cost-intensive (in money, time and resources) the treatment is.

Each DRG is assigned a numerical value, a valuation ratio (»effective cost weight«), with which the flat rate per case is calculated. To calculate the rate per case the effective cost weight is multiplied by the base case value, which varies between the various German federal states. The national average rate per case is ca. €3,300.

The G-DRG system is supplemented by a catalogue of additional fees for procedures that are especially resource intensive, which can apply to treatment of PJI. For new examination and treatment methods, which still are not fully reimbursed based on the rate per case and additional fees, special provisions apply.

2.2.3 Depiction of Reimbursements for Treatment of PJI in the G-DRG System

Treatment of PJI requires both extensive surgical debridement and targeted antibiotic therapy. There are a multitude of treatment options – such as debridement, antibiotics and implant retention (DAIR) as well as single-stage, two-stage and three-stage prosthesis exchange (Wimmer et al. 2013a) – which are grouped into different DRG case groups in the DRG system and OPS codes (◘ Tab. 2.8 and ◘ Tab. 2.9) according to the primary diagnosis T84.5 (ICD-10: infection and inflammatory reaction due to a joint prosthesis).

Debridement, Antibiotics and Implant Retention

The indication for DAIR is an acute PJI and requires the availability of antibiotics against adherent pathogens. The surgical procedure involves debridement with extensive synovectomy and replacement of all exchangeable prosthesis components (Wimmer et al. 2013b). The antimicrobial therapy sometimes entails cost-intensive bactericidal therapy and effective treatment against biofilms (at least 14 days parenteral and up to 6 months oral).

The G-DRG values for DAIR differentiate between debridement alone and debridement with an exchange of prosthesis components. The difference between the two procedures is based on the surgical expenses and implant costs with the additional replacement of components.

Single-Stage Exchange

Single-stage exchange is based on the application of bone cements impregnated with high-dose antibiotics (Zahar and Gehrke 2016). After explantation of the prosthesis and radical debridement, the wound is temporarily closed and antiseptic-soaked abdominal dressings are applied. During the same procedure, a new prosthesis is implanted along with new covering using new instruments. Essential for this procedure is the preoperative identification of pathogens since the bone cement for the revision implant must be impregnated with antibiotics based on the preoperative resistance status for high-dose topical antibiotics therapy to prevent possible residual or immediate contamination of the surface of the newly implanted prosthesis (Friesecke and Wodtke 2008).

In the G-DRG system, single-stage exchange in cases of PJI is reimbursed with the same value as a single-stage aseptic prosthesis exchange operation, the additional costs for the infection therapy not being included.

Two-Stage Exchange (With and Without Case Consolidation for Prosthesis Explantation and Re-implantation)

In contrast to single-stage exchange, explantation and replantation in two-stage exchange are performed in two temporally separate procedures. The duration of the prosthesis-free interval can vary from 2 weeks (short interval) to 12 weeks (long interval).

For billing purposes it is decisive whether both procedures (explantation and implantation) are billed as a single case (»case consolidation«) or as two separate cases. Without case consolidation the overall reimbursement is higher than with case consolidation. Local antibiotic therapy with a static or mobile antibiotic-loaded spacer system receives no additional reimbursement (◘ Fig. 2.3).

Three-Stage/Multiple-Stage Exchange (With and Without Case Consolidation of Individual Procedures)

In three-stage and multiple-stage exchanges, suppression of infection requires explantation and re-implantation as well as open revision with deep

Tab. 2.8 Representation of the individual therapy strategies for treating PJI in the G-DRG system for the knee (diagnosis: T84.5)

Procedure	DRG	Additional fee	Reimbursement[a]
Prosthesis implantation with/without component exchange			
5-823.0 Revision, exchange and explantation of a knee joint endoprosthesis: Revision (no exchange)	I12C	Does not apply	€4,723.87
5-823.19 Exchange of a unicondylar sled prosthesis, inlay exchange **or** 5-823.27 Exchange of a bicondylar surface replacement prosthesis, inlay exchange	I44B	Does not apply	€7,788.98
Single-stage exchange			
5-823.2a Exchange of a bicondylar surface replacement prosthesis by a prosthesis anchored to femoral and tibial shafts, uncemented	I04Z	ZE2016-25[b]	€10,975.38
Two-stage exchange (long interval); no case consolidation: explantation (optional with spacer implantation) and implantation			
1. Case explantation[c] 5-823.6 Explantation of a unicondylar sled prosthesis **or** 5-823.7 Explantation of a bicondylar surface replacement prosthesis **or** 5-823.a Explantation of a special/custom prosthesis Optional: 5-829.9 Spacer implantation (e.g. after explantation of an endoprosthesis)	I04Z	Does not apply	€10,975.38
2. Case implantation[c] 5-822.h0 Implantation of a knee joint endoprosthesis: Prosthesis anchored to femoral and tibial shafts: uncemented **or** 5-829.n Implantation of an endoprosthesis after prior explantation **or** 5-829.k Implantation of a modular endoprosthesis or (partial) exchange of a modular endoprosthesis in a bony defect situation Optional: 5-829.g Spacer removal	I04Z	ZE2016-25[b]	€10,975.38
Two-stage exchange (short interval); case consolidation[c]: explantation (optional with spacer) and implantation			
Explantation: 5-823. Explantation of a unicondylar sled prosthesis **or** 5-823.7 Explantation of a surface replacement prosthesis **or** 5-823.a Explantation of a special/custom prosthesis Optional: 5-829.9 Spacer implantation (e.g. after explantation of an endoprosthesis) Implantation: 5-822.h0 Implantation of a knee joint endoprosthesis: Prosthesis anchored to femoral and tibial shafts: uncemented **or** 5-829.n Implantation of an endoprosthesis after prior explantation **or** 5-829.k Implantation of a modular endoprosthesis or (partial) exchange of a modular endoprosthesis in a bony defect situation Optional: 5-829.g Spacer removal	I43A	ZE2016-25[b]	€18,049.71

Tab. 2.8 (Continued)

Procedure	DRG	Additional fee	Reimbursement[a]
Three-step (multiple-step) exchange; without case consolidation: explantation, open debridement and biopsy (optional with spacer implantation/exchange) and implantation			
1. Case explantation: 5-823.6 Explantation of a unicondylar sled prosthesis **or** 5-823.7 Explantation of a surface replacement prosthesis **or** 5-823.a Explantation of a special/custom prosthesis Optional: 5-829.9 Spacer implantation (e.g. after explantation of an endoprosthesis)	I04Z	Does not apply	€10,975.38
2. Case: open debridement with biopsy: 1-503.6 Biopsy of femur and patella, 1-503.7 Biopsy of tibia and fibula **and** 5-869.1 Extensive soft tissue debridement Optional: 5-829.f Spacer exchange	I08D	Does not apply	€8,002.06
3. Case implantation: 5-822.h0 Implantation of a knee joint endoprosthesis, prosthesis anchored to femoral and tibial shafts: uncemented. 5-829.n Implantation of an endoprosthesis after prior explantation 5-829.k Implantation of a modular endoprosthesis or (partial) exchange of a modular endoprosthesis in a bony defect situation Optional: 5-829.g Spacer removal	I04Z	ZE2016-25[b]	€10,975.38
Three-step (multiple exchange); with case consolidation: explantation, open debridement and biopsy (optional with spacer implantation/exchange) and implantation			
Explantation: 5-823.7 Explantation of a bicondylar surface replacement prosthesis Optional: 5-829.9 Spacer implantation (e.g. after explantation of an endoprosthesis) Open debridement and biopsy (optional with spacer exchange) 1-503.6 Femur and patella biopsy 1-503.7 Tibia and fibula biopsy 5-869.1 extensive soft tissue debridement Optional: 5-829.f Spacer exchange Implantation**:** 5-822.h0 Implantation of a knee joint endoprosthesis: Prosthesis anchored to femoral and tibial shafts: uncemented 5-829.n Implantation of an endoprosthesis after prior explantation 5-829.k Implantation of a modular endoprosthesis or (partial) exchange of a modular endoprosthesis in a bony defect situation Optional: 5-829.g Spacer removal	I43A	ZE2016-25[b]	€18,049.71

[a] Calculation based on the basic case value of the Clinic for Orthopedics and Trauma Surgery of the Rheinische Friedrich Wilhelm University of Bonn
[b] In cases with a bone defect, possibility of billing for supplemental reimbursement
[c] Definition of case consolidation according to § 2 of the 2016 FPV

2

Tab. 2.9 Representation of the individual therapy strategies for treating PJI in the G-DRG system for the hip (diagnosis: T84.5)

Procedure	DRG	Additional fee	Reimbursement[a]
Prosthesis implantation with/without component exchange			
5-821.0 Revision, exchange and explantation of a hip joint endoprosthesis: Revision (without exchange)	I08G	Does not apply	€4,933.68
5-821.2b Isolated exchange of inlay without socket exchange, with exchange of the femoral head	I47A	Does not apply	€8,015.17
Single-stage exchange			
5-821.43 Exchange of an (un-)cemented total endoprosthesis for total endoprosthesis, special/custom prosthesis	I03B	ZE2016-25[b]	€12,119.47
Two-stage exchange (long interval); no case consolidation[c]: explantation (optional with spacer implantation) and implantation			
1. Case explantation[c]: 5-821.7 Explantation of a total endoprosthesis Optional: 5-829.9 Spacer implantation (e.g. after explantation of an endoprosthesis)	I47B	Does not apply	€7,267.75
2. Case implantation[c]: 5-820.20 Implantation of a hip joint endoprosthesis: Total endoprosthesis, special/custom prosthesis : uncemented 5-829.n Implantation of an endoprosthesis after prior explantation 5-829.k Implantation of a modular endoprosthesis or (partial) exchange of a modular endoprosthesis in a bony defect situation Optional: 5-829.g Spacer removal	I03B	ZE2016-25[b]	€12,119.47
Two-step exchange (short interval); case consolidation: explantation (optional with spacer implantation) and implantation			
Explantation: 5-821.7 Explantation of a total endoprosthesis Optional: 5-829.9 Spacer implantation (e.g. after explantation of an endoprosthesis) Implantation: 5-820.20 Implantation of a hip joint endoprosthesis: total endoprosthesis, special/custom prosthesis: uncemented 5-829.n Implantation of an endoprosthesis after prior explantation 5-829.k Implantation of a modular endoprosthesis or (partial) exchange for a modular endoprosthesis in a bony defect situation Optional: 5-829.g Spacer removal	I03A	ZE2016-25[b]	€17,951.37
Three-step (multiple exchange); without case consolidation: explantation, open debridement and biopsy (optional with spacer implantation / exchange) and implantation			
1. Case explantation: Explantation of a total endoprosthesis Optional: 5-829.9 Spacer implantation (e.g. after explantation of an endoprosthesis)	I47B	Does not apply	€7,267.75

Tab. 2.9 (Continued)

Procedure	DRG	Additional fee	Reimbursement[a]
2. Case: open debridement with biopsy: 5-503.6 Femur and patella biopsy, 1-503.5 Pelvic biopsy, 5-869.1 Extensive soft tissue debridement Optional: 5-829.9 Spacer implantation (e.g. after explantation of an endoprosthesis)	I08D	Does not apply	€8,002.06
3. Case implantation: 5-820.20 Implantation of a hip joint endoprosthesis: total endoprosthesis, special/custom prosthesis: uncemented 5-829.n Implantation of an endoprosthesis after prior explantation 5-829.k Implantation of a modular endoprosthesis or (partial) exchange of a modular endoprosthesis in a bony defect situation Optional: 5-829.g Spacer removal	I03B	ZE2016-25[b]	€12,119.47
Three-step (multiple) exchange; with case consolidation: explantation, open debridement and biopsy (optional with spacer implantation/exchange) and implantation			
Explantation: Explantation of a total endoprosthesis Optional: 5-829.9 Spacer implantation (e.g. after explantation of an endoprosthesis) Open debridement and biopsy (optional with spacer exchange) 5-503.6 Femur and patella biopsy 1-503.5 Pelvic biopsy 5-869.1 extensive soft tissue debridement Optional: 5-829.f Spacer exchange Implantation: 5-820.20 Implantation of a hip joint endoprosthesis: total endoprosthesis, special/custom prosthesis: uncemented 5-829.n Implantation of an endoprosthesis after prior explantation 5-829.k Implantation of a modular endoprosthesis or (partial) exchange of modular endoprosthesis in a bony defect situation Optional: 5-829.g Spacer removal	I43A	ZE2016-25[b]	€17,951.37

[a] Calculation based on the basic case value of the Clinic for Orthopedics and Trauma Surgery of the Rheinische Friedrich Wilhelm University of Bonn
[b] In cases with a bone defect, possibility of billing for supplemental reimbursement
[c] Definition of case consolidation according to § 2 of the 2016 FPV

biopsy. These measures can be combined with the implantation and/or exchange of a static or mobile antibiotic-impregnated spacer system.

Here too – as in two-stage exchanges – the reimbursement depends essentially on the effect of a case consolidation (Fig. 2.3). If the individual interventions in a three-stage/multiple-stage exchange are consolidated into a single case, then the reimbursement remains the same as for two-stage exchanges with case consolidation, i.e. the third intervention (three-stage exchange) or the multiple interventions (multiple-stage exchange) are not reimbursed separately.

If each intervention is regarded as a separate case, then unlike two-stage exchanges, each revision (biopsy and extensive soft tissue debridement) is reimbursed separately. Here too, there is no separate reimbursement for local antibiotic therapy.

2.2.4 Length of Hospital Stay and Case Consolidation

Payment for length of hospital stay depends on the case group. The G-DRG system distinguishes between maximum and minimum lengths of hospital stay.

The *maximum length of hospital stay* is the length of inpatient treatment (excluding the day of discharge) that is covered by flat rate reimbursement. If this limit is exceeded, a per diem payment is made for each day beyond the limit based on the flat rate catalogue in accordance with the applicable per diem payment agreement.

The *minimum length of hospital stay* is the minimum time that inpatient treatment should last. If the length of stay is less than the minimum, the unused portion of the hospitalized days, including the »first day with discount« is deducted. In this manner, allowance is made for the lower cost and use of resource and lower costs to the patient.

In accordance with § 2 of the 2016 »Vereinbarung zum Fallpauschalensystem« for hospitals (FPV) between the German National Association of the Statutory Health Insurance system (Berlin) and the Association of Private Health Insurance (Köln) as well as the German Hospital Federation (Berlin), the case data are to be consolidated into a single case and the case reassigned to a different case rate upon readmission to the same hospital if:

1. The patient is readmitted within the maximum length of hospital stay – measured according to the number of calendar days beginning with the day of admission for the first stay – and if for the readmission the patient is assigned to the original DRG; or
2. The patient is readmitted within 30 calendar days of the first admission and is grouped in the same major diagnostic category (MDC) as for the previously reimbursable billable case rate.

An example of the conditions for a case consolidation in accordance with § 2 of the 2016 FPV is shown in ◻ Fig. 2.3.

2.2.5 Antibiotic-Impregnated Spacers

The current gold standard is two-stage exchange involving explantation of the prosthesis with targeted antibiotic therapy in the prosthesis-free interval. During the prosthesis-free interval, the systemic antibiotic therapy can be supplemented by local application of antibiotics in the form of antibiotic-impregnated bone cement spacers (Wimmer et al. 2013b).

In addition to the advantages of antibiotic-impregnated spacer systems (reduced soft tissue retraction, retention of mobility, simplified arthrolysis upon re-implantation, etc.; summarized in Sukeik and Haddad 2009), they have no reimbursement in the DRG system. Although costs can vary widely between individual measures (static vs mobile; commercially available vs custom-made spacer), costs for commercially available systems must be reimbursed.

2.2.6 Antimicrobial Coatings

Antimicrobial coatings are another tool in the prevention and treatment of PJI. An array of technical solutions (anti-adhesive surfaces, bioactive surfaces with antimicrobial properties, surfaces that release antimicrobial substances, nanostructures, bioactive surfaces that suppress biofilm formation) are tested for their effectiveness in preclinical studies (summarized in Gravius and Wirtz 2015). Market-ready products – e.g. silver coatings with their bactericidal effect – are rare (e.g. MUTARS® Silver, Implantcast, Buxtehude, Germany; Agluna, Accentus Medical Ltd., Oxfordshire, UK).

Although the available data do not confirm the clinical effectiveness of antimicrobial coating (doubts regarding the limited biocompatibility and difficult technical implementation in clinical routine), it is given no billing-relevant consideration in the DRG system. To date it has received merely a supplementary, non-revenue-enhancing code; the cost difference to, e.g. non-coated mega-implants, however, is sometimes considerable (a price difference of several hundred euro for proximal and up to several thousand euro for total femur replacement).

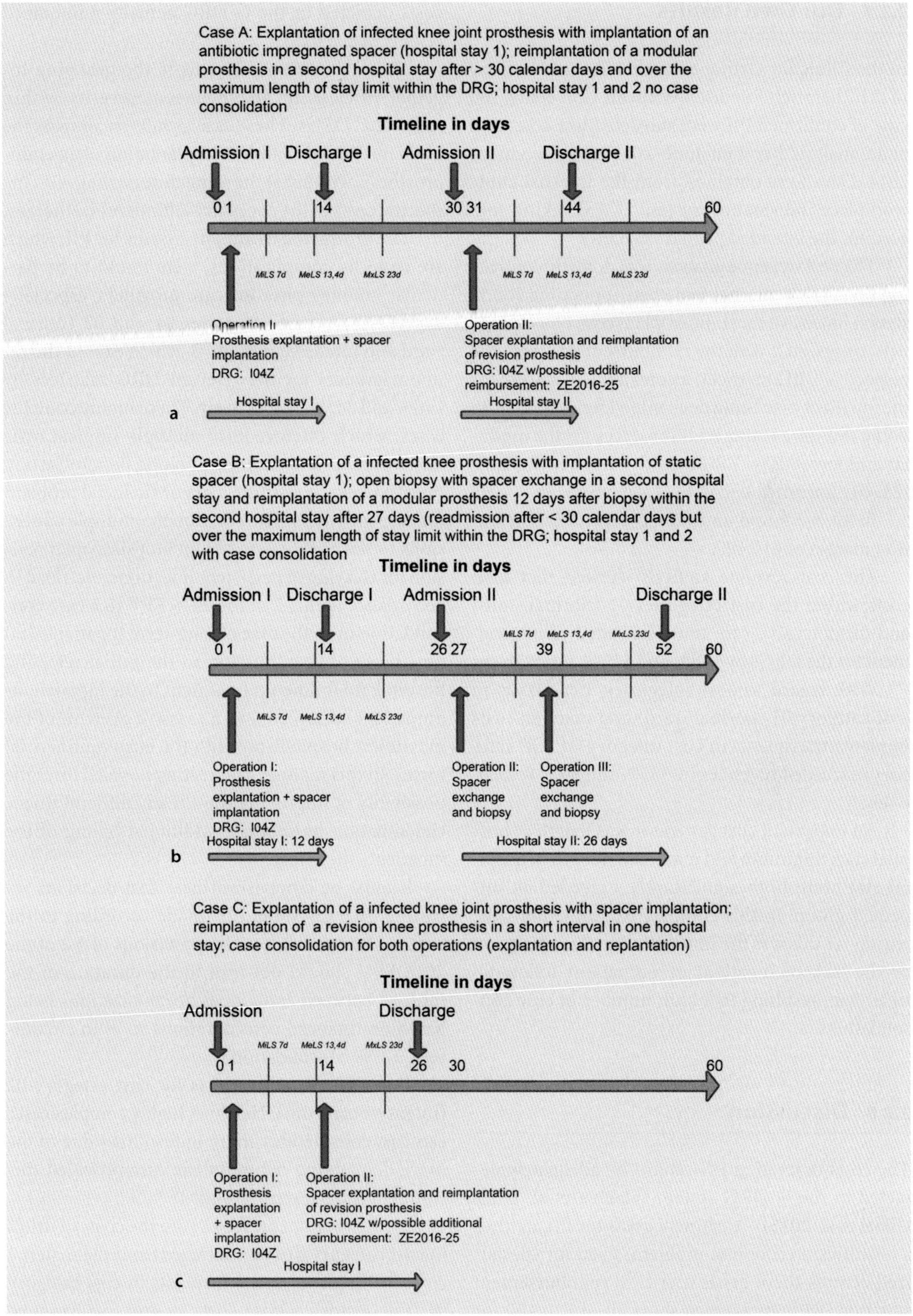

Fig. 2.3 a–c Examples of the conditions for a case consolidation in accordance with § 2 of the 2016 FPV (Vereinbarung zum Fallpauschalensystem) for hospitals

2

2.2.7 Our Own Results

In the Clinic for Orthopedics and Trauma Surgery of the Rheinisch Friedrich Wilhelm University, 160 case of confirmed PJI were subjected to a cost–revenue analysis between June 2013 and December 2014. Data were obtained from the internal clinic workplace information system (KAS) taking into account the intended primary G-DRG.

The cost–revenue analysis was done by comparing the clinic's internal real costs (operating room, station, intensive care unit, implant cost, blood products, drugs, etc.) with the reimbursements from the respective DRG matrices, a contribution margin for the inpatient case being determined for each case. In doing this the existing additional fees for the modular endoprosthesis (ZE-25) and for pelvic implants (ZE-01) were included in the calculation.

In all, we found an average negative contribution margin of €10,400.

The cost–revenue analysis showed that total costs within the cost categories 01 (normal ward) and 02 (intensive care unit) exceeded reimbursement for the DRGs by 148% and 345%, respectively.

With regard to cost categories, drug costs in cost category 01 (normal ward) and material costs implants/transplants in cost category 04 (OP category) exceeded revenues by 385% and 80%, respectively.

An important cost generator was length of hospital stay: minimum and maximum length of hospital stay were both significantly exceeded in our patient group. In this complex patient cohort, the reason for this was the impossibility of readmission or the lack of inpatient or outpatient follow-up treatment, resulting in a high number of case consolidations.

2.2.8 Discussion

The costs of treating PJI cannot be adequately depicted in the G-DRG system (Haenle et al. 2012; Göbel et al. 2015) – treatment costs for PJI are thus a health-care economic problem. Even for specialized centres there exists a critical reimbursement situation, with an average shortfall of €10,400 for our own patients – in only 12% of cases were the costs depicted in the G-DRG actually reimbursed (Göbel et al. 2015).

The main reason for this is the grouping together of cases of heterogeneous severity within individual DRGs. These case groups encompass the implantation, exchange or explantation of an endoprosthesis without at the same time dealing with the specific costs of the necessary antimicrobial therapy.

The protracted treatment courses for PJI, which are beset by complications, were found to be particular »money pits« for care providers; especially expensive are cost categories 01 and 02 (normal ward and intensive care unit), which exceed the reimbursements for the relevant DRG matrices by 148% and 345%, respectively. These highly complex cases, which often require multiple surgical revisions with accompanying antibiotic therapy lasting several weeks, constitute a major financial problem for care providers. The consequent multiple admissions to hospital (e.g. to obtain biopsies, open revision for clearing of persistent infections, etc.) lead in accordance with § 2 of the 2016 FPV to a case consolidation or in the case of long-term inpatients (no possibility of re-admission to the initial referring hospital; no follow-up treatment in the inpatient or outpatient sector, etc.) to a massive overrun of the maximum hospital stay with the ensuing financial losses. In this manner the treating hospital loses the possibility of improving the already difficult financial situation by separate additional billing of the inpatients they treat.

It must be emphasized here that decisions regarding therapy should be made according to the best medical practices. The provisions of § 2 of the 2016 FPV should not lead to the duration of the interval between individual hospitalizations being based on financial considerations so as to circumvent a case consolidation.

A similar situation exists for cost category 02 (intensive care unit). Here too, highly complex cases can cost considerably more in resources due to the more demanding nature of the care provided (including artificial respiration).

Further major cost factors are the costs of drugs in cost category 01 (normal ward) and the material costs for implants and transplants in cost category 04 (OR sector), whose costs in our cost–revenue analysis exceeded reimbursements by 385% and

Take-Home Message

- With the steadily increasing number of primary implantations, and the ongoing aging of the population, the number of PJIs can be expected to increase.
- Treatment of PJI requires both extensive surgical debridement and targeted antibiotic therapy.
- There are multiple treatment options (DAIR, single-stage, two-stage, three-stage exchange), which are grouped into different DRG case groups.
- Treatment costs for PJI are a health-care economic problem.
- The current gold standard is a two-stage exchange involving explantation of the prosthesis with targeted antibiotic therapy in the prosthesis-free interval.

80%, respectively. This reflects the fact that the additional costs incurred for the obligatory antibiotic therapy as an essential component of infection therapy in the G-DRG system are not taken adequately into account. These extra costs can vary widely, but they also require the administration of expensive reserve antibiotics/antimycotics for difficult-to-treat pathogens or polymicrobial infections (Wimmer et al. 2014, 2015). Of equal rank are PJI requiring multiple revisions or for which there is no possibility of continuing intravenous antibiotic therapy orally in the outpatient sector, which necessarily – regardless of the use of reserve anti-infectives – lead to a sizable increase in costs.

A similar problem is created by the use of temporary antibiotic-impregnated spacer systems which, despite their advantages for local antibiotic therapy, are not given cost-relevant consideration in the G-DRG system (additional costs of up to €1,200), but, nevertheless, have a positive impact on the prevention of later re-revisions. The same is true of anti-infective coatings (e.g. silver coating), which in the G-DRG are only included in a non-reimbursement relevant supplementary code.

Separate reimbursement modalities are needed that accurately reflect the increase in the costs of treating PJI and so as to compensate for the incomplete reproduction of procedures in the G-DRG system. There is a danger here that specialized centres – including university clinics and other maximum care providers – will in future no longer be able to bear the financial burden. Confronted with an increasing number of PJI (Kurtz et al. 2007) and rising cost pressures within the health-care system – also for specialized centres – such bottlenecks must be avoided and medical care in Germany cannot be reduced to providing the »less costly« options.

The providers of health care need adequate reimbursement of the costs they incur. Among the possibilities are payment of a centre surcharge or the creation of special accommodation within the DRG system. Conceivable would be continued use of separate »Fallpauschalen« that accurately reflect the particularities of proving infection therapy as part of treating PJI – e.g. secondary diagnoses that increase the PCCL, »new examination and treatment methods« (NUB) for depicting costly additional expenses (e.g. reserve antibiotics/antimycotics).

References

Friesecke C, Wodtke J (2008) Management of periprosthetic infection. Chirurg 79:777-792

Göbel P, Randau T Wimmer MD, Parbs S, Wirtz DC, Gravius S (2015) Septische Endoprothetik – der Supergau? Deutscher Kongress für Orthopädie und Unfallchirurgie 2015

Haenle M, Skripitz C, Mittelmeier W, Skripitz R (2012) Economic impact of infected total hip arthroplasty in the German diagnosis-related groups system. Orthopäde 41:467-476

Kurtz S, Ong K, Lau E et al (2007) Projections of primary and revision hip and knee arthroplasty in the United States from 2005 to 2030. JBJS(Am) 89:780-785

Lavernia C, Lee DJ, Hernandez VH (2006)The increasing financial burden of knee revision surgery in the United States. Clin Orthop Rel Res 446:221-226

Marculescu CE, Berbari EF, Hanssen AD et al (2006) Outcome of prosthetic joint infections treated with debridement and retention of components. Clin Infect Dis 42:471-478

Peersman G, Laskin R, Davis J, Peterson M (2001) Infection in total knee replacement: a retrospective review of 6489 total knee replacements. Clin Orthop Relat Res 392:15-23

Pulido L, Ghanem E, Joshi A et al (2008) Periprosthetic joint infection: the incidence, timing, and predisposing factors. Clin Orthop Rel Res 466:1710-1715

Sukeik M, Haddad FS (2009) Two-stage procedure in the treatment of late chronic hip infections--spacer implantation. Int J Med Sci 6:253-257

Trampuz A, Zimmerli W (2008) Diagnosis and treatment of implant-associated septic arthritis and osteomyelitis. Curr Infect Dis Rep 10:394-403

Vereinbarung zum Fallpauschalensystem für Krankenhäuser für das Jahr 2016. FPV vom 24.09.2015. Deutschen Krankenhausgesellschaft

Wimmer MD, Randau TM, Petersdorf S, Pagenstert GI, Weißkopf M, Wirtz DC, Gravius S (2013a) Evaluation of an interdisciplinary therapy algorithm in patients with prosthetic joint infections. Int Orthop 37:2271-2278

Wimmer MD, Vavken P, Pagenstert GI et al (2013b) Spacer usage in prosthetic joint infections does not influence infect resolution: retrospective analysis of 120 joints with two-stage exchange. Re: Clinical outcome and microbiological findings using antibiotic-loaded spacers in two-stage revision of prosthetic joint infections. Cabo J, Euba G, Saborido A, Gonzalez-Panisello M, Dominguez MA, Agullo JL, Murillo O, Verdaguer R, Ariza J. Journal of Infection 2011 Jul, 63(1)23-31. J Infect 67:82-84

Wimmer MD, Randau T, Friedrich M, Schmolders J, Vavken P, Pagenstert G, Wirtz DC, Gravius S (2014) Schwer behandelbare Keime reduzieren die Infektsanierungsrate beim zweizeitigen Prothesenwechsel bei periprothetischen Infektionen. Deutscher Kongress für Orthopädie und Unfallchirurgie 2014

Wimmer MD, Friedrich MJ, Randau TM, Ploeger MM, Schmolders J, Strauss AA, Hischebeth GT, Pennekamp PH, Vavken P, Gravius S (2015) Polymicrobial infections reduce the cure rate in prosthetic joint infections: outcome analysis with two-stage exchange and follow-up ≥two years. Int Orthop 40:1367-1373

Zahar A, Gehrke TA (2016) One-stage revision for infected total hip arthroplasty. Orthop Clin North Am 47:11-18

Clinical Aspects

K.-D. Kühn (Ed.), *Management of Periprosthetic Joint Infection*
DOI 10.1007/978-3-662-54469-3_3

3.1 Clinical Aspects of Prosthetic Joint Infection

Vincent Moretti and Javad Parvizi

3.1.1 Introduction

Prosthetic joint infection (PJI) is a rare but potentially catastrophic complication after total hip (THA) and total knee arthroplasty (TKA). Early suspicion of PJI along with an efficient evaluation and accurate diagnosis is critical to minimize patient morbidity, mortality, and the overall burden on the health-care system. Although infrequent, with an incidence of 0.39–0.97%, it is one of the most common modes of failure after joint replacement and remains a persistent challenge for the arthroplasty community (Peersman et al. 2001; Pulido et al. 2008).

The current evidence supports the notion that the burden of PJI is increasing (Trampuz and Zimmerli 2005; O'Toole et al. 2016). There are numerous explanations for this rise that include improvements in diagnostic methods for PJI and a better recognition of the role of slow-growing bacteria such as *Propionibacterium acnes* in causing PJI in cases that were previously presumed to be aseptic failures. Additionally, due to the improvements in material design and surgical techniques and the increase in life expectancy, more of the prosthetic joints remain functional, raising the lifetime chances of PJI occurring (O'Toole et al. 2016).

In this chapter, we review the pathomechanism, common clinical presentations, and suggested definitional parameters for PJI. We also discuss various diagnostic tests and review the recommendations for antibiotic prophylaxis.

3.1.2 Pathomechanism of PJI

An understanding and appreciation of bacterial pathomechanisms are imperative to preventing, recognizing, and treating PJI. Bacterial access to the joint space and subsequent initiation of infection is theorized to occur via one of three main pathways: intraoperative introduction at the time of index surgery; contiguous spread of an infection from an adjacent site; and haematogenous seeding from transient bacteraemia or a remote site of infection (Coventry 1975; Trampuz and Zimmerli 2005; Tande and Patel 2014).

PJIs occurring within 1 year of surgery are usually presumed to be from an intraoperative inoculation of bacteria (Coventry 1975; Gallo et al. 2003; Trampuz and Zimmerli 2005; Tande and Patel 2014). Mechanisms for this inoculation include fallout of aerosolized bacteria or direct contamination of the surgical site from infecting organisms on instruments, gloves, or the patient's own integument (Gallo et al. 2003; Tande and Patel 2014). Despite a multitude of preoperative and intraoperative antiseptic procedures, true complete sterilization of the skin at the operative site is impossible (Johnston et al. 1987; Ritter 1999; Savage et al. 2012). Skin at incisional edges has been found to be recolonized with bacteria within 30–180 min of antiseptic procedures (Johnston et al. 1987; Ritter 1999). Furthermore, airborne bacteria can never be fully eliminated from operating rooms as micro-organisms are constantly shed from the skin, hair, nose, and oral cavity of patients and operating room staff (Ritter 1999; Hughes and Anderson 1999). Inoculation with high-virulence organisms typically causes a rapid and early inflammatory response with clear and severe symptoms within a few weeks of surgery. Intraoperative contamination with less virulent or slow-growing organisms can result in a subtle or occult infection, with clinical manifestations not arising for 1 year or more after surgery (Tunney et al. 1998; Nguyen et al. 2002; Gallo et al. 2003).

Contiguous spread of an adjacent infection is another mechanism for PJIs occurring within the first few weeks or months of surgery (Coventry 1975; Trampuz and Zimmerli 2005; Tande and Patel 2014). In the early postoperative period a superficial surgical site infection can develop from intraoperative contamination, as described earlier, or from later access of bacteria to the incision through a draining wound, for example. If not controlled, bacteria from a superficial surgical site infection can spread deeper to the joint space owing to incompletely healed facial planes and tissue layers (Tande and Patel 2014).

Haematogenous seeding of the joint space and prosthesis is the purported source for most late PJIs that occur years after the index procedure (Coventry 1975; Schmalzried et al. 1992; Gallo et al. 2003; Trampuz and Zimmerli 2005; Tande and Patel 2014). Bacteria can gain access to the bloodstream from a remote infection in the body during periods of sepsis. Bacteraemia can also occur transiently from infections or procedural manipulations of dental, urogenital, and gastrointestinal tissues (Lindqvist and Slätis 1985; Schmalzried et al. 1992; LaPorte et al. 1999). Intravascular bacteria from scenarios such as these have been found to be able to enter the artificial joint space. Although rare, several case reports and case series document this mode of infection, with reported rates of PJI after bacteraemia being 6–40% (Lindqvist and Slätis 1985; Schmalzried et al. 1992; LaPorte et al. 1999; Murdoch et al. 2001; Uçkay et al. 2009; Sendi et al. 2011a; Tande et al. 2016).

Once in contact with the joint space and prosthesis, through any of the previously described pathways, bacteria are able to adhere to the implant and begin propagating. The actual adhesion of bacteria to foreign bodies, such as arthroplasty components, is a complex and crucial process in the pathogenesis of PJI. The adhesion process has been described in two steps or phases: an immediate, reversible, nonspecific physical phase followed by a time-dependent, irreversible, specific molecular and cellular phase (Dunne 2002; Gottenbos et al. 2002; Katsikogianni and Missirlis 2004). In phase one, Brownian motion, van der Waals forces, gravitational forces, surface electrostatic charges, and hydrophobic interactions all cooperate to attract micro-organisms to a material's surface. These physical forces predominate until the bacteria and surface are close and stable enough for the molecular and cellular interactions of phase two to take over (Dunne 2002; Gottenbos et al. 2002; Katsikogianni and Missirlis 2004). This second phase creates an irreversible attachment, predominantly mediated by adhesion receptors on the bacterial cell surface (Dunne 2002; Gottenbos et al. 2002; Katsikogianni and Missirlis 2004). These cell receptors can recognize and bind to a variety of molecular targets on the material surface in typical receptor-ligand fashion (Dunne 2002; Gottenbos et al. 2002; Katsikogianni and Missirlis 2004).

After phase two of bacterial adhesion, certain bacterial strains demonstrate an additional virulence factor: the ability to form a biofilm. An estimated 65–80% of human infections can reportedly be attributed to biofilms (Potera 1999; Tzeng et al. 2015). They are composed of layers of aggregated sessile bacterial cells surrounded and encased in a complex multifunctional extracellular matrix (ECM; ◘ Fig. 3.1) (Trampuz and Zimmerli 2005; Bauer and Grosso 2013; Tande and Patel 2014; Tzeng et al. 2015). By volume, most biofilms consist of approximately 15% cells and 85% ECM (Lawrence et al. 1991). They can be mono-microbial, consisting of only one bacterial species, or polymicrobial, consisting of multiple different bacterial types. Biofilms form when free-floating planktonic microbes come into close proximity with one another on the implant surface to begin demonstrating aggregative behaviour through extracellular cell-to-cell signalling (Trampuz and Zimmerli 2005; Elias and Banin 2012; Bauer and Grosso 2013; Tande and Patel 2014; Tzeng et al. 2015). This cell-to-cell contact and communication is critical as it allows for quorum sensing by the bacteria. Quorum sensing has been described as an elementary endocrine system in which extracellular molecules are released by bacterial cells that prompt synchronized, population-based changes in a cluster of microbes (Elias and Banin 2012; Bauer and Grosso 2013; Tande and Patel 2014). This feature allows bacterial cells to sense the local cell population density and regulate their gene expression accordingly. When local cell density is high, transcriptional changes in each in-

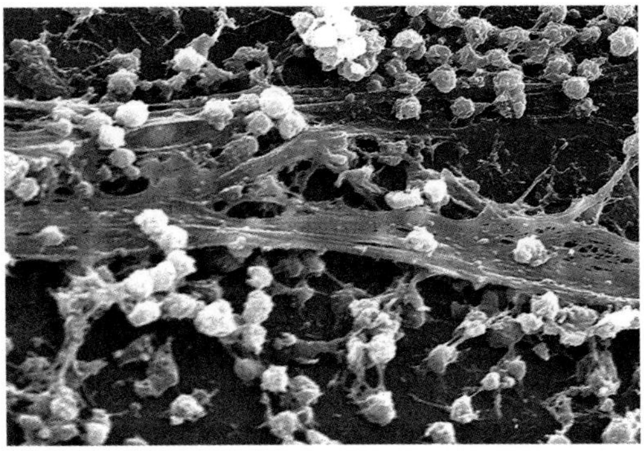

◘ **Fig. 3.1** Electron micrograph demonstrating *Staphylococcus aureus* (*round structures*) and its associated sticky, fibre-like, woven-appearing biofilm (from the CDC Public Health Image Library. Image credit: CDC/Rodney M. Donlon, PhD; Janice Carr [PHIL #7488], 2005)

dividual bacterial cell are promoted that initiate the formation and secretion of a biofilm's ECM. The composition of this ECM depends on the species of colonizing bacteria, although all consist of some form of exopolysaccharides, proteins, and extracellular DNA (Trampuz and Zimmerli 2005; Bauer and Grosso 2013; Tande and Patel 2014; Tzeng et al. 2015).

Presence in the form of biofilm affords many advantages to the infecting organism (Trampuz and Zimmerli 2005; Bauer and Grosso 2013; Tande and Patel 2014; Tzeng et al. 2015). Structural support and anchorage are provided by the ECM, which solidifies bacterial attachment to a material surface and to each other. The biofilm's ECM also provides a protective physical barrier for the bacteria against the host immune system (Thurlow et al. 2011). The barrier limits detection and response by immune cells as well as detection using the conventional laboratory tests that rely on isolation of free-floating bacteria. Additionally, the ECM barrier impedes the flow of synovial fluid through a biofilm. Decreased fluid flow leads to the rapid depletion of metabolic substances and accumulation of waste products inside the biofilm. In this environment, bacteria are encouraged to enter a slow or non-growing state that makes them up to 1,000 times more resistant to growth-dependent antimicrobial agents when compared with their planktonic equivalents (Stewart and Costeron 2001; Donla 2002). The ECM's impediment to fluid flow also limits diffusion of many antibiotics into the biofilm colony, further enhancing bacterial resistance. Another major benefit for bacteria in a biofilm is their close proximity to one another. Persistent and stable proximity between bacterial cells allows for easy exchange of plasmids, which contain extrachromosomal DNA that can include genes for antibiotic resistance and other virulence factors (Trampuz and Zimmerli 2005; Bauer and Grosso 2013; Tande and Patel 2014). For these and other reasons, even a strong and healthy host immune reaction with antibiotic support will rarely eradicate an established biofilm-based infection in a prosthetic joint.

Intracellular internalization is another mechanism by which infecting organisms are able to propagate and persist during PJI (Ellington et al. 1999; Jevon et al. 1999; Valour et al. 2013). Certain strains of bacteria, particularly staphylococci, are able to enter and survive inside osteoblasts and other host cells (Ellington et al. 1999; Jevon et al. 1999; Valour et al. 2013). This ability can help prevent the organism from being detected by both the host immune system and conventional laboratory tests. It can also protect the infecting bacteria from being exposed to antibiotics.

3.1.3 Clinical Manifestations of PJI

The clinical presentation of PJI will occasionally be obvious but it is more often subtle and non-specific, making it difficult to distinguish from aseptic failure. Commonly reported symptoms and physical signs can include joint pain, incisional erythema or drainage, joint swelling or effusion, joint warmth, fever, and a sinus tract at the involved joint (◘ Tab. 3.1) (Inman et al. 1984; Kalore et al. 2011; Sendi et al. 2011b; Tsaras et al. 2012; Peel et al. 2012; Chun et al. 2013; Lora-Tamayo et al. 2013;Tande and Patel 2014; Tornero et al. 2014; Vasso and Schiavone Panni 2015; Zajonz et al. 2015). Often the clinical manifestations and their severity will vary depending on infection mechanism, timing, organism virulence, host immunologic status, surrounding soft tissue structure, and the joint involved.

Pain is the most commonly described symptom in PJI, with a reported frequency of 42–100% (Inman et al. 1984; Kalore et al. 2011; Sendi et al. 2011b; Tsaras et al. 2012; Peel et al. 2012; Chun et al. 2013; Lora-Tamayo et al. 2013; Tande and Patel 2014; Tornero et al. 2014; Vasso and Schiavone Panni 2015; Zajonz et al. 2015). Severe pain is typically associated with high-virulence organisms and early-onset infections while mild or moderate pain can be seen in chronic low-grade PJI (Kalore et al. 2011; Chun et al. 2013; Vasso and Schiavone Panni 2015). Pain with PJI has also been seen more often in knee infections than in the hip (Zajonz et al. 2015). Incisional drainage is reported in 32–72% of PJI, although this finding may be more common in early-onset infections rather than late or chronic infections (Inman et al. 1984; Peel et al. 2012; Tornero et al. 2014). Persistent drainage, sinus tracts, and abscesses are similarly found more often in patients with early-onset perioperatively acquired or

Tab. 3.1 Common clinical signs and symptoms of periprosthetic joint infection

Sign/symptom	Frequency	Notes
Joint pain	42–100%	More common after TKA, with early-onset infections, and with high-virulence organisms
Incisional drainage	32–72%	More common with early-onset infections
Incisional erythema	41–42%	More common after TKA
Joint swelling	25–51%	More common after TKA
Fever	20–47%	More common with late-onset haematogenous infections
Chills/Rigor	45%	More common with late-onset haematogenous infections
Malaise	14%	More common with late-onset haematogenous infections

TKA total knee arthroplasty

contiguously spread infections than in those with late-onset haematogenously originated organisms (Sendi et al. 2011b; Lora-Tamayo et al. 2013; Tande and Patel 2014). Erythema at the surgical wound and swelling of the involved joint have been reported in 41–42% and 25–51% of PJI, respectively (Inman et al. 1984; Peel et al. 2012; Zajonz et al. 2015). Both of these symptoms are significantly more common at the knee than at the hip (Zajonz et al. 2015).

Constitutional signs and symptoms, such as fevers, chills or malaise, are generally seen less often than localized manifestations in PJI. The reported frequency of fever, chills, and malaise with PJI is 20–47%, 45%, and 14%, respectively (Inman et al. 1984; Sendi et al. 2011b; Peel et al. 2012; Tornero et al. 2014; Zajonz et al. 2015). In contrast to the local signs and symptoms, systemic presentations are significantly more common in patients with late-onset haematogenously originated infections (Sendi et al. 2011b; Lora-Tamayo et al. 2013).

3.1.4 Definitional Criteria/Parameters for PJI

Currently there is no official definition of PJI that has been universally established. Several organizations have recently held consensus meetings and formulated guidelines to help standardize the criteria for PJI diagnosis. These include the Musculoskeletal Infection Society (MSIS), the Infectious Disease Society of America (IDSA), and the American Academy of Orthopaedic Surgeons (AAOS) (Parvizi 2010a; Workgroup Convened by the Musculoskeletal Infection Society 2011; Osmon et al. 2013). Although the guidelines from each of these groups share many similarities, those put forth by the MSIS appear to offer the most widely accepted definition for PJI and should be familiar to all physicians who care for joint replacement patients (Workgroup Convened by the Musculoskeletal Infection Society 2011).

The MSIS criteria provide a standardized method for evaluating and establishing a suspected PJI (Workgroup Convened by the Musculoskeletal Infection Society 2011). First put forth in 2011, the MSIS definition was amended slightly in 2013 at the International Consensus Meeting on PJI (Workgroup Convened by the Musculoskeletal Infection Society 2011; Parvizi and Gehrke 2014). These modified criteria (Tab. 3.2) have been adopted by over 130 societies and organizations across the world, including the United States' Centers for Disease Control and Prevention (Parvizi and Gehrke 2014). The definition system contains both major or definitive criteria for PJI diagnosis as well as minor or supportive criteria. To establish the diagnosis, at least one of two major criteria must be present: a sinus tract in communication with the prosthesis or an identical organism identified from at least two separate periprosthetic fluid or tissue cultures. Alternatively, under the modified definition, a PJI

Tab. 3.2 Modified Musculoskeletal Infection Society criteria for diagnosing periprosthetic joint infection

Definite periprosthetic joint infection exists when at least one major criteria or three minor criteria are present:	
Major criteria	A. Sinus tract in communication with the prosthesis
	B. Isolation of identical pathogen(s) from cultures of at least two separate periprosthetic fluid or tissue samples
Minor criteria	A. Elevated serum erythrocyte sedimentation rate and serum C-reactive protein concentration
	B. Elevated synovial white blood cell count or positive result on leukocyte esterase test strip
	C. Elevated synovial neutrophil percentage on differential analysis
	D. Isolation of pathogen(s) from a culture of one periprosthetic fluid or tissue sample
	E. Greater than five neutrophils per high-power field in five high-power fields observed from histologic analysis of periprosthetic tissue at 400× magnification

diagnosis can also be established by the presence of at least three of the following five minor criteria: elevated serum erythrocyte sedimentation rate (ESR) and serum C-reactive protein concentration (CRP); elevated synovial leukocyte count or positive result on leukocyte esterase test strip; elevated synovial neutrophil percentage (PMN%); isolation of an organism in one culture of periprosthetic fluid or tissue; or greater than five neutrophils per high-power field in five high-power fields observed from histologic analysis of periprosthetic tissue at 400× magnification.

3.1.5 Diagnostic Tests

Numerous tests are available to physicians to assist them in diagnosing PJI, but no gold standard truly exists at this time. Because of the ease and low-risk nature of venous blood sampling, serum markers are an attractive and frequently utilized tool for evaluating PJI. In this realm, ESR and CRP tests are particularly ubiquitous and inexpensive. Along with their high sensitivity and specificity, these features make ESR and CRP ideal initial screening tools for PJI (Tab. 3.3 and Tab. 3.4) (Spangehl et al. 1999; Schinsky et al. 2008; Ghanem et al. 2009; Cipriano et al. 2012; Alijanipour et al. 2013). However, ESR and CRP are not direct measures of a joint infection. They are instead associated with the general level of inflammation in the body. Physicians therefore need to be aware that multiple confounding variables can lower the utility of ESR and CRP tests. Besides infections in other parts of the body, comorbidities such as obesity, cancer, diabetes, rheumatoid arthritis, gout, and any other acute or chronic inflammatory condition can alter the reliability of these tests (Shih et al. 1978; Osei-Bimpong et al. 2007; Fink et al. 2008; Liu et al. 2014). The timing for ESR and CRP testing is also important. ESR and CRP levels are routinely elevated in the immediate postoperative period and can remain elevated after surgery for up to 6 and 2 weeks, respectively (Larsson et al. 1992; Bilgen et al. 2001; Alijanipour et al. 2013). Because of this, in the early postoperative period a higher ESR and CRP threshold should be used before describing the numerical result as concerning for PJI. Although rare, it should also be noted that some PJI can exist despite normal ESR and CRP levels (McArthur et al. 2015). Organisms such as *Propionibacterium acnes*, coagulase-negative Staphylococcus, Candida, Corynebacterium, Mycobacterium, and Actinomyces are particularly known to present as seronegative infections (McArthur et al. 2015).

Similar to ESR and CRP, serum white blood cell (WBC) count and neutrophil percentage testing are inexpensive and widely available. However, serum WBC has not been found to be a reliable tool for PJI. It demonstrates a relatively low sensitivity and specificity for PJI, ranging from 20–55% to 66–96%, respectively (Larsson et al. 1992; Toossi et al. 2012). Most experts therefore consider serum WBC to be of limited diagnostic value and it has no role in the

Tab. 3.3 Reported sensitivity and specificity of serum erythrocyte sedimentation rate (ESR) for diagnosing periprosthetic joint infection

Reference	Joint	Cases (*n*)	ESR threshold (mm/h)	Sensitivity (%)	Specificity (%)
Ghanem et al. 2008	Hips	479	30 31	94 95	70 72
Cipriano et al. 2012	Hips and knees	871	32 30	87 94	67 59
Schinsky et al. 2008	Hips	201	30	97	39
Alijanipour et al. 2013	Hips and knees	1962	48.5	78	90
Spangehl et al. 1999	Hips	202	30	82	85

Tab. 3.4 Reported sensitivity and specificity of serum C-reactive protein concentration (CRP) for diagnosing periprosthetic joint infection

Reference	Joint	Cases (*n*)	CRP threshold (mg/l)	Sensitivity (%)	Specificity (%)
Ghanem et al. 2008	Hips	479	10 20.5	91 94	77 81
Cipriano et al. 2012	Hips and knees	871	15 17	86 94	83 70
Schinsky et al. 2008	Hips	201	10	94	71
Alijanipour et al. 2013	Hips and knees	1962	13.5	90	88
Spangehl et al. 1999	Hips	202	10	96	92

modified MSIS criteria for PJI (Workgroup Convened by the Musculoskeletal Infection Society 2011).

Many other possible PJI serum markers, besides ESR and CRP, are currently being evaluated. Interleukin (IL)-6, procalcitonin, monocyte chemoattractant protein-1, soluble intercellular adhesion molecule-1, and IgG to short-chain exocellular lipoteichoic acid have all shown some potential in recent studies, but more research is needed and testing is generally not yet readily available or economical at this time (Wirtz et al. 2000; Bottner et al. 2007; Shah et al. 2009; Berbari et al. 2010; Worthington et al. 2010; Drago et al. 2011; Glehr et al. 2013). IL-6 appears to show the most promise. IL-6 is released by monocytes, macrophages, fibroblasts, and lymphocytes in response to tissue trauma and infection. Its level rises and falls relatively rapidly in response to these stimuli, peaking in less than 24 h and demonstrating a mean half-life of 15 h (Selberg et al. 2000; Wirtz et al. 2000). This feature may be particularly useful in the early postoperative period since levels should return to baseline within a few days of uncomplicated total joint replacement and remain persistently elevated in cases of ongoing PJI. The sensitivity and specificity for IL-6 in PJI varies based on the threshold level selected but reportedly ranges from 81–97% to 59–91%, respectively (Berbari et al. 2010; Worthington et al. 2010; Glehr et al. 2013).

Beyond serum evaluations, synovial fluid biomarkers can also aid in the diagnosis of PJI. They can be tested on preoperative aspirates or intraoperative samples. Preoperatively obtaining synovial fluid is more invasive than serum draws, how-

Tab. 3.5 Reported sensitivity and specificity of synovial white blood cell (WBC) count for diagnosing periprosthetic joint infection

Reference	Joint	Cases (*n*)	WBC threshold (WBC/μl)	Sensitivity (%)	Specificity (%)
Schinsky et al. 2008	Hips	201	>4,200	84	93
Zmistowski et al. 2012	Knees	153	>3,000	93	94
Trampuz et al. 2004	Knees	133	>1,700	94	88
Dinneen et al. 2013	Hips and knees	75	>1,590	90	91
Ghanem et al. 2008	Knees	429	>1,100	91	88

Tab. 3.6 Reported sensitivity and specificity of synovial white blood cell neutrophil percentage (WBC%) for diagnosing periprosthetic joint infection

Reference	Joint	Cases (*n*)	WBC% threshold (%)	Sensitivity (%)	Specificity (%)
Schinsky et al. 2008	Hips	201	>80	84	82
Zmistowski et al. 2012	Knees	153	>75	93	83
Trampuz et al. 2004	Knees	133	>65	97	98
Dinneen et al. 2013	Hips and knees	75	>65	90	87
Ghanem et al. 2008	Knees	429	>64	95	95

ever, and thus most guidelines only recommend that joint aspiration and fluid analysis be performed in patients with elevated serum markers or a high clinical suspicion for PJI (Lachiewicz et al. 1996; Ali et al. 2006; Della Valle et al. 2010). Arguably the most common and valuable synovial fluid tests are WBC count and differential. Synovial WBC count has a sensitivity of 84–94% and a specificity of 88–94% (Tab. 3.5) (Trampuz et al. 2004; Ghanem et al. 2008; Schinsky et al. 2008; Zmistowski et al. 2012; Dinneen et al. 2013). Synovial WBC differential, or neutrophil percentage, has a similarly high sensitivity and specificity of 93–97% and 83–95%, respectively (Tab. 3.6) (Trampuz et al. 2004; Ghanem et al. 2008; Schinsky et al. 2008; Zmistowski et al. 2012; Dinneen et al. 2013). Both of these tests can provide rapid results, allowing for their use in an intraoperative setting. They are commonly recommended in most expert guidelines and both are included in the MSIS criteria (Workgroup Convened by the Musculoskeletal Infection Society 2011). Just as for ESR and CRP, the timing for testing synovial WBC count and differential is again important. Both levels are routinely elevated in the immediate postoperative period (Bedair et al. 2011). Therefore, in the early postoperative period a higher threshold should be used before describing the numerical result as concerning for PJI (Bedair et al. 2011). Surgeons should also be aware of the impact of metal-on-metal articulations on these tests. Most notably, synovial WBC counts can appear falsely elevated when automated counters are used since they can confuse metallic debris for a WBC. Manual counting of cell numbers can overcome this limitation and thereby preserve the test's high sensitivity and specificity in this particular population (Wyles et al. 2013).

Evaluating the leukocyte esterase (LE) level in synovial fluid has been recognized as another valuable test for PJI (Parvizi et al. 2011; Workgroup

Convened by the Musculoskeletal Infection Society 2011; Wetters et al. 2012). LE is an enzyme produced by neutrophils. The level of LE in a fluid sample, which is associated with the volume of neutrophils present, can be estimated by using a colorimetric strip. Although the LE test was originally developed to evaluate for pyuria in urine, some investigators began reporting its off-label use with synovial fluid (Parvizi et al. 2011; Wetters et al. 2012). It demonstrated a relatively high sensitivity of 81–93% and specificity of 77–100% for diagnosing PJI, which prompted its inclusion in the latest MSIS criteria (Parvizi et al. 2011; Workgroup Convened by the Musculoskeletal Infection Society 2011; Wetters et al. 2012). Major advantages of the LE test are its ease of use, low cost, and rapid results. It is one of the few readily available point-of-care tests for PJI, providing physicians with nearly immediate data in the office or operative room. However, one limitation of the LE test is that excessive blood or debris in a synovial fluid sample can interfere with the colorimetric change on the test strip (Parvizi et al. 2011; Wetters et al. 2012).

Other synovial fluid biomarkers that have been investigated include alpha-defensin, beta-defensins, CRP, procalcitonin, IL-6, and IL-1-beta (Nilsdotter-Augustinsson et al. 2007; Deirmengian et al. 2010; Jacovides et al. 2011; Saeed et al. 2013; Bingham et al. 2014; Deirmengian et al. 2014a, 2014b, 2015a, 2015b; Frangiamore et al. 2015). At this time, synovial alpha-defensin testing is the only one that has been specifically optimized and commercialized for diagnosing PJI. Alpha-defensin is an antimicrobial peptide that is produced as part of the innate immune response and secreted by neutrophils in the presence of pathogens (Ganz et al. 1985). Elevated levels of alpha-defensin have demonstrated a very high sensitivity and specificity for PJI of 97–100% and 95–100%, respectively (Bingham et al. 2014; Deirmengian et al. 2014a, 2014b, 2015a, 2015b; Frangiamore et al. 2015). Of additional interest is the finding that alpha-defensin testing appears to remain highly sensitive and specific for PJI even in patients with systemic inflammatory diseases and in patients concurrently receiving antibiotics (Deirmengian et al. 2014a).

Gram stains and cultures can be performed on synovial fluid or tissue, either from preoperative aspirates or intraoperative samples. Gram stains have long been used in the work-up for PJI. They are fast, inexpensive, and easy to perform. However, multiple studies question the utility of Gram stains owing to their very low sensitivity, which ranges from 9.8 to 35% (Della Valle et al. 1999; Parvizi et al. 2006; Johnson et al. 2010; Oethinger et al. 2011). Most experts therefore discourage the use of Gram stains and they have no role in the modified MSIS criteria for PJI (Workgroup Convened by the Musculoskeletal Infection Society 2011).

Cultures have historically been the closest test to a gold standard for diagnosing PJI. They can be an effective method for organism identification and determination of antibiotic sensitivities but have many limitations, particularly when used as a screening tool for PJI. Specificity for diagnosing PJI tends to be high at 94–100% but sensitivity is low, ranging from 44 to 94% (◘ Tab. 3.7) (Spangehl et al. 1999; Baré et al. 2006; Mikkelsen et al. 2006; Gallo et al. 2008; Gomez et al. 2012; Shanmugasundaram et al. 2014). Consequently, physicians need to be aware that a negative culture result does not confidently rule out the possibility of a PJI being present. Cultures should instead only be used to confirm the presence of infection (Spangehl et al. 1999; Ali et al. 2006; Parvizi et al. 2006). Caution should also be used before placing too much weight on a solitary positive culture, as these can be false-positives because of contamination (Atkins et al. 1998; Mikkelsen et al. 2006). Multiple samples should be obtained and analysed separately. Isolating indistinguishable micro-organisms from two or more specimens is generally considered the strongest evidence for infection and this is listed as major or definitive criteria for PJI by the modified MSIS guidelines (Workgroup Convened by the Musculoskeletal Infection Society 2011).

Improved culture yields can be achieved by acquiring tissue samples instead of fluid, placing fluid samples in blood culture vials rather than using swabs, and by immediately sending specimens for analysis (Fuller et al. 1994; von Essen 1997; Spangehl et al. 1999; Hughes et al. 2001; Toms et al. 2006; Wilson and Winn 2008; Font-Vizcarra et al. 2010; Gomez et al. 2012; Aggarwal et al. 2013; Shanmugasundaram et al. 2014). Use of blood culture vials minimizes contamination and exposure to aerobic

Tab. 3.7 Reported sensitivity and specificity of synovial fluid, swabs, or tissue cultures for diagnosing periprosthetic joint infection

Reference	Joint	Number and form of samples	Sensitivity (%)	Specificity (%)
Spangehl et al. 1999	Hips	180 tissue 168 swab	94 76	97 99
Baré et al. 2006	Knees	295 tissue	53	94
Gallo et al. 2008	Hips and knees	94 fluid	44	94
Gomez et al. 2012	Hips and knees	366 tissue 214 fluid	70 65	99 97
Shanmugasundaram et al. 2014	Knees	58 tissue 31 fluid	79 45	
Mikkelsen et al. 2006	Knees	120 tissue	46	100

environments while prompt specimen transportation prevents loss of anaerobes and other sensitive bacteria if not inoculated into specific media right away (Toms et al. 2006). The detection of slow-growing fastidious organisms such as Propionibacterium species, aerobic Gram-positive bacilli, and Peptostreptococcus species can be improved by incubating cultures for a longer duration of 14–21 days (Schäfer et al. 2008; Springer 2015). Although prolonged culture duration may raise the risk of identifying an organism which was a contaminant, studies have shown that up to 30% of infectious organism can be missed if extended culturing times are not used (Schäfer et al. 2008; Shannon et al. 2013). Sonication of explanted prosthetic implants is another method to increase the yield for isolation of infecting organisms. It has been shown to be particularly useful in patients infected with low-virulence organisms as well as those treated with antibiotics just prior to the surgery (Trampuz et al. 2007; Bjerkan et al. 2009; Monsen et al. 2009; Savarino et al. 2009). Physicians should be aware that culture yields from patients currently or recently on antibiotics are significantly diminished (Barrack et al. 1997; Malekzadeh et al. 2010). The odds of a culture negative infection increase 4.7-fold in patients on antibiotics within the previous 3 months (Malekzadeh et al. 2010). As such, many recommend that antibiotics be held for at least 2 weeks before obtaining samples for culture (Barrack et al. 1997; Ali et al. 2006; Della Valle et al. 2010). The use of local anaesthetics such as lidocaine at the time of sampling is also discouraged. These drugs have demonstrated bacteriostatic properties through the inhibition of bacterial macromolecular synthetic pathways and may potentially decrease culture yield (Schmidt and Rosenkranz 1970).

The final diagnostic tool which is readily available and commonly used is a histologic analysis of periprosthetic tissue. Histologic evidence of neutrophilic infiltration on fixed or frozen periprosthetic tissues is suggestive of an acute inflammatory process such as a PJI. The sensitivity and specificity of this test are 42–100% and 77–100%, respectively (Lonner et al. 1996; Banit et al. 2002; Musso et al. 2003; Ko et al. 2005; Wong et al. 2005; Francés et al. 2007; Morawietz et al. 2009; Bori et al. 2011). Improved sensitivity can reportedly be reached by obtaining specimens from the periprosthetic interface membrane instead of the pseudocapsule (Bori et al. 2011). Sensitivity and specificity will also vary depending on the threshold used to define a positive result, which has been anywhere from five to 23 neutrophils per high-powered field. (Lonner et al. 1996; Banit et al. 2002; Musso et al. 2003; Ko et al. 2005; Wong et al. 2005; Francés et al. 2007; Morawietz et al. 2009). The modified MSIS guidelines consider the presence of at least five neutrophils per high-powered field in at least five separate samples as minor criteria for PJI (Workgroup Convened by the Musculoskeletal Infection Society 2011). Being a maximally invasive test, it can realistically only be performed intraoperatively but it has the advantage of providing relatively rapid results. This can help a surgeon reach a decision intraoperatively regarding the likelihood of infection and either continue or alter the surgical plan accordingly. Another advantage is that the result is unlikely to be impacted by active antibiotic use since the test measures inflammation and not bacteria per se. The main disadvantage of histologic analysis is its operator dependency. A skilled pathologist is needed to properly interpret specimens. Additionally, some studies have shown that certain organisms do not consistently elicit a robust inflammatory response (Zeller et al. 2007; Bori et al. 2009). *Propionibacterium acnes* and coagulase-negative Staphylococcus are notable in this regard (Zeller et al. 2007; Bori et al. 2009).

The next generation of diagnostic tests for PJI is likely to involve molecular techniques. Several such tools are currently being developed thanks to advances in the field of molecular biology. Although most are not yet fully optimized or commercialized, they have the potential to provide tests that are rapid, economical, and highly accurate for diagnosis of PJI. These developing techniques include polymerase chain reaction (PCR), fluorescence in situ hybridization (FISH), and matrix-assisted laser desorption/ionization time-of-flight mass spectrometry (MALDI-TOF MS)(Krimmer et al. 1999; Seng et al. 2009; Achermann et al. 2010; Harris et al. 2010; Costerton et al. 2011; Gomez et al. 2012; Titécat et al. 2012; Greenwood-Quaintance et al. 2014; Melendez et al. 2014; Rak et al. 2015; Tzeng et al. 2015). In PCR, bacteria can be rapidly detected in the fluid or tissue from PJI by targeting the highly conserved 16S ribosomal RNA gene found in most microbes (Achermann et al. 2010; Gomez et al. 2012; Titécat et al. 2012; Rak et al. 2015; Tzeng et al. 2015). This targeted gene undergoes enzymatic amplification by DNA polymerase using known primers which have base-pair sequences complementary to areas near the target. Different primers can also be used to amplify known bacterial genes carrying antibiotic resistance or virulence factors. Besides costs and availability, the main drawback of PCR techniques is the potential for false positives from dead or contaminating bacteria. With the FISH technique, bacteria and even biofilms can potentially be visualized on tissue or implant sections (Krimmer et al. 1999; Costerton et al. 2011; Tzeng et al. 2015). This technique utilizes fluorescent DNA or peptide nucleic acid probes that target known bacterial genes, such as the 16S ribosomal RNA gene. Similar to the PCR primers, these probes contain base-pair sequences that are complementary to the target of interest, which allows them to hybridize. Examination with a fluorescent microscope then allows for visual detection and even localization of bacteria. Thanks to additional viability stains and the ability to visually inspect for true bacteria–host integration, FISH nearly eliminates false-positives from dead or contaminated bacteria. In MALDI-TOF MS, bacteria are first lysed through exposure to water, organic solvents and/or strong acids (Seng et al. 2009; Harris et al. 2010; Greenwood-Quaintance et al. 2014; Melendez et al. 2014). The bacteria and their extracts are then ionized and vaporized by a pulsed laser. The ionized fragments are separated, and their mass determined, through mass spectrometry. Analysing the mass differences between the fragmented ions can reportedly reveal the parent molecules and their source bacteria in PJI.

3.1.6 Antibiotic Prophylaxis

Despite our best preventative and antiseptic measure, bacteria are capable of entering a surgical incision during surgery or prior to completion of healing. Antibiotic prophylaxis is an essential tool for preventing PJI and nearly all guidelines recognize preoperative antibiotics to be a critical part of modern arthroplasty surgery (Bratzler et al. 2004; Prokuski 2008; Bratzler et al. 2013). Their benefit is clear from several historical studies that demonstrated significant decreases in surgical site infections with the use of prophylactic antibiotics (Tachjian and Compere1957; Burke 1961; Fogelberg et al. 1970).

A solitary systemic intravenous antibiotic, such as cefazolin or cefuroxime, is generally the preoperative antibiotic of choice for lower limb arthroplasty. Intravenous delivery allows for rapid and predictable distribution while the routine use of dual antibiotics has not shown any consistent

3

Take-Home Message

- Antibiotic prophylaxis is an essential tool for preventing PJI.
- Physicians should be aware of their institution's antibiogram and tailor the antibiotic choice accordingly.
- Many possible PJI serum markers, besides ESR and CRP, are currently being evaluated; interleukin (IL)-6 seems to be the most promising.
- Cultures have historically been the closest test to a gold standard for diagnosing PJI. Still, a negative culture does not rule out PJI, and therefore cultures should instead only be used to confirm the presence of infection.
- The ideal timing and duration of systemic prophylactic antibiotic use to minimize PJI remain somewhat variable and controversial.

benefit in the literature (Parvizi et al. 2010b; Tyllianakis et al. 2010; Sewick et al. 2012). First- or second-generation cephalosporins are widely used because of their activity against common orthopaedic pathogens: specifically Gram-positive bacteria and 40% of Gram-negative bacteria (Prokuski 2008; Parvizi et al. 2010b; Tyllianakis et al. 2010; Sewick et al. 2012; Bratzler et al. 2013). Alternatively, vancomycin should be considered in patients with an anaphylactic allergy to penicillin or beta-lactams, with a history of infection with methicillin-resistant staphylococcus aureus (MRSA), known to be carriers of MRSA, or known to be at high risk of MRSA infection (Parvizi et al. 2013). Physicians should be aware of their institution's antibiogram, however, and tailor the antibiotic choice accordingly. Antibiograms provide a periodic summary of an institution's bacterial isolates along with their antimicrobial susceptibilities. They are an essential tool for selecting effective prophylactic or empiric antibiotics and monitoring resistance trends within a hospital (Bauer et al. 2012).

The ideal timing and duration of systemic prophylactic antibiotic use to minimize PJI remain somewhat variable and controversial. The goal is for the antibiotic to be at an optimal concentration at the surgical site when the procedure begins. To accomplish this, most antibiotics should be infused within 1 h of incision or inflation of a tourniquet, although the actual amount of time needed for full tissue penetration varies with each antibiotic (Bratzler et al. 2004; Prokuski 2008; Steinberg et al. 2009; Bratzler et al. 2013). Some studies have also suggested that infusion within 30 min of incision is more preferable, reportedly reducing infection rates from 2.4% to 1.6% (Steinberg et al. 2009). To maintain effective concentrations in the tissue and bloodstream, antibiotics should be re-dosed during surgeries longer than 4 h, when blood loss is over 2,000 ml, or when fluid resuscitation over 2,000 ml is required (Swoboda et al. 1996; Parvizi et al. 2010b, 2013). With regards to duration, 24 h is generally considered the ideal for prophylactic antibiotic treatment. In elective, clean surgical cases there has been no consistently demonstrated benefit with the use of prolonged or long-term prophylactic antibiotics beyond this short-term 24-h period (Williams and Gustilo 1984; Heydemann and Nelson 1986; Wymenga et al. 1991). There is similarly no strong or consistent evidence at this time to support the use of local antibiotics, such as antibiotic-loaded cement, during a primary joint procedure (Hinarejos et al. 2013).

References

Achermann Y, Vogt M, Leunig M, Wüst J, Trampuz A (2010) Improved diagnosis of periprosthetic joint infection by multiplex PCR of sonication fluid from removed implants. J Clin Microbiol 48(4):1208–1214

Aggarwal VK, Higuera C, Deirmengian G, Parvizi J, Austin MS (2013) Swab cultures are not as effective as tissue cultures for diagnosis of periprosthetic joint infection. Clin Orthop Relat Res 471(10):3196–3203

Ali F, Wilkinson JM, Cooper JR, Kerry RM, Hamer AJ, Norman P, Stockley I (2006) Accuracy of joint aspiration for the preoperative diagnosis of infection in total hip arthroplasty. J Arthroplasty 21(2):221–226

Alijanipour P, Bakhshi H, Parvizi J (2013) Diagnosis of periprosthetic joint infection: the threshold for serological markers. Clin Orthop Relat Res 471(10):3186–3195

Atkins BL, Athanasou N, Deeks JJ, Crook DW, Simpson H, Peto TE, McLardy-Smith P, Berendt AR (1998) Prospective evaluation of criteria for microbiological diagnosis of

prosthetic-joint infection at revision arthroplasty. The OSIRIS Collaborative Study Group. J Clin Microbiol 36(10):2932–2939
Banit DM, Kaufer H, Hartford JM (2002) Intraoperative frozen section analysis in revision total joint arthroplasty. Clin Orthop Relat Res 401:230–238
Baré J, MacDonald SJ, Bourne RB (2006) Preoperative evaluations in revision total knee arthroplasty. Clin Orthop Relat Res 446:40–44
Barrack RL, Jennings RW, Wolfe MW, Bertot AJ (1997) The Coventry Award. The value of preoperative aspiration before total knee revision. Clin Orthop Relat Res 345: 8–16
Bauer TW, Grosso MJ (2013) The basic science of biofilm and its relevance to the treatment of periprosthetic joint infection. OKOJ 11(9)
Bauer S, Bouldouyre MA, Oufella A, Palmari P, Bakir R, Fabreguettes A, Gros H (2012) Impact of a multidisciplinary staff meeting on the quality of antibiotherapy prescription for bone and joint infections in orthopedic surgery. Med Mal Infect 42(12):603–607
Bedair H, Ting N, Jacovides C, Saxena A, Moric M, Parvizi J, Della Valle CJ (2011) The Mark Coventry Award: diagnosis of early postoperative TKA infection using synovial fluid analysis. Clin Orthop Relat Res 469(1):34–40
Berbari E, Mabry T, Tsaras G, Spangehl M, Erwin PJ, Murad MH, Steckelberg J, Osmon D (2010) Inflammatory blood laboratory levels as markers of prosthetic joint infection: a systematic review and meta-analysis. J Bone Joint Surg Am 92(11):2102–2109
Bilgen O, Atici T, Durak K, Karaeminoğullari, Bilgen MS (2001) C-reactive protein values and erythrocyte sedimentation rates after total hip and total knee arthroplasty. J Int Med Res 29(1):7–12
Bingham J, Clarke H, Spangehl M, Schwartz A, Beauchamp C, Goldberg B (2014) The alpha defensin-1 biomarker assay can be used to evaluate the potentially infected total joint arthroplasty. Clin Orthop Relat Res 472(12):4006–4009
Bjerkan G, Witsø E, Bergh K (2009) Sonication is superior to scraping for retrieval of bacteria in biofilm on titanium and steel surfaces in vitro. Acta Orthop 80(2):245–250
Bori G, Soriano A, García S, Gallart X, Mallofre C, Mensa J (2009) Neutrophils in frozen section and type of microorganism isolated at the time of resection arthroplasty for the treatment of infection. Arch Orthop Trauma Surg 129(5):591–595
Bori G, Muñoz-Mahamud E, Garcia S, Mallofre C, Gallart X, Bosch J, Garcia E, Riba J, Mensa J, Soriano A (2011) Interface membrane is the best sample for histological study to diagnose prosthetic joint infection. Mod Pathol 24(4):579–584
Bottner F, Wegner A, Winkelmann W, Becker K, Erren M, Götze C (2007) Interleukin-6, procalcitonin and TNF-alpha: markers of peri-prosthetic infection following total joint replacement. J Bone Joint Surg Br 89(1):94–99
Bratzler DW, Houck PM, et al (2004) Antimicrobial prophylaxis for surgery: an advisory statement from the National Surgical Infection Prevention Project. Clin Infect Dis 38(12):1706–1715
Bratzler DW, Dellinger EP, et al (2013) Clinical practice guidelines for antimicrobial prophylaxis in surgery. Surg Infect 14(1):73–156
Burke JF (1961) The effective period of preventive antibiotic action in experimental incisions and dermal lesions. Surgery 50:161–168
Cipriano CA, Brown NM, Michael AM, Moric M, Sporer SM, Della Valle CJ (2012) Serum and synovial fluid analysis for diagnosing chronic periprosthetic infection in patients with inflammatory arthritis. J Bone Joint Surg Am 94(7):594–600
Costerton JW, Post JC, Ehrlich GD, Hu FZ, Kreft R, Nistico L, Kathju S, Stoodley P, Hall-Stoodley L, Maale G, James G, Sotereanos N, DeMeo P (2011) New methods for the detection of orthopedic and other biofilm infections. FEMS Immunol Med Microbiol 61(2):133–140
Coventry MB (1975) Treatment of infections occurring in total hip surgery. Orthop Clin North Am 6(4):991–1003
Deirmengian C, Hallab N, Tarabishy A, Della Valle C, Jacobs JJ, Lonner J, Booth RE Jr (2010) Synovial fluid biomarkers for periprosthetic infection. Clin Orthop Relat Res 468(8):2017–2023
Deirmengian C, Kardos K, Kilmartin P, Cameron A, Schiller K, Parvizi J (2014a) Combined measurement of synovial fluid α-Defensin and C-reactive protein levels: highly accurate for diagnosing periprosthetic joint infection. J Bone Joint Surg Am 96(17):1439–1445
Deirmengian C, Kardos K, Kilmartin P, Cameron A, Schiller K, Parvizi J (2014b) Diagnosing periprosthetic joint infection: has the era of the biomarker arrived? Clin Orthop Relat Res 472(11):3254–3262
Deirmengian C, Kardos K, Kilmartin P, Gulati S, Citrano P, Booth RE Jr (2015a) The Alpha-defensin Test for Periprosthetic Joint Infection Responds to a Wide Spectrum of Organisms. Clin Orthop Relat Res 473(7):2229–2235
Deirmengian C, Kardos K, Kilmartin P, Cameron A, Schiller K, Booth RE Jr, Parvizi J (2015b) The alpha-defensin test for periprosthetic joint infection outperforms the leukocyte esterase test strip. Clin Orthop Relat Res 473(1):198–203
Della Valle CJ, Scher DM, Kim YH, Oxley CM, Desai P, Zuckerman JD, Di Cesare PE (1999) The role of intraoperative Gram stain in revision total joint arthroplasty. J Arthroplasty 14(4):500–504
Della Valle C, Parvizi J, Bauer TW, Dicesare PE, Evans RP, Segreti J, Spangehl M, Watters WC 3rd, Keith M, Turkelson CM, Wies JL, Sluka P, Hitchcock K (2010) American Academy of Orthopaedic Surgeons. Diagnosis of periprosthetic joint infections of the hip and knee. J Am Acad Orthop Surg 18(12):760–770
Dinneen A, Guyot A, Clements J, Bradley N (2013) Synovial fluid white cell and differential count in the diagnosis or exclusion of prosthetic joint infection. Bone Joint J 95-B(4):554–557
Donlan RM (2002) Biofilms: microbial life on surfaces. Emerg Infect Dis 8(9):881–890

Chun KC, Kim KM, Chun CH (2013) Infection following total knee arthroplasty. Knee Surg Relat Res 25(3):93–99
Drago L, Vassena C, Dozio E, Corsi MM, De Vecchi E, Mattina R, Romanò C (2011) Procalcitonin, C-reactive protein, interleukin-6, and soluble intercellular adhesion molecule-1 as markers of postoperative orthopaedic joint prosthesis infections. Int J Immunopathol Pharmacol 24(2):433–440
Dunne WM Jr (2002) Bacterial adhesion: seen any good biofilms lately? Clin Microbiol Rev 15(2):155–166
Elias S, Banin E (2012) Multi-species biofilms: living with friendly neighbors. FEMS Microbiol Rev 36(5):990–1004
Ellington JK, Reilly SS, Ramp WK, Smeltzer MS, Kellam JF, Hudson MC (1999) Mechanisms of Staphylococcus aureus invasion of cultured osteoblasts. Microb Pathog 26(6):317–323
Fink B, Makowiak C, Fuerst M, Berger I, Schäfer P, Frommelt L (2008) The value of synovial biopsy, joint aspiration and C-reactive protein in the diagnosis of late peri-prosthetic infection of total knee replacements. J Bone Joint Surg Br 90(7):874–878
Fogelberg EV, Zitzmann EK, Stinchfield FE (1970) Prophylactic penicillin in orthopaedic surgery. J Bone Joint Surg Am 52(1):95–98
Font-Vizcarra L, García S, Martínez-Pastor JC, Sierra JM, Soriano A (2010) Blood culture flasks for culturing synovial fluid in prosthetic joint infections. Clin Orthop Relat Res 468(8):2238–2243
Francés Borrego A, Martínez FM, Cebrian Parra JL, Grañeda DS, Crespo RG, López-Durán Stern L (2007) Diagnosis of infection in hip and knee revision surgery: intraoperative frozen section analysis. Int Orthop 31(1):33–37
Frangiamore SJ, Gajewski ND, Saleh A, Farias-Kovac M, Barsoum WK, Higuera CA (2015) α-Defensin Accuracy to Diagnose Periprosthetic Joint Infection-Best Available Test? J Arthroplasty 31(2):456–460
Fuller DD, Davis TE, Kibsey PC, Rosmus L, Ayers LW, Ott M, Saubolle MA, Sewell DL (1994) Comparison of BACTEC Plus 26 and 27 media with and without fastidious organism supplement with conventional methods for culture of sterile body fluids. J Clin Microbiol 32(6):1488–1491
Gallo J, Kolár M, Novotný R, Riháková P, Tichá V (2003) Pathogenesis of prosthesis-related infection. Biomed Pap Med Fac Univ Palacky Olomouc Czech Repub 147(1):27–35
Gallo J, Kolar M, Dendis M, Loveckova Y, Sauer P, Zapletalova J, Koukalova D (2008) Culture and PCR analysis of joint fluid in the diagnosis of prosthetic joint infection. New Microbiol 31(1):97–104
Ganz T, Selsted ME, Szklarek D, Harwig SS, Daher K, Bainton DF, Lehrer RI (1985) Defensins. Natural peptide antibiotics of human neutrophils. J Clin Invest 76(4):1427–1435
Ghanem E, Parvizi J, Burnett RS, Sharkey PF, Keshavarzi N, Aggarwal A, Barrack RL (2008) Cell count and differential of aspirated fluid in the diagnosis of infection at the site of total knee arthroplasty. J Bone Joint Surg Am 90(8):1637–1643
Ghanem E, Antoci V Jr, Pulido L, Joshi A, Hozack W, Parvizi J (2009) The use of receiver operating characteristics analysis in determining erythrocyte sedimentation rate and C-reactive protein levels in diagnosing periprosthetic infection prior to revision total hip arthroplasty. Int J Infect Dis 13(6):e444–e449
Glehr M, Friesenbichler J, Hofmann G, Bernhardt GA, Zacherl M, Avian A, Windhager R, Leithner A (2013) Novel biomarkers to detect infection in revision hip and knee arthroplasties. Clin Orthop Relat Res 471(8):2621–2628
Gomez E, Cazanave C, Cunningham SA, Greenwood-Quaintance KE, Steckelberg JM, Uhl JR, Hanssen AD, Karau MJ, Schmidt SM, Osmon DR, Berbari EF, Mandrekar J, Patel R (2012) Prosthetic joint infection diagnosis using broad-range PCR of biofilms dislodged from knee and hip arthroplasty surfaces using sonication. J Clin Microbiol 50(11):3501–3508
Gottenbos B, Busscher HJ, Van Der Mei HC, Nieuwenhuis P (2002) Pathogenesis and prevention of biomaterial centered infections. J Mater Sci Mater Med 13(8): 717–722
Greenwood-Quaintance KE, Uhl JR, Hanssen AD, Sampath R, Mandrekar JN, Patel R (2014) Diagnosis of prosthetic joint infection by use of PCR-electrospray ionization mass spectrometry. J Clin Microbiol 52(2):642–649
Harris LG, El-Bouri K, Johnston S, Rees E, Frommelt L, Siemssen N, Christner M, Davies AP, Rohde H, Mack D (2010) Rapid identification of staphylococci from prosthetic joint infections using MALDI-TOF mass-spectrometry. Int J Artif Organs 33(9):568–574
Heydemann JS, Nelson CL (1986) Short-term preventive antibiotics. Clin Orthop Relat Res 205:184–187
Hinarejos P, Guirro P, Leal J, Montserrat F, Pelfort X, Sorli ML, Horcajada JP, Puig L (2013) The use of erythromycin and colistin-loaded cement in total knee arthroplasty does not reduce the incidence of infection: a prospective randomized study in 3000 knees. J Bone Joint Surg Am 95(9):769–774
Hughes SP, Anderson FM (1999) Infection in the operating room. J Bone Joint Surg Br 81(5):754–755
Hughes JG, Vetter EA, Patel R, Schleck CD, Harmsen S, Turgeant LT, Cockerill FR 3rd (2001) Culture with BACTEC Peds Plus/F bottle compared with conventional methods for detection of bacteria in synovial fluid. J Clin Microbiol 39(12):4468–4471
Inman RD, Gallegos KV, Brause BD, Redecha PB, Christian CL (1984) Clinical and microbial features of prosthetic joint infection. Am J Med 77(1):47–53
Jacovides CL, Parvizi J, Adeli B, Jung KA (2011) Molecular markers for diagnosis of periprosthetic joint infection. J Arthroplasty 26(6 Suppl):99–103.e1
Jevon M, Guo C, Ma B, Mordan N, Nair SP, Harris M, Henderson B, Bentley G, Meghji S (1999) Mechanisms of internalization of Staphylococcus aureus by cultured human osteoblasts. Infect Immun 67(5):2677–2681
Johnson AJ, Zywiel MG, Stroh DA, Marker DR, Mont MA (2010) Should gram stains have a role in diagnosing hip arthroplasty infections? Clin Orthop Relat Res 468(9):2387–2391

Johnston DH, Fairclough JA, Brown EM, Morris R (1987) Rate of bacterial recolonization of the skin after preparation: four methods compared. Br J Surg 74(1):64

Kalore NV, Gioe TJ, Singh JA (2011) Diagnosis and management of infected total knee arthroplasty. Open Orthop J 5:86–91

Katsikogianni M, Missirlis YF (2004) Concise review of mechanisms of bacterial adhesion to biomaterials and of techniques used in estimating bacteria-material interactions. Eur Cell Mater 8:37–57

Ko PS, Ip D, Chow KP, Cheung F, Lee OB, Lam JJ (2005) The role of intraoperative frozen section in decision making in revision hip and knee arthroplasties in a local community hospital. J Arthroplasty 20(2):189–195

Krimmer V, Merkert H, von Eiff C, Frosch M, Eulert J, Löhr JF, Hacker J, Ziebuhr W (1999) Detection of Staphylococcus aureus and Staphylococcus epidermidis in clinical samples by 16S rRNA-directed in situ hybridization. J Clin Microbiol 37(8):2667–2673

Lachiewicz PF, Rogers GD, Thomason HC (1996) Aspiration of the hip joint before revision total hip arthroplasty. Clinical and laboratory factors influencing attainment of a positive culture. J Bone Joint Surg Am 78(5):749–754

LaPorte DM, Waldman BJ, Mont MA, Hungerford DS (1999) Infections associated with dental procedures in total hip arthroplasty. J Bone Joint Surg Br 81(1):56–59

Larsson S, Thelander U, Friberg S (1992) C-reactive protein (CRP) levels after elective orthopedic surgery. Clin Orthop Relat Res 275:237–242

Lawrence JR, Korber DR, Hoyle BD, Costerton JW, Caldwell DE (1991) Optical sectioning of microbial biofilms. J Bacteriol 173(20):6558–6567

Lindqvist C, Slätis P (1985) Dental bacteremia--a neglected cause of arthroplasty infections? Three hip cases. Acta Orthop Scand 56(6):506–508

Liu JZ, Saleh A, Klika AK, Barsoum WK, Higuera CA (2014) Serum inflammatory markers for periprosthetic knee infection in obese versus non-obese patients. J Arthroplasty 29(10):1880–1883

Lonner JH, Desai P, Dicesare PE, Steiner G, Zuckerman JD (1996) The reliability of analysis of intraoperative frozen sections for identifying active infection during revision hip or knee arthroplasty. J Bone Joint Surg Am 78(10):1553–1558

Lora-Tamayo J, Murillo O, Iribarren JA, Soriano A, Sánchez-Somolinos M, Baraia-Etxaburu JM, Rico A, Palomino J, Rodríguez-Pardo D, Horcajada JP, Benito N, Bahamonde A, Granados A, del Toro MD, Cobo J, Riera M, Ramos A, Jover-Sáenz A, Ariza J; REIPI Group for the Study of Prosthetic Infection (2013) A large multicenter study of methicillin-susceptible and methicillin-resistant Staphylococcus aureus prosthetic joint infections managed with implant retention. Clin Infect Dis 56(2):182–194

Malekzadeh D, Osmon DR, Lahr BD, Hanssen AD, Berbari EF (2010) Prior use of antimicrobial therapy is a risk factor for culture-negative prosthetic joint infection. Clin Orthop Relat Res 468(8):2039–2045

McArthur BA, Abdel MP, Taunton MJ, Osmon DR, Hanssen AD (2015) Seronegative infections in hip and knee arthroplasty: periprosthetic infections with normal erythrocyte sedimentation rate and C-reactive protein level. Bone Joint J 97-B(7):939–944

Melendez DP, Uhl JR, Greenwood-Quaintance KE, Hanssen AD, Sampath R, Patel R (2014) Detection of prosthetic joint infection by use of PCR-electrospray ionization mass spectrometry applied to synovial fluid. J Clin Microbiol 52(6):2202–2205

Mikkelsen DB, Pedersen C, Højbjerg T, Schønheyder HC (2006) Culture of multiple peroperative biopsies and diagnosis of infected knee arthroplasties. APMIS 114(6):449–452

Monsen T, Lövgren E, Widerström M, Wallinder L (2009) In vitro effect of ultrasound on bacteria and suggested protocol for sonication and diagnosis of prosthetic infections. J Clin Microbiol 47(8):2496–2501

Morawietz L, Tiddens O, Mueller M, Tohtz S, Gansukh T, Schroeder JH, Perka C, Krenn V (2009) Twenty-three neutrophil granulocytes in 10 high-power fields is the best histopathological threshold to differentiate between aseptic and septic endoprosthesis loosening. Histopathology 54(7):847–853

Murdoch DR, Roberts SA, Fowler Jr VG Jr, Shah MA, Taylor SL, Morris AJ, Corey GR (2001) Infection of orthopedic prostheses after Staphylococcus aureus bacteremia. Clin Infect Dis 32(4):647–649

Musso AD, Mohanty K, Spencer-Jones R (2003) Role of frozen section histology in diagnosis of infection during revision arthroplasty. Postgrad Med J 79(936):590–593

Nguyen LL, Nelson CL, Saccente M, Smeltzer MS, Wassell DL, McLaren SG (2002) Detecting bacterial colonization of implanted orthopaedic devices by ultrasonication. Clin Orthop Relat Res 403:29–37

Nilsdotter-Augustinsson A, Briheim G, Herder A, Ljunghusen O, Wahlström O, Ohman L (2007) Inflammatory response in 85 patients with loosened hip prostheses: a prospective study comparing inflammatory markers in patients with aseptic and septic prosthetic loosening. Acta Orthop 78(5):629–639

Oethinger M, Warner DK, Schindler SA, Kobayashi H, Bauer TW (2011) Diagnosing periprosthetic infection: false-positive intraoperative Gram stains. Clin Orthop Relat Res 469(4):954–960

Osei-Bimpong A, Meek JH, Lewis SM (2007) ESR or CRP? A comparison of their clinical utility. Hematology 12(4):353–357

Osmon DR, Berbari EF, Berendt AR, Lew D, Zimmerli W, Steckelberg JM, Rao N, Hanssen A, Wilson WR (2013) Infectious Diseases Society of America. Diagnosis and management of prosthetic joint infection: clinical practice guidelines by the Infectious Diseases Society of America. Clin Infect Dis 56(1):e1–e25

O'Toole P, Maltenfort MG, Chen AF, Parvizi J (2016) Projected Increase in Periprosthetic Joint Infections Secondary to Rise in Diabetes and Obesity. J Arthroplasty 31(1):7–10

Parvizi J, Ghanem E, Menashe S, Barrack RL, Bauer TW (2006) Periprosthetic infection: what are the diagnostic challenges? J Bone Joint Surg Am 88(Suppl4):138–147
Parvizi J (2010a) New CPG on diagnosing periprosthetic infections. AAOS Now
Parvizi J, Pawasarat IM, Azzam KA, Joshi A, Hansen EN, Bozic KJ (2010b) Periprosthetic joint infection: the economic impact of methicillin-resistant infections. J Arthroplasty 25(6Suppl):103–107
Parvizi J, Jacovides C, Antoci V, Ghanem E (2011) Diagnosis of periprosthetic joint infection: the utility of a simple yet unappreciated enzyme. J Bone Joint Surg Am 93(24):2242–2248
Parvizi J, Gehrke T, Chen AF (2013) Proceedings of the International Consensus on Periprosthetic Joint Infection. Bone Joint J 95-B(11):1450–1452
Parvizi J, Gehrke T (2014) International Consensus Group on Periprosthetic Joint Infection. Definition of periprosthetic joint infection. J Arthroplasty 29(7):1331
Peersman G, Laskin R, Davis J, Peterson M (2001) Infection in total knee replacement: a retrospective review of 6489 total knee replacements. Clin Orthop Relat Res 392:15–23
Potera C (1999) Forging a link between biofilms and disease. Science 283(5409):1837, 1839
Peel TN, Cheng AC, Buising KL, Choong PF (2012) Microbiological aetiology, epidemiology, and clinical profile of prosthetic joint infections: are current antibiotic prophylaxis guidelines effective? Antimicrob Agents Chemother 56(5):2386–2391
Prokuski L (2008) Prophylactic antibiotics in orthopaedic surgery. J Am Acad Orthop Surg 16(5):283-293
Pulido L, Ghanem E, Joshi A, Purtill JJ, Parvizi J (2008) Periprosthetic joint infection: the incidence, timing, and predisposing factors. Clin Orthop Relat Res 466(7):1710–1715
Rak M, Barlič-Maganja D, Kavčič M, Trebše R, Cőr A (2015) Identification of the same species in at least two intra-operative samples for prosthetic joint infection diagnostics yields the best results with broad-range polymerase chain reaction. Int Orthop 39(5):975–979
Ritter MA (1999) Operating room environment. Clin Orthop Relat Res 369:103–109
Saeed K, Dryden M, Sitjar A, White G (2013) Measuring synovial fluid procalcitonin levels in distinguishing cases of septic arthritis, including prosthetic joints, from other causes of arthritis and aseptic loosening. Infection 41(4):845–849
Savage JW, Weatherford BM, Sugrue PA, Nolden MT, Liu JC, Song JK, Haak MH (2012) Efficacy of surgical preparation solutions in lumbar spine surgery. J Bone Joint Surg Am 94(6):490–494
Savarino L, Tigani D, Baldini N, Bochicchio V, Giunti A (2009) Pre-operative diagnosis of infection in total knee arthroplasty: an algorithm. Knee Surg Sports Traumatol Arthrosc 17(6):667–675
Schäfer P, Fink B, Sandow D, Margull A, Berger I, Frommelt L (2008) Prolonged bacterial culture to identify late periprosthetic joint infection: a promising strategy. Clin Infect Dis 47(11):1403–1409
Schinsky MF, Della Valle CJ, Sporer SM, Paprosky WG (2008) Perioperative testing for joint infection in patients undergoing revision total hip arthroplasty. J Bone Joint Surg 90(9):1869–1875
Schmalzried TP, Amstutz HC, Au MK, Dorey FJ (1992) Etiology of deep sepsis in total hip arthroplasty. The significance of hematogenous and recurrent infections. Clin Orthop Relat Res 280:200–207
Schmidt RM, Rosenkranz HS (1970) Antimicrobial activity of local anesthetics: lidocaine and procaine. J Infect Dis 121(6):597–607
Selberg O, Hecker H, Martin M, Klos A, Bautsch W, Köhl J (2000) Discrimination of sepsis and systemic inflammatory response syndrome by determination of circulating plasma concentrations of procalcitonin, protein complement 3a, and interleukin-6. Crit Care Med 28(8):2793–2798
Sendi P, Banderet F, Graber P, Zimmerli W (2011a) Periprosthetic joint infection following Staphylococcus aureus bacteremia. J Infect 63(1):17–22
Sendi P, Banderet F, Graber P, Zimmerli W (2011b) Clinical comparison between exogenous and haematogenous periprosthetic joint infections caused by Staphylococcus aureus. Clin Microbiol Infect 17(7):1098–1100
Seng P, Drancourt M, Gouriet F, La Scola B, Fournier PE, Rolain JM, Raoult D (2009) Ongoing revolution in bacteriology: routine identification of bacteria by matrix-assisted laser desorption ionization time-of-flight mass spectrometry. Clin Infect Dis 49(4):543–551
Sewick A, Makani A, Wu C, O'Donnell J, Baldwin KD, Lee GC (2012) Does dual antibiotic prophylaxis better prevent surgical site infections in total joint arthroplasty? Clin Orthop Relat Res 470(10):2702–2707
Shah K, Mohammed A, Patil S, McFadyen A, Meek RM (2009) Circulating cytokines after hip and knee arthroplasty: a preliminary study. Clin Orthop Relat Res 467(4):946–951
Shanmugasundaram S, Ricciardi BF, Briggs TW, Sussmann PS, Bostrom MP (2014) Evaluation and Management of Periprosthetic Joint Infection-an International, Multicenter Study. HSS J 10(1):36–44
Shannon SK, Mandrekar J, Gustafson DR, Rucinski SL, Dailey AL, Segner RE, Burman MK, Boelman KJ, Lynch DT, Rosenblatt JE, Patel R (2013) Anaerobic thioglycolate broth culture for recovery of Propionibacterium acnes from shoulder tissue and fluid specimens. J Clin Microbiol 51(2):731–732
Shih LY, Wu JJ, Yang DJ (1987) Erythrocyte sedimentation rate and C-reactive protein values in patients with total hip arthroplasty. Clin Orthop Relat Res 225:238–246
Spangehl MJ, Masri BA, O'Connell JX, Duncan CP (1999) Prospective analysis of preoperative and intraoperative investigations for the diagnosis of infection at the sites of two hundred and two revision total hip arthroplasties. J Bone Joint Surg Am 81(5):672–683
Springer BD (2015) The Diagnosis of Periprosthetic Joint Infection. J Arthroplasty 30(6):908–911
Steinberg JP, Braun BI, et al (2009) Timing of antimicrobial prophylaxis and the risk of surgical site infections: results

from the Trial to Reduce Antimicrobial Prophylaxis Errors. Ann Surg 250(1):10–16
Stewart PS, Costerton JW (2001) Antibiotic resistance of bacteria in biofilms. Lancet 358(9276):135–138
Swoboda SM, Merz C, Kostuik J, Trentler B, Lipsett PA (1996) Does intraoperative blood loss affect antibiotic serum and tissue concentrations? Arch Surg 131(11):1165–1171
Tande AJ, Patel R (2014) Prosthetic joint infection. Clin Microbiol Rev 27(2):302–345
Tande AJ, Palraj BR, Osmon DR, Berbari EF, Baddour LM, Lohse CM, Steckelberg JM, Wilson WR, Sohail MR (2016) Clinical Presentation, Risk Factors, and Outcomes of Hematogenous Prosthetic Joint Infection in Patients with Staphylococcus aureus Bacteremia. Am J Med 129(2):221.e11–20
Tachjian MO, Compere EL (1957) Postoperative wound infections in orthopedic surgery; evaluation of prophylactic antibiotics. J Int Coll Surg 28(6Pt1):797–805
Thurlow LR, Hanke ML, Fritz T, Angle A, Aldrich A, Williams SH, Engebretsen IL, Bayles KW, Horswill AR, Kielian T (2011) Staphylococcus aureus biofilms prevent macrophage phagocytosis and attenuate inflammation in vivo. J Immunol 186(11):6585–6596
Titécat M, Loïez C, Senneville E, Wallet F, Dezèque H, Legout L, Migaud H, Courcol RJ (2012) Evaluation of rapid mecA gene detection versus standard culture in staphylococcal chronic prosthetic joint infections. Diagn Microbiol Infect Dis 73(4):318–321
Toms AD, Davidson D, Masri BA, Duncan CP (2006) The management of peri-prosthetic infection in total joint arthroplasty. J Bone Joint Surg Br 88(2):149–155
Toossi N, Adeli B, Rasouli MR, Huang R, Parvizi J (2012) Serum white blood cell count and differential do not have a role in the diagnosis of periprosthetic joint infection. J Arthroplasty 27(8Suppl):51–54.e1
Tornero E, Senneville E, Euba G, Petersdorf S, Rodriguez-Pardo D, Lakatos B, Ferrari MC, Pilares M, Bahamonde A, Trebse R, Benito N, Sorli L, del Toro MD, Baraiaetxaburu JM, Ramos A, Riera M, Jover-Sáenz A, Palomino J, Ariza J, Soriano A (2014) European Society Group of Infections on Artificial Implants (ESGIAI). Characteristics of prosthetic joint infections due to Enterococcus sp. and predictors of failure: a multi-national study. Clin Microbiol Infect 20(11):1219–1224
Trampuz A, Zimmerli W (2005) Prosthetic joint infections: update in diagnosis and treatment. Swiss Med Wkly 135(17–18):243–251
Trampuz A, Hanssen AD, Osmon DR, Mandrekar J, Steckelberg JM, Patel R (2004) Synovial fluid leukocyte count and differential for the diagnosis of prosthetic knee infection. Am J Med 117(8):556–562
Trampuz A, Piper KE, Jacobson MJ, Hanssen AD, Unni KK, Osmon DR, Mandrekar JN, Cockerill FR, Steckelberg JM, Greenleaf JF, Patel R (2007) Sonication of removed hip and knee prostheses for diagnosis of infection. N Engl J Med 357(7):654–663
Tsaras G, Osmon DR, Mabry T, Lahr B, St Sauveur J, Yawn B, Kurland R, Berbari EF (2012) Incidence, secular trends, and outcomes of prosthetic joint infection: a population-based study, olmsted county, Minnesota, 1969-2007. Infect Control Hosp Epidemiol 33(12):1207–1212
Tunney MM, Patrick S, Gorman SP, Nixon JR, Anderson N, Davis RI, Hanna D, Ramage G (1998) Improved detection of infection in hip replacements. A currently underestimated problem. J Bone Joint Surg Br 80(4):568–572
Tyllianakis ME, Karageorgos ACh, Marangos MN, Saridis AG, Lambiris EE (2010) Antibiotic prophylaxis in primary hip and knee arthroplasty: comparison between cefuroxime and two specific antistaphylococcal agents. J Arthroplasty 25(7):1078–1082
Tzeng A, Tzeng TH, Vasdev S, Korth K, Healey T, Parvizi J, Saleh KJ (2015) Treating periprosthetic joint infections as biofilms: key diagnosis and management strategies. Diagn Microbiol Infect Dis 81(3):192–200
Uçkay I, Lübbeke A, Emonet S, Tovmirzaeva L, Stern R, Ferry T, Assal M, Bernard L, Lew D, Hoffmeyer P (2009) Low incidence of haematogenous seeding to total hip and knee prostheses in patients with remote infections. J Infect 59(5):337–345
Valour F, Trouillet-Assant S, Rasigade JP, Lustig S, Chanard E, Meugnier H, Tigaud S, Vandenesch F, Etienne J, Ferry T, Laurent F; Lyon BJI Study Group (2013) Staphylococcus epidermidis in orthopedic device infections: the role of bacterial internalization in human osteoblasts and biofilm formation. PLoS One 8(6):e67240
Vasso M, Schiavone Panni A (2015) Low-grade periprosthetic knee infection: diagnosis and management. J Orthop Traumatol 16(1):1–7
von Essen R (1997) Culture of joint specimens in bacterial arthritis. Impact of blood culture bottle utilization. Scand J Rheumatol 26(4):293–300
Wetters NG, Berend KR, Lombardi AV, Morris MJ, Tucker TL, Della Valle CJ (2012) Leukocyte esterase reagent strips for the rapid diagnosis of periprosthetic joint infection. J Arthroplasty 27(8Suppl):8–11
Williams DN, Gustilo RB (1984) The use of preventive antibiotics in orthopaedic surgery. Clin Orthop Relat Res 190:83–88
Wilson ML, Winn W (2008) Laboratory diagnosis of bone, joint, soft-tissue, and skin infections. Clin Infect Dis 46(3):453–457
Wirtz DC, Heller KD, Miltner O, Zilkens KW, Wolff JM (2000) Interleukin-6: a potential inflammatory marker after total joint replacement. Int Orthop 24(4):194–196
Wong YC, Lee QJ, Wai YL, Ng WF (2005) Intraoperative frozen section for detecting active infection in failed hip and knee arthroplasties. J Arthroplasty 20(8):1015–1020
Workgroup Convened by the Musculoskeletal Infection Society (2011) New definition for periprosthetic joint infection. J Arthroplasty 26(8):1136–1138
Worthington T, Dunlop D, Casey A, Lambert R, Luscombe J, Elliott T (2010) Serum procalcitonin, interleukin-6, soluble intercellular adhesin molecule-1 and IgG to short-chain exocellular lipoteichoic acid as predictors of infection in total joint prosthesis revision. Br J Biomed Sci 67(2):71–76

Wyles CC, Larson DR, Houdek MT, Sierra RJ, Trousdale RT (2013) Utility of synovial fluid aspirations in failed metal-on-metal total hip arthroplasty. J Arthroplasty 28(5): 818–823

Wymenga AB, Hekster YA, Theeuwes A, Muytjens HL, van Horn JR, Slooff TJ (1991) Antibiotic use after cefuroxime prophylaxis in hip and knee joint replacement. Clin Pharmacol Ther 50(2):215–220

Zajonz D, Wuthe L, Tiepolt S, Brandmeier P, Prietzel T, von Salis-Soglio GF, Roth A, Josten C, Heyde CE, Ghanem M (2015) Diagnostic work-up strategy for periprosthetic joint infections after total hip and knee arthroplasty: a 12-year experience on 320 consecutive cases. Patient Saf Surg 9:20

Zeller V, Ghorbani A, Strady C, Leonard P, Mamoudy P, Desplaces N (2007) Propionibacterium acnes: an agent of prosthetic joint infection and colonization. J Infect 55(2):119–124

Zmistowski B, Restrepo C, Huang R, Hozack WJ, Parvizi J (2012) Periprosthetic joint infection diagnosis: a complete understanding of white blood cell count and differential. J Arthroplasty 27(9):1589–1593

Diagnosis

K.-D. Kühn (Ed.), *Management of Periprosthetic Joint Infection*
DOI 10.1007/978-3-662-54469-3_4

4.1 Diagnosis of Prosthetic Joint Infections

Lorenzo Drago and Elena De Vecchi

4.1.1 Introduction

Replacement of native joints contributes towards significantly improving the quality of life of millions of patients, allows for pain relief and enables recovery of joint function. Unfortunately, in some cases, the implant may fail leading to additional surgery in most patients, with notable costs to the individual's quality of life as well as to the health-care system. Causes of implant failure may be aseptic (loosening of some components of the prosthesis, dislocation, instability, adverse reaction of the host to the implant material, periprosthetic fracture, material consumption) or infective. Although affecting a minority of patients, with an estimated incidence of 1–9% after primary total arthroplasty, depending on the joint (Huotari et al. 2015), prosthetic joint infections (PJIs) require a long hospital stay, prolonged antibiotic therapy and additional surgery (Kapadia et al. 2016). Considering that the number of joint arthroplasties is estimated to rise drastically in the next 20 years, especially because of the growth of the world population and the increase in population age and in the prevalence of comorbidities such as diabetes and obesity, the absolute number of prosthetic joint infections is predicted to inevitably increase, with a sustained economic impact on the health-care system (Kurtz et al. 2012). Therefore, an accurate recognition of these infections is essential not only to ensure appropriate (systemic and local) treatment for patients with PJI, but also to avoid unnecessary therapies for patients with aseptic failure. Diagnosis is further complicated by the wide spectrum of manifestations of PJIs, which may depend on the pathogenicity and virulence of the causative organisms, the host conditions (age, comorbidities etc.), the joint involved, and the time of infection. Usually PJIs are classified according to the time to infection as »early« (within 3 months), »delayed« (after 3 months but before 24 months) and »late« infections (after 24 months; Tande and Patel 2014).

Most PJIs are caused by intraoperative contamination which leads to either early or delayed infection while haematogenous seeding is less common, seen years later in late infections. Although they have different pathogeneses, both early postoperative and haematogenous infections usually present with an acute onset. By contrast, chronic late infections may also be caused by less virulent micro-organisms, and although they are considered to be caused by intraoperative contamination, symptoms develop very slowly. Therefore, their appearance is quite similar to that of aseptic failure and they pose major challenges in the diagnosis.

Considerable efforts have been made in the recent past to improve the diagnosis of PJIs; however, to date, a gold standard has not been established. Therefore, international consensus meetings and national guidelines have proposed a multidisciplinary approach including biochemical, microbiological and histological analyses, as well as clinical findings together with radiological studies (◘ Tab. 4.1).

4.1.2 Microbiology

Biofilm-Related Infections

Biofilm is intrinsic to the pathogenesis of all kinds of prosthetic infections, including those of the joints. Biofilm bacteria can be found on hardware components, cement, bone and fibrous tissue, and detached clumps of biofilm have also been recovered in the joint fluid (Stoodley et al. 2011) and infected tissues. Biofilm is traditionally defined as a microbial community of one or more species embedded in a self-produced matrix composed of exopolysaccharides, proteins, teichoic acids, lipids and extracellular DNA (Gbejuade et al. 2015). Formation of biofilm on a prosthetic implant begins with adhesion of bacteria through their surface structures such as pili, fimbriae, flagella, and glycocalyx (Renner and Weibel 2011). This process is also mediated by non-specific factors such as surface tension, hydrophobicity and electrostatic forces (Donlan 2002). Biofilm formation is partially regulated by quorum sensing, a communication system between bacteria dependent on population density (Castillo-Juárez et al 2015). Bacterial biofilms may reach a considerable size up to a thickness of 100 mm, but more importantly, biofilm-embedded bacteria have been shown to be up to 1,000 times

Tab. 4.1 Recommendations for the diagnosis of prosthetic joint infections

Criterion	IDSA	MSIS	ICM
Sinus tract communicating with the prosthesis	Major criterion	Major criterion	Major criterion
Same micro-organisms isolated from at least two samples	Major criterion	Major criterion	Major criterion
Purulence surrounding the implant	Major criterion	Minor criterion	Minor criterion
Acute inflammation evidenced by histology	Minor criterion	Minor criterion	Minor criterion
Any micro-organism from one sample	Not included	Minor criterion	Minor criterion
A virulent micro-organism from one sample	Minor criterion	Not included	Not included
Elevated synovial fluid leukocyte and neutrophils counts	Not included	Minor criterion	Minor criterion

IDSA Infectious Diseases Society of America, *MSIS* Musculoskeletal Infection Society, *ICM* International Consensus Meeting of Philadelphia

more resistant to most antimicrobial agents when compared with the single bacterial cell (Zoubos et al. 2012; Rabin et al. 2015). Several mechanisms have been hypothesized as being responsible for the increased antimicrobial resistance: the slow or incomplete penetration of antimicrobial agents through the matrix which has also been shown to neutralize and dilute antimicrobial substances; the slow growth rate within areas of the biofilm make ineffective those antibiotics that require a certain cellular activity in order to function; and the presence of efflux pumps, with the expression of several gene-encoding efflux pumps being increased in biofilms (Percival et al. 2015). Therefore, eradication of these slow-growing biofilms with antibiotic therapy alone is often extremely difficult. On the other hand, the presence of biofilm notably complicates isolation of bacteria when conventional sampling and culture methods are used, significantly lowering the sensitivity of microbiological analysis. These issues have recently led to the development of novel strategies for the microbiological diagnosis of PJIs with the aim of removing biofilm bacteria from prosthetic implants and periprosthetic tissues (Drago et al. 2013; Janz et al. 2015; Roux et al. 2011).

4.1.3 Micro-organisms Responsible for PJIs

Staphylococcus aureus, *Staphylococcus epidermidis* and other coagulase-negative staphylococci are universally recognized as the major causative agent of PJIs, being isolated in about 50–60% of cases in similar rates (Langvatn et al. 2015; Drago et al. 2014; Holleyman et al. 2016).

While *S. aureus* has been isolated from infections occurring at any time after implantation, early or late infections caused by this bug occur more frequently than delayed ones (Senneville et al. 2011).

The term »coagulase-negative staphylococci« (CNS) defines a variegated group of staphylococci usually retrievable as normal components of the human skin, which have gained considerable attention as pathogens only in the recent past. The pathogenicity and virulence factors of CNS have been only partially explored, but biofilm production has been recognized in the majority of *S. epidermidis* strains. Globally they represent the main cause of PJIs, although their role as pathogen has to be accurately evaluated for each patient. Among them, the most frequently isolated CNS from PJIs is *S. epidermidis*, while the real isolation rate of the other CNS species varies widely, mainly due to technical difficulties in discriminating one species from another with laboratory tests. In the past few years, particular relevance has been attributed to *Staphy-*

lococcus lugdunensis, which is increasingly isolated not only from PJIs but also from osteomyelitis, endocarditis and bacteraemia. Other species encountered in PJIs are *Staphylococcus simulans*, *Staphylococcus caprae*, *Staphylococcus hominis* and *Staphylococcus warneri*. CNS are isolated at any time after prosthetic implants, although the majority of the infections due to CNS are in revision arthroplasties (Tande and Patel 2014). It could be hypothesized that some cases of implant failure classified as aseptic may be unrecognized low-grade infections due to CNS (Lovati et al. 2016), and that revision surgery may led to the development of an acute infection.

Enterococci are involved in about 3–15% of PJIs, where they are often part of early polymicrobial infections in association prevalently with staphylococci followed by *Escherichia coli* and *Pseudomonas aeruginosa*. Moreover, the high rate of polymicrobial infections, the severity of the infection and the ability of enterococci to form strong biofilms may equally influence treatment results (Tornero et al. 2014).

Streptococci are the causative agents of about 10% of PJIs, with most of them at delayed or late onset and no differences between hip and knee PJIs. A wide variety of streptococci have been identified, with Lancefield Group A, B, C and G being the most prevalent, while viridans streptococci and *Streptococcus pneumoniae* are rarely isolated (Langvatn et al. 2004; Murillo et al. 2015)

Gram-negative bacilli are responsible for about 5–23% of all PJIs especially among the elderly (Rodríguez-Pardo et al. 2014; Murillo et al. 2015; Fernandes and Dias 2013) but their isolation rate may increase up to 60% in early PJIs where they may be retrieved as co-pathogens in polymicrobial infections. *Escherichia coli* and *Pseudomonas aeruginosa* are the most frequently found pathogens followed by other Enterobacteriaceae such *Klebsiella pneumoniae* and Salmonella species (de Sanctis et al. 2014; Gupta et al. 2014). Acquisition of infection is generally haematogenous and the virulence of these bacteria contributes to a common acute presentation.

About 3–6% of PJIs are caused by anaerobes with *Propionibacterium acnes* being the most prominent species (Tande and Patel 2014). PJIs caused by anaerobes often present late after implant surgery, and have a subtle clinical presentation. *P. acnes* is the most frequently isolated anaerobe from shoulders. Among other anaerobes isolated from PJIs, especially as part of polymicrobial infections, there are Clostridia, *Bacteroides fragilis*, *Peptostreptococcus species* and *Actinomyces species*. *Clostridium difficile* and *Clostridium perfringens* are the most frequently isolated Clostridia. They are mostly responsible for early infections, but late PJIs have been also described. Anaerobic Gram-positive cocci (*Peptostreptococcus spp.* and *Finegoldia magna*) are commensal of the gastrointestinal and genito-urinary tracts and skin that have been uncommonly isolated from delayed and late PJIs. They mainly affect hip and knee prostheses that they reach through haematogenous or contiguous spread or directly during surgery. *Actinomyces* and *Bacteroides fragilis* are responsible for a limited number of generally monomicrobial infections (Shah et al. 2015).

Uncommon micro-organisms, such as Corynebacteria, *Pasteurella multocida*, and *Mycobacterium tuberculosis*, have been occasionally reported as cause of PJIs (Cazanave et al. 2012; Romanò et al. 2013; Berbari et al. 1998).

Fungi have been isolated in less than 1% of PJIs and *Candida spp.* are responsible for 80% of these infections (Dutronc et al. 2010; Bartalesi et al. 2012; see ◘ Fig. 4.1).

4.1.4 Laboratory Diagnosis

Laboratory diagnosis occupies a prominent role in the diagnosis of PJIs. In particular, the main aim is to discriminate between infection and other causes of implant failure. As previously outlined, the lack of tests with optimal sensitivity and specificity has led to the development of a multidisciplinary approach that integrates results from microbiological, biochemical and histological analyses with clinical and radiological examination. However, isolation of the pathogen and antimicrobial susceptibility testing are still considered critical to target antimicrobial therapy, thus improving patient outcome. The available laboratory tests are summarized in ◘ Tab. 4.2. Considering that alterations in serum C-reactive protein (CRP) and/or erythrocyte sedimentation rate (ESR) without other possible causes may be

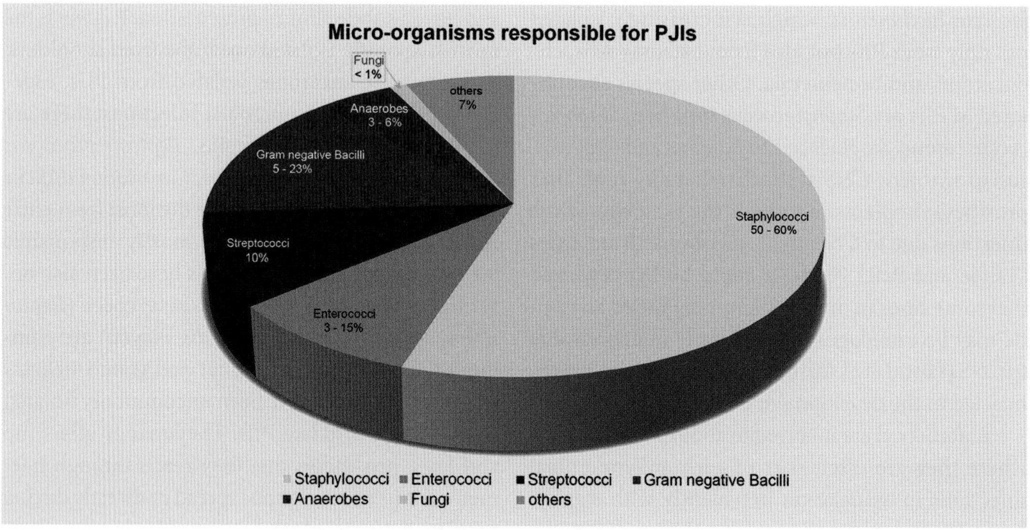

Fig. 4.1 Micro-organisms responsible for PJIs

Tab. 4.2 Most frequently used laboratory test for the diagnosis of prosthetic joint infections

Specimen	Available analysis
Synovial fluid	Culture Leukocyte count and neutrophil percentage Leukocyte esterase CRP Alpha-defensin
Periprosthetic tissue	Culture Histology of frozen section or paraffin embedded tissue
Prosthetic implants	Culture
Peripheral blood	Erythrocyte sedimentation rate CRP Interleukin-6

the first sign of a likely PJI, the diagnosis of PJIs may be carried out at pre- and intraoperative levels.

4.1.5 Microbiological Diagnosis

Preoperative Cultures

Synovial fluid culture is critical for the diagnosis of PJIs allowing for the early identification of the causative organisms with evaluation of antibiotic susceptibility in order to establish the appropriate therapy and selection of therapeutic strategy. Arthrocentesis (=joint aspiration) should be performed in all patients with suspected PJIs except in subjects with contraindications or when the diagnosis has already been established previously. However, while aspiration of the knee is a relatively simple procedure, aspiration of the hip frequently requires ultrasonographic guidance. Unfortunately, in some cases hip aspiration fails to yield a sufficient volume of liquid for further analyses, so that injection and aspiration of normal saline in the joint are needed. Aspiration must be performed under aseptic conditions. The main risks associated with the procedure are represented by contamination of the sample by skin organisms or by the inoculation of organisms into the joint. Nonetheless, joint aspiration is an invasive procedure and may cause complications (Barrack and Harris 1993).

Culture may be performed by directly inoculating the fluid into blood culture bottles or onto solid and/or liquid medium. Data on the use of blood culture bottles reveal a high variability in sensitivity ranging from 85% to 90% and a specificity of 95–100% (Levine and Evans 2001; Hughes et al. 2001; Font-Vizcarra et al. 2010). Prolonged incubation of liquid media may improve sensitivity but may also be associated with a higher isolation rate of contaminants (Font-Vizcarra et al. 2010).

Culture of preoperative arthroscopy tissue biopsies may be a valid alternative or an additional test to synovial fluid cultures. In a retrospective review of a series of patients with shoulder PJIs, results of culture periprosthetic biopsies obtained preoperatively completely overlapped those obtained from intraoperative cultures. Sensitivity and specificity were higher than those observed with fluoroscopically guided glenohumeral aspiration (Dilisio et al. 2014). Similar results were obtained for knee preoperative biopsies with a sensitivity of 100% and a specificity of 98.1% (Fink et al. 2008). By contrast, in a large population of patients with hip PJIs, the positive and negative predictive values were 81.4% and 93.1% for aspiration and 73.8% and 93.8% for tissue biopsy, respectively (Williams et al. 2004).

The presence of a sinus communicating with the implant is considered as a major criterion of PJIs in the MSIS guidelines. Nonetheless, despite swabs from the sinus tract still being considered by some clinicians as a suitable specimen for PJI diagnosis, their use is inadvisable. In fact, only a 50% concordance between cultures from the sinus and deep cultures and a higher probability to identify polymicrobial infections than deep cultures because of isolation of contaminants (particularly CNS) have been reported (Tetreault et al. 2013).

Finally, synovial fluid culture may provide a significant contribution to the preoperative diagnosis of PJIs, while culture from the sinus tract is less useful at this stage.

Intraoperative Cultures

▪ Periprosthetic Tissues

Culture of periprosthetic tissues is a valid tool for the diagnosis of PJIs and represents the predominant laboratory analysis. Samples should be collected from visible inflamed or abnormal tissue accordingly to the surgeon's opinion by using a separate scalpel. However, culture methods are not standardized, and sample processing, used media and incubation times vary widely between laboratories, so that different issues have to be considered. Despite these differences, there is general agreement on the number of samples to send to the microbiology laboratory. Generally accepted guidelines (Infectious Diseases Society of America, Musculo Skeletal Infectious Society, International Consensus Meeting of Philadelphia) recommend the collection of five to six samples with a minimum of three (Osmon et al. 2013; Zmistowski et al. 2014; Parvizi et al. 2011).

Regarding the preparation of tissue samples for microbial culture, various methods have been adopted: cutting bigger samples into smaller pieces with surgical knives, grinding with mortar and pestle, homogenization using Ballotini beads, or using a Seward Stomacher. Tissue homogenization results in the release of bacteria for the subsequent culture. This method, however, is a predominantly manual technique which is labour-intensive and may depend on individual skills and, as such, carries a high risk of contamination (Saeed 2014).

As far as culture media are concerned, few studies have addressed this issue. Most of the studies on tissue cultures employ blood or chocolate agar for growth of aerobes and a media for anaerobes, while the use of selective media (i.e. for Gram-positive cocci and Gram-negative bacilli) is optional and variable. The use of enrichment broth is still a matter of debate; several studies have shown an increase in culture sensitivity when these broths are used with an improvement particularly in isolation of propionibacteria and CNS staphylococci (Drago et al. 2015; DeHaan et al. 2013). Moreover, broths may preserve microbial vitality and when added to samples directly in the operating theatre increase sensitivity from 83 to 95% (Blackmur et al. 2014).

To date, there is no general consensus on the duration of incubation. Traditionally, plates were incubated for 2–5 days for aerobic bacteria and up to 7 days for anaerobes. However, some studies have evidenced that prolonging incubation to up to 15 days improves bacterial detection with an increase in detection rates of about 20% without significantly increasing the isolation of contaminants which were isolated at a similar rate in the first 7 days of incubation (Drago et al. 2015; Schäfer et al. 2008; Butler-Wu et al. 2011). The need for a prolonged time of incubation has been confirmed by a large study by Bemer and co-workers (Bemer et al. 2016). This means that about one fifth of PJIs patients could be missed when a short incubation time is used.

4

Sampling by Swabs

The use of swabs for sampling periprosthetic tissue as well as synovial fluid is not recommended and must be avoided. An increased risk of contamination, decreased volume of specimen for culture, and inhibition of pathogen growth have been reported as potential risks associated with the use of swabs (Rasouli et al. 2012). Moreover, a lower sensitivity has been reported for swabs when compared with sampling of tissue (53–76% vs 63–94%; Aggarwal et al. 2013; Font-Vizcarra et al. 1999).

Owing to the limited sensitivity of periprosthetic tissue culture, culture of the prosthesis may be considered as the method of choice for PJI diagnosis. The main issue with cultures of implants is related to dislodging bacteria from the implant. In fact, as previously described, bacterial growth on these devices leads to production of biofilm, which strongly encases bacteria, hampering their recovery for subsequent culture. Therefore, implants should be treated before plating to assure a high bacterial recovery. This may be obtained by mechanical, physical or chemical methods.

Mechanical methods such as scraping or vortexing have been rarely evaluated. One study using vortexing of implants for 1 min after addition of thioglycollate broth showed a sensitivity of only 40%, although its specificity was very high (99%) when a limit of 50 CFU/ml was used for considering a sample as positive (Portillo et al. 2013).

Sonication

Sonication is based on the use of long-wave ultrasound radiating into a liquid medium to dislodge micro-organisms from an inert surface by disrupting the microbial biofilm (Fig. 4.2). The first report on sonication was published in 1990 by Tunney and colleagues (Tunney et al. 1998). They analysed the impact of mild ultrasound on the release of bacteria from hip implants of 120 patients, demonstrating an increase in bacterial isolation rate when compared with tissue culture. However, this study was limited by the lack of a precise definition of PJI, and no other studies appeared until 2006 (Trampuz et al. 2006). In the 2006 study involving 78 patients, a superior sensitivity of sonication over tissue culture was reported despite a lower specificity. The lack of specificity was mainly due to the use of bags not completely sealed, which caused contamination of the bags by the water bath. The protocol was subsequently ameliorated by using rigid sealable polypropylene containers and by the vortexing of samples before sonication.

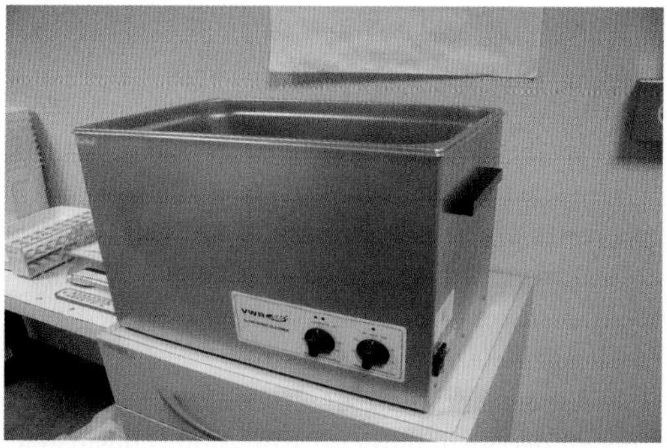

Fig. 4.2 An ultrasonic bath for sonication of prosthetic implants

With time, different authors reported some limitations of sonication, which included the risk of contamination during sample processing, the need for dedicated instrumentation, and a lower detection rate of *Staphylococcus epidermidis* compared with other methods (Bjerkan et al. 2009; Trampuz et al. 2006; Esteban et al. 2008).

The risk for isolation of contaminants (particularly of CNS) has also been evidenced in the unique study evaluating the use of blood bottles for the culture of sonicated fluid (Hao et al. 2015).

Chemical Agents

An alternative approach to dislodge bacteria from infected implants is the use of chemical agents. Sulfhydryl compounds are well known for their ability to reduce disulphide bounds between polysaccharides and neighbouring proteins and to interfere with biofilm formation.

DL-dithiothreitol (DTT) is a sulfhydryl compound which is routinely used in clinical microbiology for liquefying specimens from the respiratory tract. Its efficacy in removing bacteria from prosthetic materials has been initially studied in an in vitro model (Drago et al. 2012). In this study, the amount of bacteria retrieved from biofilm on titanium discs was comparable to that obtained after sonication of the same material and superior to bacterial cells recovered after treatment with *N*-acetyl-

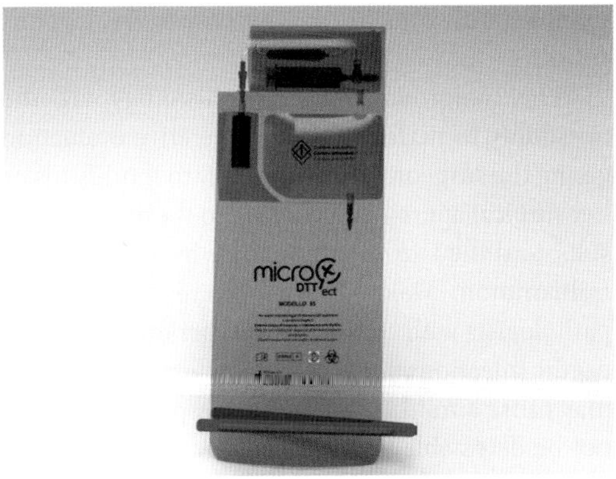

Fig. 4.3 A dithiothreitol-based device for treatment of prosthetic implants and osteoarticular tissues

cysteine and after scraping of disk surfaces. Subsequently the method was applied to prosthetic implants and compared with sonication and tissue cultures (Drago et al. 2013). After addition of a 0.1% w:v DTT solution, samples were vortexed, mechanically stirred for 15 min and centrifuged. The pellet was plated onto solid media and inoculated in enrichment broths which were incubated for 15 days. DTT showed a higher sensitivity than sonication (85.7 vs 71.4%) and the same specificity as sonication (94.1%). Differences in sensitivity were mainly due to the higher frequency of isolation of *Staphylococcus epidermidis* obtained with DTT compared with sonication.

Only a few data are available on the applicability of the aforementioned method for microbiological analysis of spacers when the revision procedure is completed in two stages. A device for the treatment of prosthetic implants and tissue samples based on the DTT method is currently under development and will be soon available on the market (Fig. 4.3). It will allow all specimens to be treated in a closed system in order to reduce contamination during sample processing.

Susceptibility Testing

The aim of microbiological analysis is to provide the clinician with data on the antimicrobial susceptibility of the causative organism. Susceptibility testing is usually performed automatically together with pathogen identification. Susceptibility is expressed as minimum inhibitory concentration (MIC) values, defined as the lowest antimicrobial concentration able to inhibit bacterial growth. However, MIC values are calculated by using bacteria grown freely in planktonic form, while bacteria responsible of PJIs usually grow as a biofilm. Therefore, in vitro susceptibility testing could not correlate with susceptibility testing of bacteria adhered on prosthetic implants embedded in a biofilm. In this context it must be underlined that biofilm bacteria may be even 1,000-fold more resistant to antibiotics than their planktonic counterparts. Therefore, susceptibility should be assessed in a different way. The term »minimum biofilm eradication concentration« (MBEC) indicates the lowest antimicrobial concentration able to prevent regrowth of the bacteria from the treated biofilm. The assay requires prolonged incubation and it is not easy to perform, thus it cannot be applied to all isolates in routine work.

4.1.6 Molecular Analysis

The characteristics of molecular methods – a high sensitivity and specificity as well as a rapid turnaround time – theoretically should be perfect for the diagnosis of PJIs. Nonetheless, their use has not been universally accepted, and some comparative studies with culture have not found significant differences between molecular and cultural methods (Rak et al. 2013; Zegaer et al. 2014). The main advantage of molecular methods is that they do not need growth of micro-organisms to detect their presence. By contrast, they can also detect the DNA of dead micro-organisms or those inadvertently left on the sample during its collection.

Essentially, two approaches have been used in the molecular diagnosis of PJIs: broad-range polymerase chain reaction (PCR) and specific PCR. The latter is tailored to detect single bacterial species or a group of closely related micro-organisms. Real-time PCR assays may yield results in a few hours, and have a sufficient limit of detection, allowing one to quantitatively detect only micro-organisms which are considered significant. In this way, contamination may be kept under control. The main limitation of specific PCR is that it detects only micro-organisms for which primers have been designed. This means that panel must include primers for micro-organisms such as *Propionibacteria* and *Corynebacteria* which are usually considered as contaminants in other infections.

Broad-range PCR facilitates the detection of a wide variety of micro-organisms. The majority of broad-range PCRs are based on amplification of the 16S rDNA, which codifies for the small ribosomal unit. This gene is composed of conserved regions common to all bacteria, and more variable regions which are specific for bacterial species. Usually detection of nucleic acid is followed by amplicon sequencing. The main limitation of these assays is the high risk of contaminating DNA. Methods developed to reduce contamination dramatically affect the test sensitivity and therefore they are not used.

Finally, although not recommended for routine use as an alternative to cultures, molecular methods may represent an additional tool in selected negative cultures from patients for whom a strong suspicion of PJI exists.

4.1.7 Histological Evaluation

Histological examination is particularly valuable when the possibility of infection is not completely confirmed or excluded after a thorough preoperative evaluation, showing a sensitivity of 50–93% and a specificity of 77–100% (Tsaras et al. 2012; Saeed 2014). Demonstration of acute inflammation – indicated by the presence of at least five neutrophils per high-power field in at least five high-power microscopic fields (400×) in fixed or frozen periprosthetic tissue samples – is considered suggestive of PJI. Alternatively, since the inflammatory response may be associated with other histological findings, a consensus classification of the periprosthetic membrane based on low-cost standard tissue processing and examination has been established (Krenn et al. 2014). It divides aseptic and septic prosthetic failure into four histological types, also describing histopathological criteria for additional significant pathologies including endoprosthetic-associated arthrofibrosis, particle-induced immunological, inflammatory, and toxic mechanisms (adverse reactions), and bone tissue pathologies. Unfortunately, this platform is not widely used by pathologists, who prefer the classic neutrophils count.

The major advantages of histology are the possibility to perform an intraoperative evaluation giving the surgeon the opportunity to modify his or her surgical approach according to the histology results, and the lack of interference by antibiotic administration. Major drawbacks are: the need for pathologists with considerable experience in orthopaedic infections; the fact that low-grade pathogens may cause a mild inflammatory response that cannot be detectable by the analysis; and the need for representative samples (periprosthetic interface membrane, or pseudocapsule) in order to avoid false-negative results.

4.1.8 Biochemical, Haematological, and Serological Diagnosis

Erythrocyte Sedimentation Rate and C-Reactive Protein

Thanks to their limited invasiveness of drawing blood as well as their rapidity and relatively low cost, ESR and CRP are the first parameters that are determined when a PJI is suspected. Their measurement is also included in procedures for PJI diagnosis (■ Tab. 4.1). Their major limitation is the low specificity, because conditions other than PJI such as inflammation, obesity or other concomitant infections may alter these parameters. By contrast, suppressive antimicrobial therapy, low-virulence pathogens (CNS, corynebacteria, propionibacteria, mycobacteria, actynomycetes) and chronic infections may cause false-negative results. Moreover, both ESR and CRP increased in the post-operative period – ESR for up to 6 weeks and CRP for up to 2 weeks – and thus their determination, particularly that of ESR, is limited in the immediate post-operative period for the diagnosis of early infections. Moreover, a serum CRP concentration higher than 100 mg/l is considered suggestive of acute infection occurring in the six post-operative weeks after primary surgery (Zmistowski et al. 2014). A combination of both parameters using a threshold of 30 mm/h and 10 mg/l for ESR and CRP, respectively, has shown a sensitivity of 96%, despite a specificity of only 56% for chronic infections, (Tande and

Patel 2014). An increase in ESR and CRP above threshold may raise the suspicion of a PJI, suggesting further investigations such as joint aspiration (Osmon et al. 2013; Zmistowski et al. 2014). If ESR and CRP are not elevated and there is no clinical suspicion of PJI, then joint aspiration is not necessary.

White Blood Cell Count

The leukocyte count and blood differential test are not reliable for the diagnosis of PJIs because of the low sensitivity and specificity; they may be more useful, however, when determined in synovial fluid (Osmon et al. 2013).

Interleukin-6 and Other Serum Inflammatory Markers

Interleukin-6 (IL-6) is released by stimulated monocytes, macrophages, fibroblasts and T2 lymphocytes. It elicits release of CRP from liver cells, so that its serum level increases faster than CRP. With a half-life of only 15 h, IL-6 could be very useful in the early post-operative period and its concentration has been shown to correlate with inflammatory activity (Wirtz et al. 2000). Available albeit limited data indicate good specificity and sensitivity (77–91% and 81–97%) when cut-off values of 9–12 pg/ml are used. Therefore, CRP and IL-6 in combination might be used as screening tests for early PJI. The major limitation in IL-6 measurement resides in the wide range of normal serum IL-6 levels, which may cause variable cut-off, and in the relative specificity of IL-6, which may increase after trauma, chronic inflammatory conditions and arthroplasty (Saeed 2014).

The role of procalcitonin (PCT) is more debated. PCT is a serum marker that increases in some conditions such as the presence of bacteria. In particular, its secretion by the mononuclear phagocytic system is stimulated by contact with lipopolysaccharides. PCT is widely used for diagnosis and for the monitoring of antibiotic therapy in sepsis and pneumonia, but contrasting data exist on its efficacy in the diagnosis of PJIs, while it seems to be more reliable in the diagnosis of septic arthritis. A wide range of sensitivity and specificity values have been described (Ettinger et al. 2015; Yuan et al. 2015; Glehr et al. 2013; Drago et al. 2011). Therefore, at the moment there are not enough data to support routine PCT evaluation in the diagnosis of PJI.

Other markers have been evaluated for the diagnosis of PJIs, such as soluble intercellular adhesion molecule-1, serum IgG to short-chain exocellular lipoteichoic acid, and soluble urokinase-type plasminogen activator receptor (suPAR), but they have not been in enough studies to allow conclusions to be drawn on their real effectiveness (Galliera et al. 2015; Worthington et al. 2010).

Synovial Analysis

The poor specificity of serum evaluation of some markers may be overcome by determining their concentration directly in synovial fluid, where the influence of inflammatory conditions may be limited. Cytokines such as IL-1β, IL-6, IL-8 and IL-17 as well as tumour necrosis factor (TNF)-α and interferon (IFN)-δ are released from macrophages in synovial fluid of patients with PJI. However, other joint inflammatory conditions like rheumatoid arthritis or vasculitis may increase production of these markers, thus limiting their potential use (Matsen Ko and Parvizi 2016). Other synovial markers seem to be more specific for infections than the aforementioned cytokines, and some of them have been more deeply investigated. Synovial CRP has a reported sensitivity and specificity of 85–87% and 71–98%, respectively, depending on the cut-off used (Omar et al. 2015; Deirmengian et al. 2014; Tetreault et al. 2014). The major advantage is that CRP measurement may be carried out on an automatic analyser, with a rapid turnaround time and limited economic cost. However, reagents available for automatic analysers have not been approved by the manufacturers for such use and not all laboratories agree to perform an analysis on biological materials for which the instrument cannot be calibrated.

Leukocyte esterase catalyses the degradation of connective tissue matrix, which is released by neutrophils recruited at the site of infections. Its presence may be easily detected by colorimetric strips, like those used for urine analysis. A change in the shade of colour indicates the occurrence of a hydrolytic reaction on the test pad. The test has been included in the criteria proposed by the International Consensus Meeting for the diagnosis of PJIs. Available data on the test performance indicate a high sensitivity and specificity, both greater than 90% (De Vecchi et al. 2016; Colvin et al. 2015; Tischler et al. 2014). The major advantages are the rapid turnaround time, which allows the test to be performed intraoperatively as an alternative to frozen section, the limited cost and no requirements for additional or dedicated instrumentation. The major limitation is represented by the interference of blood. In fact, bloody samples may lead to difficult-to-read results, since a change in the colour of the pad may be due to the sample and not to the presence of esterase. This can be partially overcome by introducing a centrifugation step and proper controls. Despite a relative prolongation of the time required for the test (about 10–15 min vs 2 min without centrifugation), an esterase reaction reading of the supernatant of the centrifuged fluids reduces the number of indeterminate samples, while maintaining an acceptable time to response even for intraoperative diagnosis.

Alpha-defensin is another synovial biomarker which is released by neutrophils upon contact with bacteria. An ELISA test specifically developed for use in synovial fluid, able to provide results in about 4–5 h, has been launched on the market. Studies evaluating its use for PJI diagnosis have shown high sensitivity and specificity (95–100% and 90–96%, respectively), comparable to or higher than those reported for leukocyte esterase (Deirmengian et al. 2014; Frangiamore et al. 2016; Deirmengian et al. 2015; Bingham et al. 2014). However, most of the studies have been carried out by the same group, and further evaluation by independent authors is expected.

Leukocyte count and blood differential tests have a high sensitivity and specificity for PJI diagnosis. The threshold for positivity varied among population and joint type. A wide range of cut-offs have been applied in the different studies, showing variable sensitivity and specificity. According to criteria defined by the Philadelphia International Consensus Meeting total leukocyte counts greater than 10,000/μl with more than 90% of neutrophils are considered as suggestive of acute PJI. Chronic infections are defined by a total leukocyte count of at least 3,000 cells per microlitre with more than 80% neutrophils. Moreover, it seems that the threshold for hip leukocyte count might be higher than for the knee, but supporting data are rather scarce. The test is easy to perform, inexpensive, rapid and affordable for all laboratories having a cell counter. Major limitations in the use of leukocyte count are blood contamination and interference by other inflammatory diseases of the joint. Contamination of the sample by blood during collection causes an increase in leukocytes count; however, if a blood sample is collected simultaneously, it is possible to normalize the count by comparing the erythrocyte count of the synovial fluid with that of the blood. Patients with rheumatoid arthritis have a higher baseline leukocyte count, and thus the proposed cut-off values must be elevated in these subjects. Moreover, failed metal-on-metal implants can interfere with leukocyte counts determined by automated counters, while no interference is observed with manual counts. Finally, synovial cell counts may increase because of haemarthrosis or post-operative inflammation, shortly after primary arthroplasty.

4.1.9 National Recommendations for Diagnosis of PJIs

Because of the complexity of PJI diagnosis and the wide variability in analytical methods used by the various centres even in the same country, the definition of a uniform diagnostic protocol is advisable. Most national recommendations for the evaluation and treatment of PJIs, such as those published in France (SPILF 2010) and Italy (AMCLI 2013), are similar to those of the ICM document (International Consensus Meeting of Philadelphia).

The Italian Association of Clinical Microbiologists (AMCLI) in 2013 defined a diagnostic algorithm for PJIs. In particular, the protocol addressed a microbiological diagnosis, which was considered the most critical point of the whole diagnostic workflow. The protocol is freely available on the association's website (http://www.amcli.it). The work-flow for the diagnosis of PJIs was divided into a pre- and intraoperative analysis and describes in detail the pre-analytic, analytic and post-analytic steps.

Take-Home Message

- Biofilm is intrinsic to the pathogenesis of all kinds of prosthetic infections, including joints infections.
- To date, an international gold standard for the diagnosis of PJI has not been established; a multidisciplinary approach including biochemical, microbiological and histological analyses, as well as clinical findings together with radiological studies, should be applied.
- The term »coagulase negative staphylococci« (CNS) defines a variegated group of staphylococci usually retrievable as normal components of the human skin; they are the main cause of PJIs.
- Some implant failures classified as aseptic may be unrecognized low-grade infections due to CNS, and revision surgery may favour development of an acute infection.
- Joint aspiration for improved diagnosis should be performed on all patients with suspected PJIs, if possible. However, the use of swabs to sample periprosthetic tissue as well as synovial fluid is not recommended and must be avoided for PJI diagnosis.
- Minimum inhibitory concentration (MIC) values are defined as the lowest antimicrobial concentration able to inhibit bacterial growth. However, MIC values are calculated by using bacteria grown freely in planktonic form, while bacteria responsible for PJIs usually grow in biofilm. Biofilm bacteria may be even 1,000-fold more resistant to antibiotics than their planktonic counterparts. Therefore, alternative methods to assess susceptibility should be used

4.1.10 Conclusion

In summary, the diagnosis of PJIs is a complex challenge for orthopaedics and requires a strict collaboration between different specialists: orthopaedists, infectious disease specialists, microbiologists, pathologists and radiologists. Diagnostic criteria have been described by national and international associations and scientific societies. On the whole, they are rather similar although they do have some peculiarities. Clinicians should be trained on how to use them, but more importantly they should know the potentials and limitations of the available tests in order to use them appropriately.

References

Aggarwal VK, Higuera C, Deirmengian G, Parvizi J, Austin MS (2013) Swab cultures are not as effective as tissue cultures for diagnosis of periprosthetic joint infection. Clin Orthop Relat Res 471(10):3196–3203

Barrack RL, Harris WH (1993) The value of aspiration of the hip joint before revision total hip arthroplasty. J Bone Joint Surg Am 75(1):66–76

Bartalesi F, Fallani S, Salomoni E, Marcucci M, Meli M, Pecile P, Cassetta MI, Latella L, Bartoloni A, Novelli A (2012) *Candida glabrata* prosthetic hip infection. Am J Orthop 41(11):500–505

Bemer P, Leger J, Tande D, Plouzeau C, Valentin AS, Jolivet-Gougeon A, Lemarie C, Kempf M, Hery-Arnaud G, Bret L, Juvin ME, Girardeau B, Corvec S, Burucoa C, the Centre de Reference des Infections Osteo-articulaires du Grand Ouest (CRIOGO) Study Team (2016) How many samples and how many culture media to diagnose a prosthetic joint infection: a clinical and microbiological prospective multicenter study. J Clin Microbiol 54(2):385–391

Berbari EF, Hanssen AD, Duffy MC, Steckelberg JM, Osmon DR (1998) Prosthetic joint infection due to *Mycobacterium tuberculosis*: a case series and review of the literature. Am J Orthop 27(3):219–227

Bingham J, Clarke H, Spangehl M, Schwartz A, Beauchamp C, Goldberg B (2014) The alpha defensin-1 biomarker assay can be used to evaluate the potentially infected total joint arthroplasty. Clin Orthop Relat Res 472(12): 4006–4009

Bjerkan G, Witsø E, Bergh K (2009) Sonication is superior to scraping for retrieval of bacteria in biofilm on titanium and steel surfaces in vitro. Acta Orthop 80(2):245–250

Blackmur JP, Tang EYH, Dave J, Simpson AHRW (2014) Use of broth cultures peri-operatively to optimize the microbiological diagnosis of musculoskeletal implant infections. Bone Joint J 96-B(11):1566–1570

Butler-Wu SM, Burns EM, Pottinger PS, Magaret AS, Rakeman JL, Matsen FA 3rd, Cookson BT (2011). Optimization of periprosthetic culture for diagnosis of *Propionibacterium acnes* prosthetic joint infection. J Clin Microbiol 49(7): 2490–2495

Castillo-Juárez I, Maeda T, Mandujano-Tinoco EA, Tomás M, Pérez-Eretza B, García-Contreras SJ, Wood TK, García-Contreras R (2015) Role of quorum sensing in bacterial infections. World J Clin Cases 3(7):575–598

Cazanave C, Greenwood-Quaintance KE, Hanssen AD, Patel R (2012) Corynebacterium prosthetic joint infection. J Clin Microbiol 50(5):1518–1523

Colvin OC, Kransdorf MJ, Roberts CC, Chivers FS, Lorans R, Beauchamp CP, Schwartz AJ (2015) Leukocyte esterase

analysis in the diagnosis of joint infection: can we make a diagnosis using a simple urine dipstick? Skeletal Radiol 44(5):673–677
de Sanctis J, Teixeira L, van Duin D, Odio C, Hall G, Tomford JW, Perez F, Rudin SD, Bonomo RA, Barsoum WK, Joyce M, Krebs V, Schmitt S (2014) Complex prosthetic joint infections due to carbapenemase-producing *Klebsiella pneumoniae*: a unique challenge in the era of untreatable infections. Int J Infect Dis 25:73–78
De Vecchi E, Villa F, Bortolin M, Toscano M, Tacchini L, Romanò CL, Drago L (2016) Leukocyte esterase, glucose and C-reactive protein in the diagnosis of prosthetic joint infections: a prospective study. Clin Microbiol Infect 22(6):555-560
DeHaan A, Huff T, Schabel K, Doung YC, Hayden J, Barnes P (2013) Multiple cultures and extended incubation for hip and knee arthroplasty revision: impact on clinical care. J Arthroplasty 28(8Suppl):59–65
Deirmengian C, Kardos K, Kilmartin P, Cameron A, Schiller K, Parvizi J (2014) Combined measurement of synovial fluid α-Defensin and C-reactive protein levels: highly accurate for diagnosing periprosthetic joint infection. J Bone Joint Surg Am 96(17):1439–1445
Deirmengian C, Kardos K, Kilmartin P, Cameron A, Schiller K, Parvizi J (2014) Diagnosing PJI: has the era of biomarkers arrived? Clin Orthop Relate Res 472(7):3254–3262
Deirmengian C, Kardos K, Kilmartin P, Gulati S, Citrano P, Booth RE Jr (2015) The Alpha-defensin test for periprosthetic joint infection responds to a wide spectrum of organisms. Clin Orthop Relat Res 473:2229–2235
Dilisio MF, Miller LR, Warner JJ, Higgins LD (2014) Arthroscopic tissue culture for the evaluation of periprosthetic shoulder infection. J Bone Joint Surg Am 96(23):1952–1958
Donlan RM (2002) Biofilms: microbial life on surfaces. Emerg Infect Dis 8(9):881–890
Drago L, Vassena C, Dozio E, Corsi MM, De Vecchi E, Mattina R, Romanò C (2011) Procalcitonin, C-reactive protein, interleukin-6, and soluble intercellular adhesion molecule-1 as markers of postoperative orthopaedic joint prosthesis infections. Int J Immunopathol Pharmacol 24(2):433–440
Drago L, Romanò CL, Mattina R, Signori V, De Vecchi E (2012) Does dithiothreitol improve bacterial detection from infected prostheses? A pilot study. Clin Orthop Relat Res 470(10):2915–2925
Drago L, Signori V, De Vecchi E, Vassena C, Palazzi E, Cappelletti L, Romanò D, Romanò CL (2013) Use of dithiothreitol to improve the diagnosis of prosthetic joint infections. J Orthop Res 31(11):1694–1699
Drago L, De Vecchi E, Cappelletti L, Mattina R, Vassena C, Romanò CL (2014) Role and antimicrobial resistance of staphylococci involved in prosthetic joint infections. Int J Artif Organs 37(5):414–421
Drago L, De Vecchi E, Cappelletti L, Vassena C, Toscano M, Bortolin M, Mattina R, Romanò CL (2015) Prolonging culture to 15 days improves bacterial detection in bone and joint infections. Eur J Clin Microbiol Infect Dis 34(9): 1809–1813
Dutronc H, Dauchy FA, Cazanave C, Rougie C, Lafarie-Castet S, Couprie B, Fabre T, Dupon M (2010) Candida prosthetic infections: case series and literature review. Scand J Infect Dis 42:890–895
Esteban J, Gomez-Barrena E, Cordero J, Martín-de-Hijas NZ, Kinnari TJ, Fernandez-Roblas R (2008) Evaluation of quantitative analysis of cultures from sonicated retrieved orthopedic implants in diagnosis of orthopedic infection. J Clin Microbiol 46(2):488–492
Ettinger M, Calliess T, Kielstein JT, Sibai J, Brückner T, Lichtinghagen R, Windhagen H, Lukasz A (2015) Circulating biomarkers for discrimination between aseptic joint failure, low-grade infection, and high-grade septic failure. Clin Infect Dis 61(3):332–341
Fernandes A, Dias M (2013) The microbiological profiles of infected prosthetic implants with an emphasis on the organisms which form biofilms. J Clin Diagn Res 7(2): 219–223
Fink B, Makowiak C, Fuerst M, Berger I, Schäfer P, Frommelt L (2008) The value of synovial biopsy, joint aspiration and C-reactive protein in the diagnosis of late peri-prosthetic infection of total knee replacements. J Bone Joint Surg Br 90(7):874–878
Font-Vizcarra L; Spangehl MJ, Masri BA, O'Connell JX, Duncan CP (1999) Prospective analysis of preoperative and intraoperative investigations for the diagnosis of infection at the sites of two hundred and two revision total hip arthroplasties. J Bone Joint Surg Am 81(5): 672–683
Font-Vizcarra L, García S, Martínez-Pastor JC, Sierra JM, Soriano A (2010) Blood culture flasks for culturing synovial fluid in prosthetic joint infections. Clin Orthop Relat Res 468(8):2238–2243
Frangiamore SJ, Gajewski ND, Saleh A, Farias-Kovac M, Barsoum WK, Higuera CA (2016) α-Defensin accuracy to diagnose periprosthetic joint infection-best available test? J Arthroplasty 31(2):456–460
Galliera E, Drago L, Marazzi MG, Romanò C, Vassena C, Corsi Romanelli MM (2015) Soluble urokinase-type plasminogen activator receptor (suPAR) as new biomarker of the prosthetic joint infection: correlation with inflammatory cytokines. Clin Chim Acta 441:23–28
Gbejuade HO, Lovering AM, Webb JC (2015) The role of microbial biofilm in prosthetic joint infections. Acta Orthoped 86(2):147–158
Glehr M, Friesenbichler J, Hofmann G, Bernhardt GA, Zacherl M, Avian A, Windhager R, Leithner A (2013) Novel biomarkers to detect infection in revision hip and knee arthroplasties. Clin Orthop Relat Res 471(8):2621–2628
Gupta A, Berbari EF, Osmon DR, Virk A (2014) Prosthetic joint infection due to Salmonella species: a case series. BMC Infect Dis doi:10.1186/s12879-014-0633-x
Hao Shen, Jin Tang, Qiaojie Wang, Yao Jiang, Xianlong Zhang (2015) Sonication of explanted prosthesis combined with incubation in BD Bactec bottles for pathogen-based diagnosis of prosthetic joint infection. J Clin Microbiol 53(3):777–781

Holleyman RJ, Baker PN, Charlett A, Gould K, Deehan DJ (2016) Analysis of causative microorganism in 248 primary hip arthroplasties revised for infection: a study using the NJR dataset. Hip Int 26(1):82–89
Hughes JG, Vetter EA, Patel R, Schleck CD, Harmsen S, Turgeant LT, Cockerill FR 3rd (2001) Culture with BACTEC Peds Plus/F bottle compared with conventional methods for detection of bacteria in synovial fluid. J Clin Microbiol 39(12):4468–4471
Huotari K, Peltola M, Jamsen E (2015) The incidence of late prosthetic joint infections. A registry based study on 112,708 primary hip and knee replacement. Acta Orthopaedica 86(3):321–325
Kapadia BH, Berg RA, Daley JA, Fritz J, Bhave A, Mont MA (2016) Periprosthetic joint infection. Lancet 387(16):386–394
Krenn V, Morawietz L, Perino G, Kienapfel H, Ascherl R, Hassenpflug GJ, Thomsen M, Thomas P, Huber M, Kendoff D, Baumhoer D, Krukemeyer MG, Natu S, Boettner F, Zustin J, Kölbel B, Rüther W, Kretzer JP, Tiemann A, Trampuz A, Frommelt L, Tichilow R, Söder S, Müller S, Parvizi J, Illgner U, Gehrke T (2014) Revised histopathological consensus classification of joint implant related pathology. Pathol Res Pract 210(12):779–786
Kurtz SM, Lau e, Watson H, Schmier JK, Parvizi J (2012) Economic burden of periprosthetic joint infection in the United States. J Arthroplasty 27(Suppl8):61–65e1
Janz V, Wassilew GI, Kribus M, Trampuz A, Perka C (2015) Improved identification of polymicrobial infection in total knee arthroplasty through sonicate fluid cultures. Arch Orthop Trauma Surg. 135(10):1453–1457
Langvatn H, Everts RJ, Chambers ST, Murdoch DR, Rothwell AG, McKie J (2004) Successful antimicrobial therapy and implant retention for streptococcal infection of prosthetic joints. ANZ J Surg 74(4):210–214
Langvatn H, Lutro O, Dale H, Schrama JC, Hallan G, Espehaug B, Sjursen H, Engesæter LB (2015) Bacterial and hematological findings in infected total hip arthroplasties in Norway assessment of 278 revisions due to infection in the Norwegian arthroplasty register. Open Orthop J 9:445–449
Levine BR, Evans BG (2001) Use of blood culture vial specimens in intraoperative detection of infection. Clin Orthop Relat Res 382:222–231
Lovati AB, Romanò CL, Bottagisio M, Monti L, De Vecchi E, Previdi S, Accetta R, Drago L (2016) Modeling *Staphylococcus epidermidis*-induced non-unions: subclinical and clinical evidence in rats. PLoS One doi:10.1371/journal.pone.0147447
Matsen Ko L, Parvizi J (2016) Diagnosis of periprosthetic infection: novel developments. Orthop Clin North Am 47(1):1–9
Murillo O, Grau I, Lora-Tamayo J, Gomez-Junyent J, Ribera A, Tubau F, Ariza J, Pallares R (2015) The changing epidemiology of bacteraemic osteoarticular infections in the early 21st century. Clin Microbiol Infect 21(3):254.e1–8
Omar M, Ettinger M, Reichling M, Petri M, Guenther D, Gehrke T, Krettek C, Mommsen P (2015) Synovial C- reactive protein as a marker for chronic periprosthetic infection in total hip arthroplasty. Bone Joint J 97-B(2):173–176
Osmon DR, Berbari EF, Berendt AR, Lew D, Zimmerli W, Steckelberg JM, Rao N, Hanssen A, Wilson WR (2013) Diagnosis and management of prosthetic joint infection: clinical practice guidelines by the Infectious Diseases Society of America. Clin Infect Dis 56(1):e1–e25
Parvizi J, Zmistowski B, Berbari EF, Bauer TW, Springer BD, Della Valle CJ, Garvin KL, Mont MA, Wongworawat MD, Zalavras CG (2011) New definition for periprosthetic joint infection: from the Workgroup of the Musculoskeletal Infection Society. Clin Orthop Relat Res 469(11):2992–2994
Percival SL, Suleman L, Vuotto C, Donelli G (2015) Healthcare-associated infections, medical devices and biofilms: risk, tolerance and control. J Med Microbiol 64(Pt4):323–334
Portillo ME, Salvadó M, Trampuz A, Plasencia V, Rodriguez-Villasante M, Sorli L, Puig L, Horcajada JP (2013) Sonication versus vortexing of implants for diagnosis of prosthetic joint infection. J Clin Microbiol 51(2):591–594
Rabin N, Zheng Y, Opoku-Temeng C, Du Y, Bonsu E, Sintim HO (2015) Biofilm formation mechanisms and targets for developing antibiofilm agents. Future Med Chem 7(4):493–512
Rak M, Barlic-Maganja D, Kavcic M, Trebse R, Cor A (2013) Comparison of molecular and culture method in diagnosis of prosthetic joint infection. FEMS Microbiol Lett 343(1):42–48
Rasouli MR, Harandi AA, Adeli B, Purtill JJ, Parvizi J (2012) Revision total knee arthroplasty: infection should be ruled out in all cases. J Arthroplasty 27(6):1239–1243.e1–2
Renner LD, Weibel DB (2011) Physicochemical regulation of biofilm formation. MRS Bull 36(5):347–355
Rodríguez-Pardo D, Pigrau C, Lora-Tamayo J, Soriano A, del Toro MD, Cobo J, Palomino J, Euba G, Riera M, Sánchez-Somolinos M, Benito N, Fernández-Sampedro M, Sorli L, Guio L, Iribarren JA, Baraia-Etxaburu JM, Ramos A, Bahamonde A, Flores-Sánchez X, Corona PS, Ariza J; REIPI group for the study of prosthetic infection (2014) Gram-negative prosthetic joint infection: outcome of a debridement, antibiotics and implant retention approach. A large multicentre study. Clin Microbiol Infect 20(11):O911–919
Romanò CL, De Vecchi E, Vassena C, Manzi G, Drago L (2013) A case of a late and atypical knee prosthetic infection by no-biofilm producer *Pasteurella multocida* strain identified by pyrosequencing. Pol J Microbiol 62(4): 435–438
Roux AL, Sivadon-Tardy V, Bauer T, Lortat-Jacob A, Herrmann JL, Gaillard JL, Rottman M (2011) Diagnosis of prosthetic joint infection by beadmill processing of a periprosthetic specimen. Clin Microbiol Infect 17(3):447–450
Saeed K (2014) Diagnostics in prosthetic joint infections. J Antimicrob Chemother 69(Suppl1): i11–19
Schäfer P, Fink B, Sandow D, Margull A, Berger I, Frommelt L (2008) Prolonged bacterial culture to identify late periprosthetic joint infection: a promising strategy. Clin Infect Dis 47(11):1403–1409

Senneville E, Joulie D, Legout L, Valette M, Dezèque H, Beltrand E, Roselé B, d'Escrivan T, Loïez C, Caillaux M, Yazdanpanah Y, Maynou C, Migaud H (2011) Outcome and predictors of treatment failure in total hip/knee prosthetic joint infections due to *Staphylococcus aureus*. Clin Infect Dis 53(4):334–340

Shah NB, Tande AJ, Patel R, Berbari EF (2015) Anaerobic prosthetic joint infection. Anaerobe 36:1–8

Société de Pathologie Infectieuse de Langue Française (SPILF); Collège des Universitaires de Maladies Infectieuses et Tropicales (CMIT); Groupe de Pathologie Infectieuse Pédiatrique (GPIP); Société Française d'Anesthésie et de Réanimation (SFAR); Société Française de Chirurgie Orthopédique et Traumatologique (SOFCOT); Société Française d'Hygiène Hospitalière (SFHH); Société Française de Médecine Nucléaire (SFMN); Société Française de Médecine Physique et de Réadaptation (SOFMER); Société Française de Microbiologie (SFM); Société Française de Radiologie (SFR-Rad); Société Française de Rheumatologie (SFR-Rhu) (2010) Recommendations for bone and joint prosthetic device infections in clinical practice (prosthesis, implants, osteosynthesis). Société de Pathologie Infectieuse de Langue Française. Med Mal Infect 40:185-211

Stoodley P, Conti SF, Demeo PJ, Nistico L, Melton-Kreft R, Johnson S, Darabi A, Ehrlich GD, Costerton JW, Kathju S (2011) Characterization of a mixed MRSA/MRSE biofilm in an explanted total ankle arthroplasty. FEMS Immunol Med Microbiol 62(1):66–74

Tande AJ, Patel R (2014) Prosthetic joint infection. Clin Microbiol Rev 27(2):302–345

Tetreault MW, Wetters NG, Aggarwal VK, Moric M, Segreti J, Huddleston JI 3rd, Parvizi J, Della Valle CJ (2013) Should draining wounds and sinuses associated with hip and knee arthroplasties be cultured? J Arthroplasty 28 (8Suppl):133–136

Tetreault MW, Wetters NG, Moric M, Gross CE, Della Valle CJ (2014) Is synovial C-reactive protein a useful marker for periprosthetic joint infection? Clin Orthop Relat Res 472(12):3997–4003

Tischler EH, Cavanaugh PK, Parvizi J (2014) Leukocyte esterase strip test: matched for musculoskeletal infection society criteria. J Bone Joint Surg Am 96(22):1917–1920

Tornero E, Senneville E, Euba G, Petersdorf S, Rodriguez-Pardo D, Lakatos B, Ferrari MC, Pilares M, Bahamonde A, Trebse R, Benito N, Sorli L, del Toro MD, Baraiaetxaburu JM, Ramos A, Riera M, Jover-Sáenz A, Palomino J, Ariza J, Soriano A, European society group of infections on artificial implants (ESGIAI) (2014) Characteristics of prosthetic joint infections due to *Enterococcus* sp. and predictors of failure: a multi-national study. Clin Microbiol Infect 20(11):1219–1224

Trampuz A, Piper KE, Hanssen AD, Osmon DR, Cockerill FR, Steckelberg JM, Patel R (2006) Sonication of explanted prosthetic components in bags for diagnosis of prosthetic joint infection is associated with risk of contamination. J Clin Microbiol 44(2):628–631

Tsaras G, Maduka-Ezeh A, Inwards CY, Mabry T, Erwin PJ, Murad MH, Montori VM, West CP, Osmon DR, Berbari EF (2012) Utility of intraoperative frozen section histopathology in the diagnosis of periprosthetic joint infection: a systematic review and meta-analysis. J Bone Joint Surg Am 94(2):1700–1711

Tunney MM, Patrick S, Gorman SP, Nixon JR, Anderson N, Davis RI, Hanna D, Ramage G (1998) Improved detection of infection in hip replacements. A currently underestimated problem. J Bone Joint Surg Br 80(4): 568–572

Yuan K, Li WD, Qiang Y, Cui ZM (2015) Comparison of procalcitonin and C-reactive protein for the diagnosis of periprosthetic joint infection before revision total hip arthroplasty. Surg Infect (Larchmt) 16(2):146–150

Williams JL, Norman P, Stockley I (2004) The value of hip aspiration versus tissue biopsy in diagnosing infection before exchange hip arthroplasty surgery. J Arthroplasty 19(5):582–586

Wirtz DC, Heller KD, Miltner O, Zilkens KW, Wolff JM (2000) Interleukin-6: a potential inflammatory marker after total joint replacement. Int Orthop 24(4):194–196

Worthington T, Dunlop D, Casey A, Lambert R, Luscombe J, Elliott T (2010) Serum procalcitonin, interleukin-6, soluble intercellular adhesin molecule-1 and IgG to short-chain exocellular lipoteichoic acid as predictors of infection in total joint prosthesis revision. Br J Biomed Sci 67(2):71–76

Zegaer BH, Ioannidis A, Babis GC, Ioannidou V, Kossyvakis A, Bersimis S, Papaparaskevas J, Petinaki E, Pliatsika P, Chatzipanagiotou S (2014) Detection of bacteria bearing resistant biofilm forms, by using the universal and specific PCR is still unhelpful in the diagnosis of periprosthetic joint infections. Front Med doi:10.3389/fmed.2014.00030

Zmistowski B, Della Valle C, Bauer TW, Malizos KN, Alavi A, Bedair H, Booth RE, Choong P, Deirmengian C, Ehrlich GD, Gambir A, Huang R, Kissin Y, Kobayashi H, Kobayashi N, Krenn V, Drago L, Marston SB, Meermans G, Perez J, Ploegmakers JJ, Rosenberg A, Simpendorfer C, Thomas P, Tohtz S, Villafuerte JA, Wahl P, Wagenaar FC, Witzo E (2014) Diagnosis of periprosthetic joint infection. J Arthroplasty 29(2Suppl):77–83

Zoubos AB, Galanakos SP, Soucacos PN (2012) Orthopedics and biofilm – what do we know? A review. Med Sci Monit 18(6):RA89–96

4.2 Diagnosis of Pathogens

Frank-Christiaan B.M. Wagenaar, Dean F.M. Pakvis, and Lars Frommelt

4.2.1 Why Are PJIs on the Rise?

The incidence of periprosthetic joint infections (PJI) ranges from 1% to 4% of all hip/knee arthroplasties (Jamsen et al. 2009, Phillips et al. 2006; Suarez et al. 2008; Kurtz et al. 2011). As the global demand for joint arthroplasty surgeries continues to rise (Kurtz et al. 2011), so will the number of PJIs. Moreover, there is an increase in patients at risk for developing a PJI. These risk factors include rheumatoid arthritis (higher life expectancy due to better anti-rheumatic medications and more frequent use of anti-rheumatic medications, especially disease modifying anti-inflammatory drugs), obesity (BMI > 30–35), diabetes mellitus (particularly poorly controlled glucose levels), male gender, prior open surgery around the joint, certain skin disorders (e.g. psoriatic skin lesions, venous stasis disease and sequelae), current infection at remote site, immunosuppressive conditions, and other comorbidities (Jamsen et al. 2009; Johnson and Bannister 1986; Dowsey and Choong 2009; Chiu et al. 2001; Yang et al. 2001; Namba et al. 2005; Minnema et al. 2004; Peersman et al. 2001; Pulido et al. 2008). Another factor why PJIs are increasing is the ever-improving diagnostic capabilities and growing global awareness of PJI. The rise in PJI poses a formidable challenge for both the patient and doctor and is an ever-increasing economic burden with PJIs costing up to five times or more than aseptic revisions (Kapadia et al. 2014; Hackett et al. 2015; Kurtz et al. 2008).

4.2.2 Which Pathogens Are Detected in PJI and What Is Their Virulence?

The prevalence of pathogens found in PJI is described in ◘ Tab. 4.3. The most common causative organisms of PJI are both commensals: These are coagulase-negative Staphylococci (CNS, of which *Staphylococcus epidermidis* is the most common species) and *Staphylococcus aureus*. The former accounts for 22.5–41% of hip/knee PJIs while the latter accounts for 26.2–35% (Phillips et al. 2006; Malhas et al. 2015; Laffer et al. 2006; Frommelt 2000; Moran et al. 2007; Stefánsdóttir et al. 2009). CNS is more often found in chronic PJI whereas *S. aureus* – being more virulent than CNS – typically causes an acute PJI (within the first 6 weeks of surgery). Next in frequency are haemolytic streptococci, *Enterococci*, *Propionibacterium acnes*, *Escherichia coli* and *Klebsiella spp*. Pathogens that are less commonly found include *Pseudomonas aeruginosa* and *Bacteroides spp*. Fungal and mycobacterial infections are the most rare PJIs and diagnosis is often delayed owing to a low level of clinical suspicion and unusual presentation. Between 2001 and 2012, Zajong et al. (2016) found a stable distribution of pathogens except for an increase in CNS related PJI.

Besides the type of pathogen, a distinction can also be made in its virulence potential. This virulence potential is determined by various factors, e.g. proteins for immune inhibition/avoidance, proteins for tissue invasion and toxins. Highly virulent pathogens that typically cause acute PJI comprise *Staphylococcus aureus* and gram-negative bacteria (e.g. *Escherichia coli, Klebsiella spp., Pseudomonas aeruginosa*). Low-virulent pathogens that typically cause chronic PJI comprise CNS (e.g. *Staphylococcus epidermidis*) and *Propionibacterium acnes*.

4.2.3 The Problem of Resistant Germs and How to Avoid Resistance

The incidence of bacterial antibiotic resistance has been increasing (Zajonz et al. 2016). Moreover, this antibiotic resistance burden varies considerably between countries but also within countries. An important causative factor is the global (ab)use of unnecessary antibiotics that is often poorly regulated by both (human and veterinarian) health-care professionals and governments. Widespread use and availability of antibiotics is almost a guarantee for resistance to an increasing amount of antibiotics. Other factors include the inability to create new antibiotics, patients with multiple comorbidities and an increase in the number of geriatric patients.

S. aureus is a harmless skin/nasal colonizer in 30% of healthy humans, which can be methicillin

Tab. 4.3 Distribution of causative pathogens of periprosthetic joint infections in hip and knee arthroplasty

Pathogen	Study								
	Berbari et al. 1998	Frommelt 2000	Phillips et al. 2006	Laffer et al. 2006	Moran et al. 2007	Stefánsdóttier et al. 2009	Zajonz et al. 2016	Malhas et al. 2015	Trampuz and Zimmerli 2005
	Number of isolated pathogens								
	N = 462	*N* = 1077	*N* = 75	*N* = 40	*N* = 267	*N* = 426	*N* = 803	*N* = 72	N/A
CNS (Gram-positive)	19	41	36	22.5	30	30.5	29	35	30–43
S. aureus (Gram-positive)	22	26.2	29	35	29.6	27.5	27	36	12–23
Other Gram-positive (esp. streptococci and enterococci)	9	8.4	19	20	13.9	17	10	11.1	12–17
Gram-negative	8	15	13	15	7.5	6	6	12.5	3–6
Anaerobes, including *P. acnes*	6	5	1	13.7	4.9	2.7	1	N/A	2–4
Other (multiple pathogens or culture negative)	36	2.5	N/A	3.3	14.1	15.9	26	N/A	20–23

N/A not available, *CNS* coagulase-negative staphylococcus sensitive or resistant. *S. aureus*-colonized patients seem to have an increased risk for a staphylococcal PJI after hip or knee arthroplasty. Screening and nasal decolonization of *S. aureus* may potentially reduce the rates of staphylococcal PJI after hip and total knee arthroplasty (Weiser and Moucha 2015). Methicillin-resistant *S. aureus* (MRSA), a subset of *S. aureus*, has unique resistance and virulence characteristics and is the most common »multi-drug resistant« (MDR) pathogen in hospitals worldwide together with methicillin-resistant *S. epidermidis* (MRSE) and the most important cause of MDR health-care-associated infections. MDR pathogens are opportunistic pathogens that are difficult to treat and associated with prolonged hospital stay but also higher costs and mortality rates (Wolkewitz et al. 2011). Other examples of multi-resistant (MR) organisms are MR-coagulase-negative staphylococci (MR-CoNS), vancomycin-resistant enterococci (VRE), MDR *Acinetobacter baumannii*, and MDR *Pseudomonas aeruginosa*. Highly resistant organisms include VRE, MDR *Acinetobacter baumannii* and MDR *Pseudomonas aeruginosa*; these pathogens have higher failure rates of septic treatment (Vasso et al. 2016). In one study, MRSA and MRSE accounted for 14% of infected total knee arthroplasties (Mittal et al. 2007). Another study reported that 34% of PJIs were caused by either MRSA or MRSE (Parvizi et al. 2009). Moreover, in septic revision surgery, Malhas et al. (2015) found resistance of CNS to both methicillin and gentamicin to be higher than with *S. aureus* and appeared to be increasing.

Several extensive reviews investigated the effectiveness of general infection control (e.g. hand hygiene and transmission-based precautions) (Muto et al. 2003; Loveday et al. 2006). However, the evidence for the effectiveness of more specific prevention methods to prevent and control MRSA has been poorly evaluated. Nevertheless, it has been included in standard prevention protocols in a majority of European countries (Kalenic et al. 2010). In 2014, a review was published by Kock et al. 2014, who evaluated the available literature between 2000 and 2012. In summary, there is good evidence supporting the role of active surveillance followed by decolonization therapy. The effectiveness of single-room isolation was mostly shown in non-controlled studies, which requires further research according to these authors. It also highlighted that several aspects should be considered when planning the implementation of preventive interventions. These aspects involve MRSA prevalence, the incidence of infections, the competing effect of standard control measures (e.g. hand hygiene), and the likelihood of transmission in the respective settings of implementation (Kock et al. 2014).

The Dutch MRSA Guideline is a specific example of a proven and cost-effective protocol aimed at preventing in-hospital MRSA transmission as much as possible. It is based on two pillars, i.e. a »search and destroy« and strict antibiotic use protocol. If followed rigorously it has been proven successful and cost effective in preventing MRSA transmission (Wertheim et al. 2004; Vos et al. 2005, 2009; van Rijen and Kluytmans 2009; van Rijen et al. 2009; Vriens et al. 2002; Wassenberg et al. 2010). However, this requires a cultural and/or national change regarding hygienic compliance and better use of antibiotics.

4.2.4 Importance of Aspiration and Tissue Biopsies

Currently, the only definitive proof of PJI is the detection of causative pathogens. All other available diagnostic modalities remain indirect measures of PJI. These modalities include basic serology (erythrocyte sedimentation rate (ESR), C-reactive protein (CRP)), synovial fluid analysis (white blood cell count (WBC), polymorphonuclear granulocyte (PMN) %, leukocyte-esterase strip and biomarkers like alpha-defensin), conventional radiographic analysis and various imaging techniques (e.g. MRI, CT scan, nuclear imaging modalities such as leukocyte/bone marrow scintigraphy, three-phase bone scanning, FDG-PET).

Even though finding a pathogen is the benchmark of current PJI diagnostics, cultures have reported sensitivity and specificity rates of 65%–94% and 81%–100%, respectively (Schafer et al. 2008). The duration of culture incubation is a particularly important factor. Schafer et al. (2008) found a pathogen detection rate of 73.6% when using a 7-day incubation period. This rate increased to 100% by prolonging the incubation period to

13 days (mostly *P. acnes*; Schafer et al. 2008). Therefore, these authors proposed a routine 14-day incubation period. This advice was also acknowledged by the International Consensus Meeting (Zmistowski et al. 2014). The difficulties in diagnosing chronic PJI have been reported by Gristina (1987). Most pathogens compete with the body's own fibroblasts in a race »to the surface«. After winning this race, many types of pathogenic bacteria form a glycocalyx containing colonies of frequently sessile bacteria. The formation of this so-called biofilm makes pathogen eradication difficult, because the bacteria inside this biofilm remain largely hidden and protected from the body's defence system. These sessile bacteria have prolonged multiplication times, which – in combination with gene suppression – may create a state of near dormancy. It has been estimated that these sessile and near-dormant bacteria are 1,000 times more resistant to antibiotics than their planktonic counterparts (Costerton et al. 1995). These pathogens only become detectable by the body's defence system when their numbers are so abundant that they extrude from the biofilm layer. Only then will they produce symptoms like pain. Next to this biofilm issue, pathogens that can be cultured in biofilm-related PJIs are defective pathogens. These viable pathogens are difficult to culture as these live in the biofilm that hinders detection. Detection can also be hindered owing to the small numbers and/or slow growth rate of some pathogens. Another challenge is to demonstrate whether the pathogen found is the true pathogen and not a contaminant, as will be discussed later in this chapter.

A PJI may still be present when cultures are negative as also defined by the most recent MSIS criteria and diagnostic work-up algorithm as formulated during the first international consensus meeting on PJI (Zmistowski et al. 2014; Parvizi et al. 2013). Cultures may remain negative because of the suboptimal sensitivity of cultures (due to various factors as described earlier and may explain the existence of the entity of a culture-negative PJI; Choi et al. 2013; Parvizi et al. 2014; Huang et al. 2012). In these cases other indirect measures of PJI are usually positive, e.g. WBC count and/or PMN%. And confusingly enough, a PJI may even be clinically present without meeting the MSIS criteria, particularly in the case of less virulent pathogens (e.g. *P. acnes*; Zmistowski et al. 2014). Especially in these cases, biomarker (e.g. alpha-defensin) and/or nucleic acid techniques (e.g. polymerase chain reaction, PCR) may show promise in increasing our capability to diagnose PJI. These modalities are not yet accepted in the routine diagnostic work-up.

Despite these remarks, to find a pathogen via synovial fluid aspiration and/or tissue biopsies, optimized practical and laboratory procedures should be used in any patient with a suspected PJI (Ochsner et al. 2014). Joint aspiration should be done as soon as possible in the case of a suspected/possible acute PJI, as timely diagnosis gives the option of simpler treatment and implant retention. In these cases the decision to surgically intervene and then start empirical antibiotic therapy can be based on the white blood cell count (WBC) and polymorphonuclear granulocyte percentage (PMN%) found in the aspirate if waiting for the culture results may negatively influence PJI treatment. These parameters (WBC and PMN%) are available within a few hours and usually offer a reasonable indication of whether a PJI is present or not. In the case of suspected/possible chronic PJI, the most challenging diagnostic PJI group, the patient should be antibiotic-free for at least 2 weeks before aspiration/biopsy. The analysis is as in suspected acute PJI, only with different cut-off values for WBC and PMN%.

The prerequisites for ensuring optimal culture procedures are optimal culture media supplemented with additional growth factors (Becton Dickinson, a growth enhancer that improves cultivation of fastidious organisms from normally sterile body fluids other than blood), and incubated using the BD BACTEC 9050 automatic blood culture system (Becton Dickinson), extended observation time (routine culture time should be 14 days, as bacteria that are recovering from a sessile state and small colony variants are very slow growing), and basic rules for detection of contamination (Schafer et al. 2008). Moreover, materials should be rapidly transported to the laboratory. This means that the (EDTA) tube for synovial fluid analysis should be in the clinical laboratory within 1 h of aspiration. Cultures (synovial fluid or intra-articular tissue biopsies) should arrive in the microbiology laboratory within 4 h of the culture procedure. The culture period could be even longer (up to 21 days) in the case of suspected PJI with low-virulence organisms (e.g. *P. acnes*, an anaerobic skin flora bacterium known for its slow growth and difficulty to culture). This period can also be considered if preoperative cultures have failed to show bacterial growth but the clinical picture is consistent with PJI (culture-negative PJI; Choi et al. 2013; Parvizi et al. 2014; Huang et al. 2012). The other important factors for ensuring optimal culture procedure are described in the subsequent text.

4.2.5 Aspiration: How Many Samples, How Much, from Where?

Joint aspiration (also known as arthrocentesis) of prosthetic joints should be performed in an optimal sterile manner, therefore preferably in the operating theatre. Some clinics perform aspirations in an outpatient clinic fashion. If this workflow is chosen it should be in a dedicated aspiration room and not in the office or patient examination room where the risk of infection is significantly higher. The goal should be to obtain as much intra-articular fluid as possible, to optimize culture gain. Methods for aspiration depend on the specific joint, e.g. hips may be aspirated via an anterior or lateral approach while knees can be approached via one of the typical arthroscopy portal positions (anteromedial or anterolateral soft spot, or the superopatellar region). A dedicated PJI physician should do this aspiration work-up to assure optimal procedure.

Basic fluid analysis should include synovial WBC count, PMN%, and several cultures (Zmistowski et al. 2014). This requires one EDTA tube (for WBC count and PMN% analysis) and culture tubes/vials (one anaerobic blood culture vial, one aerobic blood culture vial, and one tube without additives) (Ochsner et al. 2014). The fluid aspirate is distributed according to the following priorities (also in the case of small volumes; Ochsner et al. 2014):

1. EDTA tube: 1 ml (minimum) and gently invert five times immediately so as to prevent coagulation (otherwise automated cell count is impossible).
2. Blood culture vials (anaerobic and aerobic): First fill the aerobic and then the anaerobic culture vial, preferably with 2–5 ml (minimum 1 ml), after disinfection of the rubber stoppers of the vials. The authors suggest using BD BACTEC-PEDS-PLUS/F Medium (Becton Dickinson, Heidelberg, Germany) blood culture vials. This medium, originally designed to optimize blood cultures in children, has been shown to be superior when compared with standard blood culture media in both recovery and time to detection of clinically significant micro-organisms, even in low-volume samples (Morello et al. 1991). Note: Using blood culture bottles increases sensitivity. There are reports in the literature of sensitivities (50–93%) and specificities (82–97%) that vary depending on the method used (Ochsner et al. 2014).
3. Plain tube (i.e. without additives): 0.5–1 ml. Note: For bacteriological analysis (Gram stain test, original culture on aerobic, anaerobic, defective bacteria, fungi and mycobacteria).

Optional synovial fluid analysis modalities may include the leukocyte esterase strip test as adjunct to WBC count (requires one/two drops of fluid preferably without blood) (Parvizi et al. 2012; Wetters et al. 2012; Parvizi et al. 2013; Ghanem et al. 2008; Aggerwal et al. 2013), biomarker tests (usually requires only a few drops of fluid, e.g. alpha-defensin; Deirmengian et al. 2010, 2014a, 2014b), and/or nucleic acid test (NAT) techniques (e.g. PCR requires separate plain tube, indications may include small colony variant diagnostics or patients who have received prior antibiotic treatment).

4.2.6 Tissue Biopsies: How Many Samples, from Where?

In our opinion, physicians who regularly treat PJI should do this diagnostic work-up. As the likelihood of detecting the true pathogen increases by the number of biopsies, numerous biopsies should be taken to get five to six separate culture bottles with a sufficient amount of material (Atkins et al. 1998). Biopsy forceps can be used for arthroscopic biopsies, while using a scalpel to obtain open biopsies. The biopsies should be obtained from the synovial tissue, preferably close to the implant (bone–cement region), collected in sterile tubes and transferred to the microbiology laboratory within 4 h of sampling. In the laboratory, specimens should be processed immediately upon arrival. Cultivation of tissue samples can be carried out with optimized culture media suitable for fastidious germs for a period appropriate for recovering damaged or constitutional slow-growing bacteria. For the processing details, national guidelines like the British guideline (UK Standards for Microbiology Investigations 2016), which was recently updated in February 2016, may be used because of lack of consistent evidence. Preoperative PJI cultures of synovial biopsies have shown to be superior to synovial fluid cultures via aspiration; the accuracy increases from 89% to 98.6% according to Fink et al. (2008). Some biopsy material may also be collected for histological analysis, providing a skilled pathologist performs this analysis.

4.2.7 How to Differentiate Contaminations from Causative Pathogens

As described, finding a pathogen (via aspiration or biopsy) is the benchmark of PJI diagnostics. The challenge is to demonstrate whether the pathogen found is the true pathogen and not a (skin flora) contaminant. Particularly Proprionibacteria and CNS are notorious culture contaminants. We agree with the adjusted MSIS definition as formulated during the 2013 consensus meeting (Zmistowski et al. 2014), stating that a PJI is present in the case of two positive periprosthetic cultures with phenotypically identical organisms.

4.2.8 Our Diagnostic Algorithm and a Case-Based Illustration

In our institutions, following international consensus (Zmistowski et al. 2014), the diagnostic work-up revolves around striving to identify a causative pathogen in the case of suspected PJI, i.e. joint aspiration and/or biopsy (arthroscopic or open). A PJI is suspected if there is abnormal blood serology (C-reactive protein and/or erythrocyte sedimentation rate) and/or higher probability for PJI (based on history, detailed risk factor analysis, physical examination, and conventional radiography) (Zmistowski et al. 2014). Out of the various available algorithms, the authors currently prefer the algorithm as proposed during the 2013 international consensus meeting (Zmistowski et al. 2014). However, in the case of a dry tap situation but correct sampling technique (i.e. when no fluid can be obtained, a more frequent issue in hips than other joints) we favour biopsies over repeat joint aspiration. Although arthroscopic biopsies have been shown to be reliable in hip and knee arthroplasty (Fink et al. 2008, 2013) we occasionally perform a limited open approach at the surgeons' discretion. Following the consensus meeting (Zmistowski et al. 2014) we add acid-fast bacilli (AFB) and fungi cultures when a second aspiration is done. New biomarker technologies like alfa-defensin show promising results as an addition to the diagnostic modalities in PJI (Springer 2015; Deirmengian et al. 2010, 2014a, 2014b; Bingham et al. 2014; Bonanzinga et al. 2016). Currently, pending more scientific data, we do not use these biomarkers routinely. Some articles and algorithms support nuclear imaging in routine PJI diagnostics (Jutte et al. 2014; Volpe et al. 2014; Glaudemans et al. 2016; Gemmel et al. 2012) but the role of imaging techniques in PJI diagnostics remains highly debated (Zmistowski et al. 2014; Diaz-Ledezma et al. 2014). We only sporadically use nuclear imaging, i.e. in some culture-negative or complex cases or as a rule-out test. In these situations we use an algorithm analogous to that of Jutte et al. (2014).

Case 1: Early PJI (Postoperative)

A 70-year-old male patient received a total knee arthroplasty (TKA) with prompt wound healing and removal of the skin staples 14 days after surgery. The patient presented to our clinic 3 days later because a wound defect (about 10×8 mm) had formed at the beginning of the wound after a physical therapist massaged the knee for some tight sensations 2 days after removal of the skin staples (◘ Fig. 4.4). A significant seroma was released from the defect directly and some serosanguineous discharge from this wound defect since that time. Blood serology results were CRP 1 mg/l and ESR 14 mm/h. Treatment involved wound care, pressure bandage, and immobilization via a knee immobi-

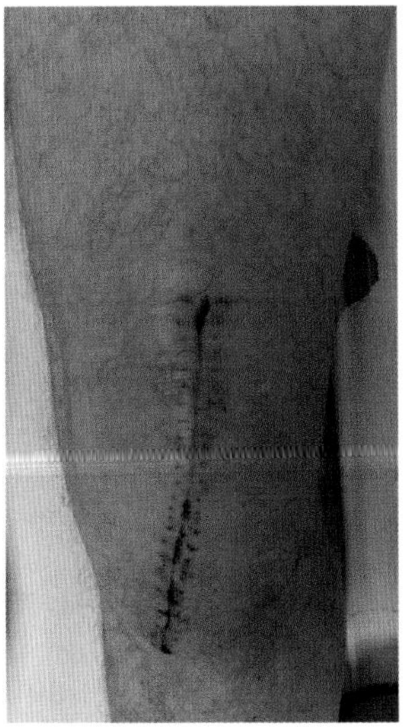

Fig. 4.4 Small wound dehiscence in upper aspect of the surgical wound after a total knee arthroplasty that occurred 2 days after removal of the skin staples (14 days after surgery)

lizer and bed rest. At 36 h later the wound discharge had rapidly worsened (more milky like and smelling) with the patient feeling ill, a fever of 39 °C, CRP of 305 mg/l but with stable vital signs. The knee was also more swollen and function was now limited owing to diffuse pain. Blood cultures and knee aspiration were done that same morning with synovial fluid showing a WBC count of 215,000 cells/μl and PMN% of 84%. An early PJI was concluded, presenting itself with an early wound-healing problem. The patient was operated on the same day (19 days after surgery), which involved a DAIR procedure (debridement, antibiotics, irrigation and retention) and wound closure with monofilament everting type sutures. Antibiotic treatment was started (we routinely start with cefazolin, with a dose according to weight). On the day of surgery, the synovial fluid aspirate showed cocci in the Gram preparate, while the next day *S. aureus* was found in cultures of the synovial fluid aspirate. In the next 2 days all six tissue samples taken during the DAIR also showed *S. aureus* that was sensitive to all antibiotics according to the antibiogram. The patient recovered well and blood serology normalized within 4 weeks. After the 2 weeks of intravenous antibiotic treatment, oral antibiotic treatment was tailored to the *S. aureus* antibiogram and consisted of ciprofloxacin and rifampicin for 10 weeks.

Case 2: Acute Haematogenous PJI

A 65-year-old female patient received a hybrid total hip arthroplasty (THA) for primary osteoarthritis of the left hip with uneventful wound healing and postoperative rehabilitation. Other medical history included aortic–femoral bifurcation prosthesis, factor VIII disease and Fontaine 2B vascular complaints of the left leg.

Eight months after the THA the patient presented to our emergency department with sudden left groin pain that had started 3 days earlier. Physical examination showed a blood pressure of 130/68, regular pulse of 103/min, respiratory rate of 14/min, 95% peripheral oxygen saturation and a core temperature of 39.2° C. The hip showed no wound or scar problems, normal passive function, but did

Exkurs

PJI diagnostics requires a high index of suspicion, but this is especially true for chronic PJI. An early PJI is generally obvious based on classic infectious clinical parameters (rubor, calor, dolor, functio laesa) and supplemental blood serology (CRP is most useful). Joint aspiration can be done but treatment usually consists of a rapid DAIR procedure. Wound healing issues have shown to increase the chance for PJI. Persisting (in our institution longer than 3–5 days) wound drainage that does not resolve with some (2–5) days of conservative treatment should be treated by surgical intervention (DAIR). Conservative treatment in our institution involves wound care, pressure bandage (hip spica for the hip) and bed rest (with a knee immobilizer for knees), but also attention to uncontrolled glucose in diabetes, malnutrition and temporarily stopping certain chronic anticoagulant home medication like coumarins. Persisting wound drainage may offer a pathway for retrograde pathogen seeding of the joint via the draining fluid but may also be the sole symptom of a developing/existing early PJI per se. The latter specifically applies to early new wound drainage. In these cases we admit the patient to the clinic and carry out a DAIR procedure if the new wound drainage remains after 48 h of conservative treatment.

reveal a positive psoas sign. Examination of the lungs, heart and abdomen were normal. Head-to-toe examination showed skin erythema in the right groin area due to obesity skin folds and an unguis incarnatus of the right hallux (present for 4 weeks). Serologic testing showed a CRP level of 250 mg/l and an ESR of 95 mm/h. Conventional radiographic examination was normal (pelvic AP and axial view). Ultrasound showed peri-articular fluid collections around the hip. Supplemental CT scanning revealed no peri-articular (hip), intra-pelvic (psoas) or intra-abdominal abnormalities.

Urinary and several blood samples were taken and the patient was admitted on our orthopaedic ward for further analysis and observation. Antibiotic treatment was started (i.v. augmentin 4 dd 1,000 mg and gentamicin 1 dd 6 mg/kg according to hospital protocol). Urinary cultures remained negative, but the blood cultures showed *S. aureus* within 24 h of culturing. Based on these findings, a cardiac ultrasound was done, showing no sign of endocarditis. We decided to do a PET-CT scan to further determine/localize a primary infection focus and investigate the THA. This scan showed a normal postoperative uptake surrounding the cementless socket and no uptake surrounding the cemented stem. In the peri-articular soft tissue we found a higher uptake than anticipated in correlation with the ultrasound and CT scan 3 days earlier. No other focus of enlarged uptake was seen on the PET-CT scan.

The patient's case was further discussed in our PJI unit and she was scheduled for DAIR with customary tissue sampling for cultures. The DAIR procedure was done 3 days after hospital admission, i.e. 9 days after the symptoms started. Findings during DAIR surgery revealed intra-articular fluid with a pocket passing to the anterior aspect of the acetabulum into the pelvic cavity. The liner and head were changed as part of the DAIR. After the DAIR her pain decreased, the psoas function restored, and the CRP and temperature quickly normalized.

The DAIR cultures showed *S. aureus* but also a haemolytic streptococcus. The patient was treated with intravenous antibiotics (flucloxacillin 12 g/24 h and rifampicine 2 dd 450 mg) based on the antibiogram. Oral antibiotics were started after 2 weeks of intravenous treatment, also tailored to the antibiogram (ciprofloxacin 2 dd 500 mg and rifampicin 2 dd 450 mg). At the latest outpatient visit all blood serology results were normal, no clinical symptoms of infection were present and still radiographic abnormalities of the THA were found.

Case 3: Acute-on-Chronic Osteomyelitis Below Tibial Component in Total Knee Arthroplasty

A 57-year-old male patient was referred to our clinic at the end of 2014 because of a painful TKA. A high tibial osteotomy was done in 1995 with prolonged postoperative wound drainage, arthroscopy in 2005 (Kellgren Lawrence grade 4 medial osteoarthritis) and a TKA in 2007. The patient was satisfied with the outcome until August 2013 when he slowly developed increasing pain on the medial side of the knee upon loading activities (e.g. walking) and also occasional pain at night. There was also swelling on the medial side of the knee. Examination revealed a painful proximal aspect tibia with local swelling and a range of motion (ROM) of 110-0-0. Further investigations showed a suspected tibial loosening (serial X-ray and bone scan, ◘ Fig. 4.5) with normal serology (CRP 2 mg/l, ESR 9 mm/h) and synovial fluid analysis that was negative for PJI (both cultures negative), WBC count < 750 cells/μl and therefore PMN% normal as it was too low for determination. However, when the patient came to the outpatient clinic for the results he reported diffuse swelling and redness coupled with increasing swelling around the tibial osteotomy scar for 4–5 days. He also mentioned having frequent night sweats for a longer period of time. Examination confirmed redness of the anteromedial side around the old osteotomy scar with small droplet of pus and abnormal blood serology results (CRP 76 mg/l, ESR 9 mm/h). On the basis of this new information we ordered a three-phase bone scan confirming our suspicion of an acute-on-chronic osteomyelitis below the tibial component. Treatment involved a two-stage septic revision. The TKA was removed the next day along with a radical debridement and static spacer. The anteromedial swelling was opened via the old osteotomy scar revealing pus and a tibial defect with the pus running up to most of the cement around the tibial stem. This wound was left open to heal via secondary healing and later VAC therapy. Cultures showed *S. aureus*, sensitive to all antibiotics except

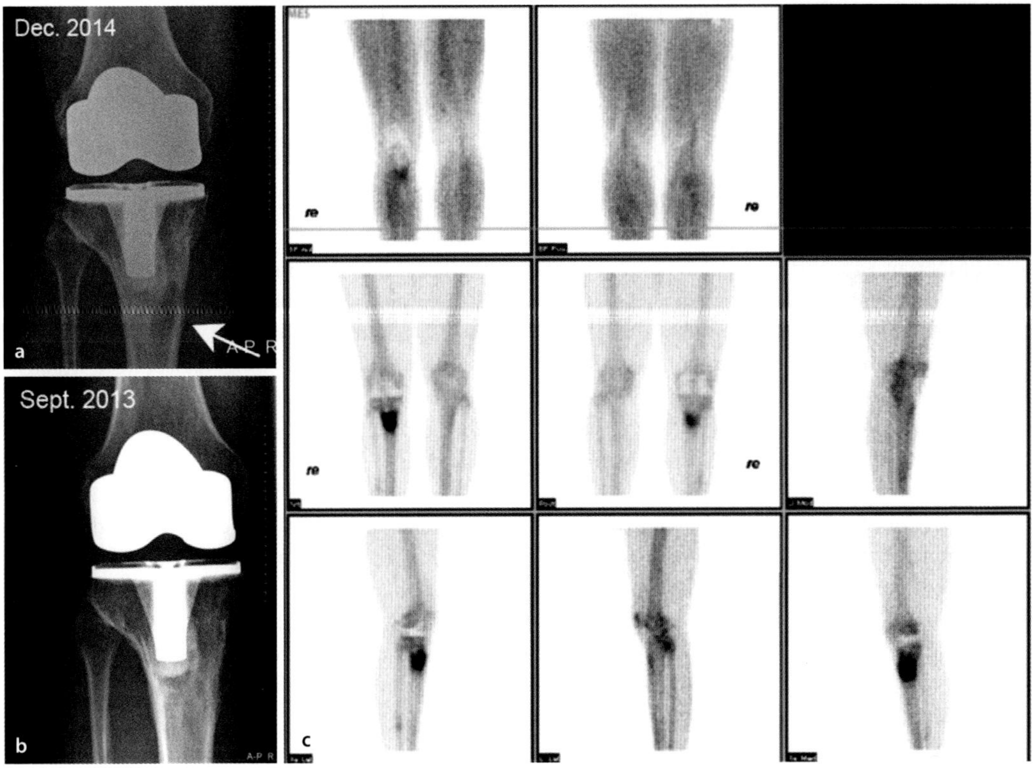

Fig. 4.5 **a,b** Development of increasing lucent region below tibial stem (*arrow*). **c** Three-phase bone scanning confirmed suspicion of chronic osteomyelitis (stress fracture unlikely given normal cortices and extent of lesion)

penicillin. Antibiotic treatment was started and, after (primary and secondary) wound healing, a rotating hinge TKA was re-implanted with uneventful healing, current infection control and patient satisfaction.

Case 4: Culture-Negative PJI

A 43-year-old female patient had a TKA placed in June 2012 and an inlay change early 2013 for instability symptoms after a fall on the knee. In September 2014 she developed acute swelling, pain, and warmth of the knee about 2 weeks after vaginal removal of the uterus. Blood serology first showed a CRP level of 12 mg/l and an ESR of 20 mm/h. This increased in the following 3 days to 110 mg/l and 35 mm/h, respectively. The clinical picture also worsened (swelling, pain and warmth). Synovial knee aspiration showed a WBC count of 21,200 cells/

Exkurs

PJI diagnostics requires a high index of suspicion, especially for chronic PJI. Joint aspiration is the basics in PJI analysis if there is abnormal blood serology (CRP and/or ESR) or a higher likelihood of infection based on patient characteristics (detailed history, risk factor analysis, physical examination and X-rays). However, normal blood serology (CRP and /or ESR) does not exclude PJI, as it may be completely normal in low-grade infections such as chronic osteomyelitis or chronic PJI.
Moreover, synovial fluid/tissue analysis may not show any signs of PJI if the infection remains contained below an orthopaedic implant, i.e. without connection with the joint itself. In these rare cases, supplemental nuclear imaging (or MRI) may be helpful.

Exkurs

Culture-negative PJI is a difficult entity, posing several questions such as what are the exact diagnostic steps, what is the optimal treatment, which antibiotic to give and for how long? And even if a PJI can be treated successfully (meaning infection control), infection treatment carries potential side effects that may lead to an incapacitating end situation. This should be extensively communicated to the patient and family from the early start of the diagnostic and treatment period.

µl, a PMN% of 84% and no signs of gout crystals. Based on the suspicion of an acute haematogenous PJI the decision was made to perform a debridement and implant retention procedure (DAIR, i.e. extensive synovectomy, lavage and liner change and start of antibiotics). However, cultures remained negative. Based on a potential culture-negative PJI the patient was kept on antibiotics for 6 weeks. Clinically, the knee symptoms and blood serology quickly normalized and for a short period the patient was even happier than before the debridement. At the 3-month outpatient clinic follow-up the patient complained about persistent symptomatic swelling of the knee. The knee was aspirated 6 months after the debridement procedure. The WBC was 6,210 cells/µl, PMN% 91%, cultures negative for all pathogens including yeast/fungi/tuberculosis; there were also no gout crystals. Arthroscopic biopsies were taken for cultures that also did not reveal any abnormalities (no pathogens, including yeast/fungi/tuberculosis) but WBC and PMN% remained abnormal (4,900 cells/µl and 95%). A Synovasure (alpha-defensin) test was also done that was positive. Given the inability to culture a pathogen but with parameters suggesting PJI (abnormal WBC, PMN% and Synovasure), three-phase bone scanning was done. This showed elevated diffuse hyperaemic bone activity and an inflammatory capsule. This combined information was discussed with an (inter)national panel of experienced revision arthroplasty colleagues and led to the conclusion that the most probable cause of the persistent symptomatic swelling was a culture-negative PJI. Therefore, a two-stage revision was performed with local loading of bone cement with antibiotics (Palacos G+C and vancomycin) and systemic antibiotics (augmentin and gentamicin for 2 weeks i.v. followed by 10 weeks of oral ciproxin/clindamycin). The knee recovered uneventfully (no complaints) but the patient developed a permanent invalidating vertigo that, after extensive evaluation, was evaluated to be caused by gentamicin-induced bilateral destruction of the vestibular organs.

4.2.9 Conclusion

PJI is an increasing problem due to ever-increasing worldwide demand for joint arthroplasty and patients that are at risk for PJI. *Staphylococcus aureus* and coagulase-negative Staphylococci are the most common pathogens but multidrug resistant PJI is an increasing problem in many countries. Various bacteria form a biofilm that can make pathogen diagnosis (and eradication) difficult because the bacteria inside this biofilm remain largely hidden and protected from the body's defence system. Thus, crucial aspects in PJI diagnostics include op-

Take-Home Message

- The number of periprosthetic joint infections (PJIs) continues to rise.
- Methicillin-resistant *S. aureus* (MRSA) has unique resistance and virulence characteristics and is the most common »multi-drug resistant« (MDR) pathogen in hospitals worldwide, together with methicillin-resistant *S. epidermidis* (MRSE), and the most important cause of MDR health-care-associated infections.
- Currently, the only definitive proof of PJI is the detection of causative pathogens. All other available diagnostic modalities remain indirect measures of PJI.
- PJI diagnostics requires a high index of suspicion, particularly for chronic PJI.

timized practical and laboratory procedures, such as sufficient amount of biopsies, coupled with additional diagnostic modalities (synovial joint fluid leukocyte count, polymorphonuclear granulocyte %) that can aid diagnostics. Optional synovial fluid analysis may include leukocyte esterase strip test and potentially biomarker tests (e.g. alpha-defensin) and/or nucleic acid test techniques.

References

Aggerwal VK, Tischler E, Ghanem E, Parvizi J (2013) Leukocyte esterase from synovial fluid aspirate: a technical note. J Arthroplasty 28(1):193–195

Atkins BL, Athanasou N, Deeks JJ, Crook DW, Simpson H, Peto TE, McLardy-Smith P, Berendt AR (1998). Prospective evaluation of criteria for microbiological diagnosis of prosthetic-joint infection at revision arthroplasty. The OSIRIS Collaborative Study Group. J Clin Microbiol 36(10):2932–2939

Berbari EF, Hanssen AD, Duffy MC, Steckelberg JM, Ilstrup DM, Harmsen WS, Osmon DR (1998) Risk factors for prosthetic joint infection: case-control study. Clin Infect Dis 27:1247–1254

Bingham J, Clarke H, Spangehl M, Schwartz A, Beauchamp C, Goldberg B (2014) The alpha defensin-1 biomarker assay can be used to evaluate the potentially infected total joint arthroplasty. Clin Orthop Relat Res 472(12):4006–4009

Bonanzinga T, Zahar A, Dütsch M, Lausmann C, Kendoff D, Gehrke T (2016) How reliable is the Alpha-defensin immunoassay test for diagnosing periprosthetic joint infection? A Prospective Study. Clin Orthop Relat Res. [Epub ahead of print]

Chiu FY, Lin CF, Chen CM, Lo WH, Chaung TY (2001) Cefuroxime-impregnated cement at primary total knee arthroplasty in diabetes mellitus. A prospective, randomized study. J Bone Joint Surg Br 83(5):691–695

Choi HR, Kwon YM, Freiberg AA, Nelson SB, Malchau H (2013) Periprosthetic joint infection with negative culture results: clinical characteristics and treatment outcome. J Arthroplasty 28(6):899–903

Costerton JW, Lewandowski Z, Caldwell DE, Korber DR, Lappin-Scott HM (1995) Microbial biofilm. Annu Rev Microbiol 49:711–745

Deirmengian C, Hallab N, Tarabishy A, Della Valle C, Jacobs JJ, Lonner J, Booth RE Jr (2010) Synovial fluid biomarkers for periprosthetic infection. Clin Orthop Relat Res 468(8):2017–2023

Deirmengian C, Kardos K, Kilmartin P, Cameron A, Schiller K, Booth RE Jr, Parvizi J (2014a) The alpha-defensin test for periprosthetic joint infection outperforms the leukocyte esterase test strip. Clin Orthop Relat Res 473(1):198–203

Deirmengian C, Kardos K, Kilmartin P, Cameron A, Schiller K, Parvizi J (2014b) Diagnosing periprosthetic joint infection: has the era of the biomarker arrived? Clin Orthop Relat Res 472(11):3254–3262

Diaz-Ledezma C, Lichstein PM, Dolan JG, Parvizi J (2014) Diagnosis of periprosthetic joint infection in medicare patients: multicriteria decision analysis. Clin Orthop Relat Res 472(11):3275–3284

Dowsey MM, Choong PF (2009) Obese diabetic patients are at substantial risk for deep infection after primary TKA. Clin Orthop Relat Res 467(6):1577–1581

Fink B, Makowiak C, Fuerst M, Berger I, Schäfer P, Frommelt L (2008) The value of synovial biopsy, joint aspiration and C-reactive protein in the diagnosis of late periprosthetic infection of total knee replacements. J Bone Joint Surg Br 90:874–878

Fink B, Gebhard A, Fuerst M, Berger I, Schäfer P (2013) High diagnostic value of synovial biopsy in periprosthetic joint infection of the hip. Clin Orthop Relat Res 471:956–964

Frommelt L (2000) Periprosthetic joint infection – bacteria and the interface between prosthesis and bone. In: Learmonth ID (ed) Interfaces in total hip arthroplasty. Springer, London Berliln Heidelberg New York, pp 153–161

Gemmel F, Van den Wyngaert H, Love C, Welling MM, Gemmel P, Palestro CJ (2012) Prosthetic joint infections: radionuclide state-of-the-art imaging. Eur J Nucl Med Mol Imaging 39(5):892–909

Ghanem E, Houssock C, Pulido L, Han S, Jaberi FM, Parvizi J (2008) Determining »True« leukocytosis in bloody joint aspiration. J Arthroplasty 23(2):182–187

Glaudemans AW, Jutte PC, Petrosillo N, Erba PA, Lazzeri E, Signore A (2016) Comment on: »Diagnosis of Periprosthetic Joint Infection: The Role of Nuclear Medicine May Be Overestimated« by Claudio Diaz-Ledezma, Courtney Lamberton, Paul Lichtstein and Javad Parvizi. J Arthroplasty 31(2):551–552

Gristina AG (1987. Biomaterial-centered infection: microbial adhesion versus tissue integration. Science 237:1588–1595

Hackett DJ, Rothenberg AC, Chen AF, Gutowski C, Jaekel D, Tomek IM, Parsley BS, Ducheyne P, Manner PA (2015) The economic significance of orthopaedic infections. J Am Acad Orthop Surg 23 Suppl:S1–7

Huang R, Hu CC, Adeli B, Mortazavi J, Parvizi J (2012) Culture-negative periprosthetic joint infection does not preclude infection control. Clin Orthop Relat Res 470(10):2717–2723

Jamsen E, Huhtala H, Puolakka T, Moilanen T (2009) Risk factors for infection after knee arthroplasty: a register-based analysis of 43,149 cases. J Bone Joint Surg Am 91(1):38–47

Johnson DP, Bannister GC (1986) The outcome of infected arthroplasty of the knee. J Bone Joint Surg Br 68(2): 289–291

Jutte P, Lazzeri E, Sconfienza LM, Cassar-Pullicino V, Trampuz A, Petrosillo N, Signore A (2014) Diagnostic flowcharts in osteomyelitis, spondylodiscitis and prosthetic joint infection. Q J Nucl Med Mol Imaging 58(1):2–19

Kalenic S, Cookson BD, Gallagher R, Popp W, Asensio-Vegas A, Assadian O, et al (2010) Comparison of recommendations in national/regional Guidelines for prevention and control of MRSA. Int J Infect Control v6:i2

Kapadia BH, McElroy MJ, Issa K, Johnson AJ, Bozic KJ, Mont MA (2014) The economic impact of periprosthetic infections following total knee arthroplasty at a specialized tertiary care center. J Arthroplasty 29(5):929–932

Kock R, Friedrich A, On Behalf Of The Original Author Group C (2014) Systematic literature analysis and review of targeted preventive measures to limit healthcare-associated infections by meticillin-resistant Staphylococcus aureus. Euro Surveill 19(37). pii: 20902

Kurtz SM, Lau E, Schmier J, Ong KL, Zhao K, Parvizi J (2008) Infection burden for hip and knee arthroplasty in the United States. J Arthroplasty 23(7):984–991

Kurtz SM, Röder C, et al (2011) International survey of primary and revision total knee replacement. Int. Ortho (SICOT) 35:1783–1789

Laffer RR, Graber P, Ochsner PE, Zimmerli W (2006) Outcome of prosthetic knee-associated infection: evaluation of 40 consecutive episodes at a single centre. Clin Microbiol Infect 12:433–439

Loveday HP, Pellowe CM, Jones SR, Pratt RJ (2006) A systematic review of the evidence for interventions for the prevention and control of meticillin-resistant Staphylococcus aureus (1996-2004): report to the Joint MRSA Working Party (Subgroup A). J Hosp Infect 63[Suppl 1]:S45–70

Malhas AM, Lawton R, Reidy M, Nathwani D, Clift BA (2015) Causative organisms in revision total hip & knee arthroplasty for infection: Increasing multi-antibiotic resistance in coagulase-negative Staphylococcus and the implications for antibiotic prophylaxis. Surgeon Oct;13(5):250–255

Minnema B, Vearncombe M, Augustin A, Gollish J, Simor AE (2004) Risk factors for surgical-site infection fol- lowing primary total knee arthroplasty. Infect Control Hosp Epidemiol 25(6):477–480

Mittal Y, Fehring TK, Hanssen A, Marculescu C, Odum SM, Osmon D (2007) Two-stage reimplantation for periprosthetic knee infection involving resis- tant organisms. J Bone Joint Surg Am 89(6):1227–1231

Moran E, Masters S, Berendt AR, McLardy-Smith P, Byren I, Atkins BL (2007) Guiding empirical antibiotic therapy in orthopaedics: the microbiology of prosthetic joint infection managed by debridement, irrigation and prosthesis retention. J Infect 55:1–7

Morello JA, Matushek SM, Dunn WM, Hinds DB (1991) Performance of a BACTEC non- radiometric medium for pediatric blood cultures. J Clin Microbiol 29:359–362

Muto CA, Jernigan JA, Ostrowsky BE, Richet HM, Jarvis WR, Boyce JM, et al (2003) SHEA guideline for preventing nosocomial transmission of multidrug-resistant strains of Staphylococcus aureus and enterococcus. Infect Control Hosp Epidemiol 24(5):362–386

Namba RS, Paxton L, Fithian DC, Stone ML (2005) Obesity and perioperative morbidity in total hip and total knee arthroplasty patients. J Arthroplasty 20(7):46–50

Ochsner PE, Borens O, Bodler P-M, Broger I, Eich G, Hefti F, Maurer T, Nötzli H, Seiler S, Suvà D, Trampuz A, Uçkay I, Vogt M, Zimmerli W (2014) Infections of the musculoskeletal system. Basic principles, prevention, diagnosis and treatment. Swiss Orthopaedics In-House Publisher, Grandvaux, Switzerland, pp. 70–94

Parvizi J, Azzam K, Ghanem E, Austin MS, Rothman RH (2009) Periprosthetic infection due to resistant staphylococci: serious problem in horizon. Clin Orthop Relat Res 467(7):1732–1739

Parvizi J, Erkocak OF, Della Valle CJ (2014) Culture-negative periprosthetic joint infection. J Bone Joint Surg Am 96(5):430-436

Parvizi J, Gehrke T, Chen AF (2013) Proceedings of the international consensus on periprosthetic joint infection. Bone Joint J 95-B:1450–1452

Parvizi J, Jacovides C, Antoci V, Ghanem E (2012) Diagnosis of periprosthetic joint infection: the utility of a simple yet unappreciated enzyme. J Bone Joint Surg Am 93(24): 2242–2248

Peersman G, Laskin R, Davis J, Peterson M (2001) Infection in total knee replacement: a retrospective review of 6489 total knee replacements. Clin Orthop Relat Res 392:15–23

Phillips JE, Crane TP, Noy M, Elliott TS, Grimer RJ (2006) The incidence of deep prosthetic infections in a specialist orthopaedic hospital. A 15-year prospective survey. J Bone Joint Surg Br 88(7):943–948

Pulido L, Ghanem E, Joshi A, Purtill JJ, Parvizi J (2008) Periprosthetic joint infection: the incidence, tim- ing, and predisposing factors. Clin Orthop Relat Res 466(7):1710–1715

Schafer P, Fink B, Sandow D, Margull A, Berger I, Fromelt L (2008) Prolonged bacterial culture to identify late periprosthetic joint infection: a promising strategy. Clin Infect Dis 47:1403–1409

Springer BD (2015) CORR Insights®: The Alpha-defensin test for periprosthetic joint infection responds to a wide spectrum of organisms. Clin Orthop Relat Res 473(7): 2236–2237

Stefánsdóttir A, Johansson D, Knutson K, Lidgren L, Robertsson O (2009) Microbiology of the infected knee arthroplasty: report from the Swedish Knee Arthroplasty Register on 426 surgically revised cases. Scand J Infect Dis. 41(11-12):831–840

Suarez J, Griffin W, Springer B, Fehring T, Mason JB, Odum S (2008) Why do revision knee arthroplasties fail? J Arthroplasty 23(6):99–103

Trampuz A, Zimmerli W (2005) Prosthetic joint infections: update in diagnosis and treatment. Swiss Med Wkly 135(17):243–251

UK Standards for Microbiology Investigations (2016) Investigations of orthopaedic implant associated infections. Issued by the Standards Unit, Microbiology Services, PHE. Bacteriology B44(2)

van Rijen MM, Bosch T, Heck ME, Kluytmans JA (2009) Meticillin-resistant Staphylococcus aureus epidemiology and transmission in a Dutch hospital. J Hosp Infect 72(4): 299–306

van Rijen MM, Kluytmans JA (2009) Costs and benefits of the MRSA Search and Destroy policy in a Dutch hospital. Eur J Clin Microbiol Infect Dis 2009; 28(10):1245–52
Vasso M, Schiavone Panni A, De Martino I, Gasparini G (2016) Prosthetic knee infection by resistant bacteria: the worst-case scenario. Knee Surg Sports Traumatol Arthrosc Feb 1. [Epub ahead of print]
Volpe L, Indelli PF, Latella L, Poli P, Yakupoglu J, Marcucci M (2014) Periprosthetic joint infections: a clinical practice algorithm. Joints 2(4):169–174
Vos MC, Ott A, Verbrugh HA (2005) Successful search-and-destroy policy for methicillin-resistant Staphylococcus aureus in The Netherlands. J Clin Microbiol 43(4):2034–2035
Vos MC, Behrendt MD, Melles DC, Mollema FP, de Groot W, Parlevliet G, Ott A, Horst-Kreft D, van Belkum A, Verburgh HA (2009) 5 years of experience implementing a methicillin-resistant Staphylococcus aureus search and destroy policy at the largest university medical center in the Netherlands. Infect Control Hosp Epidemiol 30(10):977–984
Vriens M, Blok H, Fluit A, Troelstra A, van der Werken C, Verhoef J (2002) Costs associated with a strict policy to eradicate methicillin-resistant Staphylococcus aureus in a Dutch University Medical Center: a 10-year survey. Eur J Clin Microbiol Infect Dis 21(11):782–86
Wassenberg MW, de Wit GA, van Hout BA, Bonten MJ (2010) Quantifying cost-effectiveness of controlling nosocomial spread of antibiotic-resistant bacteria: the case of MRSA. PLoS One 5(7):e11562
Weiser MC, Moucha CS (2015) The current state of screening and decolonization for the prevention of staphylococcus aureus surgical site infection after total hip and knee arthroplasty. J Bone Joint Surg Am. 97(17):1449–1458
Wetters NG, Berend KR, Lombardi AV, Morris MJ, Tucker TL, Della Valle CJ (2012) Leukocyte esterase reagent strips for the rapid diagnosis of periprosthetic joint infection. J Arthroplasty 27(8 Suppl):8-11
Wertheim HF, Vos MC, Boelens HA, Voss A, Vandenbroucke-Grauls CM, Meester MH, Kluytmans JA, van Keulen PH, Verbrugh HA (2004) Low prevalence of methicillin-resistant Staphylococcus aureus (MRSA) at hospital admission in the Netherlands: the value of search and destroy and restrictive antibiotic use. J Hosp Infect 56(4):321–325
Wolkewitz M, Frank U, Philips G, Schumacher M, Davey P (2011) Mortality associated with in-hospital bacteraemia caused by Staphylococcus aureus: a multistate analysis with follow-up beyond hospital discharge. J Antimicrob Chemother 66(2):381-386
Yang K, Yeo SJ, Lee BP, Lo NN (2001) Total knee arthroplasty in diabetic patients. J Arthroplasty 16(1):102–106
Zajonz D, Wuthe L, Rodloff AC, Prietzel T, von Salis-Soglio GF, Roth A, Heyde CE, Josten C, Ghanem M (2016) Infections of hip and knee endoprostheses : Spectrum of pathogens and the role of multiresistant bacteria. Chirurg. 87(4): 332–339
Zmistowski B, Della Valle C, Bauer TW, Malizos KN, Alavi A, Bedair H, Booth RE, Choong P, Deirmengian C, Ehrlich GD, Gambir A, Huang R, Kissin Y, Kobayashi H, Kobayashi N, Krenn V, Lorenzo D, Marston SB, Meermans G, Perez J, Ploegmakers JJ, Rosenberg A, Simpendorfer C, Thomas P, Tohtz S, Villafuerte JA, Wahl P, Wagenaar FC, Witzo E (2014) Diagnosis of periprosthetic joint infection. J Arthroplasty 29 (Suppl 1):77–83

4.3 Diagnosis of Pathogens Causing Periprosthetic Joint Infections

John Segreti

4.3.1 Introduction

Periprosthetic joint infections (PJI) are an uncommon but serious complication of total joint arthroplasty (TJA). In the United States, the burden of infection has increased during the period 1990–2004 (Kurtz et al. 2008). Infection may result in significant morbidity and functional limitation for the patient and is associated with twice the length of hospitalization and excess cost (Kurtz et al. 2008, 2012). Risk of infection is related to patient risk factors – age, obesity and rheumatoid arthritis – as well as surgical factors such as revision arthroplasty and operative time (Brause 1989; Lentino 2003). Arriving at the diagnosis may be simple in patients presenting with classic symptoms of fever and acute pain in the joint. However, many patients present with an indolent course and joint dysfunction, and establishing the diagnosis may be more challenging.

4.3.2 Diagnostic Considerations

Establishing the diagnosis of PJI utilizes a combination of synovial fluid analysis, histopathologic examination, intraoperative appearance, and bacterial cultures. New diagnostic methods, such as multiplex polymerase chain reaction (PCR) and mass spectrometry, are under development, but the utility of these highly sensitive diagnostic techniques with unknown specificity should be interpreted with caution (Rak et al. 2013). Such methods also fail to determine the antibiotic susceptibility of the identified organisms. Thus traditional microbiology remains the mainstay for identifying organisms causing PJI and determining their antimicrobial susceptibility. Only by knowing the antibiotic susceptibility of the infecting organisms can one reasonably assure administration of appropriate antibiotic therapy. Unfortunately, rates of negative intraoperative cultures range from 10% to 30%, making optimal management of these infections difficult (Shanmugasundaram et al. 2014). Therefore attempts need to be made to optimize the yield of traditional cultures.

Whenever possible, it is recommended to delay antibiotic treatment in patients with suspected PJI until cultures from the joint have been obtained (Della-Valle et al. 2011). It is widely accepted by orthopaedic surgeons that antibiotics should be withheld until aspiration has been performed to increase the odds of identifying an organism. In one study, the sensitivity of microscopy in all patients dropped from 58% to 12% when patients had received antibiotics (native knees: 46–0%, prosthetic knees: 72–27%; Hindle et al. 2012). It has been suggested that antibiotics for surgical prophylaxis are given only after sample collection, but more recent data suggest that a single dose of preoperative antibiotics does not significantly decrease the yield of cultures (Tetreault et al. 2014). Preoperative synovial fluid analysis can be an aid in diagnosis of infection and aid surgical planning (Lachiewicz et al. 1996). In a review of 220 patients undergoing total hip revision, synovial fluid white blood cell (WBC) count and neutrophil predominance were found to be sensitive and specific markers of infection; notably the WBC counts may be much lower in PJI than native joint infection (Schinsky et al. 2008; Cipriano et al. 2012). Preoperative synovial fluid cultures may be positive in up to 80% of patients with PJI (Lachiewicz et al. 1996; Spangehl et al. 1999) and can be supportive if the same pathogen is isolated at the time of surgery. Inoculating synovial fluid into blood culture media instead of using swabs for agar plating can significantly increase the yield of cultures, particularly for fastidious organisms (Fuller et al. 1994; Hughes et al. 2001).

At the time of surgery, three to six tissue samples should be obtained whenever possible and submitted for aerobic and anaerobic culture (Della Valle et al. 2011). In one retrospective study of 73 patients undergoing 77 cases of revision arthroplasties, the practice of obtaining only one intraoperative culture was compared with obtaining five separate specimens. Obtaining multiple cultures changed the microbiological diagnosis in 26 of 77 cases (34%) and antibiotic treatment in 23 of 77 cases (30%). This analysis demonstrated that obtaining multiple cultures can significantly change patient care, and suggests that one or two cultures are insufficient (DeHaan et al. 2013).

Swabs should be avoided when obtaining culture specimens. Aggarwal and colleagues found that tissue cultures had higher sensitivity, specificity, positive predictive value, and negative predictive value for diagnosing PJI than swab cultures. Swab cultures had more false-negative and false-positive results than tissue cultures (Aggarwal et al. 2013).

Cultures of sinus tracts and the surface of wounds should be avoided as they likely reflect skin colonization. Tetreault and co-workers assessed the utility of culturing draining wounds or sinuses in patients with suspected PJI. In all, 55 patients with a draining wound or sinus after total joint arthroplasty (28 knees, 27 hips) who had not received antibiotics for at least 2 weeks were prospectively studied. Superficial wound cultures were compared with intra-articular cultures to determine accuracy in isolating infecting organism(s). The superficial cultures were concordant with deep cultures in only 26 of 55 cases (47.3%) and were more likely to yield multiple bacteria. In 23 cases (41.8%), the superficial cultures would have led to a change in antibiotic regimen. Given the potential to adversely affect patient care, we recommend against obtainment of superficial cultures in patients with a draining wound or sinus following hip or knee arthroplasty (Tetreault et al. 2013).

There is evidence to support the use of sonication of prosthetic implants to improve microbiologic yield, especially in patients on prior antibiotics (Trampuz et al. 2007). However, many microbiology laboratories have been slow to adopt this practice. While many laboratories still perform Gram stains on fluid obtained from patients with suspected PJI, it has been found that intraoperative Gram staining had a sensitivity of only 27%, indicating that this test is of limited value (Morgan et al. 2009). Finally, a number of studies support incubating cultures for up to 14 days, especially for improving isolation of anaerobic bacteria (Scafer et al. 2008; Larsen et al. 2012; DeHaan et al. 2013). A known consequence of this practice, however, is that the number of probable contaminants also increases (Scafer et al. 2008).

4.3.3 Microbiology

The microbiology of PJI is a reflection of both the most common routes of infection, inoculation and haematogenous spread, as well as pathogenic properties of the infecting organism. In ◘ Tab. 4.4, the distribution of the most common microbiologic causes of infection in the prosthetic hip is shown (Maderazo et al. 1988; Lachiewicz et al. 1996; Tsukayama et al. 1996; Crockarell et al. 1998; Ure et al. 1998; Schinsky et al. 2008; Sousa et al. 2010; Cipriano et al. 2012). Gram-positive organisms, especially staphylococcal species, are common colonizers of the human skin and oral cavity and make up the majority of both early and late infections. Among Gram-negative bacteria, normal flora of the human gastrointestinal tract, such as *Escherichia coli* and *Enterobacter cloacae,* are commonly implicated. *Pseudomonas aeruginosa,* found environmentally as well as commensally, remains an important pathogen. Prosthetic hip infections with Gram-negative organisms occur more commonly in older patients and patients with older prostheses (Hsieh et al. 2009). Anaerobic bacteria, most commonly *Peptostreptococcus spp.* and *Propionibacterium acnes,* cause PJI less frequently, but are an important consideration as they require specific anaerobic culture media and longer incubation time compared with aerobic bacteria (Brook 2008).

There are myriad of unusual pathogens that have capacity to cause peri-prosthetic infections. Epidemiologic exposure and underlying immune status of the host are principal risk factors for many unusual pathogens. Unusual infections are more commonly seen in patients with underlying immunosuppression due to disease or due to treatment of disease (e.g. TNF-α-blockers). Some agents may be difficult to identify owing to specific culture media enrichment, like *Abiotrophia sp.* (previously nutritionally-variant streptococcus), *Brucella*, and *Listeria monocytogenes* (Marculescu et al. 2006a). Fungal infections of prosthetic joints are rare and generally occur in patients with underlying risk factors; *Candida* and *Aspergillus* are the most commonly implicated fungi, with endemic fungi and moulds in case reports alone (Fowler et al. 1998; Guyard et al. 2006; Marculescu et al. 2006b; Azzam et al. 2009; Gottesman-Yekutieli et al. 2011). *Mycobacterium* infection is a rare cause of prosthetic joint infection. The »rapid-growers«, such as *M. abscessus* and *M. fortuitum*, are ubiquitous in the environment and can cause PJI in patients without obvious risk factors (Eid et al. 2007). *Mycobacterium tuberculosis* (MTB) skeletal infection is the second most common manifestation of MTB disease and can present in prosthetic joint in patients with epidemiologic risk factors, and is more common in patients treated with steroids or immunosuppressants. Infection can be due to delayed local reactivation in a previously affected joint, or due to haematogenous seeding of the prosthesis during pulmonary reactivation with dissemination. Often, previous MTB infection is not known, and the diagnosis of PJI may be delayed and potentially misidentified if acid-fast-specific microbiologic studies are not performed (Tokumoto et al. 1995; Khater et al. 2007). In up to 26% of cases, despite evidence of purulence, drainage, or histopathologic diagnosis of infection, cultures fail to identify a pathogen. While fastidious or unusual organisms may seldom be responsible, prior antibiotic use is a

◘ Tab. 4.4 Rates of methicillin-susceptible and methicillin-resistant organisms vary based on local epidemiology

Microbiology of prosthetic hip infections	
Staphylococcus aureus	24–30%
Coagulase-negative staphylococci	11–51%
Streptococcal spp.	4–25%
Gram-negative pathogens	
Enteric Gram-negative rods	0–15%
Pseudomonas aeruginosa	1–11%
Enterococcus spp.	0–17%
Anaerobes	0–25%
Polymicrobial	0–8%
Culture negative	7–26%

Take-Home Message

- Antibiotic treatment in patients with suspected PJI should be delayed until cultures from the joint have been obtained.
- Obtaining multiple cultures can significantly change patient care (one or two cultures are insufficient).
- Cultures should be incubated for up to 14 days.
- Susceptibility testing is necessary in choosing appropriate antimicrobial therapy.

major risk factor for culture-negative PJI (Berbari et al. 2007; Malekzadeh et al. 2010).

Susceptibility testing is necessary in choosing appropriate antimicrobial therapy, as susceptibility can no longer be predicted based on the identification of the organism. Patterns of sensitivity/resistance are constantly changing and may vary from one geographic location to another. It is expected that this growing resistance to current antibiotics will only become more common in the future. Drug-resistant organisms limit antimicrobial options, leaving only more toxic or less potent alternatives and may be associated with higher failure rates.

References

Aggarwal VK, Higuera C, Deirmengian G, et al (2013) Swab Cultures are not as effective as tissue cultures for diagnosis of periprosthetic joint infection. Clin Orthop Relat Res 471:3196–3203

Azzam K, Parvizi J, Jungkind D, et al (2009) Microbiological, clinical, and surgical features of fungal prosthetic joint infections: a multi-institutional experience. J Bone Joint Surg Am 91(Suppl6):142–149

Berbari EF, Marculescu C, Sia I, et al (2007) Culture-negative prosthetic joint infection. Clin Infect Dis 45(9):1113–1119

Brause BD (1989) Prosthetic joint infections. Curr Opin Rheumatol 1(2):194–198

Brook I (2008) Microbiology and management of joint and bone infections due to anaerobic bacteria. J Orthop Sci 13(2):160–169

Cipriano CA, Brown NM, Michael AM, et al (2012) Serum and synovial fluid analysis for diagnosing chronic periprosthetic infection in patients with inflammatory arthritis. J Bone Joint Surg Am 94(7):594–600

Crockarell JR, Hanssen AD, Osmon DR, Morrey BF (1998) Treatment of infection with débridement and retention of the components following hip arthroplasty. J Bone Joint Surg Am 80(9):1306–1313

DeHaan A, Huff T, Schabel K, et al (2013) Multiple Cultures and Extended Incubation for Hip and Knee Arthroplasty Revision: Impact on Clinical Care. J Arthroplasty 28 (Suppl1):59–65

Della Valle C, Parvizi J, Bauer TW, DiCesare PE, Evans RP, Segreti J, Spanghel M, Waters WC 3rd, Keith M, Turkelson CM, Wies JL, Sluka P and Hitchcock K (2011) American Academy of Orthopaedic Surgeons Clinical Practice Guideline: The Diagnosis of Periprosthetic Joint Infections of the Hip and Knee. J Bone and Joint Surg Am 93(14):1355–1357

Eid AJ, Berbari EF, Sia IG, et al (2007) Prosthetic joint infection due to rapidly growing mycobacteria: report of 8 cases and review of the literature. Clin Infect Dis 45(6): 687–694

Fowler VG Jr, Nacinovich FM, Alspaugh JA, Corey GR (1998) Prosthetic joint infection due to Histoplasma capsulatum: case report and review. Clin Infect Dis 26(4):1017

Fuller DD, Davis TE, Kibsey PC, et al (1994) Comparison of BACTEC Plus 26 and 27 media with and without fastidious organism supplement with conventional methods for culture of sterile body fluids. J Clin Microbiol 32(6): 1488–1491

Gottesman-Yekutieli T, Shwartz O, Edelman A, Hendel D, Dan M (2011) Pseudallescheria boydii infection of a prosthetic hip joint--an uncommon infection in a rare location. Am J Med Sci 342(3):250–253

Guyard M, Vaz G, Aleksic I, et al (2006) [Aspergillar prosthetic hip infection with false aneurysm of the common femoral artery and cup migration into the pelvis]. Rev Chir Orthop Reparatrice Appar Mot 92(6):606–609

Hindle P, Davidson E, Biant LC (2012) Septic arthritis of the knee: the use and effect of antibiotics prior to diagnostic aspiration. Ann R Coll Surg Engl 94(5):351–355

Hsieh P-H, Lee MS, Hsu K-Y, et al (2009) Gram-negative prosthetic joint infections: risk factors and outcome of treatment. Clin Infect Dis 49(7):1036–1043

Hughes JG, Vetter EA, Patel R, et al (2001) Culture with BACTEC Peds Plus/F bottle compared with conventional methods for detection of bacteria in synovial fluid. J Clin Microbiol 39(12):4468–4471

Khater FJ, Samnani IQ, Mehta JB, Moorman JP, Myers JW (2007) Prosthetic joint infection by Mycobacterium tuberculosis: an unusual case report with literature review. South Med J 100(1):66–69

Kurtz SM, Lau E, Schmier J, et al (2008) Infection burden for hip and knee arthroplasty in the United States. J Arthroplasty 23(7):984–991

Kurtz SM, Lau E, Watson H, Schmier JK, Parvizi J (2012) Economic Burden of Periprosthetic Joint Infection in the United States. J Arthroplasty 27(8Suppl):61–65

Lachiewicz PF, Rogers GD, Thomason HC (1996) Aspiration of the hip joint before revision total hip arthroplasty. Clinical and laboratory factors influencing attainment of a positive culture. J Bone Joint Surg Am 78(5):749–754

Larsen LH, Lange J, Xu Y and Schønheyder HC (2012) Optimizing Culture Methods for Diagnosis of Prosthetic Joint Infections: A Summary of Modifications and Improvements Reported Since1995. J Med Microbiol 61(Pt3): 309–316

Lentino JR (2003) Prosthetic joint infections: bane of orthopedists, challenge for infectious disease specialists. Clin Infect Dis 36(9):1157–1161

Maderazo EG, Judson S, Pasternak H (1988) Late infections of total joint prostheses. A review and recommendations for prevention. Clin Orthop Relat Res 229:131–142

Malekzadeh D, Osmon DR, Lahr BD, Hanssen AD, Berbari EF (2010) Prior use of antimicrobial therapy is a risk factor for culture-negative prosthetic joint infection. Clin Orthop Relat Res 468(8):2039–2045

Marculescu CE, Berbari EF, Cockerill FR 3rd, Osmon DR (2006a) Unusual aerobic and anaerobic bacteria associated with prosthetic joint infections. Clin Orthop Relat Res 451:55–63

Marculescu CE, Berbari EF, Cockerill FR 3rd, Osmon DR (2006b) Fungi, mycobacteria, zoonotic and other organisms in prosthetic joint infection. Clin Orthop Relat Res 451:64–72

Morgan PM, Sharkey P, Ghanem E, et al (2009) The value of intraoperative Gram stain in revision total knee arthroplasty. J Bone Joint Surg Am 91:2124–2129

Rak M, Barli-Maganja D, Kavcic M, et al (2013) Comparison of molecular and culture method in diagnosis of prosthetic joint infection. FEMS Microbiol Lett 343:42–48

Scafer P, Fink B, Sandow D, et al (2008) Prolonged Bacterial Culture to Identify Late Periprosthetic Joint Infection: A Promising Strategy. Clin Infect Dis 47(11):1403–1409

Schinsky MF, Della Valle CJ, Sporer SM, Paprosky WG (2008) Perioperative testing for joint infection in patients undergoing revision total hip arthroplasty. J Bone Joint Surg Am 90(9):1869–1875

Shanmugasundaram S, Ricciardi BF, Briggs TWR, et al (2014) Evaluation and management of periprosthetic joint infections – an international, multicenter study. HSSJ 10(1):36–44

Sousa R, Pereira A, Massada M, et al (2010) Empirical antibiotic therapy in prosthetic joint infections. Acta Orthop Belg 76(2):254–259

Spangehl MJ, Masri BA, O'Connell JX, Duncan CP (1999) Prospective analysis of preoperative and intraoperative investigations for the diagnosis of infection at the sites of two hundred and two revision total hip arthroplasties. J Bone Joint Surg Am 81(5):672–683

Tetreault MW, Wetters NG, Aggarwal V, et al (2014) Should Prophylactic antibiotics be withheld before revision surgery to obtain appropriate cultures? Clin Orthop Relat Res 472:52–56

Tetreault MW, Wetters NG, Aggarwal VK, Moric M, Segreti J, Huddleston JI 3rd, Parvizi J, Della Valle CJ (2013) Should draining wounds and sinuses associated with hip and knee arthroplasties be cultured? J Arthroplasty 28 (8Suppl):133–136

Tokumoto JI, Follansbee SE, Jacobs RA (1995) Prosthetic joint infection due to Mycobacterium tuberculosis: report of three cases. Clin Infect Dis 21(1):134–136

Trampuz A, Piper KE, Jacobson MJ, et al (2007) Sonication of removed hip and knee prostheses for diagnosis of infection. N Engl J Med 357:654–663

Tsukayama DT, Estrada R, Gustilo RB (1996) Infection after total hip arthroplasty. A study of the treatment of one hundred and six infections. J Bone Joint Surg Am 78(4):512–523

Ure KJ, Amstutz HC, Nasser S, Schmalzried TP (1998) Direct-exchange arthroplasty for the treatment of infection after total hip replacement. An average ten-year follow-up. J Bone Joint Surg Am 80(7):961–968

Prevention

K.-D. Kühn (Ed.), *Management of Periprosthetic Joint Infection*
DOI 10.1007/978-3-662-54469-3_5

5.1 Prophylaxis for Implant-Related Infections: Current State of the Art

Willemijn Boot and H. Charles Vogely

5.1.1 Introduction

Joint replacement is a successful surgical procedure that provides pain relief, restores joint function and improves the quality of life of patients. A minority of patients will experience complications like aseptic failure or prosthetic joint infection (PJI; Tande and Patel 2014). The incidence for PJI is estimated at 1% for hip arthroplasties and between 1% and 2% for knee arthroplasties (Pulido et al. 2008; Lindeque et al. 2014; Kapadia et al. 2015). It has been reported that 60–70% of infections occur within the first 2 years of the arthroplasty (Tande and Patel 2014).

To minimize the overall incidence of infection, many methods are being investigated, for example identifying the host risk factors, patients' health modification, proper wound care, and optimizing the operative room environment (Owens and Stoessel 2008; Rezapoor et al. 2015; Shahi and Parvizi 2015). Besides these preventive measures, intraoperative systemic antibiotics are standard of care for PJI prophylaxis. Antibiotic prophylaxis is effective in reducing infection in patients following total joint replacement (Al-Buhairan et al. 2008). The Surgical Care Improvement Project guidelines (Rosenberger et al. 2011) recommend starting with antibiotics at least 1 h before surgery and stopping within 24 hours. The Clinical Practice Guidelines for Antimicrobial Prophylaxis in Surgery (Bratzler et al. 2013) recommend cefazolin for patients with total joint arthroplasty. Clindamycin and vancomycin are regarded as adequate alternatives (Bratzler et al. 2013). Vancomycin is recommended to be used for methicillin-resistant *Staphylococcus aureus* (MRSA)-colonized patients and may be included in the regimen of choice in institutions with a high prevalence of MRSA surgical site infections (Bratzler et al. 2013).

One of the obstacles related to systemic administration of antibiotics is that insufficient concentrations are reached at the preferred location. Increasing the dose is not a solution owing to the risk of systemic toxicity. One successful method is the local delivery of antibiotics. Commonly used, for example, is the combination of antimicrobial-laden bone cement with systemic antibiotics for the prevention of infection in primary arthroplasties (Bratzler et al. 2013). In a study using the Norwegian Arthroplasty Register the risk of aseptic failure or infection was lowest when antibiotics were administered both systemically and locally in bone cement (Engesaeter et al. 2003). As this method for local application of antibiotics cannot be applied for cementless implants, there is a need for improving local prophylactic methods. In the past decade, multiple studies have been performed to develop and investigate the ability to provide local infection prophylaxis at the implant surface and protect the implant material by bacterial eradication. This chapter will highlight the most current research for local prophylaxis of implant-related infections, which is divided into two major topics: local infection prophylaxis of implants, and local non-antibiotic prophylaxis of implants (■ Tab. 5.1).

5.1.2 Carriers and Coatings for Local Infection Prophylaxis

Controlled release of antibacterial agents from an implant coating allows for the administration of adequate drug concentrations around the implant site. Also, there is less risk of subjecting the body to an excessively high antibiotic load, which reduces the negative effects on healthy tissues. In order to engineer new solutions for local prophylaxis of implants, a variety of materials and methods have been researched in recent years.

■ **Tab. 5.1** Overview of topics discussed in this chapter

Carriers and coatings for local infection prophylaxis	Local infection prophylaxis of implants
Polymers	Silver
Hydroxyapatite	Novaran
Chitosan	Antimicrobial peptides
Nanoscale surfaces	
Hydrogels	

Polymers

A broad spectrum of biodegradable materials and approaches have been proposed and investigated as carriers for the local application of antibacterial agents. Synthetic materials offer advantages over biologically occurring materials. For example, synthetic polymers can be produced under controlled and reproducible conditions, and the functional properties can be easily adapted by chemical modifications (Hutmacher et al. 1996).

The biodegradable polymer poly(D,L-lactide) (PDLLA) was found to be resistant against abrasion during intramedullary implantation of a PDLLA-coated implant and allows for incorporation of antibacterials (Schmidmaier et al. 2001). An implant coating with gentamicin-loaded PDLLA resulted in an initial burst release of gentamicin followed by a slow release (Vester et al. 2010). PDLLA can also be used for multi-layer coatings to enable incorporation of multiple agents of interest. For example, incorporating gentamicin, insulin-like growth factor I (IGF-I), and bone morphogenetic protein 2 (BMP-2) in a layered PDLLA coating on Kirschner wires resulted in a release first of gentamicin, shortly afterwards IGF-I and subsequently BMP-2 (Strobel et al. 2011a, 2011b). This three-layer coating can be easily applied on any desired implant with a simple dipping technique (Strobel et al. 2011a, 2011b).

Another biodegradable polymer is poly(lactic co-glycolic acid) (PLGA). Electrospun PLGA was developed as a biodegradable localized delivery system for the controlled release of antibiotics. Electrospinning utilizes electrical forces to produce fine polymeric fibres. This can produce continuous fibres and can be used to coat titanium implants. Loading the electrospun PLGA coating with various antibiotics provides a release of the antibiotics and shows antimicrobial activity in vitro and in vivo (Li et al. 2012; Gilchrist et al. 2013; Zhang et al. 2014). Another use for PLGA is a biodegradable overcoat for protection of an antibiotic layer during surgical implantation. This coating proved to degrade in vivo to enable normal osteo-integration of the implant and to release the antibiotic, which provides an antibacterial effect (Neut et al. 2011, 2012, 2015).

Additionally, several combinations of polymers are utilized as local carrier of antibacterials. For example, poly(L-lysine)/poly(L-glutamic acid) nanofilms can be fine-tuned for the amount of antibiotic release. When coated on a stainless steel disk, the nanofilm provided in vitro antibacterial efficacy. Furthermore, the nanofilm improved osteoblast viability and proliferation in vitro (Li et al. 2010). Another combination of polymers is the biodegradable Polymer–Lipid Encapsulation MatriX (PLEX), containing, amongst others, polylactic-co-glycolic acid (PLGA). The PLEX coating provides an environment in which the antimicrobial agent can be incorporated and allows for the adjustment of the amount of drug loaded and the number of applied layers for a controlled release over time (Emanuel et al. 2012). The PLEX coating loaded with antibiotic can be released for up to 28 days in vitro and, when coated on implants, the antibiotic-loaded coating shows antibacterial prophylaxis in vivo (Metsemakers et al. 2015).

Hydroxyapatite

For the past few years, titanium implants have been coated successfully with plasma-sprayed hydroxyapatite (HA) to improve implant fixation and osteo-integration (Dumbleton and Manley 2004). Adapting this coating as a local release system for antibacterials can be used to prevent implant-related infections for uncemented implants. Unfortunately, antibiotics cannot be incorporated into plasma-sprayed coatings because of the high processing temperatures. Therefore, methods to overcome this problem are being investigated. For example, antibiotics can be co-precipitated with HA crystals to form a uniform coating on top of an implant (Stigter et al. 2004). Another method to coat implants with antibiotic-containing HA is an ink-jet technology (Alt et al. 2006). This coating was reported to have antimicrobial activity in vivo when loaded with various antibiotics (Alt et al. 2014). Peri-apatite, an HA coating that is applied on implants using a solution deposition method, can be combined with tobramycin for local infection prophylaxis. In an in vivo study, the peri-apatite coating proved to be an effective local antibacterial coating for uncemented implants and also improved the implant fixation compared with uncoated implants (Moojen et al. 2009). In a clinical study, the effectiveness of preventing an infection with a vancomycin-loaded

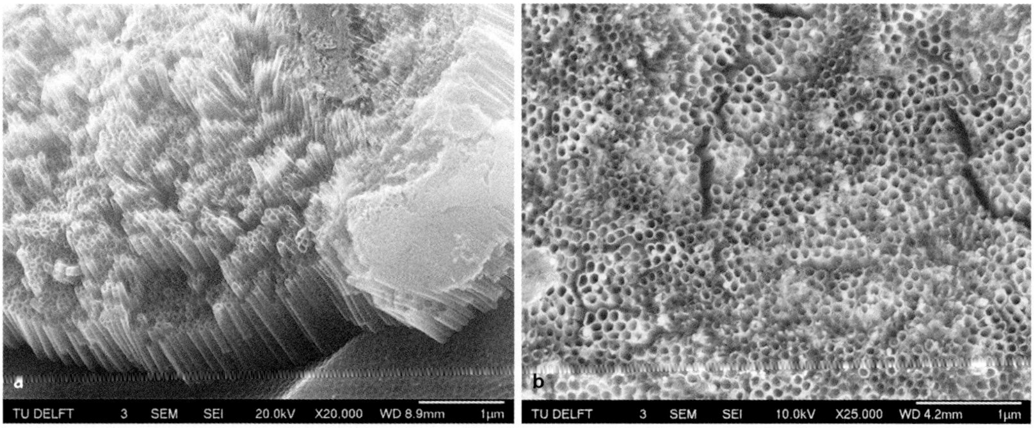

Fig. 5.1 Titanium dioxide nanotubes (**a**) and silver nanoparticles embedded in titanium dioxide nanotubes (**b**)

calcium HA was evaluated in patients with non-cemented total knee arthroplasty. A paste was made with HA and vancomycin and a thin layer was spread on the surface of the implants. After a mean period of 5 years, the treatment group showed significantly fewer infections than the non-treated group (Assor 2010).

Chitosan

Chitosan is a polysaccharide that can be degraded by the body's own enzymes. Dehydrated chitosan films have the ability to rehydrate and absorb soluble agents of interest (Nunthanid et al. 2001). This ability enables the films to be loaded during surgery and can be customized to fit the patient's needs. Vancomycin-loaded chitosan proved to reduce infection in vitro as a coating on titanium foils, without showing adverse effects on an MG-63 osteoblast-like cell line (Ordikhani 2014). Furthermore, chitosan loaded with daptomycin or vancomycin showed antibacterial activity against *S. aureus* in vitro (Smith et al. 2010).

Nanoscale Surfaces

Over the past years, the biocompatible properties of nanoscale surfaces have been investigated (Fig. 5.1). Self-organized nanotubes on the surface of titanium dioxide (TiO_2) implants can be formed by a relatively simple electrochemical oxidation reaction of a titanium substrate under a specific set of environmental conditions. Varying the voltages and anodizing times can generate different nanotopographical features (Amin et al. 2015). The key advantage is that the morphology of the nanotubes can be adapted to improve cell adhesion, spreading, growth and differentiation of cells. Mesenchymal stem cells show a size-dependent reaction to these nanoscale surfaces (Bauer et al. 2009). Another advantage is that the nanotubes can be used as a container for local delivery of antimicrobial agents. Investigations of silver nanoparticle-filled titanium nanotubes found a high bacteriostatic rate of 99.99% (Wang et al. 2013). Furthermore, the material showed good cytocompatibility, and the osteoblast adhesion to the titanium was increased compared with pure titanium (Wang et al. 2013). Antimicrobial peptide-loaded TiO_2 nanotubes could effectively reduce the amount of viable bacteria (~99.9%) in vitro and reduce bacterial adherence to the surface (Ma et al. 2012; Kazemzadeh-Narbat et al. 2013).

Hydrogels

Hydrogels are polymeric materials with a high water content that can be used as a delivery vehicle for antibacterial agents. Being able to choose an agent of interest during the surgery provides the advantage of versatility. A resorbable hydrogel (Fig. 5.2), composed of covalently linked hyaluronic acid and polylactic acid, was tested for its capability to deliver various antibiotic and anti-biofilm agents in vitro (Drago et al. 2014). The hydrogel provided a burst release of the antibacterial agents in vitro within the first few hours and all of the tested agents

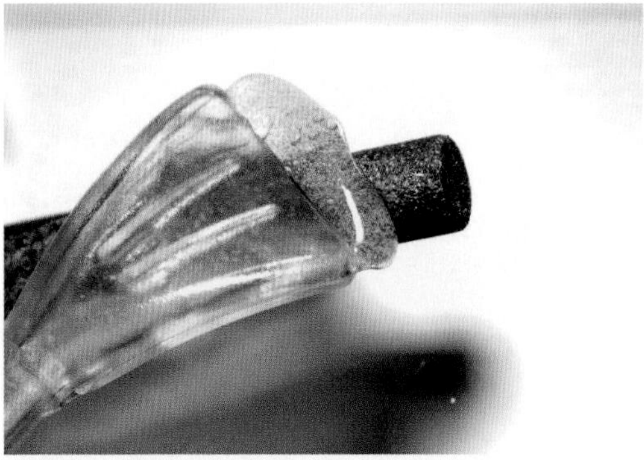

Fig. 5.2 The resorbable hydrogel, composed of hyaluronic acid and polylactic acid, applied on a sandblasted titanium rod

were delivered in medium within 96 h. The hydrogel proved to be bactericidal and exerted an antibiofilm effect in vitro in combination with different antibacterials.

5.1.3 Local Non-antibiotic Prophylaxis of Implants

The use of antibiotics to treat bacterial infections has resulted in resistant bacterial strains. Methicillin-resistant *S. aureus* and methicillin-resistant *S. epidermidis* are two commonly isolated organisms from PJIs (Pulido et al. 2008). The ability of these micro-organisms to adapt their resistance patterns renders antibiotics useless for treatment of bacterial infections. These infections can often not be treated adequately, which results in longer hospitalizations and higher costs (Parvizi et al. 2010). It is very important that alternative antibacterial strategies are researched and developed.

Silver

It has been known for a long time that silver and other metals have antimicrobial activity (Klasen 2000). The mechanism behind the antimicrobial activity is based on multiple modes of action. Free silver ions can enter the bacterial cells and cause the DNA to precipitate, causing the cells to lose the ability to multiply (Feng et al. 2000). Furthermore, silver can react with the bacterial membrane and cause structural damage (Jung et al. 2008). Inside the bacterial cells, silver ions can bind to proteins and interfere with the respiratory chain enzymes to inhibit growth (Feng et al. 2000; Jung et al. 2008; Gordon et al. 2010). The antibacterial effect of silver was found to be dependent on particle size. Smaller nanoparticles exert more antimicrobial and cellular toxicity (Dasgupta et al. 2015). As Gram-positive bacteria have thicker cell walls which inhibit silver nanoparticles to cross the cell membrane, a higher concentration is needed to prevent bacterial growth than for Gram-negative bacteria (Feng et al. 2000; Jung et al. 2008).

Investigations of silver nanoparticle-loaded bone cement demonstrated a significant reduction of biofilm formation on the surface of the cement; however, it showed no activity against planktonic bacteria (Slane et al. 2015). In vitro antibacterial tests of bone cement loaded with silver, either as silver nitrate solution or in the solid phase as silver phosphate salt, showed anti-adhesion and anti-biofilm properties, without having any toxic effects on human bone marrow stromal cells (Jacquart et al. 2013). Pauksch et al. demonstrated in an in vitro study a similar biocompatibility for nanosilver-loaded bone cement on primary human mesenchymal stem cells compared with plain bone cement or loaded with gentamicin (Pauksch et al. 2014).

Direct coating of stainless steel implants with silver nanoparticles has been shown to inhibit bacterial adhesion and biofilm formation in vitro and reduced implant-related infection in an implant-related femur infection in rats. No cytotoxicity was seen in vitro for human bone marrow stromal cells, and osteogenic differentiation was reported to be promoted (Qin et al. 2015). In a clinical study where 51 patients received a silver-coated proximal femur or tibia replacement, a decrease in periprosthetic infections was seen from 17.6% to 5.9% compared with a retrospective cohort of patients with non-coated titanium implants. Although this difference was not statistically significant, clinical outcomes were improved in the group with silver-coated implants as no patient required amputation after infection, whereas more than half of the control patients who developed an infection required amputation (Hardes et al. 2010).

Novaran

Tamai et al. evaluated an inorganic antimicrobial as antibacterial coating. Novaran is a commercially available inorganic antimicrobial made from glass, with zinc as the functional material, and is heat resistant to almost 1,000°C. The antimicrobial effect is caused by dissolving the Zn^{2+} metal ions, which has an antibacterial effect. Coating titanium alloy (Ti6Al4V) plates with Novaran showed good efficiency against *S. aureus* and *P. aeruginosa* in vitro (Tamai et al. 2009).

Antimicrobial Peptides

Antimicrobial peptides (AMPs) are an important part of the innate immune system, particularly at mucosal surfaces that form the barrier between the host and the environment. AMPs are mainly produced by neutrophils and epithelial cells and have a broad-spectrum activity against bacteria, fungi, and enveloped viruses in vitro (Zanetti 2004; Bechinger and Salnikov 2012; Fjell et al. 2012). These peptides are usually small and interact with the cell membranes of micro-organisms to cause depolarization, destabilization, and permeabilization (Hancock and Rozek 2002). Thereafter, the micro-organisms will lyse and die. The membrane-active peptide Tet213 has demonstrated antibacterial effects by reducing growth and biofilm formation of clinical *S. aureus* isolates in vitro (Zhao et al. 2015). The synthetic peptide OP-145 is developed based on the sequence of an autologous peptide, LL-37, that is suggested to be involved in the host defence in mucosa. OP-145 showed effective bactericidal activity towards *S. aureus* and is able to neutralize bacterial lipopolysaccharide and lipoteichoic acid in vitro (Nell et al. 2005; Haisma et al. 2014). The afore-mentioned PLEX coating, initially developed for the delivery of doxycycline, was evaluated for the controlled release of OP-145 in an in vivo implant infection model. The PLEX–OP-145 coating provided adequate antibacterial activity and successfully eradicated infection in the majority of infected animals (de Breij et al. 2015). As both compounds are safe for clinical use, this technique could be rapidly translated for human use.

Another promising alternative for antibiotics are membrane-active cationic steroid antimicrobials, called ceragenins. Ceragenins were synthetically developed to mimic endogenous antimicrobial peptides and have a broad spectrum of antibacterial activity (Bucki et al. 2007). Sinclair et al. evaluated the antimicrobial potential of cationic steroidal antimicrobial-13 (CSA-13; Sinclair et al. 2012). In addition to direct bactericidal activity, high concentrations of CSA-13 cause the bacterial membrane to depolarize, which results in cell death (Epand et al. 2010). Sinclair et al. showed in an in vivo study in sheep that periprosthetic infections could be prevented by coating the implants with CSA-13 without inhibiting bone growth onto the implant surface (Sinclair et al. 2013).

5.1.4 Conclusion

As no local options for infection prophylaxis are currently available for uncemented implants, a system that provides a local, controlled release of antibacterial agents over a certain period of time can prove to be advantageous for the prevention of implant-related infections. Furthermore, due to the emergence of antibiotic resistance in bacteria worldwide, alternatives for antibiotics are needed. Therefore, research has been focusing for the past few years on new methods to encapsulate and release antimicrobial compounds, and on alternative sources of antibiotics that can be loaded into them. An ideal prophylactic coating should meet various criteria such as resistance to mechanical stress, nontoxicity, exert no inhibitory effect on bone formation, and offer a controlled release of the loaded antimicrobial agent. Although the methods and materials discussed in this chapter are promising, and some are even already available for clinical use like the biodegradable hydrogel as a CE-marked medical device (Drago et al. 2014), further research is needed for the ideal next-generation local infection prophylaxis that can be used for a wide variety of orthopaedic implants.

Take-Home Message

- For PJI prophylaxis, across-the-board systemic antibiotics are used. Because these reach insufficient concentrations locally, the prosthesis must be further protected.
- In cemented prostheses, antibiotic-loaded bone cement is used. However, adequate alternatives for cementless prostheses need to be found.
- These alternatives can be divided into two general categories:
  - Carriers and coatings (coating implants with substances that contain or carry and release active agents).
  - Non-antibiotic prophylaxis (alternative substances to antibiotics which also show sufficient antimicrobial activity).

5

References

AlBuhairan B, Hind D, Hutchinson A (2008) Antibiotic prophylaxis for wound infections in total joint arthroplasty: a systematic review. J Bone Joint Surg (Br) 90(7):915-919

Alt V, Bitschnau A, Osterling J, Sewing A, Meyer C, Kraus R, et al (2006) The effects of combined gentamicin-hydroxyapatite coating for cementless joint prostheses on the reduction of infection rates in a rabbit infection prophylaxis model. Biomaterials 27(26):4627-4634

Alt V, Kirchhof K, Seim F, Hrubesch I, Lips KS, Mannel H, et al (2014) Rifampicin-fosfomycin coating for cementless endoprostheses: antimicrobial effects against methicillin-sensitive Staphylococcus aureus (MSSA) and methicillin-resistant Staphylococcus aureus (MRSA). Acta Biomater 10(10):4518-4524

Amin Yavari S, Chai YC, Bottger AJ, Wauthle R, Schrooten J, Weinans H, et al (2015) Effects of anodizing parameters and heat treatment on nanotopographical features, bioactivity, and cell culture response of additively manufactured porous titanium. Mater Sci Eng C Mater Biol Appl 51:132-138

Assor M (2010) Noncemented total knee arthroplasty with a local prophylactic anti-infection agent: a prospective series of 135 cases. Canadian J Surg 53(1):47-50

Bauer S, Park J, Faltenbacher J, Berger S, von der Mark K, Schmuki P (2009) Size selective behavior of mesenchymal stem cells on ZrO(2) and TiO(2) nanotube arrays. Integr Biology (Camb) 1(8-9):525-532

Bechinger B, Salnikov ES (2012) The membrane interactions of antimicrobial peptides revealed by solid-state NMR spectroscopy. Chem Phys Lipids 165(3):282-301

Bratzler DW, Dellinger EP, Olsen KM, Perl TM, Auwaerter PG, Bolon MK, et al (2013) Clinical practice guidelines for antimicrobial prophylaxis in surgery. Am J Health Syst Pharm 70(3):195-283

Bucki R, Sostarecz AG, Byfield FJ, Savage PB, Janmey PA (2007) Resistance of the antibacterial agent ceragenin CSA-13 to inactivation by DNA or F-actin and its activity in cystic fibrosis sputum. J Antimicrob Chemother 60(3):535-645

Dasgupta N, Ranjan S, Rajendran B, Manickam V, Ramalingam C, Avadhani GS, et al (2016) Thermal co-reduction approach to vary size of silver nanoparticle: its microbial and cellular toxicology. Environ Sci Pollut Res Int 23(5):4149-4163

de Breij A, Riool M, Kwakman PH, de Boer L, Cordfunke RA, Drijfhout JW, et al (2016) Prevention of Staphylococcus aureus biomaterial-associated infections using a polymer-lipid coating containing the antimicrobial peptide OP-145. J Control Rel 222:1-8

Drago L, Boot W, Dimas K, Malizos K, Hansch GM, Stuyck J, et al (2014) Does implant coating with antibacterial-loaded hydrogel reduce bacterial colonization and biofilm formation in vitro? Clin Orthop Relat Res 472(11):3311-3323

Dumbleton J, Manley MT (2004) Hydroxyapatite-coated prostheses in total hip and knee arthroplasty. J Bone Joint Surg (Am) 86(11):2526-2540

Emanuel N, Rosenfeld Y, Cohen O, Applbaum YH, Segal D, Barenholz Y (2012) A lipid-and-polymer-based novel local drug delivery system--BonyPid: from physicochemical aspects to therapy of bacterially infected bones. J Control Release 160(2):353-361

Engesaeter LB, Lie SA, Espehaug B, Furnes O, Vollset SE, Havelin LI (2003) Antibiotic prophylaxis in total hip arthroplasty: effects of antibiotic prophylaxis systemically and in bone cement on the revision rate of 22,170 primary hip replacements followed 0-14 years in the Norwegian Arthroplasty Register. Acta Orthop Scand 74(6):644-651

Epand RF, Pollard JE, Wright JO, Savage PB, Epand RM (2010) Depolarization, bacterial membrane composition, and the antimicrobial action of ceragenins. Antimicrob Agents Chemother 54(9):3708-3713

Feng QL, Wu J, Chen GQ, Cui FZ, Kim TN, Kim JO (2000) A mechanistic study of the antibacterial effect of silver ions on Escherichia coli and Staphylococcus aureus. J Biomed Mater Res 52(4):662-668

Fjell CD, Hiss JA, Hancock RE, Schneider G (2012) Designing antimicrobial peptides: form follows function. Nat Rev Drug Discov 11(1):37-51

Gilchrist SE, Lange D, Letchford K, Bach H, Fazli L, Burt HM (2013) Fusidic acid and rifampicin co-loaded PLGA nanofibers for the prevention of orthopedic implant associated infections. J Control Release 170(1):64-73

Gordon O, Slenters TV, Brunetto PS, Villaruz AE, Sturdevant DE, Otto M, et al (2010) Silver coordination polymers for prevention of implant infection: Thiol interaction, impact on respiratory chain enzymes, and hydroxyl radical induction. Antimicrob Agents Chemother 54(10): 4208-4218

Haisma EM, de Breij A, Chan H, van Dissel JT, Drijfhout JW, Hiemstra PS, et al (2014) LL-37-derived peptides eradicate multidrug-resistant Staphylococcus aureus from thermally wounded human skin equivalents. Antimicrob Agents Chemother 58(8):4411-4419

Hancock RE, Rozek A (2002) Role of membranes in the activities of antimicrobial cationic peptides. FEMS Microbiol Lett 206(2):143-149

Hardes J, von Eiff C, Streitbuerger A, Balke M, Budny T, Henrichs MP, et al (2010) Reduction of periprosthetic infection with silver-coated megaprostheses in patients with bone sarcoma. J Surg Oncol 101(5):389-395

Hutmacher D, Hurzeler MB, Schliephake H (1996) A review of material properties of biodegradable and bioresorbable polymers and devices for GTR and GBR applications. Int J Oral Maxillofac Implants 11(5):667-678

Jacquart S, Siadous R, Henocq-Pigasse C, Bareille R, Roques C, Rey C, et al (2013) Composition and properties of silver-containing calcium carbonate-calcium phosphate bone cement. J Mater Sci Mater Med 24(12):2665-2675

Jung WK, Koo HC, Kim KW, Shin S, Kim SH, Park YH (2008) Antibacterial activity and mechanism of action of the silver ion in Staphylococcus aureus and Escherichia coli. Appl Environ Microbiol 74(7):2171-2178

Kapadia BH, Berg RA, Daley JA, Fritz J, Bhave A, Mont MA (2015) Periprosthetic joint infection. Lancet 387:386-394

Kazemzadeh-Narbat M, Lai BF, Ding C, Kizhakkedathu JN, Hancock RE, Wang R (2013) Multilayered coating on titanium for controlled release of antimicrobial peptides for the prevention of implant-associated infections. Biomaterials 34(24):5969-5977

Klasen HJ (2000) Historical review of the use of silver in the treatment of burns. I. Early uses. Burns 26(2):117-130

Li H, Ogle H, Jiang B, Hagar M, Li B (2010) Cefazolin embedded biodegradable polypeptide nanofilms promising for infection prevention: a preliminary study on cell responses. J Orthop Res 28(8):992-999

Li LL, Wang LM, Xu Y, Lv LX (2012) Preparation of gentamicin-loaded electrospun coating on titanium implants and a study of their properties in vitro. Arch Orthop Trauma Surg 132(6):897-903

Lindeque B, Hartman Z, Noshchenko A, Cruse M (2014) Infection after primary total hip arthroplasty. Orthopedics 37(4):257-265

Ma M, Kazemzadeh-Narbat M, Hui Y, Lu S, Ding C, Chen DD, et al (2012) Local delivery of antimicrobial peptides using self-organized TiO2 nanotube arrays for peri-implant infections. J Biomed Material Res A 100(2):278-285

Metsemakers WJ, Emanuel N, Cohen O, Reichart M, Potapova I, Schmid T, et al (2015) A doxycycline-loaded polymer-lipid encapsulation matrix coating for the prevention of implant-related osteomyelitis due to doxycycline-resistant methicillin-resistant Staphylococcus aureus. J Control Release 209:47-56

Moojen DJF, Vogely HC, Fleer A, Nikkels PGJ, Higham PA, Verbout AJ, et al (2009) Prophylaxis of infection and effects on osseointegration using a tobramycin-periapatite coating on titanium implants – an experimental study in the rabbit. J Orthop Res 27(6):710-716

Nell MJ, Tjabringa GS, Wafelman AR, Verrijk R, Hiemstra PS, Drijfhout JW, et al (2006) Development of novel LL-37 derived antimicrobial peptides with LPS and LTA neutralizing and antimicrobial activities for therapeutic application. Peptides 27(4):649-660

Neut D, Dijkstra RJ, Thompson JI, van der Mei HC, Busscher HJ (2011) Antibacterial efficacy of a new gentamicin-coating for cementless prostheses compared to gentamicin-loaded bone cement. J Orthop Res 29(11):1654-1661

Neut D, Dijkstra RJ, Thompson JI, van der Mei HC, Busscher HJ (2012) A gentamicin-releasing coating for cementless hip prostheses-Longitudinal evaluation of efficacy using in vitro bio-optical imaging and its wide-spectrum antibacterial efficacy. J Biomed Materials Res Part A 100(12): 3220-3226

Neut D, Dijkstra RJ, Thompson JI, Kavanagh C, van der Mei HC, Busscher HJ (2015) A biodegradable gentamicin-hydroxyapatite-coating for infection prophylaxis in cementless hip prostheses. Eur Cell Mater 29:42-55

Nunthanid J, Puttipipatkhachorn S, Yamamoto K, Peck GE (2001) Physical properties and molecular behavior of chitosan films. Drug Dev Ind Pharm 27(2):143-157

Ordikhani F (2014) Characterization and antibacterial performance of electrodeposited chitosan-vancomycin composite coatings for prevention of implant-associated infections. Mater Sci Eng C Mater Biol Appl 41: 240-248

Owens CD, Stoessel K (2008) Surgical site infections: epidemiology, microbiology and prevention. J Hosp Infect 70[Suppl 2]:3-10

Parvizi J, Pawasarat IM, Azzam KA, Joshi A, Hansen EN, Bozic KJ (2010) Periprosthetic joint infection: the economic impact of methicillin-resistant infections. J Arthroplasty 25[6 Suppl]:103-107

Pauksch L, Hartmann S, Szalay G, Alt V, Lips KS (2014) In vitro assessment of nanosilver-functionalized PMMA bone cement on primary human mesenchymal stem cells and osteoblasts. PloS One 9(12):e114740

Pulido L, Ghanem E, Joshi A, Purtill JJ, Parvizi J (2008) Periprosthetic joint infection: the incidence, timing, and predisposing factors. Clin Orthop Relat Res 466(7): 1710-1715

Qin H, Cao H, Zhao Y, Jin G, Cheng M, Wang J, et al (2015) Antimicrobial and osteogenic properties of silver-ion-implanted stainless steel. ACS Appl Mater Interfaces 7(20):10785-10794

Rezapoor M, Parvizi J (2015) Prevention of periprosthetic joint infection. J Arthrop 30(6):902-907

Rosenberger LH, Politano AD, Sawyer RG (2011) The surgical care improvement project and prevention of post-operative infection, including surgical site infection. Surg Infect 12(3):163-168

Schmidmaier G, Wildemann B, Stemberger A, Haas NP, Raschke M (2001) Biodegradable poly(D,L-lactide) coating of implants for continuous release of growth factors. J Biomed Mat Res 58(4):449-455
Shahi A, Parvizi J (2015) Prevention of periprosthetic joint infection. Arch Bone Joint Surg 3(2):72-81
Sinclair KD, Pham TX, Farnsworth RW, Williams DL, Loc-Carrillo C, Horne LA, et al (2012) Development of a broad spectrum polymer-released antimicrobial coating for the prevention of resistant strain bacterial infections. J Biomed Mater Res A 100(10):2732-2738
Sinclair KD, Pham TX, Williams DL, Farnsworth RW, Loc-Carrillo CM, Bloebaum RD (2013) Model development for determining the efficacy of a combination coating for the prevention of perioperative device related infections: a pilot study. J Biomed Mater Res B Appl Biomater 101(7):1143-1153
Slane J, Vivanco J, Rose W, Ploeg HL, Squire M (2015) Mechanical, material, and antimicrobial properties of acrylic bone cement impregnated with silver nanoparticles. Mater Sci Eng C Mater Biol Appl 48:188-196
Smith JK, Bumgardner JD, Courtney HS, Smeltzer MS, Haggard WO (2010) Antibiotic-loaded chitosan film for infection prevention: A preliminary in vitro characterization. J Biomed Materials Res B Appl Biomater 94(1):203-211
Stigter M, Bezemer J, de Groot K, Layrolle P (2004) Incorporation of different antibiotics into carbonated hydroxyapatite coatings on titanium implants, release and antibiotic efficacy. J Control Release 99(1):127-137
Strobel C, Schmidmaier G, Wildemann B (2011a) Changing the release kinetics of gentamicin from poly(D,L-lactide) implant coatings using only one polymer. Int J Artif Organs 34(3):304-316
Strobel C, Bormann N, Kadow-Romacker A, Schmidmaier G, Wildemann B (2011b) Sequential release kinetics of two substances from one-component polymeric coating on implants. J Control Release 156:37-45
Tamai K, Kawate K, Kawahara I, Takakura Y, Sakaki K (2009) Inorganic antimicrobial coating for titanium alloy and its effect on bacteria. J Orthop Sci Assoc 14(2):204-209
Tande AJ, Patel R (2014) Prosthetic joint infection. Clin Microbiol Rev 27(2):302-345
Vester H, Wildemann B, Schmidmaier G, Stockle U, Lucke M (2010) Gentamycin delivered from a PDLLA coating of metallic implants: In vivo and in vitro characterisation for local prophylaxis of implant-related osteomyelitis. Injury 41(10):1053-1059
Wang Z, Sun Y, Wang D, Liu H, Boughton RI (2013) In situ fabrication of silver nanoparticle-filled hydrogen titanate nanotube layer on metallic titanium surface for bacteriostatic and biocompatible implantation. Int J Nanomed 8:2903-2916
Zanetti M (2004) Cathelicidins, multifunctional peptides of the innate immunity. J Leuk Biol 75(1):39-48
Zhang L, Yan J, Yin Z, Tang C, Guo Y, Li D, et al (2014) Electrospun vancomycin-loaded coating on titanium implants for the prevention of implant-associated infections. Int J Nanomed 9:3027-3036
Zhao G, Zhong H, Zhang M, Hong Y (2015) Effects of antimicrobial peptides on Staphylococcus aureus growth and biofilm formation in vitro following isolation from implant-associated infections. Int J Clin Exp Med 8(1):1546-1551

5.2 Prophylaxis During Total Hip and Knee Replacement

Jason Chan and Paul Partington

5.2.1 Introduction

Total hip replacement (THR) and total knee replacement (TKR) are two of the most commonly performed procedures in orthopaedic practice and are considered to be cost effective and safe. Periprosthetic joint infection (PJI) is an infrequent but major complication. Over a 5-year period between April 2010 and March 2015, the cumulative incidence of surgical site infection (SSI), which includes PJI for THR and TKR was 0.7% and 0.6%, respectively in England (Public Health England 2015). However, the management of these infected prostheses is associated with significant morbidity and expense.

Multiple patient and surgical factors are implicated in causing PJI (◘ Tab. 5.2; Parvizi and Gehrke 2013). The most common organisms responsible for causing PJI are shown in ◘ Fig. 5.3 (Public Health England 2015). In this chapter, we review the various strategies to reduce the risk of PJI and how they influence practice in our unit at Northumbria Healthcare NHS Foundation Trust (NHFT).

5.2.2 Patient Risk Factors

A multidisciplinary team can optimise the following factors in order to reduce the risk of PJI (Johnson et al. 2013).

Diabetes Mellitus

Diabetic patients undergoing hip and knee replacement surgery are at increased risk of developing post-operative wound infection (Mraovic et al.

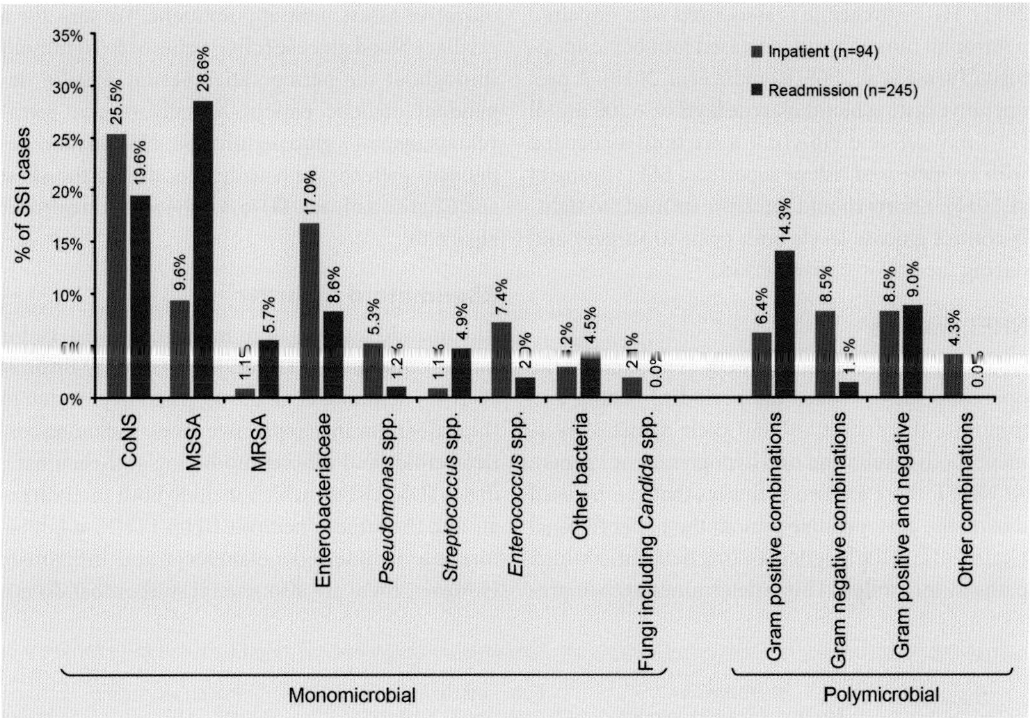

Fig. 5.3 Distribution of micro-organisms reported as causing surgical site infection (*SSI*) in hip and knee prosthesis surgery, by detection method, NHS hospitals, England, 2014/2015. *CoNS* coagulase-negative staphylococci, *MSSA* methicillin-sensitive, *MRSA* methicillin-resistant *S. aureus*. (Reproduced from Public Health England, 2015, Surveillance of Surgical Site Infections in NHS Hospitals in England 2014/2015, with permission from Public Health England)

Tab.5.2 Risk factors for surgical site infection

Patient factors	Operative factors
Systemic:	ASA score >2
Obesity	Long duration
Diabetes	Poor surgical technique
Immunosuppression	Contaminated or dirty wound
Smoking	Lack of systemic antibiotic prophylaxis
Rheumatoid arthritis	Lack of local antibiotics/antiseptic
Psoriasis	Hypothermia
Poor nutritional status	Poor diabetic control
Advanced age	MSSA/MRSA colonization
Local:	
Previous arthroplasty	
Arthroplasty following fracture	
Type of joint	
Perioperative wound complications	

2011). Hyperglycaemia is associated with impaired neutrophil function and increased monocyte apoptosis (Turina et al. 2005; Komura et al. 2010). A preoperative fasting blood glucose level of ≥ 200 mg/dl (11.1 mmol/l) and HbA1c ≥ 8 are both associated with an increased risk of superficial SSI (Hwang et al. 2015). Efforts should therefore be made to tightly control glucose levels both prior to surgery and during the perioperative period.

NHFT Practice

Diabetic patients are listed as early as possible on the operating list to reduce the period of fasting and minimise the period without their diabetes treatment (both insulin and oral hypoglycaemic agents). At NHFT, there are two pathways that can be used during the perioperative period; the patient's usual treatment and the length of fasting determine which pathway they follow. This is determined at their preoperative assessment appointment. We aim for a capillary blood glucose (cBG) value of 6–10 mmol/l throughout the perioperative period. Insulin dependent diabetic patients usually receive intravenous insulin / glucose infusion. Non-insulin dependent patients are usually allocated to the »Fast and Check« pathway. ◘ Fig. 5.4 shows our treatment algorithm.

Rheumatoid Arthritis

Rheumatoid arthritis is an independent risk factor for infection in joint replacement surgery (Bozic et al. 2012; Schrama et al. 2010). This may be due to the use of immunosuppressive agents including corticosteroids and disease-modifying anti-rheumatic drugs (DMARDs), which include both methotrexate and the tumour necrosis factor (TNF)-α inhibitors, e.g. leflunomide, etanercept and infliximab. However, there are also several studies that do not

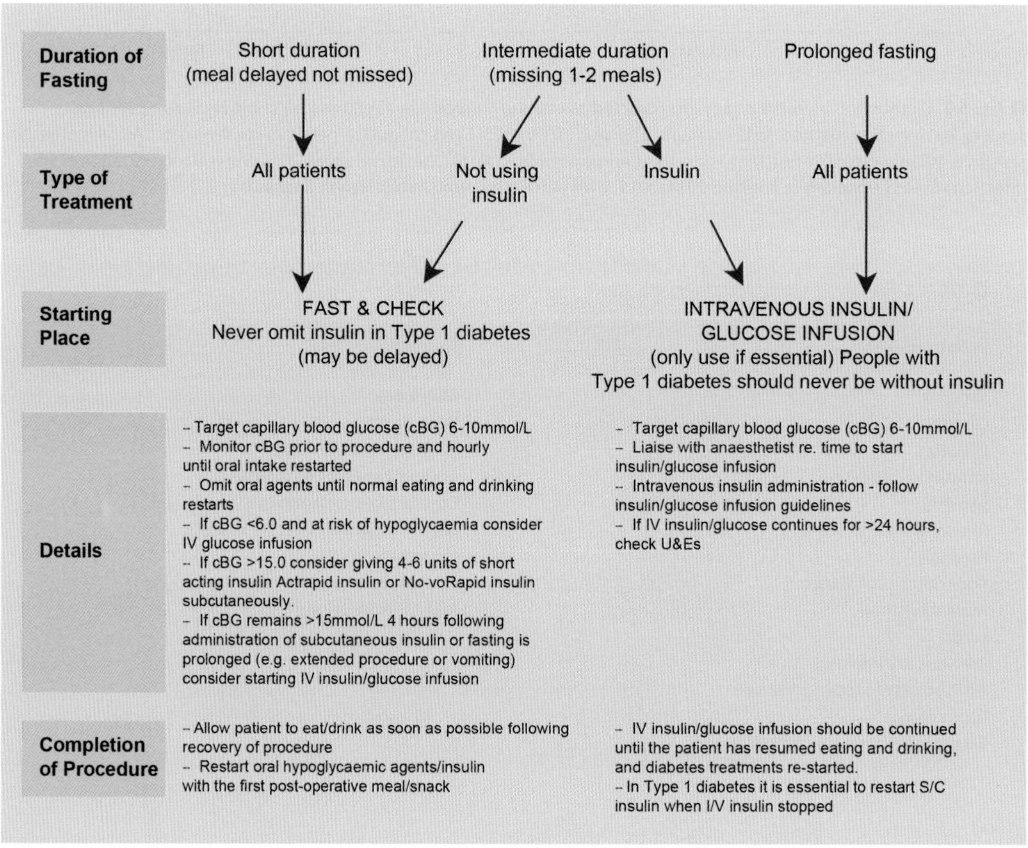

◘ **Fig. 5.4** Perioperative management of diabetic patients in Northumbria Healthcare Foundation Trust (NHFT)

Tab. 5.3 Common TNF-α inhibitors and recommendations when to stop before surgery

Medication	Half-life	Recommendation
Leflunomide	2 weeks	Stop 6 weeks before surgery
Etanercept	4.3 days	Stop 1.5 weeks before surgery
Infliximab	8–10 days	Stop 3 weeks before surgery
Rituximab	21 days	Stop 2 months before surgery

show an increased infection risk with continuing use of DMARDs (Grennan et al. 2001; Dixon et al. 2007; Bibbo et al. 2004). The recent consensus statement recommends that all DMARDs including methotrexate are stopped prior to surgery and recommenced 2 weeks later (Parvizi and Gehrke 2013). The British Society for Rheumatology (BSR) guidelines suggest that methotrexate does not need to be stopped prior to joint replacement and if TNF-α inhibitors are planned to be discontinued preoperatively, the potential benefit of preventing infection post-operatively must be balanced against the risk of developing a perioperative flare of disease. TNF-α inhibitors should be stopped 5–20 days before surgery (3–5 times the drug's half-life) and can be restarted when the wound has healed with no signs of infection (Luqmani et al. 2009; Ding et al. 2010; Tab.5.3).

NHFT Practice

We do not stop methotrexate preoperatively. However, for patients on TNF-α inhibitors, their cases are always discussed with the rheumatology team and in the majority of cases, the TNF-α inhibitor is stopped.

Obesity

There is good evidence demonstrating that obesity (defined as body mass index [BMI] ≥ 30 kg/m^2) is associated with an increased risk of poor wound healing, SSI and PJI (Namba et al. 2005, 2012; Chen et al. 2013; Dowsey and Choong 2009; Malinzak et al. 2009). The reasons for this include increased operative time and complexity of surgery, poorer vascularization of the subcutaneous layer, increased need for blood transfusion and the presence of other comorbidities such as diabetes. These patients are also at increased risk of having their prophylactic dose of antibiotics under-diagnosed and this should be taken into account with the anaesthetist (Freeman et al. 2011).

NHFT Practice

It is important that this group of patients is adequately counselled preoperatively about the risk–benefit of elective joint replacement and told that they are at increased risk of post-operative complications. In super obese patients (BMI ≥ 50 kg/m^2), we would recommend referral for bariatric surgery prior to hip or knee replacement as the SSI rate is 3.5 times lower if they have had bariatric surgery first (Kulkarni et al. 2011).

Malnutrition

Malnutrition is associated with increased risk of adverse events following hip and knee replacement including poor wound healing and persistent wound discharge resulting in increased susceptibility to infection (Lavernia et al. 1999; Nicholson et al. 2012).

NHFT Practice

Any patient suspected of malnutrition would be referred to a local dietician service in primary care for nutritional advice and supplementation with high protein, vitamin and mineral supplements. This would continue during the perioperative period as well. However, we do not routinely measure nutritional parameters such as serum albumin, pre-albumin, transferrin and lymphocyte count.

Smoking

Current smokers undergoing hip and knee placement surgery are more likely to develop SSI and PJI (Singh et al. 2011; Kwiatkowski et al. 1996; Moller et al. 2003). Former smokers are less likely to develop post-operative complications and this is related to longer periods of smoking cessation (Myers et al. 2011; Sorensen 2012).

NHFT Practice

We routinely assess for patients' smoking habits and offer strategies to help them stop. This includes referring them to our trust-based smoking cessation service if necessary. It has been shown that even if this is started 6–8 weeks before joint replacement surgery, it results in fewer wound healing complications and reoperations and a shorter length of stay (Moller et al. 2002).

Screening and Decolonization

Nasal carriers of *Staphylococcus aureus* are harbouring a potential source of bacteria for the development of post-operative SSI (Kalmeijer et al. 2000). There is extensive evidence in the orthopaedic and general surgery literature that screening and decolonization of these nasal carriers of *S. aureus* at pre-assessment reduces the number of associated SSIs (Hacek et al. 2008; Schweizer et al. 2013).

SSIs with methicillin-resistant *S. aureus* (MRSA) cost 1.5 times more to treat compared with sensitive organisms (Parvizi et al. 2010). Since April 2009, a national MRSA screening programme for all planned NHS surgeries in the United Kingdom has been implemented with a positive result leading to decolonization treatment (Department of Health 2008).

NHFT Practice

In addition to routine MRSA screening, we also screen for methicillin-sensitive *S. aureus* (MSSA). It has been found that 20% of patients are nasal carriers of MSSA and decolonization of positive carriers is associated with a nearly 60% reduction of hospital-acquired *S. aureus* infections from 7.7% to 3.4% when compared with placebo (Bode et al. 2010). As a result, hospitals in the United Kingdom are now introducing similar screening and decolonising programmes for MSSA. ◘ Fig. 5.5 shows our screening protocol and treatment algorithm.

Preoperative Anaemia

A prospective cohort study of 225 patients undergoing THR showed that preoperative anaemia was associated with increased post-operative infection and that this effect is attributed to an increase in blood transfusion requirements post-operatively (Myers et al. 2004). The risk of infection increases with more units of allogeneic blood transfused (Steinitz et al. 2001). Post-operative transfusion requirements are reduced by correcting preoperative anaemia.

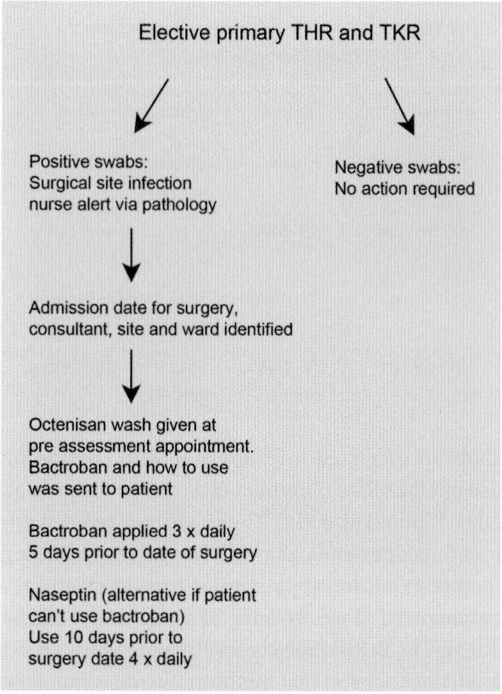

◘ **Fig. 5.5** Screening for methicillin-sensitive *Staphylococcus aureus* (MSSA) and methicillin-resistant *Staphylococcus aureus* (MRSA) at Northumbria Healthcare Foundation Trust (NHFT). *THR* total hip replacement, *TKR* total knee replacement

NHFT Practice

All patients undergoing elective THR and TKR surgery are screened for anaemia with preoperative measurements of serum haemoglobin, iron and ferritin levels. Correction of preoperative anaemia usually consists of oral administration of iron for 1 month if their ferritin levels are within normal limits. Intravenous iron therapy should be considered in patients with impaired renal function. Haemoglobin levels are checked again 28 days after treatment. Patients with significant iron deficiency anaemia with low ferritin levels are referred back to their General Practitioner for further investigations and their surgery is postponed.◘ Fig. 5.6 shows our treatment algorithm.

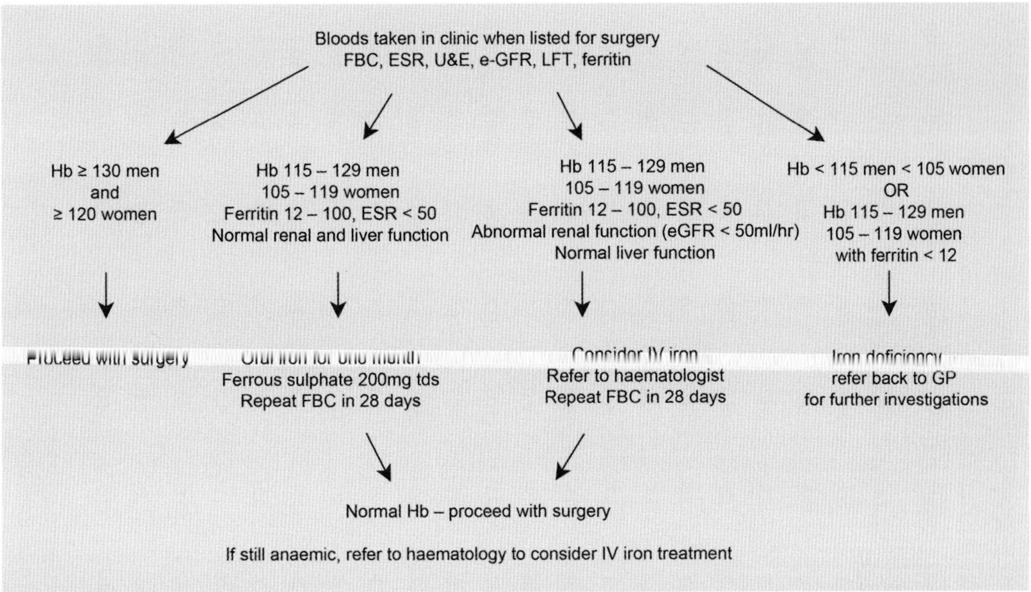

Fig. 5.6 Preoperative anaemia treatment algorithm at Northumbria Healthcare Foundation Trust (NHFT). *FBC* full blood count, *ESR* erythrocyte sedimentation rate, *U&E* urea and electrolytes, *GFR* glomerular filtration rate, *LFT* liver function tests, *Hb* haemoglobin (values in mg/dl)

5.2.3 Perioperative Surgical Risk Factors

Patient Preparation Prior to Theatre

Factors taken into consideration include the timing of the patient's admission, washing with soap on the morning of surgery to reduce skin organisms and hair removal.

NHFT Practice

Patients are now admitted on the day of surgery to reduce the risk of colonization with hospital-acquired resistant organisms on their skin. Whilst waiting on the ward, they are pre-warmed with a HotDog® warming blanket (Augustine Temperature Management) to avoid hypothermia intraoperatively and whilst in the recovery suite. This strategy has been shown to reduce the risk of infection in general surgery by 65% in a randomized controlled trial (Melling et al. 2001). If hair removal is required, it is done in the theatre with an electric clipper to prevent skin abrasions, which could increase the bacterial cell count.

Antibiotic Prophylaxis

The use of parenteral prophylactic antibiotics is now common practice in all surgical subspecialties and has been identified as the most important factor in reducing the risk of PJI following THR and TKR surgery (Classen et al. 1992; Prokuski et al. 2011; Hanssen et al. 1994). A meta-analysis of seven studies demonstrated that using prophylactic antibiotics reduced the relative risk of a post-operative wound infection by 81% and the absolute risk by 8% (AlBuhairan et al. 2008).

The antibiotic chosen for prophylaxis should cover the common organisms known to cause PJI, take into account local patterns of antibiotic resistance and be cost effective.

A cross-sectional study performed in England analysed 189,858 elective primary THR and TKR and 1,116 SSIs from the Public Health England SSI database to examine the spectrum of organisms responsible for SSI (Hickson et al. 2015). In all, 73.8% of these SSIs had monomicrobial aetiology and the remaining 26.2% were polymicrobial. The data on causative organisms are shown in Tab. 5.4. Of these cases, 57%were attributed to *Staphylococcus*

Tab. 5.4 Micro-organisms reported as causing surgical site infection (SSI) following hip or knee prosthesis surgery, April 2010 to March 2013 (reproduced from Hickson et al. 2015, with permission from the author)

		London		Midland and East of England		North of England		South of England		England (total)	
No.	%	*n*	%	*n*	%	*n*	%	*n*	%	*n*	%
All SSI isolates	MSSA	25	20.2	88	27.2	87	26.9	91	29.2	291	26.9
	MRSA	3	2.4	24	7.4	8	2.5	10	3.2	45	4.2
	CoNS	39	31.5	73	22.5	85	26.3	79	25.3	276	25.5
	Enterobacteria	20	16.1	52	16.0	58	18.0	39	12.5	169	15.6
	Other bacteria[a]	10	8.1	35	10.8	26	8.0	40	12.8	111	10.2
	Enterococcus	11	8.9	20	6.2	31	9.6	17	5.4	79	7.3
	Streptococcus	5	4.0	24	7.4	17	5.3	21	6.7	67	6.2
	Pseudomonas	11	8.9	6	1.9	11	3.4	14	4.5	42	3.9
	Fungi	0	0.0	2	0.6	0	0.0	1	0.3	3	0.3
	Total	124	100	324	100	323	100	312	100	1083	100
Deep or organ space SSI isolates	CoNS[a]	23	31.5	51	24.6	71	30.5	64	27.2	209	27.9
	MSSA	18	24.7	50	24.2	62	26.6	54	23.0	184	24.6
	MRSA	1	1.4	13	6.3	3	1.3	8	3.4	25	3.3
	Enterobacteria	12	16.4	34	16.4	40	17.2	35	14.9	121	16.2
	Other bacteria[b]	5	6.8	20	9.7	19	8.2	32	13.6	76	10.2
	Enterococcus	5	6.8	18	8.7	18	7.7	13	5.5	54	7.2
	Streptococcus	3	4.1	18	8.7	12	5.2	19	8.1	52	7.0
	Pseudomonas	6	8.2	2	1.0	8	3.4	9	3.8	25	3.3
	Fungi	0	0.0	1	0.5	0	0.0	1	0.4	2	0.3
	Total	73	100	207	100	233	100	235	100	748	100

[a] The majority of this group comprised diphtheroids/Corynebacterium spp. (40%) followed by unidentified organisms (31%)
[b] The majority of this group comprised diphtheroids/Corynebacterium spp. (42%) followed by unidentified organisms (28%)
MSSA methicillin-sensitive *S. aureus*, *MRSA* methicillin-resistant *S. aureus*, *CoNS* coagulase-negative staphylococci

species and the seven commonest organisms accounted for 89% of cases. There is some statistically significant variation of some organisms between regions, with London having a higher burden of *Pseudomonas* and the Midlands and East of England having a higher burden of MRSA. However, no reason could be identified for this variation.

The same study surveyed 145 hospitals in England about their antibiotic prophylaxis regimens for THR and TKR and showed a wide variation in practice across the country with regards to routine prophylaxis, penicillin allergy prophylaxis and high-risk MRSA prophylaxis (◘ Fig. 5.7, ◘ Fig. 5.8, ◘ Fig. 5.9).

Such a wide variation exists because there is not enough evidence to suggest that one class of antibiotic is superior to another, and within the cephalosporin class, there is no difference between the generations. It would not be feasible to conduct randomized controlled trial as PJI is a rare event; power calculations have worked out that in order to demonstrate a reduction in infection from 2% to 1% at 90% power, 3,000 patients need to be recruited into each group (Periti et al. 1998).

The recent international consensus statement recommends the use of a first- or second-generation cephalosporin as the first-line choice for antibiotic prophylaxis in THR and TKR, which is now common practice in North America but certainly not the case in England (Parvizi and Gehrke 2013).

With regards to timing of intravenous prophylactic antibiotic administration, the National Institute of Health and Care Excellence (NICE) recommends a single dose on induction of anaesthesia with a repeat dose if the operation lasts longer than the antibiotic's half-life or if there is significant blood loss (National Institute for Health and Clinical Excellence 2008). The American Academy of Orthopaedic Surgeons (AAOS) recommendation is for antibiotics to be administered 1 h before skin incision and not to continue for longer than 24 h (American Academy of Orthopaedic Surgeons 2004). Continuing antibiotics for 3 days instead of 24 h post-operatively does not lead to reduced rates of PJI (Mauerhan et al. 1994).

NHFT Practice

Our unit's guidelines for antibiotic prophylaxis in THR and TKR surgery have been developed in con-

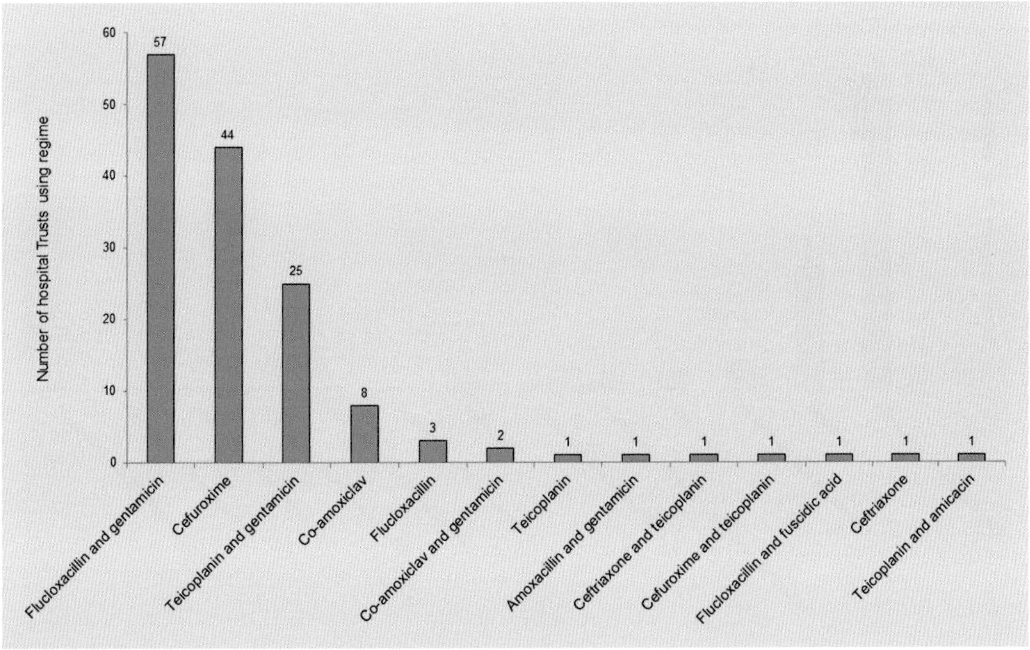

◘ **Fig. 5.7** Graph showing the routine prophylactic antibiotic regimens for patients undergoing hip and knee replacement (reproduced from Hickson et al. 2015, with permission from the author)

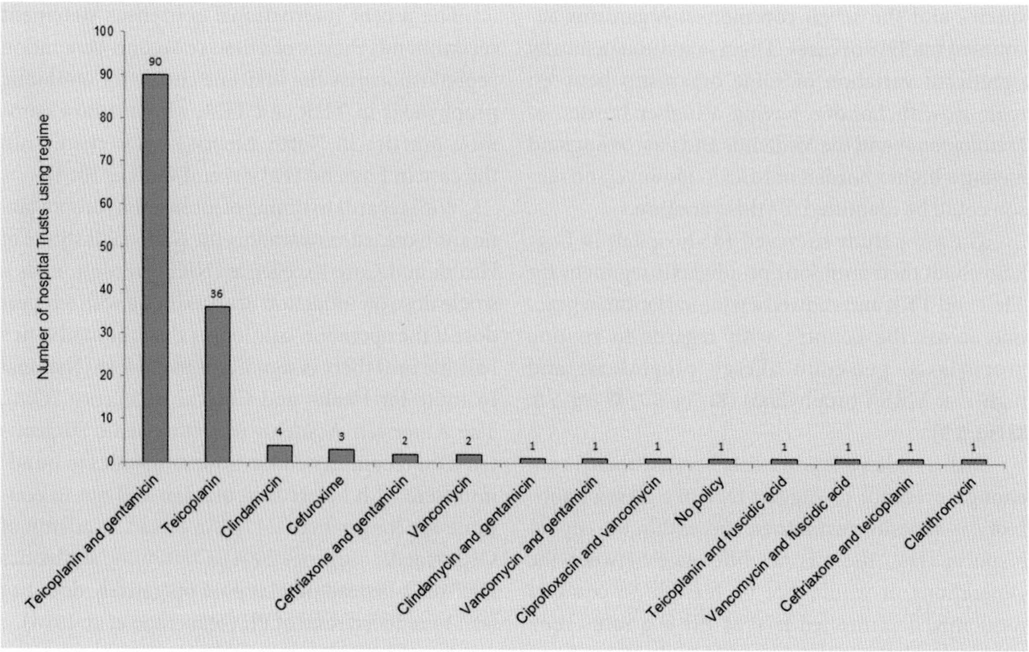

Fig. 5.8 Graph showing prophylactic antibiotic regimens in patients with penicillin allergy (reproduced from Hickson et al. 2015, with permission from the author)

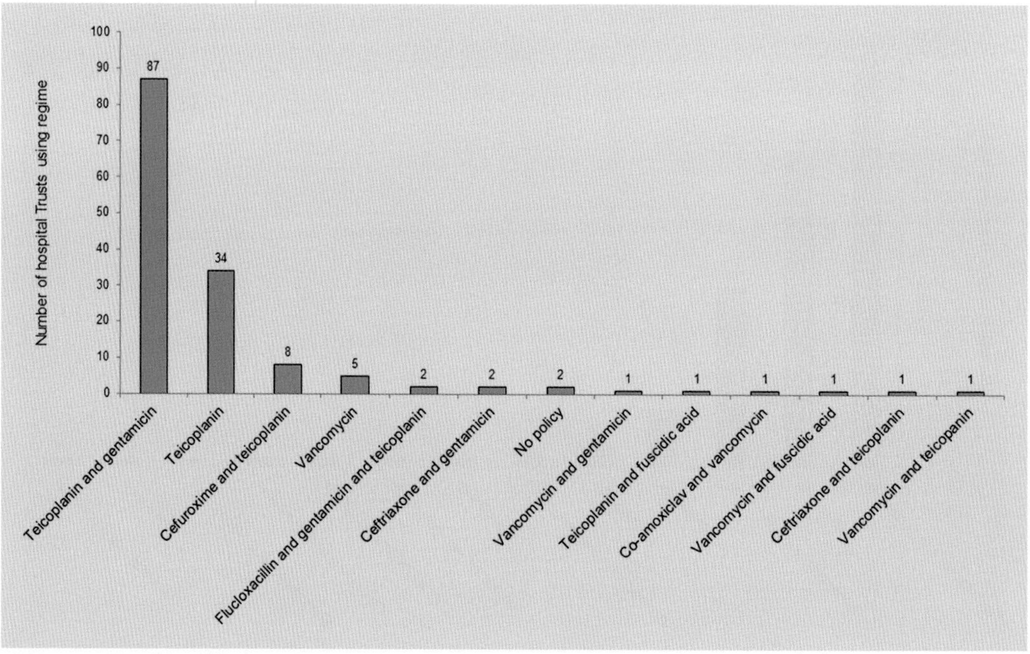

Fig. 5.9 Graph showing prophylactic antibiotic regimens for patients at high risk of MRSA colonization (reproduced from Hickson et al. 2015, with permission from the author)

junction with our medical microbiology colleagues and are summarized in ◘ Tab. 5.5. Routine primary THR/TKR and aseptic revision cases, receive a single dose of intravenous teicoplanin (400 mg) and gentamicin (3 mg/kg). Patients with chronic kidney disease receive aztreonam (1 g) instead of gentamicin. The antibiotics are administered following administration of the spinal anaesthetic and before inflation of the tourniquet in TKR cases. They are not continued in the post-operative period.

Our rationale for choosing this combination is that both teicoplanin and gentamicin are highly active against MRSA and it is a good combination in patients with penicillin allergy. Teicoplanin also has high activity against MSSA, whilst gentamicin is active against Enterobacteriacae and Pseudomonas. However, there is the risk of developing acute kidney injury (AKI) with this combination of antibiotics. We do not use cephalosporins as they are ineffective against MRSA, Enterobacteriacae and Pseudomonas and may not be effective against coagulase-negative Staphylococci (Hickson et al. 2015). Cephalosporins are also associated with the development of *Clostridium difficile* infection (CDI), but this is seen mainly in elderly inpatients and trauma patients rather than elective THR and TKR cases (Jenkins et al. 2010; Al-Obaydi et al. 2010).

All infected revision cases are discussed with the medical microbiology team to develop a customized antibiotic plan for each individual patient. The choice of antibiotic used depends on whether the infective organism is known and if a single or multiple organisms cause the infection.

Antibiotic-Loaded Bone Cement

The use of antibiotic loaded bone cement (ALBC) is common practice throughout Europe for both primary and revision hip and knee replacement surgery. Owing to its heat stability, aminoglycoside antibiotics, e.g. gentamicin, are added to the cement to provide local prophylaxis.

Deep infection rates are reduced with the use of ALBC, although superficial wound infection rates were not significantly reduced in a meta-analysis of over 6,000 joint replacements (Wang et al. 2013). The Norwegian Arthroplasty Registry has shown that patients who receive both systemic and local (in bone cement) antibiotics have the lowest

◘ **Tab. 5.5** Summary of prophylactic antibiotic regimens in patients undergoing total hip and knee replacement at Northumbria Healthcare Foundation Trust

Surgical procedure	Systemic antibiotic prophylaxis regimen	Local bone cement regimen
Primary THR or TKR	Gentamicin 3 mg/kg + teicoplanin 400 mg	Palacos® R+G
Revision THR or TKR (non-infected)	Gentamicin 3 mg/kg + teicoplanin 400 mg (unless alternative regimen recommended by microbiology team) Continue teicoplanin only post-operatively until culture results known; treatment then stopped or rationalized	Copal® G+C
First-stage revision of infected THR or TKR	Gentamicin 3 mg/kg + teicoplanin 400 mg (unless alternative regimen recommended by microbiology team) Continue teicoplanin only post-operatively until culture results known; treatment then stopped or rationalized	Copal® G+C Discuss with microbiology team about adding further antibiotics to the cement
Second-stage revision of infected THR or TKR	Gentamicin 3 mg/kg + teicoplanin 400 mg (unless alternative regimen recommended by microbiology team) Continue teicoplanin only post-operatively until culture results known; treatment then stopped or rationalized	Copal® G+C Discuss with microbiology team about adding further antibiotics to the cement

rate of revision due to infection (Engesaeter et al. 2003).

NHFT Practice

In primary hip and knee replacement, we routinely use Palacos® R+G (Heraeus), which contains gentamicin for local prophylaxis. In cases of aseptic revision, we use Copal® G+C (Heraeus), which contains both gentamicin and clindamycin. Infected revision cases are discussed on an individual basis with the medical microbiology team with regards to the addition of extra antibiotics, e.g. vancomycin, to the standard Copal® G+C.

5

5.2.4 Theatre Etiquette

At the first International Consensus Meeting on Periprosthetic Joint Infection in 2013, the only question which received unanimous 100% agreement was: »Should operating room traffic be kept to a minimum?« (Parvizi and Gehrke 2013). It is well known that frequently opening theatre doors leads to increased bacterial counts in the airborne environment (Scaltriti et al. 2007). As a result, all necessary equipment including instruments and implants should be kept in the theatre to minimize theatre traffic.

Surgical Site Preparation

The aim of preoperative skin antisepsis preparation is to decontaminate and reduce the number of organisms. The commonest skin preparations are based on either iodine or chlorhexidine.

Iodine preparations work by penetrating the bacterial cell wall to oxidise and substitute microbial contents with free iodine. This disrupts nucleic acid and protein synthesis. Povidone iodine (PI) is an example of an iodophor where iodine molecules are bound to a polymer (povidone).

Chlorhexidine gluconate (CHG) is a positively charged molecule that binds to negatively charged phospholipids in the bacterial cell wall causing it to rupture resulting in lysis.

Both PI and CHG come in either aqueous or alcoholic preparations. Alcohol-based preparations work by denaturing cell wall proteins and rely on evaporation to work properly.

A randomized trial of 849 patients undergoing general surgery procedures where skin preparation was performed with either alcoholic chlorhexidine or aqueous povidone-iodine showed a lower rate of infection in the alcoholic chlorhexidine group (Darouiche et al. 2010).

There is currently no evidence to suggest which is the best skin preparation agent for THR and TKR, although this is being addressed in a number of trials (Peel et al. 2014). However, there is an argument for using alcohol-based preparations.

NHFT Practice

We perform a »prewash« in the anaesthetic room using Hibiscrub followed by 2% chlorhexidine in alcohol. This is followed by a second skin preparation in the theatre itself using 2% chlorhexidine in alcohol. However, there is no evidence in the literature for this »double prep« technique.

5.2.5 Theatre Design (Laminar Flow) and Its Effect on Body Temperature

The biggest contributor to infection following THR and TKR surgery is airborne contaminants from human skin. One billion skin squames (cells) are shed daily and 10% of these carry bacteria (Lidwell 1988; Whyte 1988; Noble 1975).

Laminar flow ventilation systems are now used as standard practice in orthopaedic ultra clean air theatres performing THR and TKR in the United Kingdom. These use high-efficiency particulate air filters that remove particles larger than 0.3 µm whereas conventional (plenum) theatres only remove particles larger than 5 µm. Laminar flow systems allow up to 300 air exchanges an hour resulting in less than 10 colony-forming units (CFU) per square metre. Plenum theatres only have 20 air exchanges an hour and have up to 50 CFUs per square metre.

The use of laminar air flow and prophylactic antibiotics have both independent and additive effects in reducing SSI after THR and TKR surgery (Lidwell et al. 1982, 1987). However, there have been studies showing an increase in SSI using laminar air flow even after adjusting for other variables (Brandt et al. 2008; Hooper et al. 2011). As a result, these

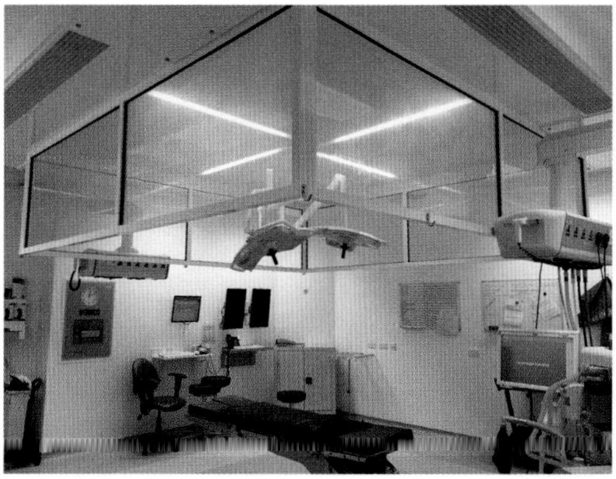

■ **Fig. 5.10** Laminar airflow theatre at Northumbria Healthcare Foundation Trust (NHFT)

authors have questioned whether the extra costs of using laminar flow can be justified.

Laminar air flow increases heat loss in patients resulting in perioperative hypothermia. This results in peripheral vasoconstriction, decreased tissue perfusion and an increased risk of infection. It is also associated with increased blood loss, cardiac events, transfusion requirements and length of stay (Sessler 2001; Sessler and Akca 2002).

NHFT Practice

All of our primary and revision THR and TKR are performed in laminar air flow theatres (■ Fig. 5.10). NICE guidelines in England emphasise the importance of maintaining normothermia during surgery (National Institute of Health and Clinical Excellence 2016). However, instead of forced air warming (FAW) devices, we use conductive warming devices, e.g. HotDog® warming blankets (Augustine Temperature Management) to avoid hypothermia intraoperatively. It has been shown that if FAW devices are used, air from outside the laminar flow canopy can be drawn into the operative area leading to higher infection rates than if conductive devices are used (McGovern et al. 2011).

5.2.6 Conclusion

Infection following THR and TKR surgery has disastrous consequences for both the patients who experience severe morbidity and the healthcare professionals for whom there is a major burden on resources. Adopting a multidisciplinary team approach can reduce the risk of infection (■ Tab. 5.6). Medical comorbidities can be optimized and measures taken to reduce skin contamination and colonization with pathogens before surgery. During the perioperative period, theatre design and etiquette and the use of prophylactic antibiotics are of paramount importance. Both patients and all health-care staff must be educated in raising awareness about PJI and actively participate in its prevention.

■ **Tab. 5.6** Methods for reducing surgical site infection in joint replacement (reproduced from Johnson et al. 2013, with permission from the author)

Risk factor	Summary
Patient factors	
Diabetes mellitus	Aggressive glucose control
Rheumatoid arthritis	DMARDs and methotrexate should not be stopped Perioperative steroids are generally not required Balance the risks and benefits of stopping anti-TNF – stop at 3–5 half-lives preoperative, restart after wound healing and no evidence of infection Nitrous oxide should be avoided in patients on methotrexate
Obesity	Dietician input to encourage weight loss Adjust perioperative antibiotic doses appropriately In super-obese consider bariatric surgery prior to surgery
Smoking	Consider a smoking cessation programme
Carrier screening	MRSA and MSSA screening based on local guidelines, and decolonise prior to admission

Tab. 5.6 (Continued)

Risk factor	Summary
Preoperative factors	
Patient preparation	Shower on day of surgery If shaving required, use electric clippers on day of surgery Avoid oil-based skin moisturisers
Antibiotics	Prophylactic antibiotics should be given as early as possible in the anaesthetic room (antibiotic type dependent on local guidelines) Administer antibiotics at least 5 min prior to tourniquet inflation If cementation is required, antibiotic-impregnated type should be used
Perioperative factors	
Theatre	Use laminar flow where possible Keep theatre door opening to a minimum
Personnel	Hand wash with antiseptic surgical solution, using a single-use brush or pick for the nails Before subsequent operations, hands should be washed with either an alcoholic hand rub or an antiseptic surgical solution Double glove and change gloves regularly Polypropylene non-woven gowns with adequate mask and hat coverage
Skin preparation	Use an alcohol pre-wash followed by a 2% chlorhexidine–alcohol scrub solution
Anaesthetic	Maintain normothermia Maintain normovolaemia A higher inspired oxygen concentration perioperatively and for 6 h post-operative may be of benefit
Drapes	Use of iodine-impregnated incise drapes may be of benefit (in patients without allergy)
Blood transfusion	Optimise preoperative haemoglobin If possible, transfusion should be avoided intraoperatively and if anticipated should be given more than 48 h prior to surgery Anti-fibrinolytics may indirectly reduce SSI by reducing the need for transfusion
Post-operative factors	
Dental procedures	Insufficient evidence to recommend the use of prophylactic antibiotics for patients undergoing routine dental procedures following joint replacement

DMARDs disease-modifying anti-rheumatic drugs, *TNF* tumour necrosis factor, *MRSA* methicillin-resistant *Staphylococcus aureus*, *MSSA* methicillin-sensitive *Staphylococcus aureus*, *SSI* surgical site infection

Take Home Message

To prevent PJI, the Northumbria Healthcare (Hospital) screens and deals with two types of risk factors:

1. Patient risk factors
   - Diabetes
   - Obesity
   - Smoking
   - Preoperative anaemia
   - Rheumatoid arthritis
   - Malnutrition
   - Nasal carriers of *Staphylococcus aureus* (MRSA)
2. Preoperative surgical risk factors:
   - Patient preparation
   - Antibiotic-loaded bone cement
   - Surgical site preparation
   - Theatre design
   - Antibiotic prophylaxis

References

AlBuhairan B, Hind D, Hutchinson A (2008) Antibiotic prophylaxis for wound infections in total joint arthroplasty: a systematic review. J Bone Joint Surg (Br) 90B:915-919

Al-Obaydi W, Smith CD, Foguet P (2010) Changing prophylactic antibiotic protocol for reducing Clostridium difficile-associated diarrhoeal infections. J Orthop Surg (Hong Kong) 18:320-323

American Academy of Orthopaedic Surgeons (2004) Recommendations for the use of intravenous antibiotic prophylaxis in primary total joint arthroplasty, 2004. Retrieved from http:// www.aaos.org/about/papers/advistmt/1027.asp. (date last accessed 17 January 2016)

Bibbo C, Goldberg JW (2004) Infectious and healing complications after elective orthopaedic foot and ankle surgery during tumor necrosis factor-alpha inhibition therapy. Foot Ankle Int 25(5):331-335

Bode LG, Kluytmans JA, Wertheim HF, et al (2010) Preventing surgical-site infections in nasal carriers of Staphylococcus aureus. N Engl J Med 362:9-17

Bozic KJ, Lau E, Kurtz S, et al (2012) Patient-related risk factors for periprosthetic joint infection and postoperative mortality following total hip arthroplasty in Medicare patients. J Bone Joint Surg Am 94(9):794-800

Brandt C, Hott U, Sohr D, Daschner F, Gastmeier P, Ruden H (2008) Operating room ventilation with laminar airflow shows no protective effect on the surgical site infection rate in orthopedic and abdominal surgery. Ann Surg 248:695–700

Chen J, Cui Y, Li X, et al (2013) Risk factors for deep infection after total knee arthroplasty: a meta-analysis. Arch Orthop Trauma Surg 133(5):675-687

Classen DC, Evans RS, Pestotnik SL, Horn SD, Menlove RL, Burke JP (1992) The timing of prophylactic administration of antibiotics and the risk of surgical-wound infection. N Engl J Med 326(5):281-286

Darouiche RO, Wall MJ, Itani KM, et al (2010) Chlorhexidine-alcohol versus povidone- iodine for surgical-site antisepsis. N Engl J Med 362:18–26

Department of Health (2008) MRSA Screening: Operational Guidance 2008. Retrieved from http:// www.dh.gov.uk/prod_consum_dh/groups/dh_digitalassets/documents/digitalas- set/dh_092845.pdf (date last accessed 17 January 2016)

Ding T, Ledingham J, Luqmani R, Westlake S, Hyrich K, Lunt M, et al (2010) BSR and BHPR rheumatoid arthritis guidelines on safety of anti-TNF therapies. Rheumatology (Oxford) 49(11):2217-2219

Dixon WG LM, Watson KD, Hyrich KL, Symmons DP (2007) Anti-TNF therapy and the risk of serious post-operative infection: results from the BSR Biologics register (BSRBR). Ann Rheum Dis 66[Suppl II]:118

Dowsey MM, Choong PF (2009) Obese diabetic patients are at substantial risk for deep infection after primary TKA. Clin Orthop Relat Res 467(6):1577-1581

Engesaeter LB, Lie SA, Espehaug B, et al (2003) Antibiotic prophylaxis in total hip arthroplasty: effects of antibiotic prophylaxis systemically and in bone cement on the revision rate of 22,170 primary hip replacements followed 0-14 years in the Norwegian Arthroplasty Register. Acta Orthop Scand 74:644–651

Freeman JT, Anderson DJ, Hartwig MG, Sexton DJ (2011) Surgical site infections following bariatric surgery in community hospitals: a weighty concern? Obes Surg 21(7):836-840

Grennan DM, Gray J, Loudon J, Fear S (2001) Methotrexate and early postoperative complications in patients with rheumatoid arthritis undergoing elective orthopaedic surgery. Ann Rheum Dis 60(3):214-217

Hacek DM, Robb WJ, Paule SM, Kudrna JC, Stamos VP, Peterson LR (2008) Staphylococcus aureus nasal decolonization in joint replacement surgery reduces infection. Clin Orthop Relat Res 466(6):1349-1355.

Hanssen AD, Osmon DR (1994) Prevention of deep wound infection after total hip arthroplasty: the role of prophylactic antibiotics and clean air technology. Semin Arthroplasty 5(3):114-121

Hickson CJ, Metcalf D, Elgohari S, Oswald T, Masters JP et al (2015) Prophylactic antibiotics in elective hip and knee arthroplasty. An analysis of organisms reported to cause infections and national survey of clinical practice. Bone Joint Res 4:181-189

Hooper GJ, Rothwell AG, Frampton C, Wyatt MC (2011) Does the use of laminar flow and space suits reduce early deep infection after total hip and knee replacement?: the ten-year results of the New Zealand Joint Registry. J Bone Joint Surg (Br) 93B:85–90

Hwang JS, Kim SJ, Bamne AB, Na YG, Kim TK (2015) Do glycemic markers predict occurrence of complications after total knee arthroplasty in patients with diabetes? Clin Orthop Rel Res 473(5):1726-1731

Jenkins PJ, Teoh K, Simpson PM, et al (2010) Clostridium difficile in patients undergoing primary hip and knee replacement. J Bone Joint Surg (Br) 92B:994-998

Johnson R, Jameson SS, Sanders RD, et al (2013) Reducing surgical site infection in arthroplasty of the lower limb: A multi-disciplinary approach. Bone Joint Res 2:58-65

Kalmeijer MD, van Nieuwland-Bollen E, Bogaers-Hofman D, de Baere GA (2000) Nasal carriage of Staphylococcus aureus is a major risk factor for surgical-site infections in orthopedic surgery. Infect Control Hosp Epidemiol 21(5):319-323

Komura T, Sakai Y, Honda M, Takamura T, Matsushima K, Kaneko S (2010) CD14+ monocytes are vulnerable and functionally impaired under endoplasmic reticulum stress in patients with type 2 diabetes. Diabetes 59(3): 634-643

Kulkarni A, Jameson SS, James P, Woodcock S, Muller S, Reed MR (2011) Does bariatric surgery prior to lower limb joint replacement reduce complications? Surgeon 9(1):18-21

Kwiatkowski TC, Hanley EN, Jr., Ramp WK (1996) Cigarette smoking and its orthopedic consequences. Am J Orthop (Belle Mead NJ) 25(9):590-597

Lavernia CJ, Sierra RJ, Baerga L (1999) Nutritional parameters and short term outcome in arthroplasty. J Am Coll Nutr 18(3):274-278
Lidwell OM, Lowbury EJ, Whyte W et al (1982) Effect of ultraclean air in operating rooms on deep sepsis in the joint after total hip or knee replacement: a randomised study. Br Med J (Clin Res Ed) 285(6344):10-14
Lidwell OM, Elson RA, Lowbury EJ, et al (1987) Ultraclean air and antibiotics for prevention of postoperative infection: a multicenter study of 8,052 joint replacement operations. Acta Orthop Scand 58:4-13
Lidwell OM (1988) Air, antibiotics and sepsis in replacement joints. J Hosp Infect 11[Suppl C]:18-40
Luqmani R, Hennell S, Estrach C, Basher D, Birrell F, Bosworth A, et al (2009) British Society for Rheumatology and British Health Professionals in Rheumatology guideline for the management of rheumatoid arthritis (after the first 2 years). Rheumatology (Oxford) 48(4):436-439
Malinzak RA, Ritter MA, Berend ME, Meding JB, Olberding EM, Davis KE (2009) Morbidly obese, diabetic, younger, and unilateral joint arthroplasty patients have elevated total joint arthroplasty infection rates. J Arthroplasty 24 [6 Suppl]:84-88
Mauerhan DR, Nelson CL, Smith DL, et al (1994) Prophylaxis against infection in total joint arthroplasty: one day of cefuroxime compared with three days of cefazolin. J Bone Joint Surg (Am) 76A:39-45
McGovern PD, Albrecht M, Belani KG, et al (2011) Forced-air warming and ultra-clean ventilation do not mix: an investigation of theatre ventilation, patient warming and joint replacement infection in orthopaedics. J Bone Joint Surg (Br) 93B:1537-1544
Melling AC, Ali B, Scott EM, Leaper DJ (2001) Effects of preoperative warming on the incidence of wound infection after clean surgery: a randomised controlled trial. Lancet 358(9285):876-880
Moller AM, Villebro N, Pedersen T, Tonnesen H (2002) Effect of preoperative smoking intervention on postoperative complications: a randomised clinical trial. Lancet 359(9301):114-117
Moller AM, Pedersen T, Villebro N, Munksgaard A (2003) Effect of smoking on early complications after elective orthopaedic surgery. J Bone Joint Surg Br 85(2):178-181
Mraovic B, Donghun S, Jacovides C, Parvizi J (2011) Perioperative hyperglycemia and postoperative infection after lower limb arthroplasty. J Diabetes Sci Technol 5(2): 413-418
Myers E, O'Grady P, Dolan AM (2004) The influence of preclinical anaemia on outcome following total hip replacement. Arch Orthop Trauma Surg 124(10):699-701
Myers K, Hajek P, Hinds C, McRobbie H (2011) Stopping smoking shortly before surgery and postoperative complications: a systematic review and meta-analysis. Arch Intern Med 171(11):983-989
Namba RS, Paxton L, Fithian DC, Stone ML (2005) Obesity and perioperative morbidity in total hip and total knee arthroplasty patients. J Arthroplasty 20[7 Suppl 3]:46-50
Namba RS, Inacio MC, Paxton EW (2012) Risk factors associated with surgical site infection in 30,491 primary total hip replacements. J Bone Joint Surg Br 94(10):1330-1338
National Institute for Health and Clinical Excellence (2008) Surgical site infection: prevention and treatment of surgical site infection, 2008. Retrieved from http://www.nice.org.uk/ nicemedia/pdf/CG74NICEGuideline.pdf. (date last accessed 17 January 2016)
National Institute of Health and Clinical Excellence (2016) NICE Clinical Guidelines. Perioperative hypothermia: Management of inadvertent perioperative hypothermia in adults. Retrieved from http://www.nice.org.uk/guidance/index.jsp?action=byID&o=11639 (date last accessed 24 January 2016)
Nicholson JA, Dowrick AS, Liew SM (2012) Nutritional status and short-term outcome of hip arthroplasty. J Orthop Surg (Hong Kong) 20(3):331-335
Noble WC (1975) Dispersal of skin microorganisms. Br J Dermatol 93:477–485
Parvizi J, Pawasarat IM, Azzam KA, Joshi A, Hansen EN, Bozic KJ (2010) Periprosthetic joint infection: the economic impact of methicillin-resistant infections. J Arthroplasty 25[6 Suppl]:103-107
Parvizi J, Gehrke T (2013) Proceedings of the International Consensus Meeting on Periprosthetic Joint Infection. Retrieved from http://www.bjj.boneandjoint.org.uk/content/jbjsbr/suppl/2013/11/12/95-B.11.1450.DC1/Proceedings_of_the_International_Consensus_Meeting_on_Periprosthetic_Joint_Infection.pdf (date last accessed 17 January 2016)
Peel TN, Cheng AC, Buising KL, Dowsey MM, Choong PF (2014) Alcoholic Chlorhexidine or Alcoholic Iodine Skin Antisepsis (ACAISA): protocol for cluster randomised controlled trial of surgical skin preparation for the prevention of superficial wound complications in prosthetic hip and knee replacement surgery. BMJ Open 4:e005424
Periti P, Mini E, Mosconi G (1998) Antimicrobial prophylaxis in orthopaedic surgery: the role of teicoplanin. J Antimicrob Chemother 41:329-340
Prokuski L, Clyburn TA, Evans RP, Moucha CS (2011) Prophylactic antibiotics in orthopaedic surgery. Instructional Course Lectures 60:545-555
Public Health England. Surveillance of Surgical Site Infections in NHS Hospitals in England 2014/15 (2015) Retrieved from https://www.gov.uk/government/uploads/system/uploads/attachment_data/file/484874/Surveillance_of_Surgical_Site_Infections_in_NHS_Hospitals_in_England_report_2014-15.pdf (date last accessed 17 January 2016)
Scaltriti S, Cencetti S, Rovesti S, Marchesi I, Bargellini A, Borella P (2007) Risk factors for particulate and microbial contamination of air in operating theatres. J Hosp Infect 66:320-326
Schrama JC, Espehaug B, Hallan G, et al (2010) Risk of revision for infection in primary total hip and knee arthroplasty in patients with rheumatoid arthritis compared with osteoarthritis: a prospective, population-based study on 108,786 hip and knee joint arthroplasties from the

5

Norwegian Arthroplasty Register. Arthritis Care Res (Hoboken) 62(4):473-479
Schweizer M, Perencevich E, McDanel J, et al (2013) Effectiveness of a bundled intervention of decolonization and prophylaxis to decrease Gram positive surgical site infections after cardiac or orthopedic surgery: systematic review and meta-analysis. BMJ 346:f2743
Sessler DI (2001) Complications and treatment of mild hypothermia. Anesthesiology 95:531-543
Sessler DI, Akca O (2002) Nonpharmacological prevention of surgical wound infections. Clin Infect Dis 35:1397-1404
Singh JA, Houston TK, Ponce BA, et al (2011) Smoking as a risk factor for short-term outcomes following primary total hip and total knee replacement in veterans. Arthritis Care Res (Hoboken) 63(10):1365-1374
Sorensen LT (2012) Wound healing and infection in surgery. The clinical impact of smoking and smoking cessation: a systematic review and meta-analysis. Arch Surg 147(4): 373-383
Steinitz D, Harvey EJ, Leighton RK, Petrie DP (2001) Is homologous blood transfusion a risk factor for infection after hip replacement? Can J Surg 44:355-358
Turina M, Fry DE, Polk HC, Jr (2005) Acute hyperglycemia and the innate immune system: clinical, cellular, and molecular aspects. Crit Care Med 33(7):1624-1633
Wang J, Zhu C, Cheng T, Peng X, Zhang W, Qin H, et al (2013) A systematic review and meta-analysis of antibiotic-impregnated bone cement use in primary total hip or knee arthroplasty. PLoS One 8(12):e82745
Whyte W (1988) The role of clothing and drapes in the operating room. J Hosp Infect 11[Suppl C]:2-17

5.3 Strategies for Preventing Infections in Total Hip and Total Knee Arthroplasty

Christopher W. Jones, Ben Clark, and Piers Yates

5.3.1 Introduction

In a tertiary orthopaedic referral unit with a subspecialty interest in the diagnosis and management of prosthetic joint infections (PJI), we have aimed to establish a multidisciplinary, evidence-based approach for the prevention, diagnosis, treatment and long-term management of infected arthroplasties.

The strategies for reducing the risk of infection in total hip arthroplasty (THA) and total knee arthroplasty (TKA) can be broken down into three key time periods: preoperatively, intraoperatively, and post-operatively. Each of these three areas will be detailed individually prior to an illustrative case study.

Preoperatively, we aim to optimize the patient's medical risk factors, screen the patient for concurrent infectious processes, decolonize the patient if colonized with *Staphylococcus aureus,* and provide timely and appropriate antibiotic prophylaxis. Intraoperatively, the vital importance of maintaining a sterile field, providing ultraclean air flow, adopting strict gowning and gloving protocols, and ensuring robust sterilization procedures has long been recognized. Post-operatively, wound care regimens, drain management and inpatient care protocols have all been shown to play important roles.

5.3.2 Preoperative Management

Despite numerous publications in this area, there remains a startling gulf between what factors the literature has consistently proven as important and those factors believed to be important by orthopaedic surgeons worldwide (Merollini et al. 2013). Preoperative risk stratification has identified several key risk factors, in particular obesity (body mass index [BMI] >35; hazard ratio [HR]: 1.47), diabetes mellitus ([DM]; HR: 1.28) and multiple medical comorbidities (American Society of Anesthesiologists [ASA] ≥3, HR: 1.65) (Namba et al. 2013). There is evidence that optimization of nutrition, diabetic control, cardiac risk factors, smoking cessation and anaemia can decrease the risk of PJI (Everhart et al. 2013). In our unit we attempt to address each of the reversible preoperative risk factors individually utilizing a multidisciplinary approach.

Risk Factor Identification and Optimization at Pre-admission Clinic

Identification of patent risk factors and pre-emptive optimization of a patient's cardiac, respiratory and endocrine co-morbidities are undertaken in an outpatient pre-admission clinic (PAC) setting with appropriate medical referrals and follow-up. The PAC plays a vital role in the preparation for complex arthroplasty surgery. Our standard PAC assessment protocol and routine preoperative medication regimen are summarized briefly in ◘ Tab. 5.7 and ◘ Tab. 5.8.

Tab. 5.7 Pre-admission clinic screening protocol

1	Preoperative blood tests: full blood count, urea and electrolytes (U&E, EUC), blood sugar level and group and hold
2	Preoperative radiographs of the operative joint in template views with calibration ball and prosthesis templating
3	Preoperative electrocardiogram for men over 50 and women over 60, or patients with a history of cardiac disease
4	Preoperative medication review
5	Preoperative midstream urine analysis in symptomatic patients
6	Venous thrombo-embolism (VTE) assessment
7	Assessment of skin integrity and signs of active infection

Tab. 5.8 tandard perioperative medication regimen

– Oral aperients nightly, Movicol or Coloxyl Senna
– Celecoxib 100–200 mg p.o. for 6 weeks, unless contraindicated
– Tranexamic acid 1 g p.o. 1 h before surgery
– Cease aspirin 7 days and non-steroidal anti-inflammatory drugs (NSAIDs) 2 days preoperatively (unless significant cardiovascular (CVS) disease when aspirin can be continued)

Obesity has been consistently demonstrated to be a major risk factor for PJI with the overall risk of infection directly proportional to BMI (BMI >35, odds ratio [OR]:1.5; BMI >39, OR: 9; BMI >50, OR: 23; (Namba et al. 2013). Likewise, malnutrition (lymphocyte count <1,500 cells/mm^3, albumin <5 g/dl and transferrin <500 mg/dl) has been independently shown to have a 5–7 times increased wound complication rate (Huang et al. 2013). Obese or malnourished patients are referred to dieticians for further optimization of their weight loss and nutritional status.

Uncontrolled *diabetes* (HbA1C >6.5%) and raised preoperative blood glucose level (BGL >7.0 mmol/l) are independent infection risks (adjusted odds ratio: 1.83–2.28); however, there remains no definite threshold with which to establish a clear preoperative recommendation for glycaemic control (Adams et al. 2013). In our unit all diabetic patients are reviewed by the endocrinology service for optimized glycaemic control and diabetic education aiming for HbA1C <6.0%.

Smoking impairs collagen synthesis and immune function and compromises oxygen supply to surgical site. Even in the short term, smoking-induced changes are partially reversible and smoking cessation programs 6–8 weeks prior to surgery reduce complications, especially wound-related issues (Mills et al. 2011). We utilize a multimodal smoking cessation program consisting of patient education, cognitive behavioural therapy and pharmacological intervention.

Active infection is a contraindication to arthroplasty surgery, and the presence of even minor skin and soft tissue infections should prompt a deferment until the infection has been appropriately managed. Likewise chronic skin diseases, such as psoriasis and eczema, are associated with increased colonization with potentially pathogenic bacteria, and management must be optimized prior to arthroplasty surgery.

The risk of infection following surgery is increased in patients receiving immunomodulatory therapy, such as long-term steroids, chemotherapy, and disease-modifying agents for rheumatological conditions. The use of tumour necrosis factor alpha (TNF-α) inhibitors, e.g. etanercept, infliximab, and adalimumab, is not uncommon in patients requiring arthroplasty, and these agents have been associated with an increase in post-operative infections

(OR: 2.47; Goodman et al. 2016). As such, discussions with treating physicians should take place in these circumstances, with medical therapy being ceased or modified prior to operation if possible, or surgery deferred.

Screening and Decolonization

Screening for *Staphylococcus aureus* colonization, followed by decolonization and bundled preoperative intranasal mupirocin and appropriate perioperative antibiotic prophylaxis have been shown to reduce the incidence of PJI. It has been reported, however, that these interventions do not reduce risk back to a non-carrier level (Kim et al. 2010; Moroski et al. 2015). In our centre, all patients are screened for methicillin-susceptible (MSSA) or methicillin-resistant *S. aureus* (MRSA) colonization via polymerase chain reaction (PCR) testing of nasal swabs using the *GenExpert* platform, which has a rapid turnaround (<2 h) and enables targeted eradication agents to be provided on the same day. If MSSA or MRSA is identified, the patient is prescribed mupirocin 2% nasal ointment twice a day for 3 days prior to the operation, and for 2 days post-operatively. Additionally, a chlorhexidine 4% body wash (including hair) daily for 5 days prior to the operation and on the day of operation is performed. If the patient has a known allergy or resistance to mupirocin we use nitrofurazone 0.2% nasal ointment (recommended for high-level mupirocin-resistant strains).

Urine Screening and Prophylaxis

The efficacy of preoperative urine screening in arthroplasty populations has been the subject of considerable study with no convincing linkage between asymptomatic bacteriuria and PJI (Bouvet et al. 2014). Current recommendations advise against the routine screening of mid-stream urinalysis (MSU) and prophylactic treatment of asymptomatic bacteriuria (Bouvet et al. 2014). All patients are directly questioned for urinary symptoms at PAC, with MSU screening undertaken for patients with symptomatic urinary tract infection (UTI) or a strong history of UTI. Directed antibiotic treatment is then initiated based on the results of microscopy, culture and sensitivities and patients are secondarily screened via MSU prior to their surgery date.

Patient and Skin Preparation

Preoperatively all arthroplasty patients undergo a skin preparation regimen consisting of hair removal with clippers, and decontamination with chlorhexidine-impregnated skin wipes. Hair removal using clippers close to the time of surgery minimizes skin trauma and potential bacterial contamination and has been shown to be superior to shaving with razor blades (Alexander et al. 2011; Tanner et al. 2011). Chlorhexidine-impregnated skin wipes are then used in a whole-body fashion from »chin-to-toe« with repeated topical applications the evening before and morning of surgery. This has been shown to be more effective than showering with chlorhexidine soaps and superior to iodine (Zywiel et al. 2011).

5.3.3 Intraoperative Management

Surgical Staff Hand Washing

We utilize standard surgical hand-washing techniques in keeping with international guidelines (World Health Organization [WHO], Australian College of Perioperative Nurses [ACORN], Centre for Disease Control and Prevention [CDC]). Following standard hand washing with antibacterial soap and water for the first scrub of the day, a 70% alcoholic hand rub (Skinman 90 Soft N Antiseptic Hand Rub) is topically applied prior to sterile gowning and gloving (Parienti et al. 2002; Zywiel et al. 2011).

Patient Skin Preparation and Draping

Fastidious aseptic skin preparation is necessary to render the incision site free from dirt and microorganisms, thus reducing the possibility of infection and maintaining a sterile field around the surgical site. We utilize chlorhexidine combined with alcohol as it has been shown to be superior to other combinations (Darouiche et al. 2010). We pre-prep using alcoholic chlorhexidine as we are setting up in the theatre. The definitive preparation solution is then applied in a circular motion from the site of the incision to the periphery thereby mechanically removing and chemically cleaning of any microorganisms. The preparation solution is applied and allowed to air dry prior to commencement of draping, which allows sufficient contact time of the antiseptic solution to achieve maximum effectiveness and for complete evaporation of the alcohol-based solution to reduce the possibility of a surgical fire (Zywiel et al. 2011).

Disposable multi-layered plastic adhesive drapes should be used with caution as there is some evidence that they may actually increase infection due to the formation of moisture pockets (Webster et al. 2015). If a sterile stockinette is used to cover the foot, it should not be rolled proximal to the surgical site (Boekel et al. 2012; Marvil et al. 2014). The stockinette is secured with circumferential wrap and adhesive (Boekel et al. 2012; Marvil et al. 2014). Iodine-impregnated incise drapes (3M Loban™) are applied over the surgical incision site as the final barrier layer (Webster et al. 2015).

5

Theatre Ventilation

Within the operative theatre we aim to reduce all traffic to an essential minimum, and keep surgical time as low as possible, as surgery longer than 2 h increases infection rates significantly (Willis-Owen et al. 2010; Parvizi et al. 2013a). Lamina flow theatre ventilation systems capable of exchanging the total volume of air in a room >300×/h are utilized in order to reduce airborne particulate count. Although recent papers seem to suggest that these may actually increase infection rates in joint replacements, the reasons for this are still very unclear. It is possible that the ultraclean airflow is disrupted and contaminated by the forced airflow heaters, and we make sure these are not turned on until the patient is fully draped (Breier et al. 2011; Evans 2011; Hooper et al. 2011). Whilst there are conflicting data regarding body exhaust suits, we favour their use as a personal protective barrier for surgeons if nothing else (Hooper et al. 2011).

Glove Changes

There is excellent evidence to demonstrate that the surgeon's gloves are most frequently contaminated after draping and that perforation and contamination are significantly lower in gloves changed at 20-min intervals (McCue et al. 1981). Double gloves have also been shown to significantly reduce perforations (Al-Maiyah et al. 2005). The highest degree of contamination is seen on the index finger of the primary surgeon, with 76% of gloves removed just before cementing being contaminated (Al-Maiyah et al. 2005). Based on this evidence we utilize the glove change protocol outlined in ◘ Tab. 5.9.

◘ **Tab. 5.9** Gloving protocol

– Double glove for all arthroplasty cases
– Glove change after draping
– Glove changes every 20 min
– Glove change prior to cementing
– Glove change prior to handling prosthesis – avoid direct prosthesis handling/skin contact

Wound Lavage

Following the implantation of the prosthetic components, further irrigation with aqueous antiseptics seems reasonable, but we have little hard evidence to back up their use. The protocol outlined by Brown et al. (2012) demonstrated a decrease in PJI from 0.97% to 0.15%. Alternatively, chlorhexidine 0.4% in 1-l normal saline can be used (especially in the setting of iodine allergy; Brown et al. 2012).

This simple algorithm is as follows:

1. Dilute betadine soak 0.35% for 3 min after prosthesis implantation
2. Pulsatile lavage 1 l NaCl solution
3. Painting of skin with 10% betadine before final subcuticular closure

Blood Transfusion

Allogeneic blood transfusion following arthroplasty has been clearly demonstrated as a significant risk factor for PJI, more than doubling the risk (0.75% no transfusion vs 1.67% allogeneic transfusion; Innerhofer et al. 2005; Friedmann et al. 2014; Newman et al. 2014). Furthermore, the medical benefits of low transfusion thresholds have not been proven (Newman et al. 2014). Preoperatively, all patients are screened at the PAC for iron studies, with low results triggering an automatic referral for iron supplementation. On the day of surgery, tranexamic acid 1 g orally is administered 1 h prior to surgery with a second dose administered post-operatively at 4 h. During surgery tourniquets are released before closure of the wound if used at all, with attention paid to meticulous haemostasis and drains are rarely, if ever, required. Our unit maintains a strict transfusion protocol developed in conjunction with our haematology colleagues; transfusion is only considered for Hb <70g/l in asymptomatic patients and Hb <80g/l in symptomatic patients or those with high risk of ischaemic events. When symptomatic post-operative anaemia is encountered iron infusions are combined with single-unit allogeneic blood transfusions prior to repeat anaemia screening.

5.3.4 Antibiotic Prophylaxis

Clear effectiveness has been demonstrated across a multitude of studies for the benefits of preoperative antibiotic prophylaxis in the prevention of PJI with an 8% reduction in overall surgical site infection and an 81% reduction in relative risk for PJI using first- or second-generation cephalosporins in primary uncomplicated arthroplasty (AlBuhairan et al. 2008). The aim of prophylactic therapy is to eliminate potential pathogens that may have contaminated the surgical site during the procedure. As such, the timing of administration is important and adequate concentrations of antibiotic must be present in blood, tissue, and bone at the time of incision. Antibiotic infusions should therefore be commenced within 60 min before incision and prior to tourniquet inflation. We routinely use a single dose of 2 g cefazolin with no further routine doses (Parvizi et al. 2013b). During complex cases with operation in excess of 2× the half-life of the antibiotic agent (or >2 h), or in cases with significant blood loss or blood product use, a repeat dose is administered.

The routine use of vancomycin for preoperative prophylaxis is not recommended. However, for complex primary or revision arthroplasty surgery, and/or MRSA colonization, the addition of vancomycin has proven efficacious, reducing the infection rate in MRSA carriers from 4.21% to 0.89% (AlBuhairan et al. 2008). The dose of vancomycin used is determined by the patient's weight (15mg/kg with a maximum dose of 2,000 mg). If the patient has a documented history of immediate hypersensitivity reaction to penicillins, vancomycin is an appropriate alternative to cefazolin.

It is important to maintain close links with the institution's infectious disease physicians and/or microbiologists. In our institution, which manages a population with a low incidence of carriage of multi-drug-resistant Gram-negative bacteria, the use of cefazolin prophylaxis is adequate when performing complex primary or revision arthroplasty. In institutions with high rates of resistant Gram-negative organisms, it may be appropriate to use antibiotics with activity against these organisms when performing such operations, e.g. i.v. piperacillin-tazobactam or meropenem. If a patient has previously been treated for a prosthetic joint infection, antimicrobial therapy should be tailored to ensure the previous infecting organism is covered. In patients undergoing revision surgery when an infection has not been excluded, input from and infectious disease physicians and/or microbiologist should be sought to determine antimicrobial choice and duration.

From a practical point of view, it is essential to liaise closely with the perioperative nursing and anaesthetic staff to ensure that all perioperative antibiotic dosing schedules are strictly adhered to and that appropriate antibiotics have been systemically administered prior to tourniquet elevation and skin incision. Ideally, intravenous antibiotics are initiated upon admission to the hospital on the day of admission prior to the patient being transported to theatre. Incorporation and verification of antibiotic administration into the time-out protocol before the commencement of surgery has demonstrated an improvement in compliance from 65% to 99.1% and has therefore been incorporated into our institution's practice (Rosenberg et al. 2008).

In conjunction with anaesthetic, infectious disease and microbiology colleagues, our unit has developed a robust evidence-based algorithm for administering preoperative antibiotic prophylaxis for all arthroplasty cases. This is consistent with the current Australian Therapeutic Guidelines (Therapeutic Guidelines: Antibiotics 2014). The standard and revision arthroplasty antibiotic prophylaxis regimens are presented in ◘ Tab. 5.10 and ◘ Tab. 5.11.

A large number of studies have been performed comparing durations of prophylactic antibiotics following arthroplasty and the overwhelming majority do not show any benefit in prolonged therapy. The

Tab. 5.10 Standard arthroplasty antibiotic prophylaxis protocol (Dyer et al. 2009)

Standard regimen	MRSA-colonized (known or suspected)	Severe penicillin or other lactam allergy
Cefazolin 2 g i.v. (3 g if body mass >120 kg) administered within the 60 min (ideally 15–30 min) before surgical incision THEN further re-dosing as required: Cefazolin 2 g i.v. (3 g i.v. if weight >120 kg) to be given at 2 h if surgery continues	As per standard regimen PLUS addition of: <60 kg: vancomycin 1 g i.v. infusion over 60 min ≥60 kg: vancomycin 1.5 g i.v. infusion over 90 min ≥120kg: vancomycin 2 g i.v. infusion over 120 min Begin within 1 h before surgery	<60 kg: vancomycin 1 g i.v. infusion over 60 min ≥60 kg: vancomycin 1.5 g i.v. infusion over 90 min ≥120 kg: vancomycin 2 g i.v. infusion over 120 min Begin within 1 h before surgery

Tab. 5.11 Revision arthroplasty antibiotic prophylaxis protocol (Dyer et al. 2009)

Standard regimen	MRSA-colonized (known or suspected)	Severe penicillin or other lactam allergy
Cefazolin 2 g i.v. (3 g if body mass >120 kg) PLUS <60 kg: vancomycin 1 g i.v. infusion over 60 min ≥60 kg: vancomycin 1.5 g i.v. infusion over 90 min ≥120 kg: vancomycin 2 g i.v. infusion over 120 min Start after operative specimens have been taken Continue treatment until microbiology results are finalized	Cefazolin 2 g i.v. (3 g if body mass >120 kg) PLUS <60 kg: vancomycin 1 g i.v. infusion over 60 min ≥60 kg: vancomycin 1.5 g i.v. infusion over 90 min ≥120 kg: vancomycin 2 g i.v. infusion over 120 min Start after operative specimens have been taken Continue treatment until microbiology results are finalized	Ciprofloxacin 400 mg 12 hourly PLUS <60 kg: vancomycin 1 g i.v. infusion over 60 min ≥60 kg: vancomycin 1.5 g i.v. infusion over 90 min ≥120 kg: vancomycin 2 g i.v. infusion over 120 min Start after operative specimens have been taken Continue treatment until microbiology results are finalized

Australian Therapeutic Guidelines recommends antibiotics are not continued beyond 24 h of surgical incision because of a lack of evidence (Therapeutic Guidelines: Antibiotics 2014). It is also stated that prolonged dosing increases the risk of subsequent infection with resistant pathogens or *Clostridium difficile*. The American Academy of Orthopaedic Surgeons guidelines also recommend that antibiotic administration should not exceed the 24-h post-operative period, and prophylactic antibiotics should therefore be discontinued within 24 h of surgery.

5.3.5 Antibiotic-Impregnated Cement

The benefits of antibiotic-impregnated cement are now widely acknowledged in THA and perhaps also in TKA (Bohm et al. 2014; Hinarejos et al. 2015). By slow elution a high concentration of antibiotics in the effective joint space can be maintained over days to weeks, and has led some authors to suggest that this may be independently as beneficial as prophylactic intravenous antibiotics (AlBuhairan et al. 2008). For all cemented arthroplasties in our unit we utilize PALACOS® R+G (Heraeus Medical) or Antibiotic Simplex® P with tobramycin (Stryker Kalamazoo, USA) as per surgeon preference. For one- or two-stage revision arthroplasty in the setting of PJI, infectious diseases advice is sought regarding the antibiotic sensitivities of the pathogen and the optimal agent for incorporation into bone cement spacers/prostheses.

5.3.6 Post-operative Management

Post-operative management in our high-volume arthroplasty unit is largely protocol driven with standardize wound care, drain, bladder/bowel and thrombo-prophylaxis regimens aimed at minimizing both PJI and other arthroplasty-related complications.

Wound Care Regimen

On the first post-operative day, all outer bandages/dressings are removed with the sterile waterproof theatre dressing left intact. Adhesive dressings are used to reinforce wounds as required. Dressings are taken down completely and changed prior to discharge most typically on day three post-operatively. If there is persistent wound ooze over 48–72 h post-operatively, we have a low threshold for taking back to the theatre for irrigation, debridement and repeat closure (Galat et al. 2009). Antibiotic prophylaxis is re-instituted in the setting of that rare event.

Drain Management

All drains are removed day one post-operatively at approximately 24 h. Likewise we attempt to remove all intravenous cannulae and indwelling urinary catheters as soon as possible. There is no evidence to support the continued administration of prophylactic antibiotics whilst surgical drains remain, nor is there evidence to support their use whilst a urinary catheter is in situ. Antibiotic prophylaxis (gentamicin) is provided in the instance that urinary retention requires re-catheterization.

Follow-up

We maintain a strict follow-up protocol with all wounds reviewed 10–14 days post-operatively for signs of superficial infection, dehiscence or deep vein thrombosis.

5.3.7 Conclusion

Proven strategies to decrease the risk of infection in THA and TKA include the preoperatively medical optimization of patients, identification and eradication of *Staphylococcus aureus* colonization (MSSA and MRSA), fastidious perioperative skin preparation, selection and timing of prophylactic antibiotic and the avoidance of allogeneic blood transfusions.

5.3.8 Case Study

Case 1: Pre-admission Clinic

- **History**

A 67-year-old male patient with advanced hip osteoarthritis was referred for right total hip replacement. There was a past medical history of ischaemic heart disease, obesity (BMI = 31), hypertension and diabetes mellitus type II (HbA1C 9.6%). The patient was seen in the pre-admission clinic for routine preoperative assessment. Screening for MRSA was positive from the nasal swab. There were no urinary symptoms and therefore no MSU was required.

- **Management**

1. Eradication therapy:
   - Prescribed mupirocin 2% nasal ointment twice a day for 3 days prior to the operation, and for 2 days post-operatively
   - Prescribed chlorhexidine 4% body wash (including hair) daily for 5 days prior to the operation and on the day of operation
2. Antibiotic prophylaxis:
   - Cefazolin 2 g at time of induction
   - Vancomycin 1 g slow infusion over 1 h prior to surgery
   - No further antibiotics required
3. Endocrine consultation
   - Commencement of basal/bolus insulin regimen
   - Dietician consultation
   - Vitamin supplementation
4. Dietary modification
   - Weight loss program

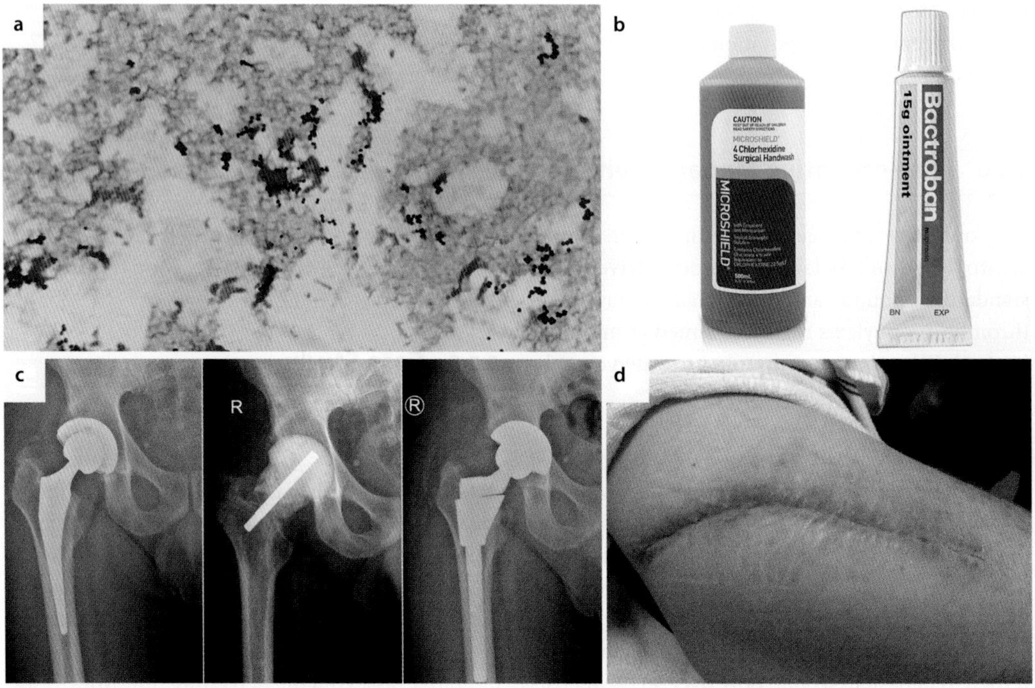

Fig. 5.11 **a** Photomicrograph of Gram-stained methicillin-resistant *Staphylococcus aureus* (MRSA) on culture plate demonstrating classic grape-like clusters of Gram-positive cocci amongst pink-stained tissue substrate and inflammatory cells. **b** Chlorhexidine 4% preoperative body wash and Bactroban nasal ointment. **c** Standard radiographs of a typical two-stage revision arthroplasty for infection. Initial prosthesis implanted 4 years previously with a late haematogenous MSSA infection; antibiotic cement spacer after first-stage revision; after 6 weeks of intravenous antibiotics and normal inflammatory markers a second-stage reconstruction was undertaken with a large trabecular metal acetabular component to accommodate central acetabular defect and uncemented modular femoral component. **d** Clinical photo of healed hip wound 2 weeks post-operatively following second-stage revision total hip arthroplasty corresponding to radiographs in **c**

■ Outcome

Uncomplicated arthroplasty was undertaken 1 month after PAC assessment. MRSA swabs were clear on admission after eradication therapy. Improved glycaemic control (HbA1c 7.6%) and weight loss (BMI = 28) were seen at further follow-up. Arthroplasty was performing well at the 2-year mark (Fig. 5.11).

■ Conclusion

The pre-admission clinic provides a unique opportunity to intervene prior to surgery. A multidisciplinary approach can reduce infection risk in arthroplasty and improve multiple aspects of a patient's health.

Take-Home Message

Measures for infection prevention in THA/TKA need to take place at three different time periods:

- Preoperatively:
  - Identify and deal with risk factors
  - Screening for (nasal/urinary) infections
  - Skin preparation
- Intraoperatively:
  - OR preparation
  - OR routines
  - Antibiotics
- Post-operatively:
  - Wound care
  - Drain management
  - Follow-up

References

Adams AL, Paxton EW, Wang JQ, Johnson ES, Bayliss EA, Ferrara A, Nakasato C, Bini SA, Namba RS (2013) Surgical outcomes of total knee replacement according to diabetes status and glycemic control, 2001 to 2009. Jf Bone Joint Surg 95:481-487

AlBuhairan B, Hind D, Hutchinson A (2008) Antibiotic prophylaxis for wound infections in total joint arthroplasty: a systematic review. J Bone Joint Surg Br 90(7):915-919

Alexander JW, Solomkin JS, Edwards MJ (2011) Updated recommendations for control of surgical site infections. Annal Surg 253(6):1082-1093

Al-Maiyah M, Bajwa A, Mackenney P, Port A, Gregg PJ, Hill D, Finn P (2005) Glove perforation and contamination in primary total hip arthroplasty. J Bone Joint Surg Br 87(4):556-559

Boekel P, Blackshaw R, Van Bavel D, Riazi A, Hau R (2012) Sterile stockinette in orthopaedic surgery: a possible pathway for infection. ANZ J Surg 82(11):838-843

Bohm E, Zhu N, Gu J, de Guia N, Linton C, Anderson T, Paton D, Dunbar M (2014) Does adding antibiotics to cement reduce the need for early revision in total knee arthroplasty? Clin Orthop Relat Res 472(1):162-168

Bouvet C, Lübbeke A, Bandi C, Pagani L, Stern R, Hoffmeyer P, Uçkay I (2014) Is there any benefit in pre-operative urinary analysis before elective total joint replacement? Bone Joint J 96b(3):390-394

Breier AC, Brandt C, Sohr D, Geffers C, Gastmeier P (2011) Laminar airflow ceiling size: no impact on infection rates following hip and knee prosthesis. Infect Control Hosp Epidemiol 32(11):1097-1102

Brown NM, Cipriano CA, Moric M, Sporer SM, Della Valle CJ (2012) Dilute betadine lavage before closure for the prevention of acute postoperative deep periprosthetic joint infection. J Arthroplasty 27(1):27-30

Darouiche RO, Wall MJ Jr, Itani KM, Otterson MF, Webb AL, Carrick MM, Miller HJ, Awad SS, Crosby CT, Mosier MC, Alsharif A, Berger DH (2010) Chlorhexidine–alcohol versus povidone– iodine for surgical-site antisepsis. N Engl J Med 362:18-26

Dyer J, McGechie D, Yates P (2009) Fremantle Antibiotic and Immunisation Guidelines. D.o.O. Surgery (Ed). 2009. Infection Control Unit, Fremantle Hospital

Evans RP (2011) Current concepts for clean air and total joint arthroplasty: laminar airflow and ultraviolet radiation: a systematic review. Clin Orthop Relat Res 469(4):945-953

Everhart JS, Altneu E, Calhoun JH (2013) Medical comorbidities are independent preoperative risk factors for surgical infection after total joint arthroplasty. Clin Orthop Relat Res 471:3112-3119

Friedman R, Homering M, Holberg G, Berkowitz SD (2014) Allogeneic blood transfusions and postoperative infections after total hip or knee arthroplasty. J Bone Joint Surg Am 96(4):272-278

Galat DD, McGovern SC, Larson DR, Harrington JR, Hanssen AD, Clarke HD (2009) Surgical treatment of early wound complications following primary total knee arthroplasty. J Bone Joint Surg Am 91(1):48-54

Goodman SM, Menon I, Christos PJ, Smethurst R, Bykerk VP (2016) Management of perioperative tumour necrosis factor alpha inhibitors in rheumatoid arthritis patients undergoing arthroplasty: a systematic review and meta-analysis. Rheumatology (Oxford) 55(3):573-582

Hinarejos, P, Pau Guirro, Lluis Puig-Verdie, Raul Torres-Claramunt, Joan Leal-Blanquet, Juan Sanchez-Soler, Joan Carles Monllau (2015) Use of antibiotic-loaded cement in total knee arthroplasty. World J Orthop 6(11):877-885

Hooper GJ, Rothwell AG, Frampton C, Wyatt MC (2011) Does the use of laminar flow and space suits reduce early deep infection after total hip and knee replacement?: the ten-year results of the New Zealand Joint Registry. J Bone Joint Surg Br 93(1):85-90

Huang R, Greenky M, Kerr GJ, Austin MS, Parvizi J (2013) The effect of malnutrition on patients undergoing elective joint arthroplasty. J Arthroplasty 28 [Suppl 1]:21-24

Innerhofer P, Klingler A, Klimmer C, Fries D, Nussbaumer W (2005) Risk for postoperative infection after transfusion of white blood cell-filtered allogeneic or autologous blood components in orthopedic patients undergoing primary arthroplasty. Transfusion 45(1):103-110

Kim DH Spencer M, Davidson SM, Li L, Shaw JD, Gulczynski D, Hunter DJ, Martha JF, Miley GB, Parazin SJ, Dejoie P, Richmond JC (2010) Institutional prescreening for detection and eradication of methicillin-resistant Staphylococcus aureus in patients undergoing elective orthopaedic surgery. J Bone Joint Surg 92:1820-1826

Marvil SC, Tiedeken NC, Hampton DM, Kwok SC, Samuel SP, Sweitzer BA (2014) Stockinette application over a non-prepped foot risks proximal contamination. J Arthroplasty 29(9):1819-1822

McCue SF, Berg EW, Saunders EA (1981) Efficacy of double-gloving as a barrier to microbial contamination during total joint arthroplasty. J Bone Joint Surg Am 63(5): 811-813

Merollini K, Zheng H, Graves N (2013) Most relevant strategies for preventing surgical site infection after total hip arthroplasty: Guideline recommendations and expert opinion. Am J Infect Control 41:221-226

Mills E, Eyawo O, Lockhart I, Kelly S, Wu P, Ebbert JO (2011) Smoking cessation reduces postoperative complications: a systematic review and meta analysis. Am J Med 124(2):144-154

Moroski NM, Woolwine S, Schwarzkopf R (2015) Is preoperative staphylococcal decolonization efficient in total joint arthroplasty. J Arthrop 30:444-446

Namba RS, Inacio MCS, Paxton EW (2013) Risk factors associated with deep surgical site infections after primary total knee arthroplasty an analysis of 56,216 knees. J Bone Joint Surg 95:775-782

Newman ET, Watters TS, Lewis JS, Jennings JM, Wellman SS, Attarian DE, Grant SA, Green CL, Vail TP, Bolognesi MP (2014) Impact of perioperative allogeneic and autologous blood transfusion on acute wound infection follow-

ing total knee and total hip arthroplasty. J Bone Joint Surg Am 96(4):279-284
Parienti JJ, Thibon P, Heller R, Le Roux Y, von Theobald P, Bensadoun H, Bouvet A, Lemarchand F, Le Coutour X, Antisepsie Chirurgicale des mains Study Group (2002) Hand-rubbing with an aqueous alcoholic solution vs traditional surgical hand-scrubbing and 30-day surgical site infection rates: a randomized equivalence study. JAMA 288(6):722-727
Parvizi J, Gehrke T, Chen AF (2013a) Proceedings of the international consensus on periprosthetic joint infection. Bone Joint J 95b(11):1450-1452
Parvizi J, Cavanaugh PK, Diaz-Ledezma C (2013b) Periprosthetic knee infection: ten strategies that work. Knee Surg Relat Res 25(4):155-164
Rosenberg AD, Wambold D, Kraemer L, Begley-Keyes M, Zuckerman SL, Singh N, Cohen MM, Bennett MV (2008) Ensuring appropriate timing of antimicrobial prophylaxis. J Bone Joint Surg Am 90(2):226-232
Tanner J, Norrie P, Melen K (2011) Preoperative hair removal to reduce surgical site infection. Cochrane Database of Systematic Reviews 11
Therapeutic Guidelines: Antibiotics (2015) Version 15, AE Group (Ed) 2014. Therapeutic Guidelines Limited, Melbourne, Australia
Webster J, Alghamdi A (2015) Use of plastic adhesive drapes during surgery for preventing surgical site infection. Cochrane Database of Systematic Reviews 4
Willis-Owen CA, Konyves A, Martin DK (2010) Factors affecting the incidence of infection in hip and knee replacement: an analysis of 5277 cases. J Bone Joint Surg Br 92(8): 1128-1133
Zywiel MG, Daley JA, Delanois RE, Naziri Q, Johnson AJ, Mont MA (2011) Advance pre-operative chlorhexidine reduces the incidence of surgical site infections in knee arthroplasty. Int Orthop (SICOT) 35:1001-1006

5.4 Treatment of Bone and Joint Infection: Clinical Practice at the Centre de Référence des Infections Ostéo-Articulaires Complexes (CRIOAc) Lyon, France

Anthony Viste, Florent Valour, Yannick Herry, Frederic Laurent, Vincent Ronin, Isabelle Bobineau, Frédéric Aubrun, Sébastien Lustig, and Tristan Ferry

5.4.1 Introduction

In France, there are more than 2,000 hospitals characterized by three types of providers: public hospitals, private not-for-profit clinics and private for-profit clinics. The responsibility for hospital planning is shared between the Central Ministry of Health and the Regional Health Agencies (Agences Régionales de Santé, ARSs). Based on the Regional Health Schemes, the ARSs establish target agreements with hospitals to define the services, volumes, and responsibilities for each hospital in their area so as to ensure that population needs are covered.

Since 2004, French hospital care is funded through activity tariffs, based on diagnosis-related groups (DRGs). DRG-based financing includes public, private not-for-profit and private for-profit hospitals as long as they are formally accredited by the National Health Authority (HAS). In the same year, general practitioners (*médecin traitant*) were announced as gatekeepers to refer their patient to specialists, if indicated. In 2008, HAS selected nine dedicated university clinics allotted throughout seven geographical regions to act as reference centres, especially for patients with complex bone- and implant-related infections. In 2011, another 15 corresponding centres were allocated to the existing reference centres around their neighbourhood. All these centres are specialized in complex medical cases, with additional equipment and financing. Most importantly, difficult orthopaedic infections such as bone and periprosthetic joint infection (BPJI) are treated in an institutional multi-doctor team (MDT) approach that is co-ordinated by one of the three officially announced treating doctors: the infectious disease specialist, the clinical microbiologist, and the septic orthopaedic surgeon.

The care of patients with bone and joint infection is a public health concern. The prerequisite for adequate treatment of complex bone and joint infections is considered to be the responsibility of the Health Ministry in France. Concerned patients need to be informed about the emergency of their symptoms, they are assisted and advised by their informed doctor, or alternatively by the Health Government Internet website. A national BPJI database collects treatment data and serves as a disease-specific national registry. This planned structure addresses the control of nosocomial infections or infections caused by medical interventions. Such implementation of regional reference centres, like the centres de Référence des Infections Ostéo-articulaires complexes (CRIOAcs) for the management of chronic and difficult-to-treat pathologies (e.g. BPJI), assures horizontal and vertical equity in patient care.

5.4.2 Centre de Référence des Infections Ostéo-Articulaires Complexes (CRIOAc)

Implant-associated BJIs (e.g. PJI or osteosynthesis-associated BJIs) are nosocomial infections and eradication of the pathogen is always challenging in infected patients. Therefore, teamwork in tertiary care centres is required to determine optimal medico-surgical strategies and to limit treatment failure, motor disabilities and risk for amputation. Indeed, these BJIs are associated with a high morbidity, mortality and economic cost, rendering their management a priority.

As a result, in France, the Direction Générale de l'Offre de Soins (DGOS) of the French Health Ministry (Ministère des Affaires sociales et de la Santé) has approved nine regional reference centres, also called CRIOAc for »*Centre de Référence des Infections Ostéo-Articulaires Complexes*«. Each CRIOAc works with two or three associated university hospitals, totalling 24 university hospitals spread over the French territory located in Lyon, Paris, Boulogne-Billancourt, Lille-Tourcoing, Rennes, Tours, Toulouse, Marseille and Nancy (http://www.sante.gouv.fr/centres-de-reference-interregionaux-pour-la-prise-en-charge-des-infections-osteo-articulaires-complexes.html).

> CRIOAcs have several missions, and cover in particular the management of complex BJIs, which are defined by the following criteria:
> I. Patients with severe comorbidities; and/or
> II. Patients with medicinal allergy; and/or
> III. Patients infected with a multidrug-resistant pathogen; and/or
> IV. Patients who require a large bone resection and/or reconstruction.

CRIOAcs also promote education and research in the field of BJI. Members of all these BJI specialized centres in France (◘ Fig. 5.12), including the CRIOAc Lyon (◘ Fig. 5.13), meet at least twice per week with a multidisciplinary team consisting of infectious disease specialists, surgeons and microbiologists to discuss the individual treatment of each patient with complex BJI. The following complex cases were managed at the CRIOAc Lyon in 2015.

5.4.3 Late Acute Staphylococcus aureus Hip PJI: When Antimicrobial-Related Toxicity Interferes and Leads to Complexity

A 70-year-old man, with a history of diabetes mellitus and left total hip arthroplasty implanted 15 years earlier, was admitted for febrile left hip pain with chills for 5 days. His C-reactive protein (CRP) level was at 390 mg/l and the white blood cell count was 20,000/mm^3. A left hip X-ray disclosed an acetabular and trochanteric osteolysis (◘ Fig. 5.14a). Computed tomography (CT) scan confirmed prosthesis loosening (◘ Fig. 5.14b), with a voluminous abscess in the ilio-psoas muscle of 77×35 mm (◘ Fig. 5.14c). Blood cultures rapidly turned positive for methicillin-sensitive *Staphylococcus aureus* (MSSA).

Despite the diagnosis of late acute haematogenous hip PJI, a multidisciplinary team meeting argued for surgical management consisting in prosthesis removal (◘ Fig. 5.14d) for the following reasons:

> **First**, and despite the absence of literature data, a severe septic presentation often requires an aggressive surgical strategy in order to rapidly reduce the bacterial inoculum.
> **Second**, the quality of soft tissue structures and the remaining bone stock impacts the prognosis (Crockarell et al. 1998; Marculescu et al. 2006). Consequently, the presence of a sinus tract or voluminous abscess should lead one to consider implant retention in favour of a two-stage revision strategy (Osmon et al. 2013).
> **Third**, in addition to the increased risk of haematogenous seeding on orthopaedic devices (30–40%), compared with other pathogens (5%; Murdoch et al.

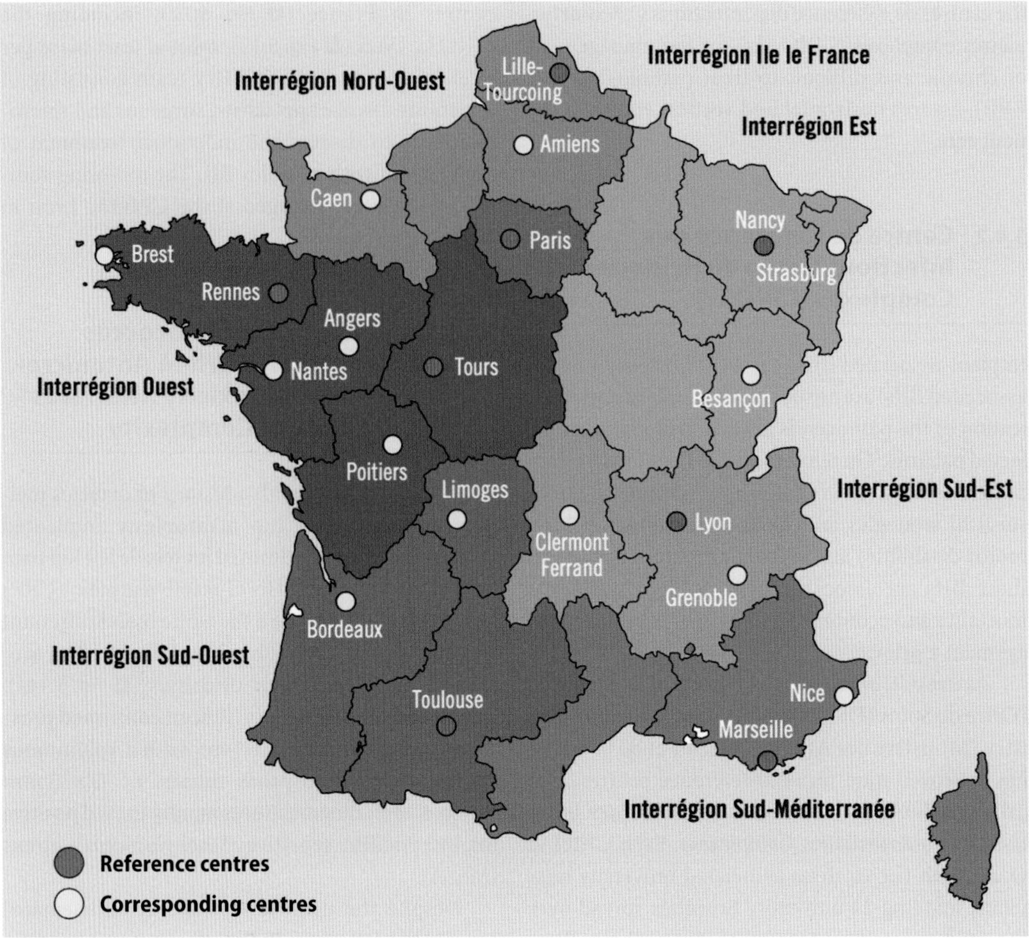

Fig. 5.12 CRIOAcs in France

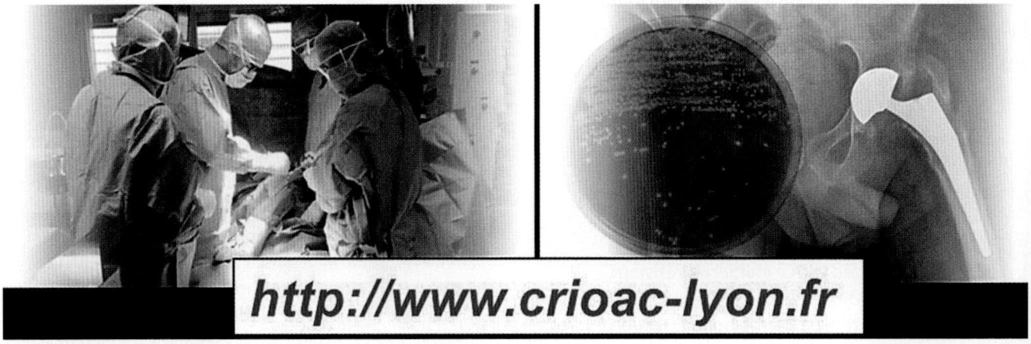

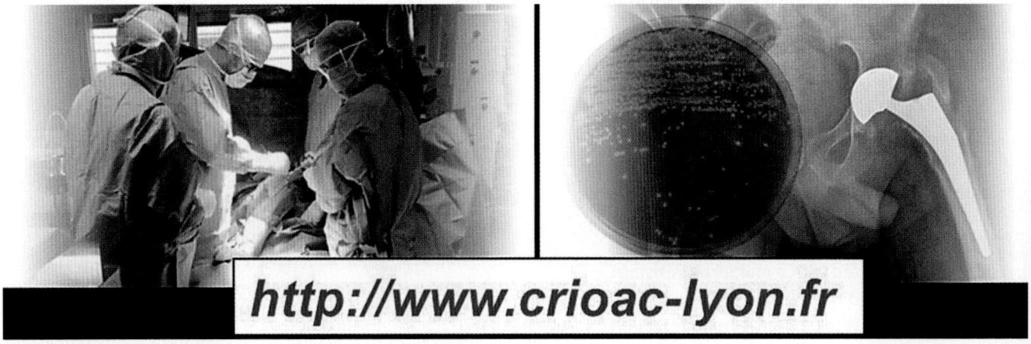

Fig. 5.13 Homepage of CRIOAc Lyon

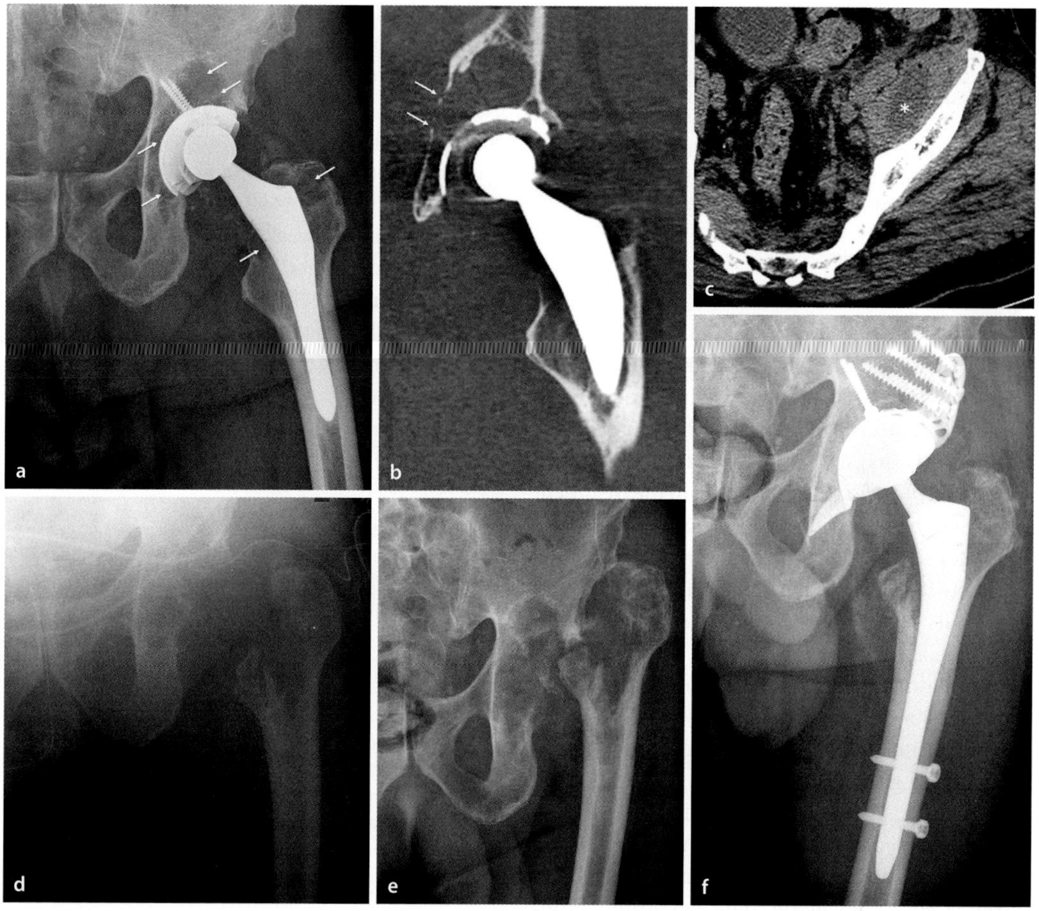

Fig. 5.14a–f Late acute haematogenous *Staphylococcus aureus* hip prosthetic joint infection. **a** Left hip X-ray disclosing an acetabular and trochanteric osteolysis (*arrows*). **b** Computed tomography scan confirming prosthesis loosening with osteolysis (*arrows*). **c** Computed tomography scan showing a 77×35-mm abscess in the ilio-psoas muscle (*asterisk*). **d** Left hip X-ray performed immediately after prosthesis removal. **e** Left hip X-ray performed 3 months after prosthesis removal. **f** Left hip X-ray performed after prosthesis re-implantation

2001; Sendi et al. 2011; Uckay et al. 2009), *S. aureus* has been associated with implant retention and one-stage exchange failures (Marculescu et al. 2006; Byren et al. 2009; Lora-Tamayo et al. 2013). This is especially the case in the setting of acute haematogenous PJI (Konigsberg et al. 2014), owing to numerous staphylococcal virulence factors and the ability of *S. aureus* to adhere and invade bone tissue, which causes persistent infections (Ferry et al. 2005).

Regarding medical therapy, administration of a combination of oxacillin and gentamicin was started immediately, which constitutes the reference antimicrobial regimen for acute MSSA PJI associated with bacteraemia. Lip swelling occurred after an oxacillin infusion on day 2. Beta-lactams are the first cause of antimicrobial-related adverse events (AE) during treatment of staphylococcal BJI (Valour et al. 2014), notably causing allergic reactions (Lagace-Wiens and Rubinstein 2012). This severe adverse event led to us switching the antimicrobial regimen to vancomycin and gentamicin. Although combination therapy is actually recommended for such situations, the treatment is problematic because:

1. The treatment of MSSA bacteraemia and BJI by a glycopeptide instead of beta-lactam represents a risk factor for treatment failure (Salgado et al. 2007, Kim et al. 2008).
2. The association of these two nephrotoxic molecules increases the risk of glycopeptide-induced renal failure from 5% to 15–35% (Elyasi et al. 2012). Indeed, the patient presented with vancomycin/gentamicin-induced acute renal failure (glomerular filtration rate, 30 ml/min).

In the absence of other validated alternatives, antimicrobial therapy was finally switched to daptomycin and ciprofloxacin, allowing for the improvement of renal function and blood culture sterilization. New molecules such as daptomycin in the treatment of BJI must be used with caution. Since it was initially developed for the treatment of skin and soft tissue infection (SSTI), little information is available regarding its bone diffusion and optimal dosing, and the tolerance of long-term use of higher dosages than recommended in SSTI is incompletely known (Malizos et al. 2015). Consequently, the unlabelled use of such molecules in BJI requires an experience physician to give clear information to the patient. After 17 days, the patient presented with daptomycin-induced acute eosinophilic pneumonia (diffuse alveolar and interstitial radiological opacities, hypoxemia, eosinophil blood count 2,600/mm^3, bronchoalveolar lavage fluid showing 10% of eosinophils). The patient's condition improved in a few days thanks to daptomycin withdrawal and corticoid therapy. Cefazolin and rifampin were finally administered with good tolerance and efficacy.

Prosthesis re-implantation could be performed 6 weeks later (◘ Fig. 5.14e and f). Indeed, short-term re-implantation (2 weeks) has a low likelihood of success in such situations, especially in *S. aureus* PJI (Rand and Bryan 1983). The antimicrobial therapy was eventually stopped 3 months later. At the follow-up 1 year later, the patient was doing well, without any clinical, radiological or biological signs of recurrent infection.

This case report highlights:
- The management of late acute haematogenous PJI, which can be complex because of local conditions
- The high rate of antimicrobial-related adverse events, reaching 25% in some series of MSSA BJI, with 15% of severe adverse events (Valour et al. 2014)
- The subsequent importance of a multidisciplinary approach, aiming for an optimal surgical and medical management, including choice of surgical strategy, monitoring of treatment tolerance, and prescription of alternate and unlabelled antimicrobial therapy in the case of patients with multiple drug intolerance or multidrug-resistant pathogens.

Timing	Surgery	Antibiotics	Adverse events
Day 0	THA removal	Oxacillin + gentamicin	–
Day 2	–	Vancomycin + gentamicin	Betalactam-induced lip swelling
Day 5	–	Daptomycin + ciprofloxacin	Vancomycin- and gentamicin-induced acute renal failure
Day 9	–	Daptomycin + clindamycin	Fluoroquinolon-induced encephalopathy
Day 22	–	Cefazolin + rifampin	Daptomycin-induced acute eosinophilic pneumonia
Day 45	THA reimplantation	–	–
Day 130	–	Antimicrobial therapy stop	–

5.4.4 A Complex Chronic Propionibacterium acnes Infection Treated with Girdlestone Procedure and Suppressive Antimicrobial Therapy

A 78-year-old man complained of having pain in his left hip. His history began in 1991 when he fell from a height and broke his left acetabulum. After acute osteosynthesis, a total hip arthroplasty (THA) was implanted 2 years later. Owing to wear, he underwent revision after 13 years with an early complication: femoral fracture treated by osteosynthesis and stem replacement. One year later, he was still suffering from pain: greater trochanter and diaphysis pseudarthrosis with femoral loosening were diagnosed. A revision was done by transfemoral osteotomy and a cemented long stem was implanted. At 6 days after surgery, he had isolated fever of unknown aetiology. All his functions resumed satisfactorily. After 6 years after, he complained of pain due to acetabular protrusion on X-rays (◘ Fig. 5.15a). His CRP level was of 40 mg/l. A LeukoScan showed bipolar septic loosening and abscess around the THA.

Prosthesis removal required femorotomy and, unfortunately, two screws had to be left broken in the acetabulum because the surgeons were unable to extract them (◘ Fig. 5.15b). After the surgery, probabilistic antimicrobial therapy was initiated: piperacillin-tazobactam and vancomycin. *Propionibacterium acnes* (*P. acnes*) was detected in all samples. The antimicrobial therapy was replaced by high doses of amoxicillin administered intravenously.

A large haematoma complicated the post-operative period with deglobulization, treated by debridement and radiological embolization. After this, a proximal deep venous thrombosis was diagnosed and treated by curative anticoagulation and inferior vena cava filter. Six weeks after the explantation, intravenous amoxicillin was replaced by oral clindamycin. Because of all these complications, the patient was not re-operated, and chronic suppressive antibiotic therapy with clindamycin was prescribed. At the 2-year follow-up after surgery, clindamycin was still well tolerated, and the patient was able to walk without pain, using a right compensatory shoe and a crutch (◘ Fig. 5.15c).

Resection arthroplasty (Girdlestone procedure) is a salvage procedure for uncontrolled infections (Kantor et al. 1986) or patients with poor health conditions. Poor function and leg length discrepancy (3–10 cm) with need of walking supports are frequent (Grauer et al. 1989; Castellanos et al. 1998), as well as general complications (Malcolm et al. 2015). Resection arthroplasty is reserved for very elective cases (Schroder et al. 1998).

> In our particular case, the patient had two major complications:
> - A large haematoma treated by re-operation and embolization and a major thrombosis leading to implantation of an inferior vena cava filter. These complications put this patient at a too-high risk for a subsequent surgery.
> - Explantation of the broken screws would have been required before re-implantation.

Thus, we opted for resection arthroplasty to avoid life-threatening surgery.

Suppressive antimicrobial therapy should be considered to control infection when curative treatment is no longer possible. Micro-organisms must be identified that should be sensitive to antibiotics. In our case, it helped to control infection for 2 years before the treatment was stopped. Suppression of infection is often used when the prosthesis is left in place (Rao et al. 2003), with the risk of adverse effects (Tsukayama et al. 1991). This was not the case with our patient, but this major infection needed to be treated effectively.

Timing	Surgery	Antibiotics	Adverse events
Day 0	THA removal	Piperacillin/tazobactam + vancomycin	Deglobulization (hematoma) + proximal deep venous thrombosis
Day 14	–	Amoxicillin	-
Day 45	–	Suppressive antibiotic therapy: Clindamycin	-

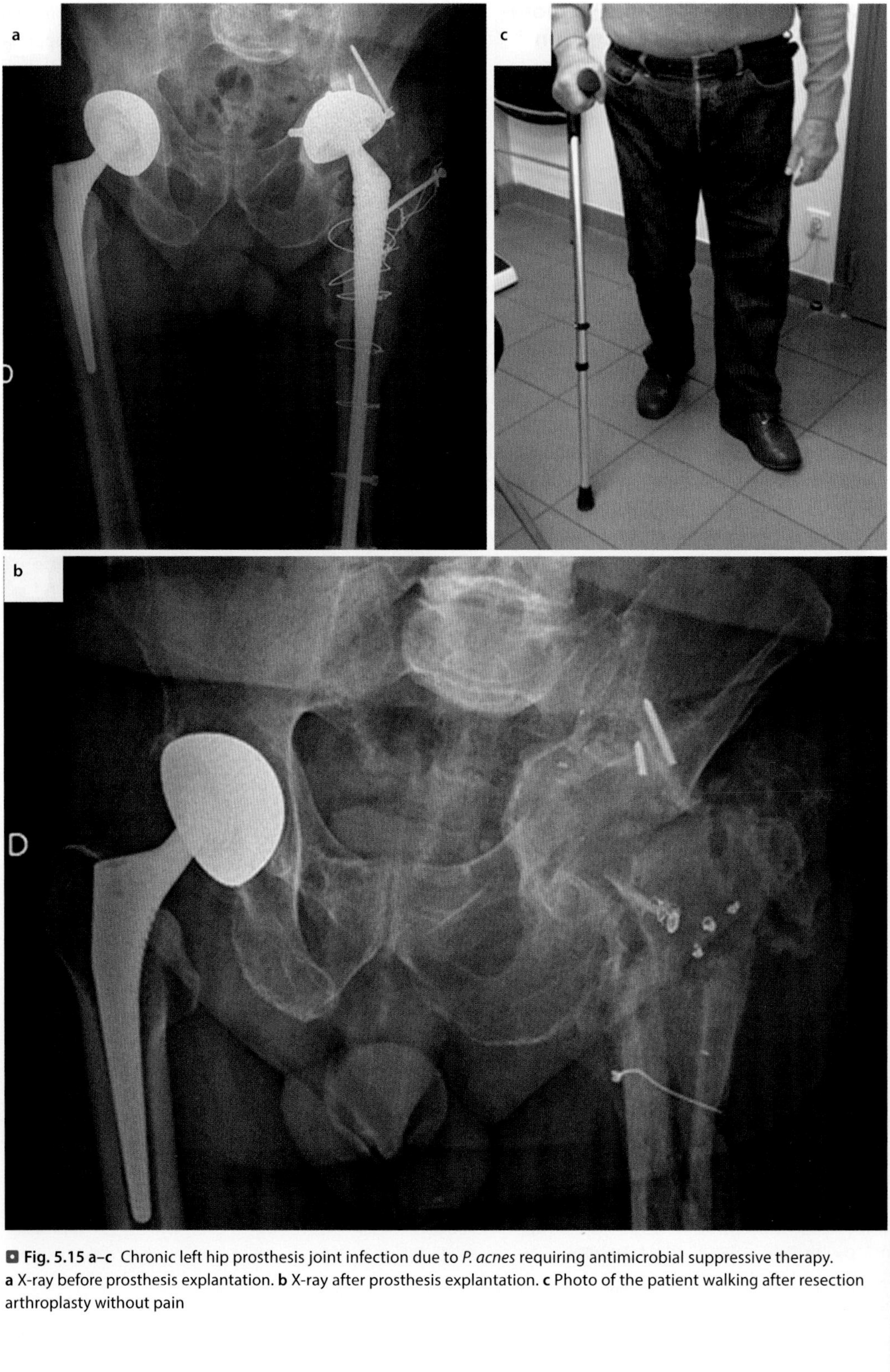

Fig. 5.15 a–c Chronic left hip prosthesis joint infection due to *P. acnes* requiring antimicrobial suppressive therapy. **a** X-ray before prosthesis explantation. **b** X-ray after prosthesis explantation. **c** Photo of the patient walking after resection arthroplasty without pain

5.4.5 Sequential Management of an Infected THA in a Young Patient

A 20-year-old female patient came to France for a suspected infected right THA. When she was 12 years old, she sustained a femoral fracture and underwent two operations in Albania and was treated for unknown reasons with amoxicillin-clavulanic acid for 2 months. In France, chronic THA infection was suspected and LeukoScan and aspiration showed signs of infection. The THA was removed and a spacer was placed (◘ Fig. 5.16a). Imipenem-cilastatin, ofloxacin and vancomycin were administered. *Proteus mirabilis* was found in the samples, and the antimicrobial therapy was changed to piperacillin-tazobactam and ofloxacin. The patient's course 1 month later was not favourable, with wound discharge and abscess, and she was managed in the CRIOAc Lyon. The spacer was removed, a new debridement was performed, and an articulated spacer loaded with gentamicin (Palacos® R+G; 0.5g per dose; intravenous cefoxitin (8 g/day) and oral ofloxacin (800 mg/day) was inserted (◘ Fig. 5.16b). At this time, *P. mirabilis*, *Staphylococcus warneri* and *P. acnes* were found in cultures. The patient was treated with intravenous cefoxitin and oral ofloxacin. The clinical course of the patient 3 months later was favourable and antimicrobial therapy was stopped. Thereafter, the patient was prepared for the revision surgery. A new exchange of the spacer was performed several weeks after antimicrobial discontinuation, and the proximal end of the femur was removed (◘ Fig. 5.16c). Empirical antimicrobial therapy was prescribed, and was withdrawn on day 15, as no persistent infection was diagnosed (no organism was found in cultures). Thus, since the clinical course was still favourable, 2 months later revision was performed using a massive hip prosthesis. The patient had good functional results (◘ Fig. 5.16d).

Management of this multi-step surgery has to be multidisciplinary. In this case, multiple surgeries were required to control the infection, after which revision surgery could be performed. At the beginning of the management, the history of the infection was uncertain: antibiotic therapy was given during primary surgery at a different hospital without knowing why it was given and for which organism.

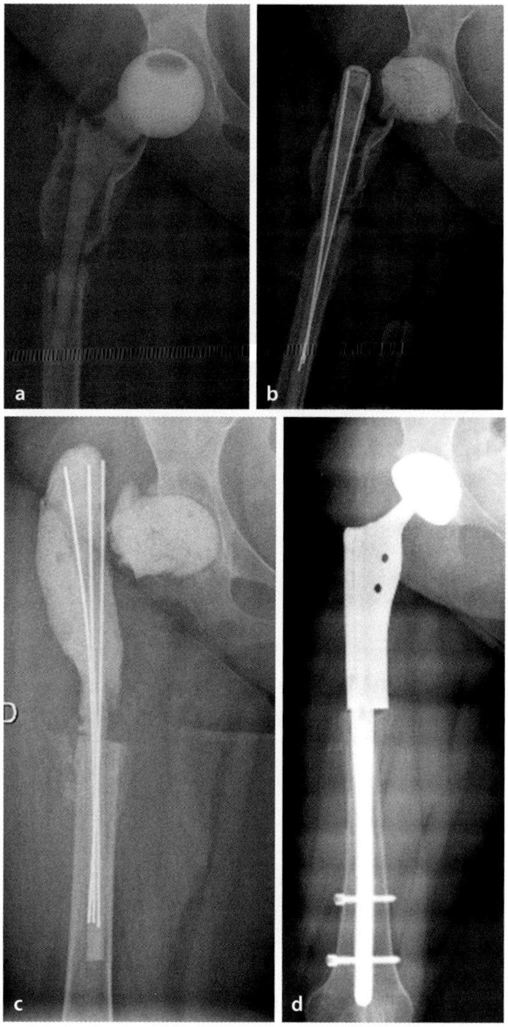

◘ **Fig. 5.16 a–d** Persistent right hip prosthesis joint infection despite prosthesis removal requiring a multistep management before re-implantation. **a** X-ray after prosthesis explantation, showing the infected first spacer. **b** X-ray after explantation of the first spacer, debridement, and insertion of a gentamicin-loaded reinforced articulated new spacer. **c** X-ray after last spacer exchange (gentamicin-loaded reinforced articulated spacer) and proximal femoral resection of the femur to exclude any persistent infection and to prepare the patient for the massive re-implantation. **d** X-ray after the re-implantation of the massive right hip prosthesis

Thus, one has to be very careful in taking care of patients with an unclear past medical history of infection. As the infectious process was not controlled after prosthesis explantation, a new debridement with change of the spacer was required. A persistent infection due to the initial *P. mirabilis* was diagnosed, with superinfection as a complication since *S. warneri* and *P. acnes* also grew in cultures. Infection was finally controlled with adapted antimicrobial therapy after the spacer change. Then, to be sure that the infection was cured and to exclude any persistent infection, we prepared the patient for re-implantation with another step after withdrawing antimicrobial treatment, which consisted in bone resection, bone biopsies and replacement of the gentamicin-loaded spacer. As no organism grew in cultures, re-implantation was successful.

Timing	Surgery	Antibiotics	Adverse events
Day 0	THA removal + spacer	Imipenem/cilastatin + ofloxacin + vancomycin	–
Day 14	–	Piperacillin/tazobactam + ofloxacin	Wound discharge + abcess
Day 30	Debridement + spacer exchange	Cefoxitin + ofloxacin	–
Day 110	Spacer exchange + proximal femur ablation	?	–
Day 180	Megaprosthesis	?	–

5.4.6 Three-Step Sequential Management for Knee Arthroplasty After Severe Ballistic Injury

Management of knee bone loss after gunshot trauma requires a multidisciplinary approach. One case of knee arthroplasty after devastating ballistic trauma is reported. Treatment comprised several steps: sampling, bone resection, reinforced cement spacer, latent sepsis control, and prosthetic reconstruction. The patient showed no neurovascular disorder and had a functioning extensor mechanism. At follow-up of at least 5 years, results were satisfactory, with return to unaided walking and International Knee Society (IKS) score was 74 points. In light of this observation, knee reconstruction arthroplasty using a sequential strategy can provide satisfactory functional outcome after severe ballistic trauma (Seng and Masquelet 2013).

A 58-year-old man had a hunting accident in 2009 involving low-energy ballistic trauma (http://social-sante.gouv.fr/systeme-de-sante-et-medico-social/), with Gustilo III open fracture of the distal right femur. Initial examination found no neurovascular lesions. Emergency lavage and wound care were performed, with osteosynthesis by external fixator; the bone defect was filled with antibiotic-laden cement. Revision surgery was needed for infection at 3 months (◘ Fig. 5.17a). Thorough radiological assessment was conducted before considering reconstruction surgery: magnetic resonance imaging (MRI) to check extensor mechanism integrity (◘ Fig. 5.17b), and computed tomography (CT) angiography to check the vascular axes. The external fixator was removed 9 months post-trauma and samples were taken (Step 1). Step 2 was implemented 6 weeks later, with bone cuts in healthy tissues (9 cm femoral and 1 cm tibial resection using a dedicated cut guide) and insertion of a non-reinforced antibiotic-laden cement spacer (Palacos® R+G) (◘ Fig. 5.17c). The post-operative course featured thrombocytopoenia induced by heparin, with superior vena cava and left common femoral vein thrombosis, which resolved completely. The patient was re-operated on at 2 months because of spacer fracture, which was replaced by a reinforced model (◘ Fig. 5.17d).

A rotating hinge reconstruction prosthesis (RHK, OSS™, Biomet®) was finally implanted in November 2010, with probabilistic antibiotic-laden cement (Step 3; ◘ Fig. 5.17e; ◘ Tab. 5.12). At the 5-year follow-up, the patient could walk without canes, with 2 cm compensation for lower-limb length discrepancy (◘ Fig. 5.17f+g). Range of motion was 0–0–100°. The International Knee Society (IKS) score was 74.

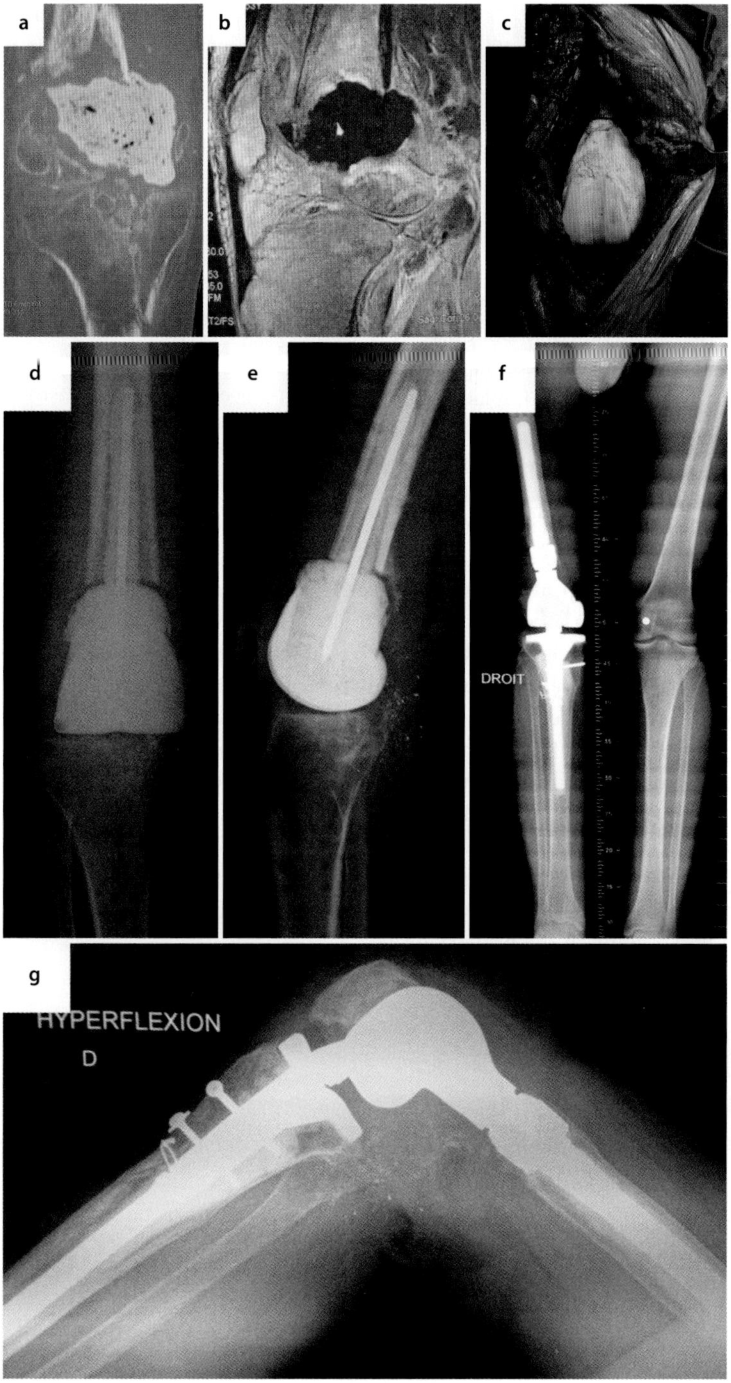

Fig. 5.17 a–g Multiple-step sequential management following severe ballistic injury responsible for complex BJI. **a** CT scan showing complex fracture of femur and tibia, major bone defect, cement spacer in place for several months. **b** MRI showing extensor system integrity. **c** Non-reinforced antibiotic-laden cement spacer to maintain limb length. **d** Anteroposterior and **e** lateral X-ray showing the reinforced cement spacer. **f** Whole-knee X-ray at 5-year follow-up. **g** Lateral X-ray in maximal flexion at 5-year follow-up

Tab. 5.12 Sequential management after severe ballistic injury

Step 1	Material removal, samples
Step 2	Bone cuts, samples, reinforced cement antibiotic-laden spacer
Step 3	Samples and arthroplasty

5

The main objective of total knee replacement in ballistic trauma is to restore function. Bone loss secondary to the trauma and septic resection indicates multi-step surgery with constrained implants (Morgan et al. 2005). Results with these prostheses are generally good (Holl et al. 2012), with recovery of unaided walking and complete extension. In devastating ballistic trauma, the range of motion remains lower than with similar first-line or revision implants in a non-septic context (Calori et al. 2014). Management of ballistic trauma should be multidisciplinary. Medically, sepsis is inevitable and requires teamwork with infectious disease specialists. Knee replacement should be performed only after bacteriologic analysis and effective antibiotic therapy of sufficient duration (Bernard et al. 2010). Surgically, skill in plastic surgery (negative pressure, flap, etc.) is mandatory (Hou et al. 2011). Nevertheless, the morbidity rate is high (Holl et al. 2012). Prolonged antibiotherapy may prove toxic in such cases, which should be taken into account in the primary decision-making.

The treatment strategy for severe ballistic trauma to the knee is not described in the literature. We have drawn up a management protocol for this situation in which severe joint destruction (Dougherty et al. 2009) requires surgical reconstruction (Calori et al. 2014).

A three-step surgical strategy is implemented after the acute phase;

- Step 1 comprises hardware removal and sampling.
- Step 2 comprises septic surgery, with bone cuts and positioning of a reinforced cement antibiotic-laden spacer, as widely practiced in implant revision surgery (Classen et al. 2014; Nickinson et al. 2012).
- Step 3 is arthroplasty, performed after a time interval, when infection control has been achieved.

Contra-indications to arthroplasty comprise neurovascular disorder and extensor system tear (Biau et al. 2006). Risk of sepsis is high (Bae et al. 2005; Suzuki et al. 2011) and requires bacteriological analysis, with at least 6 weeks of adapted antibiotic therapy before considering implantation. The three-step strategy was drawn up owing to this major risk of infection. A second bone cut step limits risk of sepsis at implantation, delayed until samples prove sterile or antibiotic therapy adapted to bacteriological findings has been initiated.

Timing	Surgery	Antibiotics	Adverse event
Day 0	Lavage wound care External fixator	Ceftriaxone gentamicin	
Day 14	Lavage	Ceftriaxone ofloxacin	Effusion on pins
Day 167	External fixator ablation		
Day 195	Bone cuts Antibiotic-laden cement spacer	Ceftriaxone teicoplanin ofloxacin vancomycin fosfomycin rocephin teicoplanin	
Day 256	Reinforced cement spacer	Teicoplanin	Fracture of the spacer
Day 465	Reimplantation	Teicoplanin	

5.4.7 A Patient with Relapsing »Aseptic« Tibial Pseudarthrosis

A 57-year-old man had a motorcycle accident on a public highway in 2012 with Gustilo II open fracture of the distal right leg. After debridement and wound closure, an intramedullary nail was inserted in the tibia and the fibula was fixed by a plate. In September 2013, tibia non-union was treated by a one-stage surgery: removal of the nail, bone grafting of the tibia defect and plate osteosynthesis. All intraoperative samples were found sterile after cultures. At the end of 2013, mechanical pain reappeared. No fistula was noticed. On X-rays, three screws were found to be broken (◘ Fig. 5.18a). Therefore, relapsing pseudarthrosis was diagnosed (◘ Fig. 5.18a). A two-stage strategy with bone resection, also called »Masquelet« technique (induced membrane) (Mauffrey et al. 2015), was proposed. In the first stage, debridement and resection of the diseased bone were performed, multiple bone specimens were sent to the bacteriology laboratory and the bone was stabilized with an external fixator and a cement spacer Subsequently, piperacillin-tazobactam (12g per day) and vancomycin (2g per day) were given as initial empirical therapy (◘ Fig. 5.18b). MSSA and *P. acnes* grew from several bacterial samples, but exclusively in anaerobic liquid media at day 14. The patient experienced acute kidney failure and a rash under the initial empirical therapy, which was instantly replaced by daptomycin and rifampin. A neutropoenia related to rifampin was then diagnosed, and the patient was switched to ofloxacin. Daptomycin and ofloxacin administration was continued for 3 months after the first surgical stage. Two weeks after this antibiotic window, the second stage was carried out: spacer removal, bone biopsies, large autologous bone graft (from the iliac crest

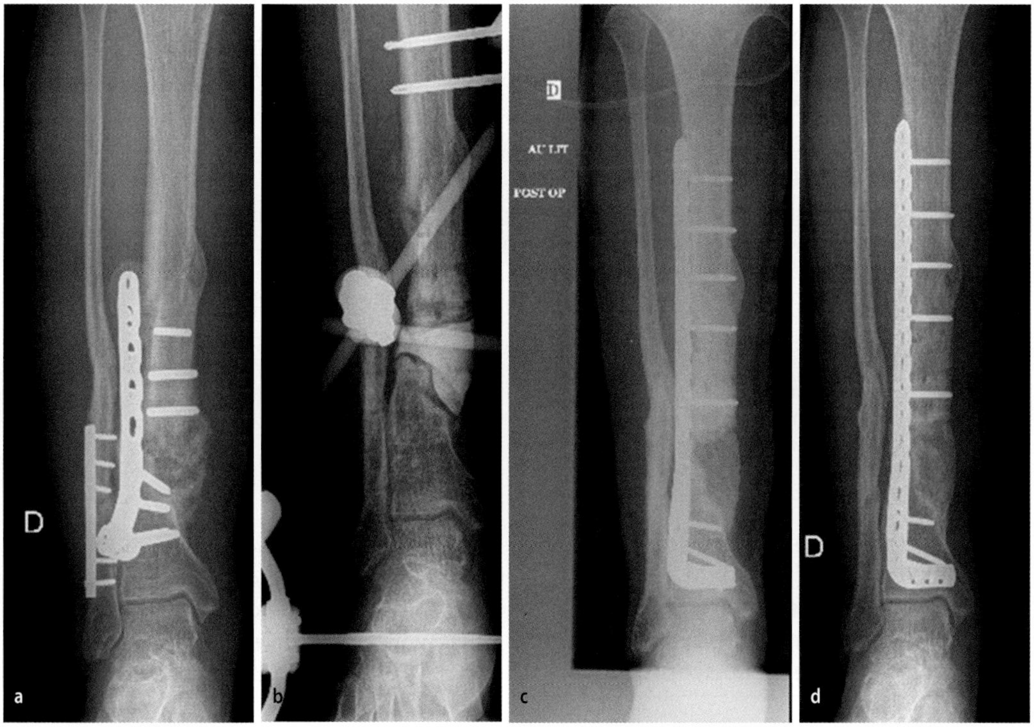

◘ **Fig. 5.18 a–d** Relapsing pseudarthrosis of the right tibia requiring a »Masquelet« two-stage surgery. **a** X-ray showing relapsing pseudarthrosis with three broken screws. **b** X-ray after the first-stage surgery (bone resection, bone sampling and external fixation). **c** X-ray after the second-stage surgery (bone grafting and plate osteosynthesis). **d** X-ray 18 months after the second-stage surgery showing bone union in a patient who could walk without pain bone) and osteosynthesis with a locking plate (◘ Fig. 5.18c). An empirical antimicrobial therapy with high doses of daptomycin (8 mg/kg/day) and ofloxacin was prescribed, and was rapidly stopped as the bacterial culture did not reveal any pathogen. Eighteen months following the second-stage surgery, the patient could walk without any pain and X-rays showed a well-united bone (◘ Fig. 5.18d).

Recurrent pseudarthrosis is mostly associated with chronic infection. In these patients, bacteria usually grow slowly in culture, and sometimes exclusively in anaerobic media. Performing multiple bone biopsies (at least five) and seeding these samples in solid and liquid media for a total culture duration of 14 days are crucial to identify the pathogen in such clinical situations (Schäfer et al. 2008). In this case, *S. aureus*, which is not an exclusive anaerobic bacterium, grew exclusively at day 14 in liquid media. No pathogen was found during the previous one-stage surgery, as these important conditions were probably not respected. This two-stage strategy is particularly adequate in patients with pseudarthrosis, and the second stage can be performed at 6 weeks under antimicrobial therapy in the case of non-relapsing pseudarthrosis. In the case described here, the second stage was performed at 3 months and after a 2-week antibiotic window, as the patient presented with relapsing pseudarthrosis. Daptomycin is not labelled for the treatment of BJI. Daptomycin has been proposed as an alternative therapeutic option in patients with staphylococcus or enterococcus PJI in the recent Infectious Diseases Society of America (IDSA) guidelines (6 mg/kg/day; Osmon et al. 2013). However, as bone penetration of daptomycin is limited, some authors proposed higher doses in BJI (i.e. 8 mg/kg/day). We recently published our experience concerning the use of high doses of daptomycin in patients with BJI (Roux et al. 2016). Prolonged high-dose daptomycin therapy was effective in patients with complex BJI, but eosinophilic pneumonia was recorded at a higher than expected incidence. Moreover, we demonstrated inter-individual and intra-individual variability in daptomycin clearance, which was significantly higher in male than in female patients. We also observed significant intra-individual changes in daptomycin clearance, which was uncorrelated with changes in renal function, suggesting that therapeutic drug monitoring is important in patients with BJI treated with daptomycin (Goutelle et al. 2016).

Timing	Surgery	Antibiotics	Adverse events
J0	Masquelet technique: 1st stage with external fixator + cement spacer	Piperacillin/tazobactam + vancomycin	Acute kidney failure + cutaneous rash
J10		Daptomycin + rifampicin	Neutropenia
J 32		Daptomycin + ofloxacin	
J105	Masquelet technique: 2nd stage with bone grafting and locking plate	Daptomycin + ofloxacin	

5.4.8 Preoperative Preventing Strategies of Surgical Site Infection in a Patient with Scheduled Revision Arthroplasty for Mechanical Prosthesis Loosening

A 68-year-old woman was referred by her general practitioner for a mechanical right painful hip arthroplasty 17 years after undergoing cementless primary right hip replacement. The patient also had a left hip arthroplasty without any pain. The evaluation showed prosthesis loosening with no further arguments for an infection (see ◘ Fig. 5.19). Total hip revision was scheduled.

The pre-anaesthesia consultation scheduled 1 month before surgery identified some risk factors related to the surgery: obesity with a body mass index (BMI) estimated at 41, recent history of diabetes mellitus, American Society of Anesthesiologists (ASA) Score = 2, and prosthetic joint revision

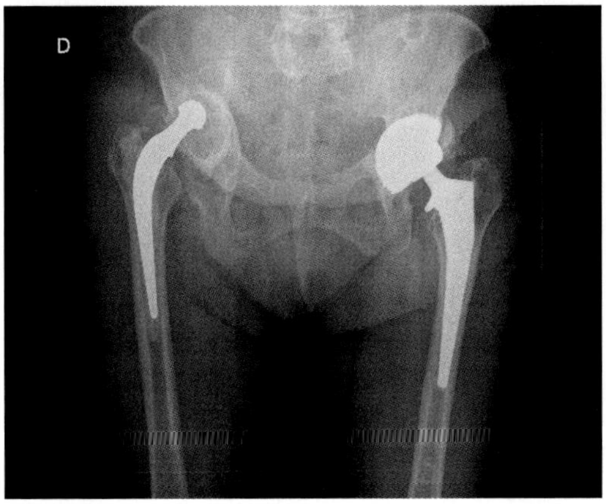

Fig. 5.19 Prosthesis loosening with no signs of infection

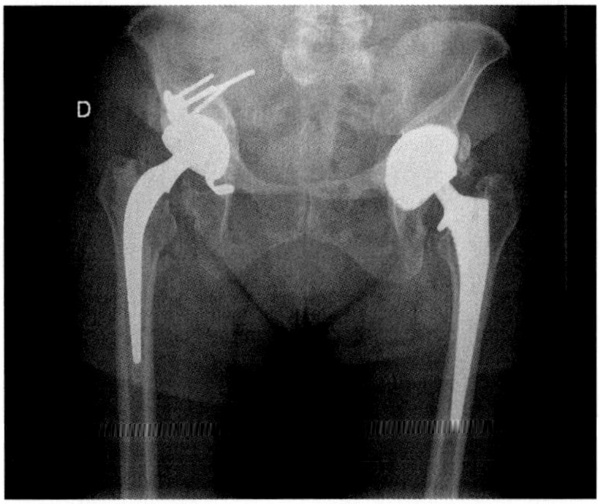

Fig. 5.20 Revision using prosthesis with gentamicin-impregnated cement

(Haute Autorité de Santé 2014). An interview did not identify allergies to drugs or foods. According to our national (La Société Française d'Anesthésie et Réanimation [SFAR] Société Française de Chirurgie Orthopédique et Traumatologique [SoFCOT] 2010) and American (Bratzler et al. 2013) guidelines, and with respect to the low prevalence of methicillin-resistant *Staphylococcus aureus* (MRSA) infections in our institution, cefazolin monotherapy was chosen as primary strategy for antimicrobial prophylaxis. Thus, we targeted the most frequent pathogen involved in early (methicillin-susceptible *S. aureus*, *Streptococci*, *Enterobacteriaceae*) or delayed (*P. acnes*) PJI in our institution. However, doses had to be doubled given the patient's BMI: 4 g in the preoperative period (at least 30 min before incision) and two additional post-operative doses of 2 g (8 and 16 h after surgery). Moreover, this patient could be a nasal carrier of MRSA, which could be an additional risk of post-operative surgical site infection. Recent data suggest that the risk for these *S. aureus* infections can be decreased by screening patients for nasal carriage of *S. aureus* and decolonizing carriers during the preoperative period with chlorhexidine bath and application of mupirocin in nostrils 5 days before the surgery (Schweizer et al. 2015). This procedure has clearly demonstrated its effectiveness in thoracic surgery, but not in orthopaedic surgery, which is why it is currently not recommended in France. However, the clinical practice in our institution includes the *S. aureus* decolonization treatment prior to joint arthroplasty for patients who have a history of *S. aureus* skin and soft tissue infection and/or bone and joint infection. The patient was admitted to hospital on the day before the surgery. The French national guidelines for patients' preoperative preparation ask for a minimum of one preoperative shower, with no recommendation concerning the use of an antiseptic scrub or not. Systematic shampooing is not recommended (head off the intervention site; SF2H 2013).

Based on our surgeons' experience and significant findings in the past (Garibaldi 1988; Hayek et al. 1987; Paulson 1993), two showers with an antiseptic scrub (the day of admission and the morning before the intervention) are required at our centre, which is controlled by the paramedical staff before the patient is transferred to the operating room.

During the patient's second systematic pre-anaesthesia interview, which is conducted during the pre-induction step, the patient finally remembered the occurrence of a rash immediately after taking amoxicillin prescribed by her general practitioner for a sore throat 10 years previously. No investigation of a potential penicillin hypersensitivity was conducted and no more AB exposition had been performed yet. Despite the low risk of cross-reactivity with cefazolin, the antimicrobial prophylaxis was switched to vancomycin monotherapy, with 15 mg/kg for 1 h of continuous intravenous infusion before incision (max. 2 g), which resulted in a satisfactory renal function. A second post-operative injection with the same dose was administered after 12 h (SFAR SoFCOT 2010; Bratzler et al. 2013). The French national societies of anaesthesiology and infectology debate the addition of gentamicin to vancomycin in antimicrobial prophylaxis to target Enterobacteriaceae, since vancomycin is only active on Gram-positive bacteria. The comparative analysis of our prospective local surveillance of surgical site infections in orthopaedics, our bacterial ecology and the antimicrobial prophylaxis recorded, as well as the risk for gentamicin renal toxicity indicate that the systematic addition of gentamicin to vancomycin should not be recommended. Instead of vancomycin, clindamycin could be used for patients with a beta-lactam allergy at the dose of 600 mg before incision, with two additional post-operative doses of 600 mg (8 and 16 h after surgery). However, clindamycin does not have any activity against Enterobacteriaceae.

On the day of surgery, the patient is transferred to the operative room and the paramedical staff begin the preoperative skin preparation. The first step, scrubbing the operative site, is optional and not necessary if the skin is free of gross contamination (e.g. dirt, soil, or any other debris). Next, two alcohol-containing antiseptic agents are applied successively (one in the preparation room, one in the operating room), allocating sufficient time for drying after each application.

For the revision, a cemented prosthesis was used with a gentamicin-impregnated cement (see ◘ Fig. 5.20). As is known, the rate of post-operative infection is higher in revision procedures compared with primary arthroplasty. Therefore, we chose to use gentamicin-impregnated cement (Palacos® R+G) for revision in our institution.

▪ **Acknowledgements**

Lyon Bone and Joint Infection Study Group: Coordinator: Tristan Ferry; **Infectious Diseases Specialists** – Tristan Ferry, Florent Valour, Thomas Perpoint, André Boibieux, François Biron, Patrick Miailhes, Florence Ader, Agathe Becker, Sandrine Roux, Claire Philit, Fatiha Daoud, Johanna Lippman, Evelyne Braun, Christian Chidiac, Yves Gillet, Laure Hees; **Surgeons** – Sébastien Lustig, Philippe Neyret, Yannick Herry, Romain Gaillard, Antoine Schneider, Michel-Henry Fessy, Anthony Viste, Philippe Chaudier, Romain Desmarchelier, Thibault Vermersch, Sébastien Martres, Franck Trouillet, Cédric Barrey, Francesco Signorelli, Emmanuel Jouanneau, Timothée Jacquesson, Ali Mojallal, Fabien Boucher, Hristo Shipkov, Mehdi Ismail, Joseph Chateau; **Anesthesiologists** – Frédéric Aubrun, Isabelle Bobineau, Caroline Macabéo; **Microbiologists** – Frederic Laurent, François Vandenesch, Jean-Philippe Rasigade, Céline Dupieux; **Nuclear Medicine** – Isabelle Morelec, Marc Janier, Francesco Giammarile; **PK/PD specialists** – Michel Tod, Marie-Claude Gagnieu, Sylvain Goutelle; **Prevention of infection** – Vincent Ronin, Solweig Gerbier-Colomban, Thomas Benet; **Clinical Research Assistant** – Eugénie Mabrut

Take-Home Message

- The guideline for adequate treatment of complex bone and joint infections is the responsibility of the health government, whose activities are monitored by the ministry and adjusted if necessary.
- The incidence of complex BPJI is low, but is associated with high morbidity, motor disability, cost and mortality. Further wandering patients often undergo numerous suboptimal surgeries.
- Regional reference centres for difficult-to-treat pathologies, like CRIOAcs for the management of BPJI, assure equity in patient care.
- Micro-organisms must be identified and be sensitive to antibiotics.
- In clinical practice, the preoperative prevention of surgical site infections is by:
  a. anasal screening and decolonization to decrease *S. aureus* infections
  b. two showers with antiseptic scrub
- The antimicrobial prophylaxis should be adjusted to the medical history of the patient

References

Bae DK, Yoon KH, Kim HS, Song SJ (2005) Total knee arthroplasty in stiff knees after previous infection. J Bone Joint Surg Br 87:333-336

Bernard L, Legout L, Zurcher-Pfund L, Stern R, Rohner P, Peter R et al (2010) Six weeks of antibiotic treatment is sufficient following surgery for septic arthroplasty. J Infect 61:125-132

Biau D, Faure F, Katsahian S, Jeanrot C, Tomeno B, Anract P (2006) Survival of total knee replacement with a megaprosthesis after bone tumor resection. J Bone Joint Surg Am 88:1285-1293

Bratzler DW, Dellinger EP, Olsen KM, Perl TM, Auwaerter PG, et al (2013) Clinical practice guidelines for antimicrobial prophylaxis in surgery. Am J Health Syst Pharm 70(3):195-283

Byren I, Bejon P, Atkins BL, Angus B, Masters S, McLardy-Smith P, Gundle R, Berendt A (2009) One hundred and twelve infected arthroplasties treated with 'DAIR' (debridement, antibiotics and implant retention): antibiotic duration and outcome. J Antimicrob Chemother 63:1264-1271

Calori GM, Colombo M, Malagoli E, Mazzola S, Bucci M, Mazza E (2014) Megaprosthesis in post-traumatic and periprosthetic large bone defects: issues to consider. Injury 45(6):S105-S110

Castellanos J, Flores X, Llusa M, Chiriboga C, Navarro A (1998) The Girdlestone pseudarthrosis in the treatment of infected hip replacements. Int Orthop 22(3): 178-181

Centres de reference interregionaux pour la prise en charge des infections osteo articulaires complexes (2016) Ministère des Affaires sociales et de la Santé, France. http://www.sante.gouv.fr/centres-de-reference-interregionaux-pour-la-prise-en-charge-des-infections-osteo-articulaires-complexes.html

Classen T, von Knoch M, Wernsmann M, Landgraeber S, Loer F, Jager M (2014) Functional interest of an articulating spacer in two-stage infected total knee arthroplasty revision. Orthop Traumatol Surg Res 100:409-412

CRIOAc Lyon (2016) Le Centre de Référence des Infections Ostéo-articulaires Complexes, France. http://www.crioac-lyon.fr

Crockarell JR, Hanssen AD, Osmon DR, Morrey BF (1998) Treatment of infection with debridement and retention of the components following hip arthroplasty. J Bone Joint Surg Am 80:1306-1313

Dougherty PJ, Vaidya R, Silverton CD, Bartlett C, Najibi S (2009) Joint and long-bone gunshot injuries. J Bone Joint Surg Am 91:980-997

Elyasi S, Khalili H, Dashti-Khavidaki S, Mohammadpour A (2012) Vancomycin-induced nephrotoxicity: mechanism, incidence, risk factors and special populations. A literature review. Eur J Clin Pharmacol 68:1243-1255

Ferry T, Perpoint T, Vandenesch F, Etienne J (2005) Virulence determinants in Staphylococcus aureus and their involvement in clinical syndromes. Curr Infect Dis Rep 7:420-428

Garibaldi RA (1988) Prevention of intraoperative wound contamination with chlorhexidine shower and scrub. J Hosp Infect 11(Suppl B):5-9

Grauer JD, Amstutz HC, O'Carroll PF, Dorey FJ (1989) Resection arthroplasty of the hip. J Bone Joint Surg Am 71(5):669-678

Goutelle S, Roux S, Gagnieu MC, Valour F, Lustig S, Ader F, Laurent F, Chidiac C, Ferry T (2016) Pharmacokinetic variability of daptomycin during prolonged therapy for bone and joint infections. Antimicrob Agents Chemother 60(5):3148-3151

Haute Autorité de Santé (2014) Recommandation de bonne pratique. Prothèses de hanche ou de genou: diagnostic et prise en charge de l'infection dans le mois suivant l'implantation. Saint-Denise, France. http://www.has-sante.fr/portail/jcms/c_1228574/fr/prothese-de-hanche-ou-de-genou-diagnostic-et-prise-en-charge-de-l-infection-dans-le-mois-suivant-l-implantation

Hayek LJ, Emerson JM, Gardner AM (1987) A placebo-controlled trial of the effect of two preoperative baths or showers with chlorhexidine detergent on postoperative wound infection rates. J Hosp Infect 10:165-172

Holl S, Schlomberg A, Gosheger G, Dieckmann R, Streitbuerger A, Schulz D et al (2012) Distal femur and proximal tibia replacement with megaprosthesis in revision knee arthroplasty: a limb-saving procedure. Knee Surg Sports Traumatol Arthrosc 20:2513-2518

Hou Z, Irgit K, Strohecker KA, Matzko ME, Wingert NC, DeSantis JG et al (2011) Delayed flap reconstruction with vacuum-assisted closure management of the open IIIB tibial fracture. J Trauma 71:1705-1708

Kantor GS, Osterkamp JA, Dorr LD, Fischer D, Perry J, Conaty JP (1986) Resection arthroplasty following infected total hip replacement arthroplasty. J Arthroplasty 1(2): 83-89

Kim SH, Kim KH, Kim HB et al (2008) Outcome of vancomycin treatment in patients with methicillin-susceptible Staphylococcus aureus bacteremia. Antimicrob Agents Chemother 52:192-197

Konigsberg BS, Della Valle CJ, Ting NT, Qiu F, Sporer SM (2014) Acute hematogenous infection following total hip and knee arthroplasty. J Arthroplasty 29:469-472

Lagace-Wiens P, Rubinstein E (2012) Adverse reactions to beta-lactam antimicrobials. Expert Opin Drug Saf 11:381-399

Lora-Tamayo J, Murillo O, Iribarren JA, Soriano A, Sanchez-Somolinos M, Baraia-Etxaburu JM, Rico A, Palomino J, Rodriguez-Pardo D, Horcajada JP, Benito N, Bahamonde A, Granados A, del Toro MD, Cobo J, Riera M, Ramos A, Jover-Saenz A, Ariza J (2013) A large multicenter study of methicillin-susceptible and methicillinresistant *Staphylococcus aureus* prosthetic joint infections managed with implant retention. Clin Infect Dis 56:182-194

Malcolm TL, Gad BV, Elsharkawy KA, Higuera CA (2015) Complication, Survival, and Reoperation Rates Following Girdlestone Resection Arthroplasty. J Arthroplasty 30(7):1183-1186

Malizos K, Sarma J, Seaton RA, Militz M, Menichetti F, Ricchio G, Gaudias J, Trostmann U, Pathan R, Hamed K (2015) Daptomycin for the treatment of osteomyelitis and orthopaedic device infections: a real-world clinical experience from a European registry. Eur J Clin Microbiol Infect Dis 35:111-118

Marculescu CE, Berbari EF, Hanssen AD, Steckelberg JM, Harmsen SW, Mandrekar JN, Osmon DR (2006) Outcome of prosthetic joint infections treated with debridement and retention of components. Clin Infect Dis 42:471-478

Mauffrey C, Hake ME, Chadayammuri V, Masquelet AC (2015) Reconstruction of long bone infections using the induced membrane technique: tips and tricks. J Orthop Trauma 30(6):e188-193

Morgan H, Battista V, Leopold SS (2005) Constraint in primary total knee arthroplasty. J Am Acad Orthop Surg 13:515-524

Murdoch DR, Roberts SA, Fowler VG, Jr, Shah MA, Taylor SL, Morris AJ, Corey GR (2001) Infection of orthopedic prostheses after *Staphylococcus aureus* bacteremia. Clin Infect Dis 32:647-649

Nickinson RS, Board TN, Gambhir AK, Porter ML, Kay PR (2012) Two stage revision knee arthroplasty for infection with massive bone loss. A technique to achieve spacer stability. Knee 19:24-27

Osmon DR, Berbari EF, Berendt AR, Lew D, Zimmerli W, Steckelberg JM, Rao N, Hanssen A, Wilson WR (2013) Diagnosis and management of prosthetic joint infection: clinical practice guidelines by the Infectious Diseases Society of America. Clin Infect Dis 56(1):e1-e25

Paulson DS (1993) Efficacy evaluation of a 4% chlorhexidine gluconate as a full-body shower wash. Am J Infect Control 21(4):205-209

Rand JA, Bryan RS (1983) Reimplantation for the salvage of an infected total knee arthroplasty. J Bone Joint Surg Am 65:1081-1086

Rao N, Crossett LS, Sinha RK, Le Frock JL (2003) Long-term suppression of infection in total joint arthroplasty. Clin Orthop Relat Res 414:55-60

Roux S, Valour F, Karsenty J, Gagnieu MC, Perpoint T, Lustig S, Ader F, Martha B, Laurent F, Chidiac C, Ferry T; Lyon BJI Study group (2016) Daptomycin > 6 mg/kg/day as salvage therapy in patients with complex bone and joint infection: cohort study in a regional reference center. BMC Infect Dis 16(1):83

Salgado CD, Dash S, Cantey JR, Marculescu CE (2007) Higher risk of failure of methicillin-resistant Staphylococcus aureus prosthetic joint infections. Clin Orthop Relat Res 461:48-53

Schäfer P, Fink B, Sandow D, Margull A, Berger I, Frommelt L (2008) Prolonged bacterial culture to identify late periprosthetic joint infection: a promising strategy. Clin Infect Dis 47(11):1403-1409

Schroder J, Saris D, Besselaar PP, Marti RK (1998) Comparison of the results of the Girdlestone pseudarthrosis with reimplantation of a total hip replacement. Int Orthop 22(4):215-218

Schweizer ML, Chiang HY, Septimus E, Moody J, Braun B, Hafner J, Ward MA, Hickok J, Perencevich EN, Diekema DJ, Richards CL5 Cavanaugh JE, Perlin JB, Herwaldt LA (2015) Association of a bundled intervention with surgical site infections among patients undergoing cardiac, hip, or knee surgery. JAMA 313(21):2162-2171

Sendi P, Banderet F, Graber P, Zimmerli W (2011) Periprosthetic joint infection following *Staphylococcus aureus* bacteremia. J Infect 63:17-22

Seng VS, Masquelet AC (2013) Management of civilian ballistic fractures. Orthop Traumatol Surg Res 99:953–958

SFAR SoFCOT ORTHORISQ (2010) Recommandations. Antibioprophylaxie en chirurgie orthopédique et traumatologique. La Société Française d'Anesthésie et Réanimation, Paris, France. http://www.orthorisq.fr/rc/fr/orthorisq/htm/Article/2011/20110225-215945-892/src/htm_fullText/fr/AntibioprophylaxieSFARORTHORISQCIPRET(1).pdf

Société Française d'Hygiène Hospitalière (SF2H) (2013) Mise à jour de la conférence de consensus Gestion préopératoire du risque infectieux. Hygiene, Saint-Sébastien-sur-Loire, France. http://nosobase.chu-lyon.fr/recommandations/sfhh/2013_gestion_preoperatoire_SF2H.pdf

Suzuki G, Saito S, Ishii T, Motojima S, Tokuhashi Y, Ryu J (2011) Previous fracture surgery is a major risk factor of infection after total knee arthroplasty. Knee Surg Sports Traumatol Arthrosc 19:2040-4

Tsukayama DT, Wicklund B, Gustilo RB (1991) Suppressive antibiotic therapy in chronic prosthetic joint infections. Orthopedics 14(8):841-4

Uckay I, Lubbeke A, Emonet S, Tovmirzaeva L, Stern R, Ferry T, Assal M, Bernard L, Lew D, Hoffmeyer P (2009) Low incidence of haematogenous seeding to total hip and knee prostheses in patients with remote infections. J Infect 59:337-345

Valour F, Karsenty J, Bouaziz A, Ader F, Tod M, Lustig S, Laurent F, Ecochard R, Chidiac C, Ferry F (2014) Antimicrobial-related severe adverse events during treatment of bone and joint infection due to methicillin-susceptible Staphylococcus aureus. Antimicrob Agents Chemother 58:746-755

Treatment

K.-D. Kühn (Ed.), *Management of Periprosthetic Joint Infection*
DOI 10.1007/978-3-662-54469-3_6

6.1 Treatment of PJI: Overview

Tamon Kabata and Hiroyuki Tsuchiya

6.1.1 Introduction

The total joint arthroplasty (TJA) of the limb is a very effective treatment of degenerative and inflammatory diseases of the joint. The demand for TJAs is increasing with the aging of the population. The number of surgical site infections (SSIs) following TJA is growing, too (National Joint Registry 2013). The incidence of SSI is reported to be about 0.2–1.1% for primary total hip arthroplasty (THA) and about 1–2% for primary total knee arthroplasty (TKA; Urquhart et al. 2010; Illingworth et al. 2013). SSI is a serious complication and difficult to treat once it occurs. Although this is an issue where efforts should be made to find a solution, it is still difficult to completely prevent the SSI, which occurs with certain probabilities.

Periprosthetic joint infection (PJI) is a generic term that covers intraoperative bacterial infection during TJA, infection that spreads from a local infected site, haematogenous infection, and recurrent infection after suppurative arthritis; it does not include superficial infection (Della Valle et al. 2004). The Centers for Disease Control and Prevention/National Healthcare Safety Network (CDC/NHSN) defined SSIs as follows: Superficial incisional SSI is defined as infection that occurs within 30 days of an operative procedure, and deep incisional SSI and organ/space SSI are defined as infection that occurs within 90 days of an operative procedure. The CDC/NHSN includes early PJI in organ/space SSI (Mangram et al. 1999). One of the traditional diagnostic criteria of PJI has been defined by Berbari and coworkers as follows:

> » If two or more cultures of joint aspirates or cultures of intraoperative specimens yielded the same micro-organism, purulence surrounding the prosthesis was observed at the time of debridement or removal of the prosthesis, acute inflammation consistent with infection was present during histopathologic examination, or a sinus tract that communicated with the prosthesis was present (Berbari et al. 1998).

Recently, the CDC/NHSN proposed the diagnostic criteria shown in ◘ Tab. 6.1 (CDC/NHSN Surveillance Definition for Specific Types of Infections 2015).

PJI has a significant impact on the mortality of patients. The mortality rate from PJI at 1 year after revision surgery is said to be fivefold higher than that from aseptic loosening at 1 year after revision surgery (Zmistowski et al. 2013). Thus, appropriate treatment and diagnosis are required.

6.1.2 Patient Factors That Increase the Risk of PJI

Bacterial infection precedes the onset of PJI. The risk is represented in the following equation: bacterial load × virulence ÷ host resistance.

This indicates that not only the causative bacteria but also the host characteristics have a great influence on the risk of onset of PJI. Patient-related risk factors include age, gender, height, weight, primary disease, underlying disease, preoperative complications, history of antibiotics used in the 3 months before surgery, history of infusion and oral administration of steroid, usage of anti-rheumatic drugs, smoking before surgery, total protein volume, and albumin levels (Masaoka et al. 2009). Large-scale studies in the United States indicated that the significant risk factors in THA are rheumatic disease, obesity, coagulopathy and preoperative anaemia, and that significant risk factors in TKA are congestive heart failure, chronic pulmonary disease, preoperative anaemia, diabetes, depression, renal disease, pulmonary circulation disorders, obesity, rheumatologic disease, psychoses, metastatic tumour, peripheral vascular disease and valvular disease (Bozic et al. 2012a, 2012b). Non-patient-related factors are years of experience of the surgeon, types of prostheses, usage of bone cement, tourniquet use, usage of bone allograft, operative time, blood loss, necessity of autologous transfusion, use of drain, intraoperative prophylactic antibiotics, laminar air flow, the number of people present in the operative room during the surgery and the wearing of space suits. The results of the Japanese Orthopaedic Association project showed that the infection rate is higher in the fol-

Tab. 6.1 Definition of periprosthetic joint infection (from CDC/NHSN 2015)

Periprosthetic joint infection (following HPRO and KPRO only)
Joint or bursa infections must meet at least one of the following criteria:
1. Two positive periprosthetic specimens (tissue or fluid) with at least one matching organism, identified by a culture or non-culture-based microbiologic testing method that is performed for purposes of clinical diagnosis and treatment (e.g. not active surveillance culture/testing, ASC/AST)
2. A sinus tract communicating with the joint
3. Having *three* of the following minor criteria: a. Elevated CRP (>100 mg/l) *and* ESR (>30 mm/h) b. Elevated synovial fluid white blood cell count (>10,000 cells/ml) *OR++ (or greater)* change on leukocyte esterase test strip of synovial fluid c. Elevated synovial fluid polymorphonuclear neutrophil percentage (PMN% >90%) d. Positive histological analysis of periprosthetic tissue (>5 PMNs per high-power field) e. Organism identified from a single positive periprosthetic (tissue or fluid) by culture or non-culture-based microbiologic testing method that is performed for purposes of clinical diagnosis and treatment (e.g. not ASC/AST)

lowing situations: the years of experience of the surgeon is less than 10 years and more than 40 years, the usage of tumour prosthesis and monopolar head prosthesis, usage of non-antibiotic-loaded bone cement, allograft bone transplant, longer operative time, greater blood loss. As for the auto-transfusion, the infected group of patients had a higher rate of transfusion. Significant differences were not observed for the other factors (Masaoka et al. 2009). Some European and American registries have reported similar results in recent years. One of the interesting differences between these results and those of the Japanese studies is that the use of laminar air flow and space suits increased the infection rates (Evans 2011; Hooper et al. 2011). The reason for the increased infection rate by laminar air flow and space suits has not been elucidated.

6.1.3 How to Deal with PJIs in the Clinical Setting

The first step in treating infection is making the diagnosis. It is critical to make an accurate diagnosis promptly when PJI occurs. Information should be gathered immediately about the causative bacteria, the elapsed time since the occurrence of the infection (PJI staging), the severity and the risk factors of the patient (host).

The American Academy of Orthopaedic Surgeons (AAOS) published an algorithm for the diagnosis of PJI in 2010 (Fig. 6.1, Fig. 6.2; Della Valle et al. 2010). This algorithm proposes that the first screening is conducted by the quantification of the erythrocyte sedimentation rate/C-reactive protein (ESR/CRP). If these inflammatory markers are positive, specific tests with aspiration of the joint fluid are recommended as the second step. The Infectious Disease Society of America (ISDA) also proposed a clinical practice guideline for PJI diagnosis in 2013 (Osmon et al. 2013). In 2011 the Musculoskeletal Infection Society (MSIS)announced criteria for a stricter diagnosis of PJI (Parvizi et al. 2011), and in 2014 the CDC/NHSN put forward their PJI diagnosis criteria (CDC/NHSN Surveillance Definition for Specific Types of Infections 2015). They introduced two major criteria:

1. Two positive periprosthetic specimens identified by culture or non-culture-based microbiologic testing methods
2. A sinus tract communicating with the joint

The following minor criteria were also included:
- Positive inflammatory markers (CRP/ESR)
- Elevated synovial fluid white blood cell count
- Elevated synovial fluid neutrophil count
- Positive histology analysis
- Organisms identified from a single positive periprosthetic sample (*tissue or fluid*) by culture or non-culture-based microbiologic testing methods (Tab. 6.1).

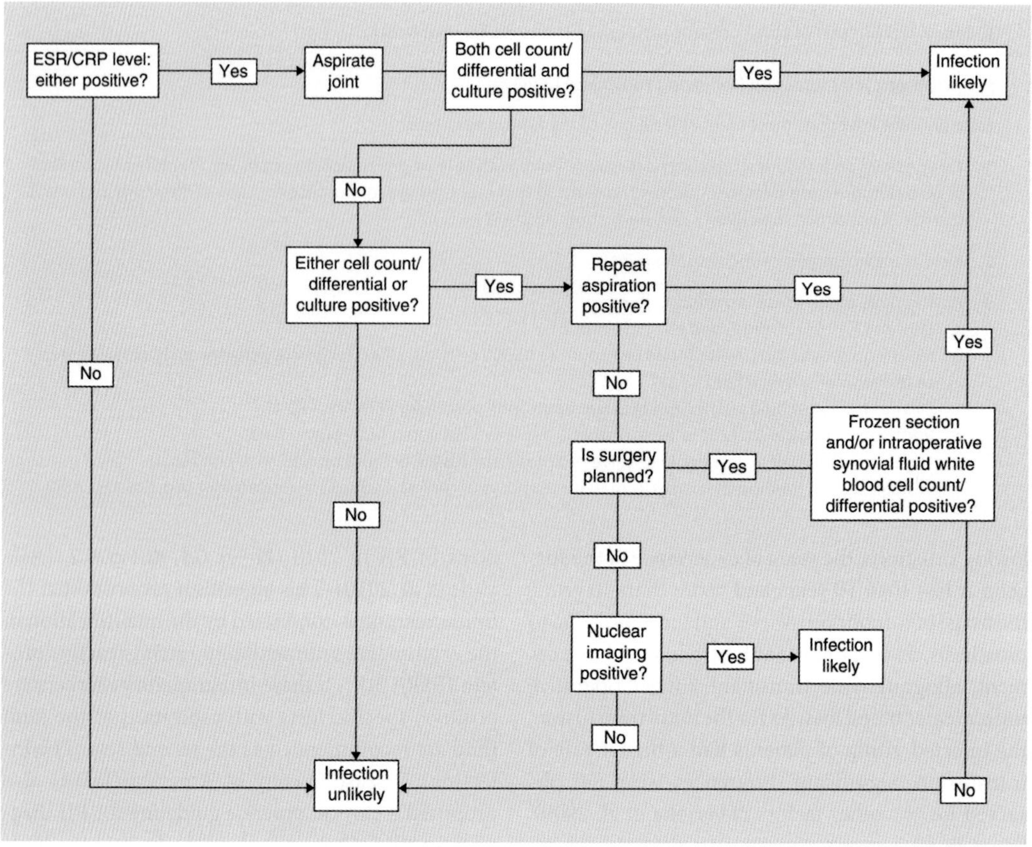

Fig. 6.1 American Academy of Orthopaedic Surgeons algorithm for patients with higher probability of hip or knee periprosthetic joint infection (from Della Valle et al. 2010)

The diagnosis of PJI can be made when one of the major criteria is met or three of the minor criteria are met. This means that although the diagnosis of PJI used to be made with one positive sample in the microbiologic culture test, the current consensus indicates that a single positive result is not sufficient. Although positive serum inflammatory markers (CRP/ESR) and quantification of white blood cells (WBCs) and neutrophils in the joint fluid used to be regarded as evaluations with low specificity, the current consensus admits that these tests are important for the diagnosis.

However, the diagnosis of PJI cannot always be made exclusively with these algorithms and diagnostic guidelines. It is not rare that causative bacteria cannot be identified. Sometimes CRP or ESR levels do not indicate inflammatory reactions. Occasionally, loosening seems to be aseptic loosening but is in fact low-grade septic loosening. The final diagnosis of PJI has to be made by a surgeon or an attending physician with their clinical judgement of each individual case, based on the comprehensive evaluation of the following:

- Clinical symptoms
- Local symptoms
- Blood tests
- Radiographs
- Microbiologic analysis
- Intraoperative findings
- Histological findings

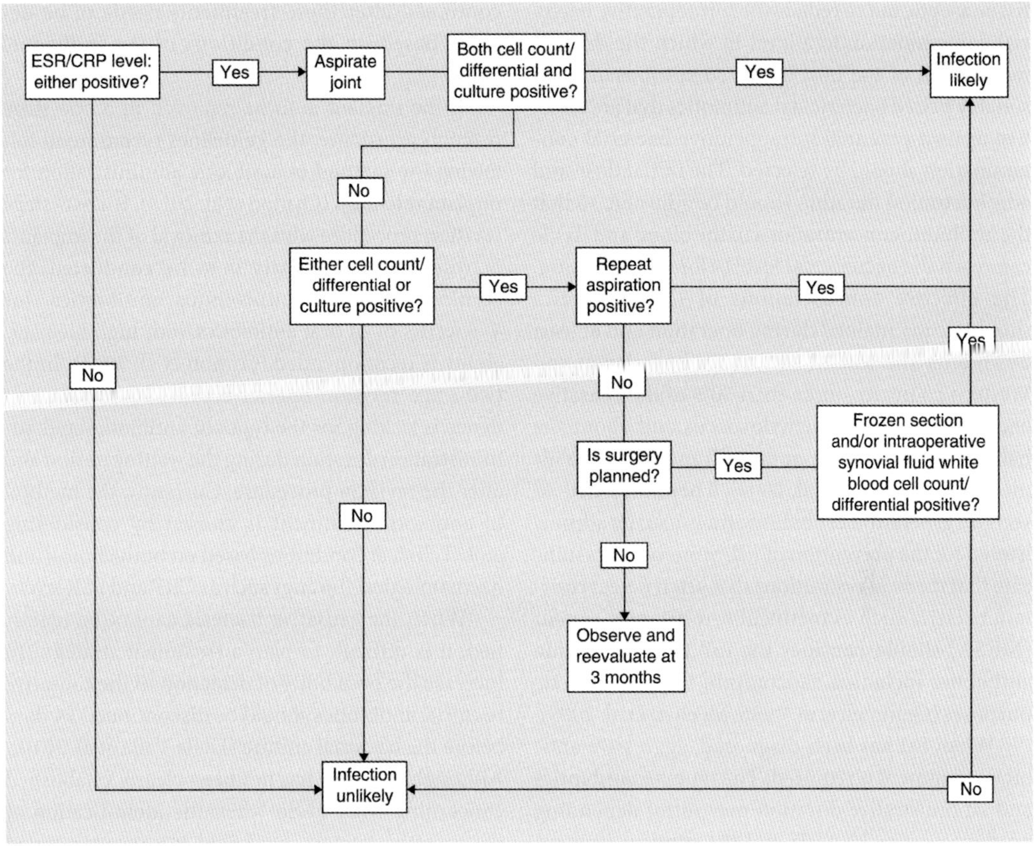

Fig. 6.2 American Academy of Orthopaedic Surgeons algorithm for patients with lower probability of hip or knee periprosthetic joint infection; wk weeks (from Della Valle et al. 2010)

Detection of the causative bacteria is critical for selecting the appropriate treatment strategy and antibiotics. However, it is not always easy. False-negative test results can occur when the causative bacteria need a special environment for growth, antibiotics have already been administered and the biofilm has been formed. The following recommendations should help improve the identification rate of the causative bacteria: multiple aspirations should be performed, samples should be collected from as many sites as possible (at least three) during the operative procedures, and the administration of antibiotics should be discontinued 14 days before bacterial culture (Trampuz et al. 2007; Della Valle et al. 2010). Recent reports indicate that polymerase chain reaction (PCR) and ultra-sonication are effective in detecting the causative bacteria (Trampuz et al. 2007; Kobayashi et al. 2009).

6.1.4 Which Antibiotics in Which Situations?

In the CDC/NHSN classification of surgical sites, most orthopaedic surgeries are classified as clean operative procedures (class 1). However, PJI is classified as a contaminated operative procedure (class 4; Mangram et al. 1999). The prophylactic antibiotics used against PJI in class 1 operations should be clearly distinguished from the antibiotics administered to treat class 4 cases.

The purpose of prophylactic use of antibiotics during operations is not to make the surgical site tissue aseptic but to reduce the intraoperative bacterial contamination to a level in which the defence mechanism of the host is not compromised. Reasonably priced bactericidal antibiotics that are effective against potential intraoperative bacterial contamination should be selected. The initial dose and administration duration should be adjusted, so that the antibiotic concentrations in the blood and tissue can reach the bactericidal level before skin incision. The effective concentrations of the antibiotics should be maintained during operation and at least 2–3 h after the wound closure. In both Japan and Western countries, more than 50% of the causative bacteria of PJIs are staphylococcus and about the half are *Staphylococcus aureus* (Trampuz and Widmer 2006; Masaoka et al. 2009). Therefore, first- or second-generation cephalosporin is usually administered for the prevention of PJI. Some authors indicate that medical institutions that often detect resistant bacteria such as methicillin-resistant *S. aureus* (MRSA) should consider the use of glycopeptide antibiotics including vancomycin for prophylactic purposes (Gemmell et al. 2006; Meehan et al. 2009).

When PJI has been diagnosed, aggressive antibiotic treatment is required. The types of antibiotics and administrative duration may differ depending on the causative bacteria and the surgical strategy, e.g. one-stage or two-stage revision procedure, and if the implant is to be retained or not.

The Infectious Diseases Society of America (IDSA) guidelines recommend that, in the case of *S. aureus* infection and implant retention, antibiotics that are effective against the causative bacteria should be selected and administered intravenously for 2–6 weeks, followed by 3–6 months of oral administration in combination with rifampicin. Rifampicin can more easily penetrate the biofilm and may possibly promote the removal of bacteria from the surface of the implant (Zimmerli et al. 1998). Regarding the treatment against other bacteria, it is recommended to use antibiotics to which the causative bacteria are susceptible in combination with the administration of intravenous antibiotics for 4–6 weeks or of oral antibiotics with high bioavailability (Osmon et al. 2013). In any case, clinical and laboratory monitoring for efficacy and toxicity is advisable. Whether or not chronic oral antimicrobial suppressive therapy should be continued after these treatments needs to be decided based on the conditions of the individual cases.

If the implant is to be removed in a one-stage revision procedure, the guidelines recommend following the method of antibiotic administration for implant retention (Osmon et al. 2013). If a two-stage revision procedure with the removal of the implants or resection arthroplasty is to be conducted, the administration of intravenous antibiotics for 4–6 weeks or of oral antibiotics with high bioavailability is recommended (Osmon et al. 2013). In the two-stage revision operative procedure, clear evidence is lacking for the types of antibiotics and administration duration during the waiting period and after the revision procedure. Currently, the method of antibiotic treatment is chosen by considering global clinical conditions based on both clinical and haematological findings such as CRP and ESR levels.

When the causative bacteria cannot be identified, it is difficult to plan a treatment strategy. To increase the possibility of detection of the causative bacteria, antibiotics should be discontinued 14 days before the bacterial culture (Della Valle et al. 2010). Although evidence has not been clearly established concerning what to do when the identification of the causative bacteria has failed, it is recommended that acute haematogenous infections should initially be treated with a combination of cefazolin and gentamicin therapy. All chronic and acute postoperative infections with Gram-positive bacteria and all cases in which a Gram staining fails to identify bacteria should be managed with vancomycin. Some reports indicate that infections with Gram-negative bacteria should be managed with a third- or fourth-generation cephalosporin, and that infections with mixed Gram-positive and Gram-negative bacteria should be managed with a combination of vancomycin and a third- or fourth-generation cephalosporin (Fulkerson et al. 2006).

6.1.5 Criteria for One-Stage Revisions, Two-Stage Revisions, and Other Procedures

There are two types of revision procedures for PJI: one-stage revisions and two-stage revisions. Generally, one-stage revisions are preferred in Europe and two-stage revisions in the United States and Japan (Zimmerli et al. 2004; Masaoka et al. 2009; Osmon et al. 2013). The two-stage revision is regarded the gold standard as it can resolve infection with higher probability. The disadvantages of two-stage revisions are the necessity for a long waiting period and two or more operative procedures. These could be a significant burden for elderly patients and compromised hosts. Therefore, less invasive one-stage revisions should be considered when certain criteria are met.

Zimmerli et al. proposed a standard algorithm for the selection of one-stage, two-stage revisions or other methods (◘ Fig. 6.4; Zimmerli et al. 2004). In the IDSA guidelines, the criteria for implant retention are similar to those indicated by Zimmerli et al. (◘ Fig. 6.5, ◘ Fig. 6.6), but criteria for one-stage exchange are stricter. The seven criteria are as follows:

1. The PJI should be of the THA.
2. There should be good soft tissue.
3. The identity of the organisms should be determined preoperatively.
4. There should be good bone stock.
5. The organisms should be susceptible to oral agents with high oral bioavailability.
6. Antibiotic-impregnated bone cement should be used for fixation.
7. No bone grafting is required (◘ Fig. 6.6; Osmon et al. 2013).

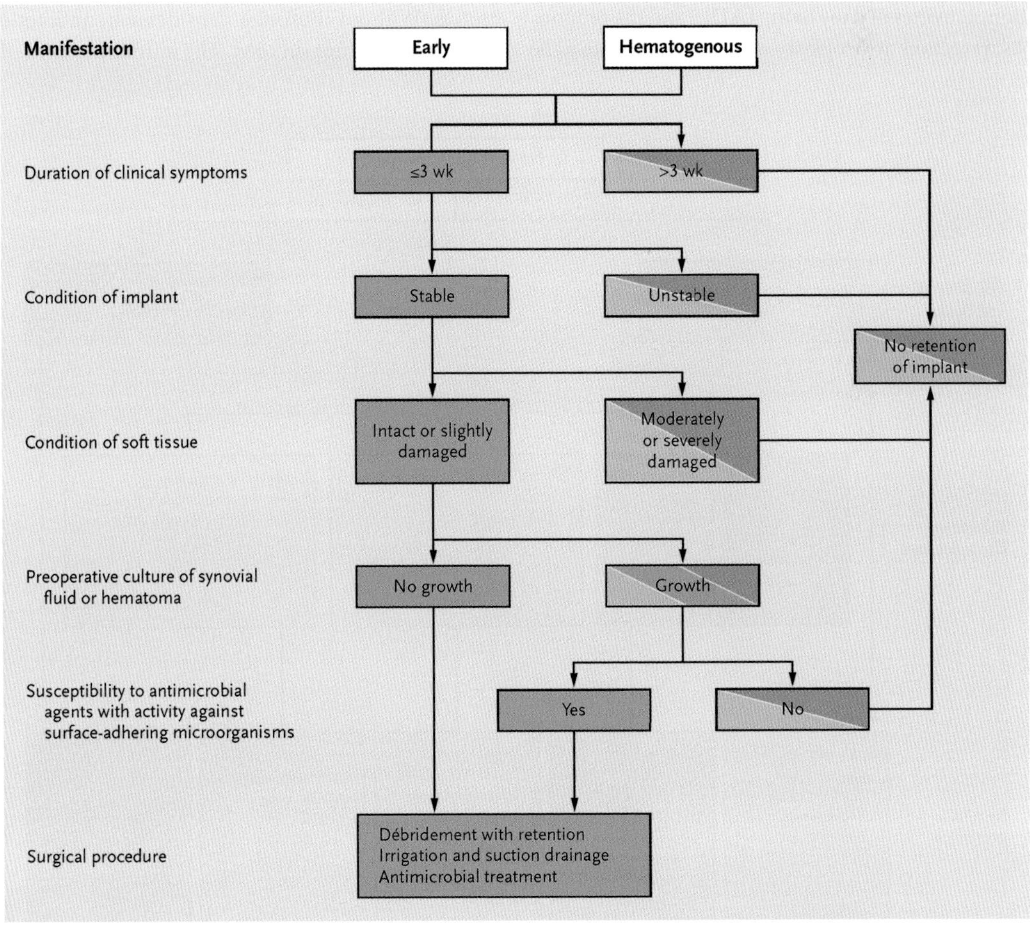

◘ **Fig. 6.3** Algorithm for the treatment of early or haematogenous infection associated with a prosthetic joint (from Zimmerli et al. 2004)

Some authors recommended two-stage revisions when the causative bacteria are multi-drug resistant, as in case of MRSA and methicillin-resistant *S. epidermidis* (MRSE), or if it is a Gram-negative organism (Jackson and Schmalzried 2000; Zimmerli et al. 2004). Nevertheless, some authors reported 80–90% success rates for one-stage revisions (Loty et al. 1992; Raut et al. 1994; Rudelli et al. 2008). Clear evidence has not been established on the indication of one-stage and two-stage revision procedures. Various opinions have been reported about the difference in the re-infection rates between one-stage and two-stage revision surgeries, but no definite conclusions have been drawn yet (Masaoka et al. 2009; Osmon et al. 2013; Kunutsor et al. 2015, 2016).

If revision surgery is considered not to be beneficial for a patient based on his/her systemic condition, activities of daily living (ADL) and the prognosis, resection arthroplasty and amputation may be selected. If the operative procedure itself is considered not to provide any benefit to a patient, suppression therapy, in which only antibiotic treatment is conducted, could be one of the treatment options (◘ Fig. 6.3, ◘ Fig. 6.7; Zimmerli et al. 2004; Osmon et al. 2013). In suppression therapy, combination antibiotic therapy is at first conducted for 3 months to resolve the infection, followed by long-term antibiotic administration to suppress any recurrence (Rao et al. 2003).

6.1.6 Role and Value of Irrigation and Surgical Debridement

The basics of the PJI treatment are aggressive debridement and administration of appropriate antibiotics. Without thorough debridement, antibiotic treatment does not succeed. The immune system of

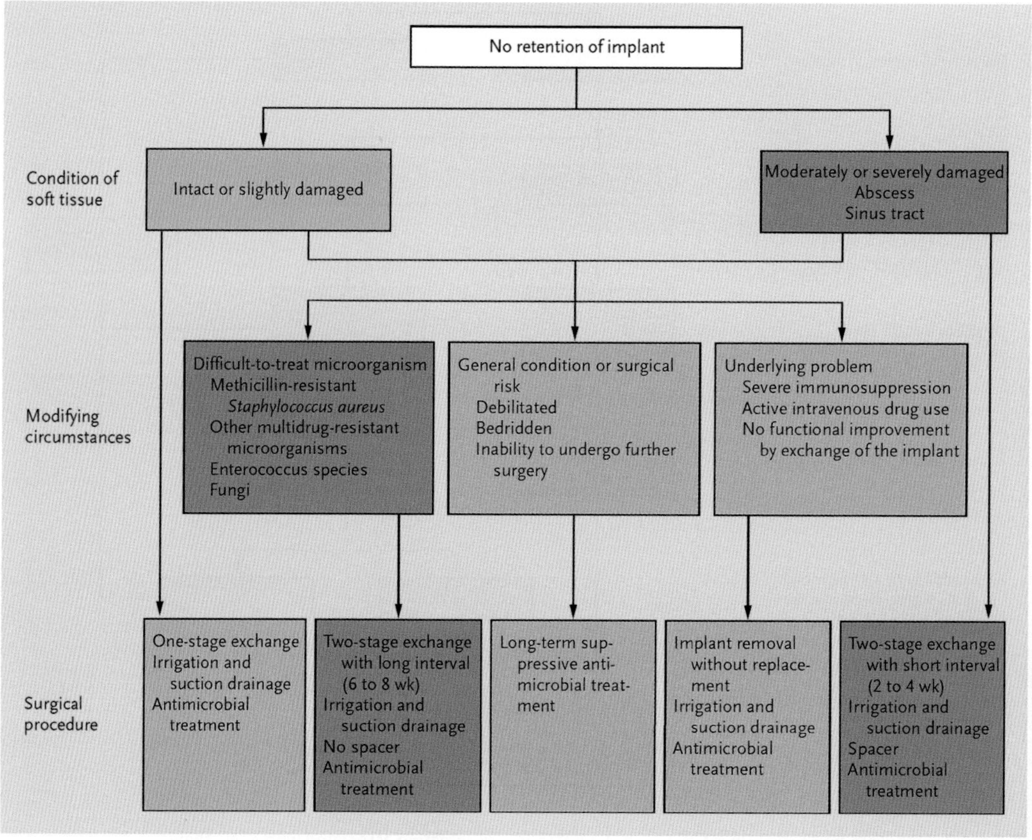

◘ **Fig. 6.4** Algorithm for the treatment of patients with infections not qualifying for implant retention (from Zimmerli et al. 2004)

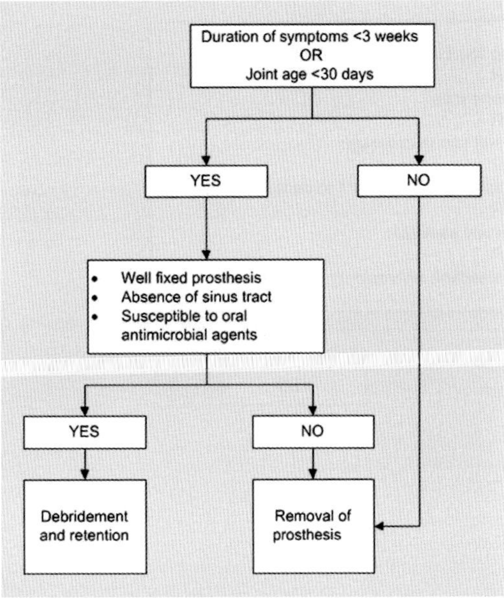

Fig. 6.5 Management of prosthetic joint infection (from Osmon et al. 2013)

the body and antibiotics to which organisms are susceptible are effective against planktonic cells and adherent bacteria on solid surface. However, the immune system and the antibiotics do not work against organisms that have formed biofilm. Regardless of the removal of the implant, an aggressive debridement of the peri-articular tissues should be done to reduce the bio-burden of the pathogens and to improve the efficiency of the patient's immune system and the efficacy of the antibiotics against the surviving pathogens. Thus, all non-bleeding soft or osseous tissues should be removed.

Irrigation conducted with aggressive debridement is effective in diluting contamination and non-viable tissues. A larger volume of irrigation fluid can achieve a higher degree of dilution; nevertheless, the appropriate volume of irrigation fluid is not yet defined. There is little consensus regarding the use of low-pressure (<15 lb/in^2) or high-pressure (>45 lb/in^2) lavage (Alijanipour et al. 2014). Some reports in the literature describe that SSI/PJI can be reduced when antibiotics or detergents, e.g. castile soap, benzalkonium chloride or povidone-iodine, are mixed with the irrigation fluid (Alijanipour et al. 2014). However, no definite conclusion has been made yet. Povidone-iodine may be the most promising chemical agent. Ten of 15 studies (11 randomized controlled trials and four prospective comparative studies) in a systematic review of different surgical specialties (two studies of spine

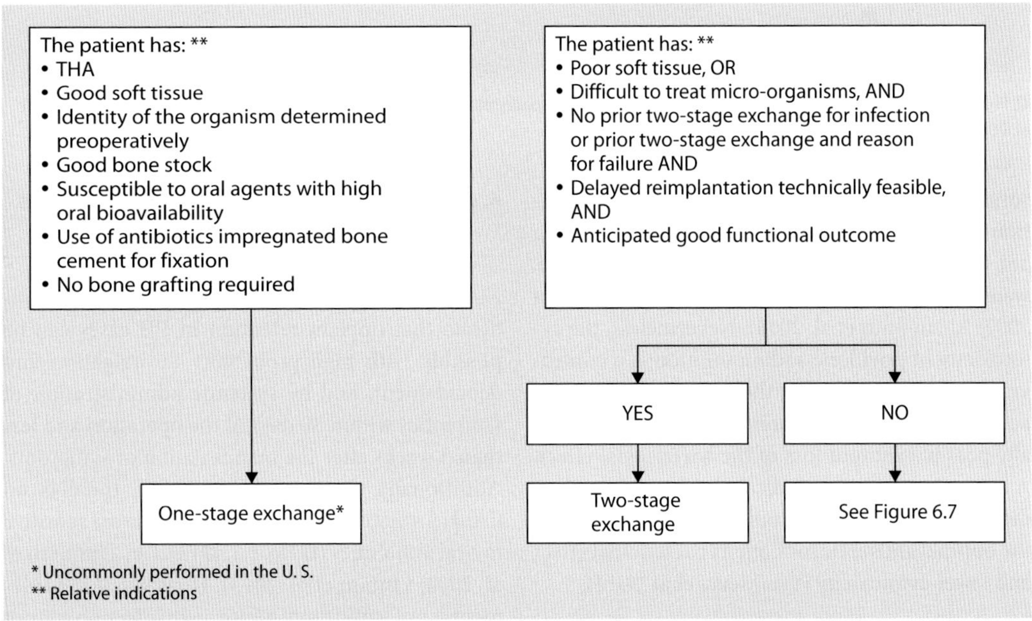

Fig. 6.6 Management of prosthetic joint infection: removal of the prosthesis (from Osmon et al. 2013)

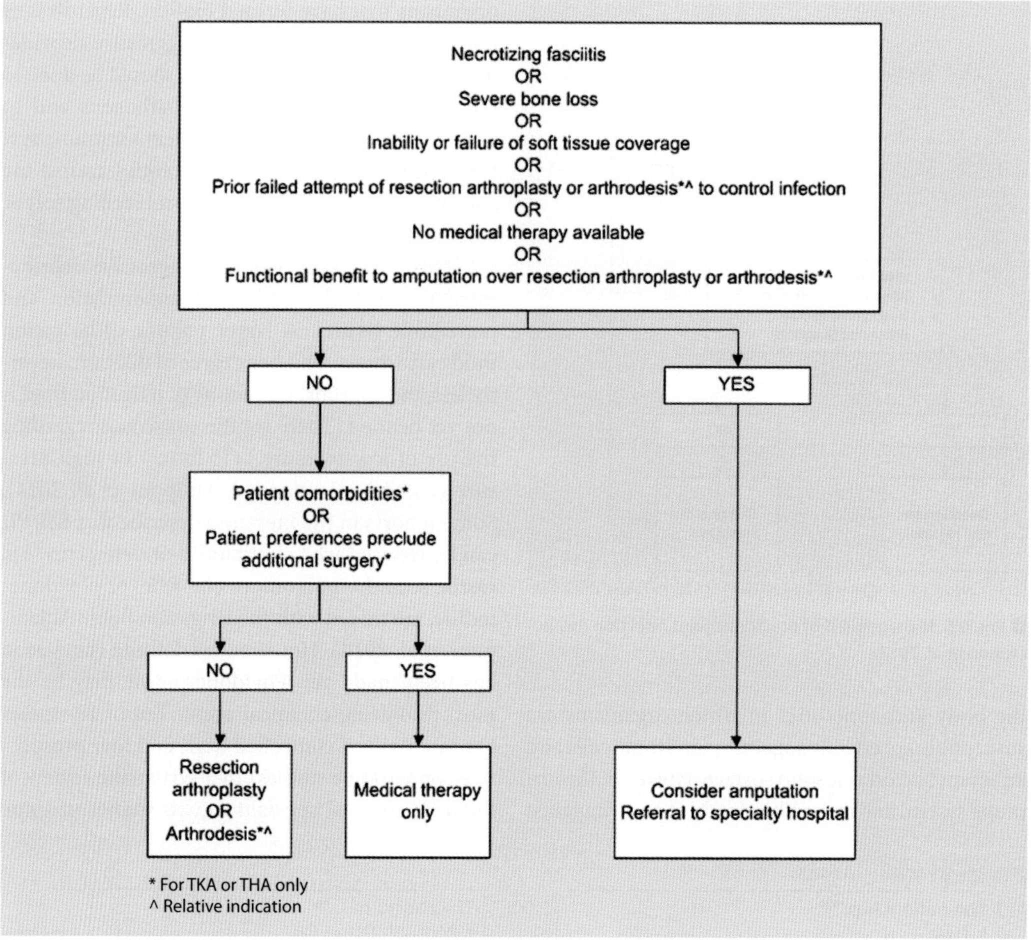

Fig. 6.7 Management of prosthetic joint infection when patients are not a candidate for new prosthesis (from Osmon et al. 2013)

surgery) demonstrated that povidone-iodine irrigation was significantly more effective at preventing SSI than the comparative interventions of saline, water, or no irrigation (Chundamala and Wright 2007; Alijanipour et al. 2014). Nevertheless, the cytotoxicity of povidone-iodine solution is a controversial issue. By reducing the concentration of the active compound, reduction of cytotoxicity is usually possible without loss of the bactericidal effect. A recent in vivo study indicated that povidone-iodine diluted to a concentration of 1.3 g/l could be the optimal antiseptic for both its bactericidal effect and lower cytotoxicity (van Meurs et al. 2014).

6.1.7 Revision Criteria when Implants Are Retained

Zimmerli's algorithm and the ISDA guidelines indicate that implant retention in PJI cases can be possible with high probability by irrigation and debridement, and by systemic administration of antibiotics within 30 days of the operation and less than 3 weeks after the manifestation of symptoms. Additionally, there is no loosening, there is no fistula formation and causative bacteria are sensitive to oral antibiotics (Fig. 6.3, Fig. 6.6; Zimmerli et al. 2004; Osmon et al. 2013). However, if debridement is not sufficiently performed, infection cannot be resolved even when these criteria are met. Even though appropriate antibiotics are selected, their effectiveness would be limited as long as focal infection and biofilm remain. If infection does not resolve locally and haematologically within 4–6 weeks of the irrigation and debridement, re-debridement or implant removal should be promptly performed.

6.1.8 What Is the Clinical Implication of ALAC in PJI Revision Procedures?

Buchholz and Engelbrecht first reported on antibiotic-loaded acrylic bone cement (ALAC) in 1970 (Buchholz and Engelbrecht 1970). Since then, ALAC has been used globally for the prevention of SSI in primary joint replacement surgery and one-state/two-stage revisions of PJI. ALAC accounts for more than 60% of bone cements on the European market, and the ratio is growing (National Joint Registry 2013).

Penetration of the intravenous/oral antibiotics is not always good in the medullary canal, where the bone cement is filled. When an implant is removed because of a PJI, a large dead space is formed in the joint cavity, which can be a hotbed of bacterial growth. ALACs can locally release antibiotics for a certain time and thus create a zone of bacterial growth inhibition. During the duration of antibiotic release, ALAC can maintain a higher antibiotic concentration in the bone and joint cavity than intravenous antibiotic administration. However, the detailed mechanism of the slow release of antibiotics from the bone cement has yet to be elucidated.

ALAC can be applied for two purposes: prevention of infection in primary procedures and treatment of infection in PJI. Commercially available ALAC is usually employed for primary procedures (National Joint Registry 2013). For revision procedures in PJI, the type of antibiotic and the dose need to be individualized for each patient based on the organism profile and antibiogram (if available), as well as on the patient's renal function and allergy profile.

ALAC utilized to treat infection in two-stage revision procedures of PJI cases should be able to release high-concentration antibiotics to the infected site. When antibiotic release is finished, ALAC needs to be removed from the body. Therefore, the mechanical characteristics of ALAC, in other words its cement strength, do not have many clinical implications. On the other hand, in one-stage/two-stage revisions, cements used for the definite fixation of the implant should have sufficient mechanical strength. The mechanical strength of bone cements should meet the International Organization for Standardization (ISO) 5833 (Pelletier et al. 2009). If too many antibiotics are mixed, the cement cannot be used because of decreased strength. If a sufficient amount of antibiotic is not mixed, the cement is not effective against infection. Heat resistance, slow-release properties and mechanical strength need to be considered for the selection of antibiotics. Aminoglycoside is usually chosen and impregnated in most commercially available ALACs. Some have tobramycin 0.5 g or gentamicin 0.5–1 g per 40 g cement. With the increase of MRSA infections in recent years, the use of vancomycin has also increased. Vancomycin is a glycopeptide antibiotic gradually released over the long term and its effectiveness in combination with aminoglycoside has been reported (Persson et al. 2006). Some antibiotics become deactivated during the exothermic setting of polymethyl methacrylate (PMMA) cement and, hence, cannot be used in spacers. A list of all available antibiotics and the organisms against which they are active is provided (◘ Tab. 6.2; Citak et al. 2014).

Some experimental studies suggest that the types and amount of antibiotics to be mixed, the cement/antibiotics ratio and the surface area of ALACs could influence the elution (Bayston and Milner 1982; Greene et al. 1998; Seeley et al. 2004). Although high-level evidence about the best waiting period in the two-stage revision using ALACs is missing, it is generally believed that antibiotic release continues for several weeks after the placement of ALAC (Masri et al. 1998; Bertazzoni et al. 2004, Anagnostakos et al. 2009).

For the two-stage revision for PJI, there are different ways of filling ALAC: filling bead-shaped ALAC in the dead space, inserting spacer-type ALAC and placing both of these. There are two types of spacers: articulating spacers and static (non-articulating) spacers. Articulating spacers will enable range of motion (ROM) exercise and partial loading during the waiting period, and can mini-

Tab. 6.2 Available antibiotics and anti-fungals that can be used in the spacer (from Citak et al. 2014)

Antibiotic group	Type of antibiotic	Activity against	Dose per 40 g cement (g)
Aminoglycoside	Tobramycin	Gram-negative bacteria such as Pseudomonas	1–4.8
Aminoglycoside	Gentamicin	Gram-negative bacteria, *Escherichia coli*, Klebsiella and particularly *Pseudomonas aeruginosa*; also aerobic bacteria (not obligate/facultative anaerobes)	0.25–4.8
Cephalosporin, 1st-gen	Cefazolin	Gram-positive infections, limited Gram-negative coverage	1–2
Cephalosporin, 2nd-gen	Cefuroxime	Reduced Gram-positive coverage, improved Gram-negative coverage	1.5–2
Cephalosporin, 3rd-gen	Cefotaxime	Gram-negative bacteria, particularly Pseudomonas	2
Cephalosporin, 4th-gen	Ceftaroline	Gram-negative bacteria, no activity against Pseudomonas	2
Fluoroquinolone	Ciprofloxacin	Gram-negative organisms including activity against Enterobacteriaceae	2–4
Glycopeptide	Vancomycin	Gram-positive bacteria, including methicillin-resistant organisms	0.2–3
Linosamide	Clindamycin	Gram-positive cocci, anaerobes	0.5–4
Macrolide	Erythromycin	Aerobic Gram-positive cocci and bacilli	1–2
Polymyxin	Colistin	Gram-negative	0.24
β-Lactam	Piperacillin not available Piptazobactam	Enterobacteria, and anaerobes	4–8
β-Lactam	Aztreonam	Only Gram-negative bacteria	4
β-Lactamase inhibitor	Tazobactam	Gram-negative bacteria (particularly Pseudomonas) Enterobacteria, and anaerobes in combination with Piperacillin	0.5
Oxazolidinones	Linezolid	Multi-drug-resistant Gram-positive cocci such as MRSA	1.2
Carbapenem	Meropenem	Gram-positive and Gram-negative bacteria, anaerobes, Pseudomonas	0.5–4
Lipopeptide	Daptomycin	Only Gram-positive organisms	2
Anti-fungal	Amphotericin	Most fungi	200
Anti-fungal	Voriconazole	Most fungi	300–600 mg

Take-Home Message

- PJI has a significant impact on the mortality of patients.
- Several diagnostic criteria and algorithms for the diagnosis of PJI were proposed, which are clinically helpful.
- The detection of the causative bacteria is critical for creating the treatment strategy and for selecting antibiotics.
- The basics of PJI treatment is »aggressive« debridement and administration of appropriate antibiotics.
- The two-stage revisions are regarded to be the gold standard, and one-stage revisions are not usually recommended when the causative bacteria is multi-drug-resistant bacteria or Gram-negative organisms.
- For better treatment of PJI, each patient should be evaluated carefully for an individualized treatment strategy, and stricter systemic management and meticulous operative procedure should be required.

mize the decrease in ADL. Although articulating spacers are reported to have better joint function during the waiting period than static (non-articulating) spacers, no difference is reported regarding the post-operative function. Some authors indicated that there is no difference in the effectiveness against PJI between the two spacers (Citak et al. 2014).

6.1.9 Risk Patients: How Would You Adapt Your Revision Strategy?

PJI in immunosuppressed patients (patients with immunosuppressant medications or with immune dysfunction) and those affected by severe diabetes mellitus, poor general status and morbid obesity have a higher risk of re-infection even when appropriate treatment is performed (Houdek et al. 2015). It is difficult to make revision strategies for these high-risk patients, since high-level evidence is currently lacking on what is the most effective treatment strategy. Each patient should be evaluated carefully to prepare an individualized treatment strategy. Stricter systemic management and a more meticulous operative procedure than for regular PJI are required. One of the future options for these patients can be the use of antibacterial surface-treated implants (Tsuchiya et al. 2012; Shirai et al. 2014; Eto et al. 2015; Kabata et al. 2015). The antibacterial surface-treated implants could possibly inhibit biofilm formation on the implant surface for a certain period after operation and may lead to better responses to the post-operative antibiotic treatment.

References

Alijanipour P, Karam J, Llinás A, Vince KG, Zalavras C, Austin M, Garrigues G, Heller S, Huddleston J, Klatt B, Krebs V, Lohmann C, McPherson EJ, Molloy R, Oliashirazi A, Schwaber M, Sheehan E, Smith E, Sterling R, Stocks G, Vaidya S (2014) Operative environment. J Orthop Res 32(Suppl1):60–80

Anagnostakos K, Wilmes P, Schmitt E, Kelm J (2009) Elution of gentamicin and vancomycin from polymethylmethacrylate beads and hip spacers in vivo. Acta Orthop 80(2):193–197

Bayston R, Milner RD (1982) The sustained release of antimicrobial drugs from bone cement. An appraisal of laboratory investigations and their significance. J Bone Joint Surg Br 64(4):460–464

Berbari EF, Hanssen AD, Duffy MC, Steckelberg JM, Ilstrup DM, Harmsen WS, Osmon DR (1998) Risk factors for prosthetic joint infection: case-control study. Clin Infect Dis 27(5): 1247–1254

Bertazzoni Minelli E, Benini A, Magnan B, Bartolozzi P (2004) Release of gentamicin and vancomycin from temporary human hip spacers in two-stage revision of infected arthroplasty. J Antimicrob Chemother 53(2):329–334

Bozic KJ, Lau E, Kurtz S, Ong K, Rubash H, Vail TP, Berry DJ (2012a) Patient-related risk factors for periprosthetic joint infection and postoperative mortality following total hip arthroplasty in Medicare patients. J Bone Joint Surg Am 94(9):794–800

Bozic KJ, Lau E, Kurtz S, Ong K, Berry DJ (2012b) Patient-related risk factors for postoperative mortality and periprosthetic joint infection in medicare patients undergoing TKA. Clin Orthop Relat Res 470(1):130–137

Buchholz HW, Engelbrecht H (1970) [Depot effects of various antibiotics mixed with Palacos resins]. Chirurg 41(11):511–515

CDC/NHSN Surveillance Definitions for Specific Types of Infections (2016) Georgia, USA. Retrieved from http://www.cdc.gov/nhsn/pdfs/pscmanual/17pscnosinfdef_current.pdf

Chundamala J, Wright JG (2007) The efficacy and risks of using povidone-iodine irrigation to prevent surgical site infection: an evidence-based review. Can J Surg 50(6):473–481

Citak M, Argenson JN, Masri B, Kendoff D, Springer B, Alt V, Baldini A, Cui Q, Deirmengian GK, del Sel H, Harrer MF, Israelite C, Jahoda D, Jutte PC, Levicoff E, Meani E, Motta F, Pena OR, Ranawat AS, Safir O, Squire MW, Taunton MJ, Vogely C, Wellman SS (2014) Spacers. J Arthroplasty 29(2Suppl):93–99

Della Valle CJ, Zuckerman JD, Di Cesare PE (2004) Periprosthetic sepsis. Clin Orthop Relat Res 420:26–31

Della Valle C, Parvizi J, Bauer TW, Dicesare PE, Evans RP, Segreti J, Spangehl M, Watters WC 3rd, Keith M, Turkelson CM, Wies JL, Sluka P, Hitchcock K, American Academy of Orthopaedic Surgeons (2010) Diagnosis of periprosthetic joint infections of the hip and knee. J Am Acad Orthop Surg 18(12):760–770

Eto S, Kawano S, Someya S, Miyamoto H, Sonohata M, Mawatari M (2015) First Clinical Experience With Thermal-Sprayed Silver Oxide-Containing Hydroxyapatite Coating Implant. J Arthroplasty 31(7):1498–1503

Evans RP (2011) Current concepts for clean air and total joint arthroplasty: laminar airflow and ultraviolet radiation: a systematic review. Clin Orthop Relat Res 469(4):945–953

Fulkerson E, Valle CJ, Wise B, Walsh M, Preston C, Di Cesare PE (2006) Antibiotic susceptibility of bacteria infecting total joint arthroplasty sites. J Bone Joint Surg Am 88(6):1231–1237

Gemmell CG, Edwards DI, Fraise AP, Gould FK, Ridgway GL, Warren RE (2006) Joint Working Party of the British Society for Joint Working Party of the British Society for Antimicrobial Chemotherapy, Hospital Infection Society and Infection Control Nurses Association. Guidelines for the prophylaxis and treatment of methicillin-resistant Staphylococcus aureus (MRSA) infections in the UK. J Antimicrob Chemother 57(4):589–608

Greene N, Holtom PD, Warren CA, Ressler RL, Shepherd L, McPherson EJ, Patzakis MJ (1998) In vitro elution of tobramycin and vancomycin polymethylmethacrylate beads and spacers from Simplex and Palacos. Am J Orthop 27(3):201–205

Hooper GJ, Rothwell AG, Frampton C, Wyatt MC (2011) Does the use of laminar flow and space suits reduce early deep infection after total hip and knee replacement?:the ten-year results of the New Zealand Joint Registry. J Bone Joint Surg Br 93(1):85–90

Houdek MT, Wagner ER, Watts CD, Osmon DR, Hanssen AD, Lewallen DG, Mabry TM (2015) Morbid obesity: a significant risk factor for failure of two-stage revision total hip arthroplasty for infection. J Bone Joint Surg Am 97(4):326–332

Illingworth KD, Mihalko WM, Parvizi J, Sculco T, McArthur B, el Bitar Y, Saleh KJ (2013) How to minimize infection and thereby maximize patient outcomes in total joint arthroplasty: a multicenter approach: AAOS exhibit selection. J Bone Joint Surg Am doi:10.2106/JBJS.L.00596

Jackson WO, Schmalzried TP (2000) Limited role of direct exchange arthroplasty in the treatment of infected total hip replacements. Clin Orthop Relat Res 381: 101–105

Kabata T, Maeda T, Kajino Y, Hasegawa K, Inoue D, Yamamoto T, Takagi T, Ohmori T, Tsuchiya H (2015) Iodine-Supported Hip Implants: Short Term Clinical Results. Biomed Res Int doi:10.1155/2015/368124

Kobayashi N, Inaba Y, Choe H, Aoki C, Ike H, Ishida T, Iwamoto N, Yukizawa Y, Saito T (2009) Simultaneous intraoperative detection of methicillin-resistant Staphylococcus and pan-bacterial infection during revision surgery: use of simple DNA release by ultrasonication and real-time polymerase chain reaction. J Bone Joint Surg Am 91(12):2896–2902

Kunutsor SK, Whitehouse MR, Blom AW, Beswick AD (2015) Re-Infection Outcomes following One- and Two-Stage Surgical Revision of Infected Hip Prosthesis: A Systematic Review and Meta-Analysis. PLoS One doi:10.1371/journal.pone.0139166

Kunutsor SK, Whitehouse MR, Lenguerrand E, Blom AW, Beswick AD, INFORM Team (2016) Re-infection outcomes following one- and two-stage surgical revision of infected knee prosthesis: a systematic review and meta-analysis. PLoS One 11(3):e0151537

Loty B, Postel M, Evrard J, Matron P, Courpied JP, Kerboull M, Tomeno B (1992) One stage revision of infected total hip replacements with replacement of bone loss by allografts. Study of 90 cases of which 46 used bone allografts. Int Orthop 16(4):330–338

Mangram AJ, Horan TC, Pearson ML, Silver LC, Jarvis WR (1999) Guideline for prevention of surgical site infection, 1999. Hospital Infection Control Practices Advisory Committee. Infect Control Hosp Epidemiol 20(4):250–278

Masaoka T, Yamamoto K, Ishii Y, Iida H, Matsuno T, Satomi K, Teshima R, Torisu T, Miyaoka H, Suguro T, Saotome K, Shinomiya K, Kawahara K, Imakiire A (2009) Epidemiology of orthopaedic surgical site infection. Japanese othopaedic association project. Rinshoseikeigeka 44(10):975–980

Masri BA, Duncan CP, Beauchamp CP (1998) Long-term elution of antibiotics from bone-cement: an in vivo study using the prosthesis of antibiotic-loaded acrylic cement (PROSTALAC) system. J Arthroplasty 13(3):331–338

Meehan J, Jamali AA, Nguyen H (2009) Prophylactic antibiotics in hip and knee arthroplasty. J Bone Joint Surg Am 91(10):2480–2490

National Joint Registry (2013) 10th annual report. Hemel Hempstead. Retrieved from http://www.njrcentre.org.uk/njrcentre/Reports,PublicationsandMinutes/Annualreports/tabid/86/Default.aspx

Osmon DR, Berbari EF, Berendt AR, Lew D, Zimmerli W, Steckelberg JM, Rao N, Hanssen A, Wilson WR (2013) Infectious Diseases Society of America. Diagnosis and management of prosthetic joint infection: clinical practice guidelines by the Infectious Diseases Society of America. Clin Infect Dis 56(1):e1–e25

Parvizi J, Zmistowski B, Berbari EF, Bauer TW, Springer BD, Della Valle CJ, Garvin KL, Mont MA, Wongworawat MD, Zalavras CG (2011) New definition for periprosthetic joint infection: from the Workgroup of the Musculoskeletal Infection Society. Clin Orthop Relat Res 469(11):2992–2994

Pelletier MH, Malisano L, Smitham PJ, Okamoto K, Walsh WR (2009) The compressive properties of bone cements containing large doses of antibiotics. J Arthroplasty 24(3):454–460

Persson C, Baleani M, Guandalini L, Tigani D, Viceconti M (2006) Mechanical effects of the use of vancomycin and meropenem in acrylic bone cement. Acta Orthop [illegible]

Rao N, Crossett LS, Sinha RK, Le Frock JL (2003) Long-term suppression of infection in total joint arthroplasty. Clin Orthop Relat Res 414:55–60

Raut VV, Siney PD, Wroblewski BM (1994) One-stage revision of infected total hip replacements with discharging sinuses. J Bone Joint Surg Br 76(5):721–724

Rudelli S, Uip D, Honda E, Lima AL (2008) One-stage revision of infected total hip arthroplasty with bone graft. J Arthroplasty 23(8):1165–1177

Seeley SK, Seeley JV, Telehowski P, Martin S, Tavakoli M, Colton SL, Larson B, Forrester P, Atkinson PJ (2004) Volume and surface area study of tobramycin- polymethylmethacrylate beads. Clin Orthop Relat Res 420:298–303

Shirai T, Tsuchiya H, Nishida H, Yamamoto N, Watanabe K, Nakase J, Terauchi R, Arai Y, Fujiwara H, Kubo T (2014) Antimicrobial megaprostheses supported with iodine. J Biomater Appl 29(4):617–623

Trampuz A, Widmer AF (2006) Infections associated with orthopedic implants. Curr Opin Infect Dis 19(4):349–356

Trampuz A, Piper KE, Jacobson MJ, Hanssen AD, Unni KK, Osmon DR, Mandrekar JN, Cockerill FR, Steckelberg JM, Greenleaf JF, Patel R (2007) Sonication of removed hip and knee prostheses for diagnosis of infection. N Engl J Med 357(7):654–663

Tsuchiya H, Shirai T, Nishida H, Murakami H, Kabata T, Yamamoto N, Watanabe K, Nakase J (2012) Innovative antimicrobial coating of titanium implants with iodine. J Orthop Sci 17(5):595–604

Urquhart DM, Hanna FS, Brennan SL et al (2010) Incidence and risk factors for deep surgical site infection after primary total hip arthroplasty: a systematic review. J Arthroplasty 25(8):1216–1222

van Meurs SJ, Gawlitta D, Heemstra KA, Poolman RW, Vogely HC, Kruyt MC (2014) Selection of an optimal antiseptic solution for intraoperative irrigation: an in vitro study. J Bone Joint Surg Am 96(4):285–291

Zimmerli W, Widmer AF, Blatter M, Frei R, Ochsner PE (1998) Role of rifampin for treatment of orthopedic implant-related staphylococcal infections: a randomized controlled trial. Foreign-Body Infection (FBI) Study Group. JAMA 279(19):1537–1541

Zimmerli W, Trampuz A, Ochsner PE (2004) Prosthetic-joint infections. N Engl J Med 351(16):1645–1654

Zmistowski B, Karam JA, Durinka JB, Casper DS, Parvizi J (2013) Periprosthetic joint infection increases the risk of one-year mortality. J Bone Joint Surg Am 95(24):2177–2184

6.2 Treatment of Orthopaedic Septic Revisions at the Medical University of Graz

Florian Amerstorfer and Mathias Glehr

6.2.1 Introduction

Prosthetic joint infection (PJI) requires operative treatment with additional antibiotic therapy in the majority of cases. Infection control by eradication of the pathogen is the main goal in PJI treatment. This may be achieved by removal of the whole infected periprosthetic tissue with retention of the prosthesis, one- or two-stage exchange, resection arthroplasty, arthrodesis, and amputation.

6.2.2 Diagnosis and Classification

To achieve a satisfactory result in the management of PJI, a correct diagnosis is the main goal. A summary of the diagnostic criteria published by a workgroup convened by the Musculoskeletal Infection Society (MSIS) in 2011 is provided in ◻ Tab. 6.3, which may help towards getting an accurate diagnosis.

Many classification systems have been published and described in the literature. Most of the staging systems consider the time of infection onset and provide a basis for decision-making on operative treatment. McPherson et al. (2002) published a staging system for periprosthetic hip infections, which not only considers the time of infection onset, but also the local status as well as the medical and immune health status of the patient.

For microbiological diagnosis of prosthetic joint infection, five or six specimen should be taken during revision surgery from tissue surrounding the implant and then separated into two samples, one for microbiological, the other one for histological analysis (◻ Fig. 6.8; Atkins et al. 1998). Furthermore, sonication of removed prosthesis should be performed (Trampuz et al. 2007).

Tab. 6.3 Definition of PJI

1. Draining sinus tract (communication with prosthesis) OR
2. Pathogen, isolated by culture from two or more separate tissue or fluid samples OR
3. Four of the six criteria exist: a) Elevated serum erythrocyte sedimentation rate and C-reactive protein (CRP) concentration b) Elevated synovial white blood cell count c) Elevated synovial polymorphonuclear percentage (PMN%) d) Presence of purulence in the affected joint e) Isolation of a microorganism in one culture of periprosthetic tissue or fluid f) Greater than five neutrophils per high-power field in five high-power fields observed from histologic analysis of periprosthetic tissue at ×400 magnification

6

6.2.3 Treatment and Algorithms

In our department, surgical procedure is based on the infection type as well as the local and medical immune health status of the patient in accordance to the McPherson staging system (Tab. 6.4). In addition to operative treatment, systemic antimicrobial therapy must be performed through parenteral infusion at the beginning, followed by oral antibiotics.

In order to increase high local antibiotics when using antibiotic-loaded cement, in one-stage as well as two-stage exchange, a novel surgical technique, called superficial vancomycin coating (SVC) of bone cement, was established (Fig. 6.9).

This special technique was developed to increase the local antibiotic concentration without the fear of systemic side effects such as nephrotoxicity or ototoxicity during vancomycin therapy, especially with concurrent administration of aminoglycosides (Goetz and Sayers 1993).

Debridement with Retention of Prosthesis

Debridement and antibiotic therapy with implant retention (DAIR) may be performed in patients with an early postoperative infection (< 4 postoperative weeks), stable implants and no compromising factors regarding health (e.g. diabetes, renal failure requiring dialysis, immunosuppressive therapy or malignancy) and local status (e.g. fistula, abscess). Furthermore, the causative micro-organism, if known at the time of operation, should be susceptible to multiple antimicrobials. All mobile parts have to be exchanged during the surgical procedure after extensive debridement.

One-Stage Exchange

A one-stage exchange is defined as a single operation with removal of the whole prosthesis, followed by accurate debridement and re-implantation of a new endoprosthesis. In order to achieve high local con-

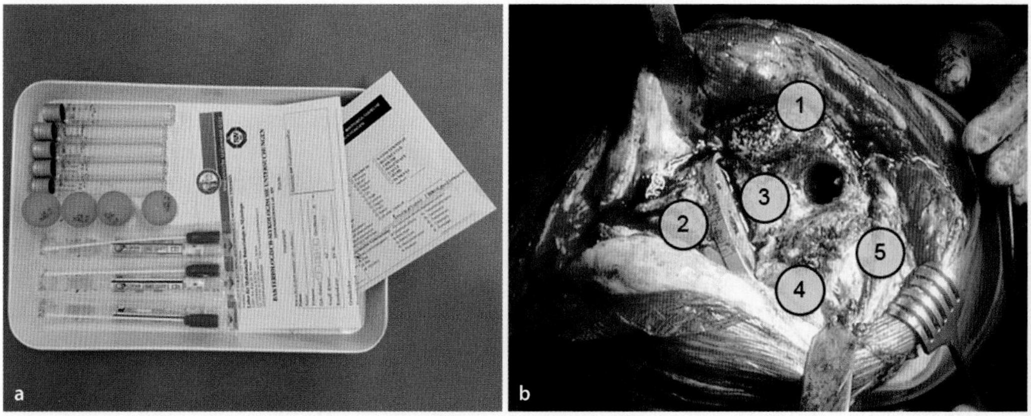

Fig. 6.8 Five to six specimens should be taken during revision surgery for microbiological and histological analysis (**a**) from different places showing macroscopic inflammatory changes (**b**)

Tab. 6.4 Staging system for prosthetic joint infection published by McPherson et al. (2002)

Infection type	Systemic host grade	Local extremity grade
I: Early postoperative infection (<4 postoperative weeks)	A: Uncompromised	1. Uncomplicated
II: Haematogenous infection (<4 weeks' duration)	B: Compromised (1 or 2 compromising factors)	2. Compromised (1 or 2 compromising factors)
III: Late chronic infection (> weeks' duration)	C: Significant compromise (>2 compromising factors) or one of:	3. Significant compromise (>2 compromising factors)
	- absolute neutrophil count <1 000	
	- CD4 T cell count <100	
	- intravenous drug abuse	
	- chronic infection at another site	
	- dysplasia or neoplasm of the immune system	
	Compromising factors:	Compromising factors:
	- age > 80 years	- active infection present for more than 3–4 months
	- immunosuppressive drugs	- multiple incisions with skin bridges
	- alcoholism	- soft tissue loss from prior trauma
	- malignancy	- subcutaneous abscess >8 cm^2
	- chronic dermatitis or cellulites	- synovial cutaneous fistula
	- pulmonary insufficiency	- prior peri-articular fracture or trauma of a joint
	- chronic indwelling catheter	- prior local irradiation
	- renal failure requiring dialysis	- vascular insufficiency to extremity
	- chronic malnutrition	
	- systemic inflammatory disease	
	- current nicotine use	
	- systemic immune compromise	
	- diabetes	
	- hepatic insufficiency	

centrations of antimicrobial agents, antibiotic-loaded polymethylmethacrylate (PMMA) cement may be used according to the antimicrobial susceptibility profile (Kühn 2014). If Gram-positive bacteria cause the infection, SVC may be used additionally to further increase the local antibiotic concentration and thereby minimize the risk of reinfection.

The benefits of a one-stage exchange are: (a) only one operation, (b) faster recovery due to earlier mobility, and (c) reduced health-care costs.

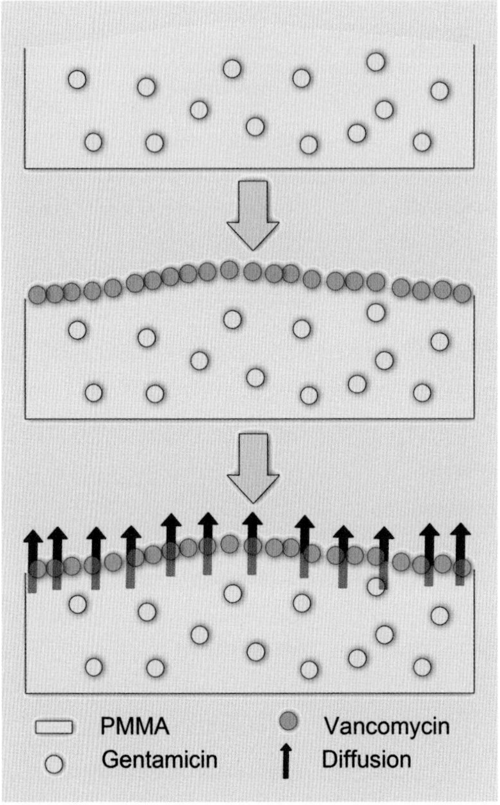

Fig. 6.9 Superficial vancomycin coating of bone cement: After the bone cement is mixed and placed in the correct position, vancomycin powder is pressed manually onto the surface of the cement, just before it completely hardens. *PMMA* polymethylmethacrylate

Many studies have shown almost similar outcome comparing one- and two-stage exchange procedures (Tande and Patel 2014); however, a one-stage procedure may be performed in patients with an acute haematogenous (primary arthroplasty > 4 weeks and symptoms < 4 weeks' duration) infection and only one or two compromising systematic medical and immune status factors.

Two-Stage Exchange

A two-stage exchange arthroplasty remains the gold standard for chronic periprosthetic joint infection treatment (Insall et al. 1983, Goldman et al. 1996, Mahmud et al. 2012), although there are country-specific preferences. In patients with haematogenous or chronic infections with sepsis, difficult or antibiotic-resistant micro-organism, or more than two compromising systemic medical and immune status factors, a two-stage exchange procedure may be indicated. After the whole implants are removed, extensive debridement and wound flushing are performed. The removed implants are sonicated in saline to get rid of micro-organisms from the surface, followed by culture of the sonication fluid (Fig. 6.10b). A temporary spacer, either static or mobile, is inserted (Fig. 6.10c). Re-implantation is performed after 4–6 weeks. Frozen sections during operation exclude persistent infection before re-implantation (Fig. 6.10e).

Depending on the present soft tissue, bone and ligamentous status, cemented constrained implants with or without metaphyseal sleeves may be used in knee arthroplasty revision surgery in order to restore function and stability (Fig. 6.10f).

The disadvantages of a two-stage exchange procedure are: (a) second operation accompanied by higher morbidity risk, (b) longer total hospital stay duration, and (c) loss of function with impairment of quality of life for several weeks.

Arthrodesis

In cases of massive bone and soft tissues destruction due to multiple previous operations, implantation of another prosthesis may be impossible. In these cases arthrodesis of the knee is one of the last options to save the lower extremity, can result in a stable and functional extremity and is preferable to amputation (Fig. 6.11). Besides internal or external fixation, plates as well as intramedullary fixation through the knee with a modular nail have been described in the literature (MacDonald et al. 2006).

Resection Arthroplasty

Complete implant removal without re-implantation may be performed in patients with failed hip arthroplasty, in patients with multiple operations with compromised local or host grade status, and in those in whom re-implantation of a prosthesis or an arthrodesis is impossible.

It often results in poor functionality due to leg shortening because of the muscle tension. Thus, resection arthroplasty without re-implantation is reserved for old and bedridden patients or patients with spinal paralysis (Fig. 6.12).

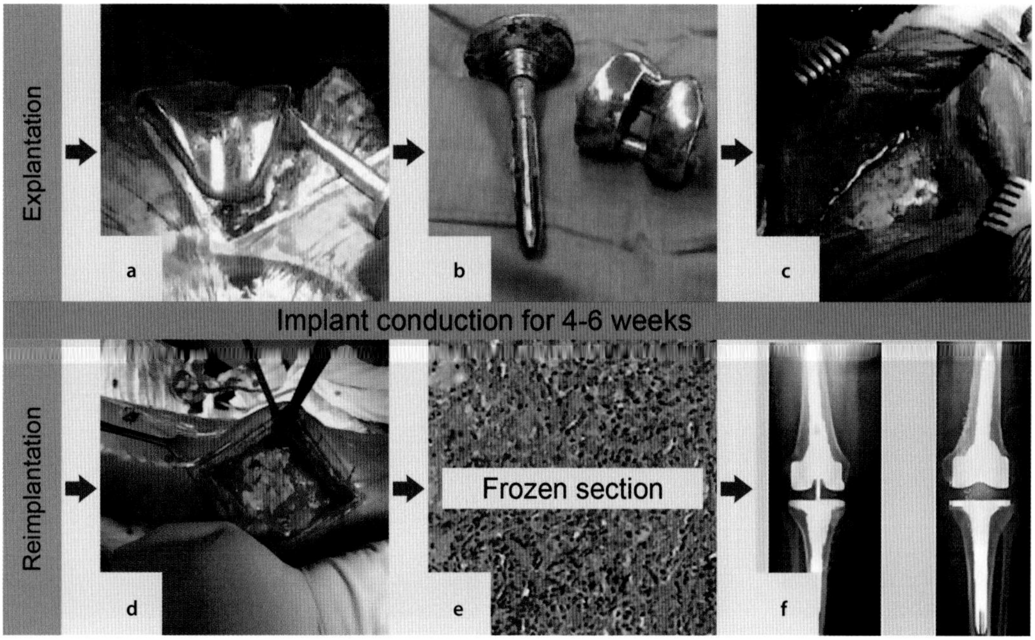

Fig. 6.10 Two-stage exchange procedure after infected total knee arthroplasty. **a–c** Implant removal and debridement of surrounding infected tissue and insertion of a static spacer as an antibiotic delivery device in order to achieve high local antimicrobial concentrations. **d–f** Re-implantation of prosthesis takes place after 4–6 weeks. During spacer removal, frozen section of surrounding soft tissue may rule out persistent or re-infection

Permanent Fistula

In patients with persistent infections, multiple previous operations and the request to save the limb, creating an iatrogenic permanent fistula is a therapeutic option (Fig. 6.13).

Furthermore, in patients who are in no condition for surgery, these operations may be performed under local anaesthesia. Disadvantages of this treatment are the extensive care required of the general practitioner (regular follow-ups to keep open the sinus) as well as the high rates of fistula closure, which may lead to septicaemia.

Amputation/Exarticulation

Amputation or exarticulation of the upper or lower extremity is the last surgical option for patients who have undergone multiple previous operations and in whom insertion of an arthrodesis is impossible owing to the presence of chronic infection and severe bone loss (Fig. 6.14). Furthermore, in patients with uncontrollable sepsis, amputation may be performed as an emergency procedure to save the patient's life.

Take-Home Message

- After correct diagnosis, different treatment options are possible, with increasing gravity: debridement with retention of prosthesis, one-stage or two-stage exchange, arthrodesis, permanent fistula, resection arthroplasty, and amputation.
- Superficial vancomycin coating of bone cement is an effective and safe way to increase the local antibiotic concentration.

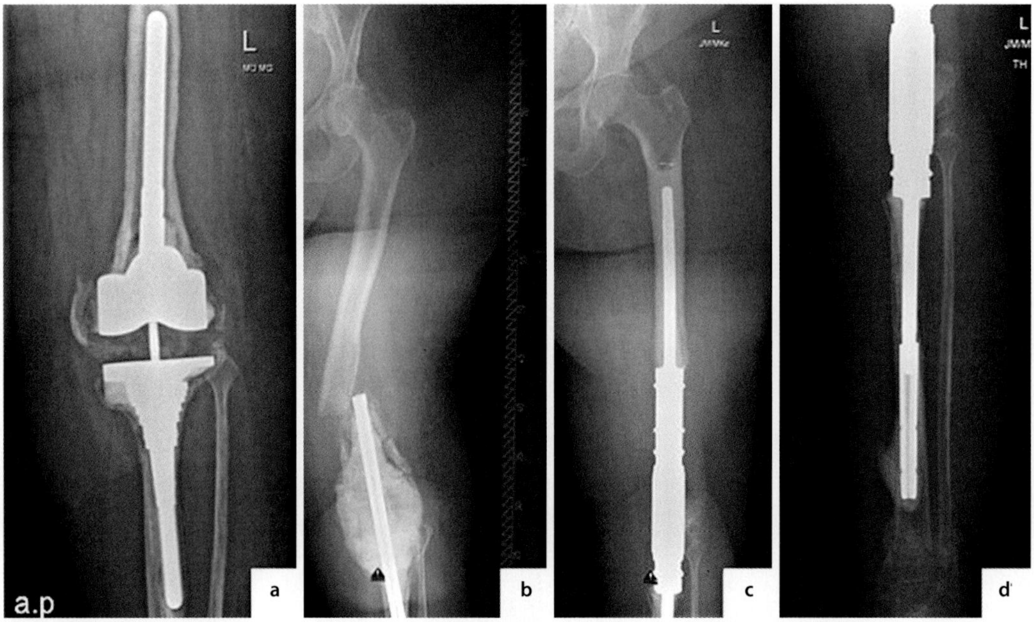

Fig. 6.11 Arthrodesis fixation after multiple previous operations: A 75-year-old woman who suffered from failed knee arthroplasty due to infection was primarily treated with a two-stage revision surgery. Four years later a chronic infection with mixed flora (*Staphylococcus aureus* and *Enterococcus faecalis*) occurred with massive soft tissue damage and bone loosening (**a**). Again, a two-stage exchange surgery was performed and a static cement spacer with a nail was inserted after the implants were removed. One month later, the patient suffered from a distal femur fracture (**b**). Because of the massive soft tissue and bone damage, an arthrodesis nail was inserted (**c, d**)

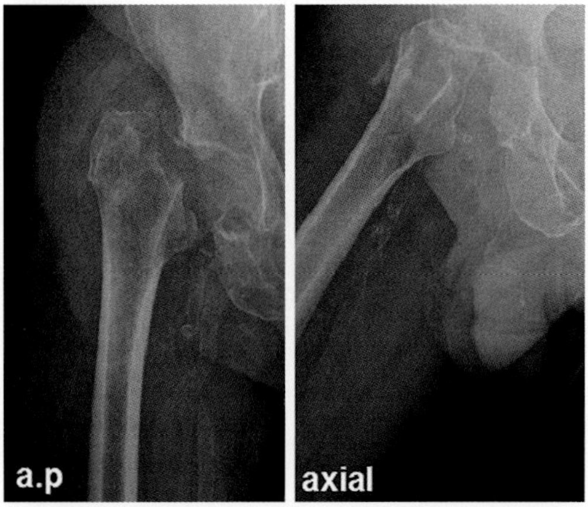

Fig. 6.12 Girdlestone hip: The X-ray shows a Girdlestone situation of an old bedridden patient who suffered from a prosthetic joint infection of the right hip (*ap* anteroposterior)

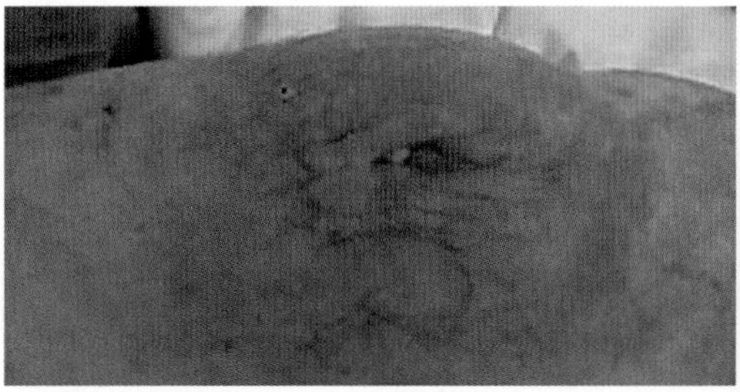

Fig. 6.13 Iatrogenic chronic fistula: A 74-year-old patient suffered from multiple infections after knee arthroplasty. An iatrogenic fistula was created, which resulted in limb salvage and moderate, pain-free range of motion with flexion up to 90°

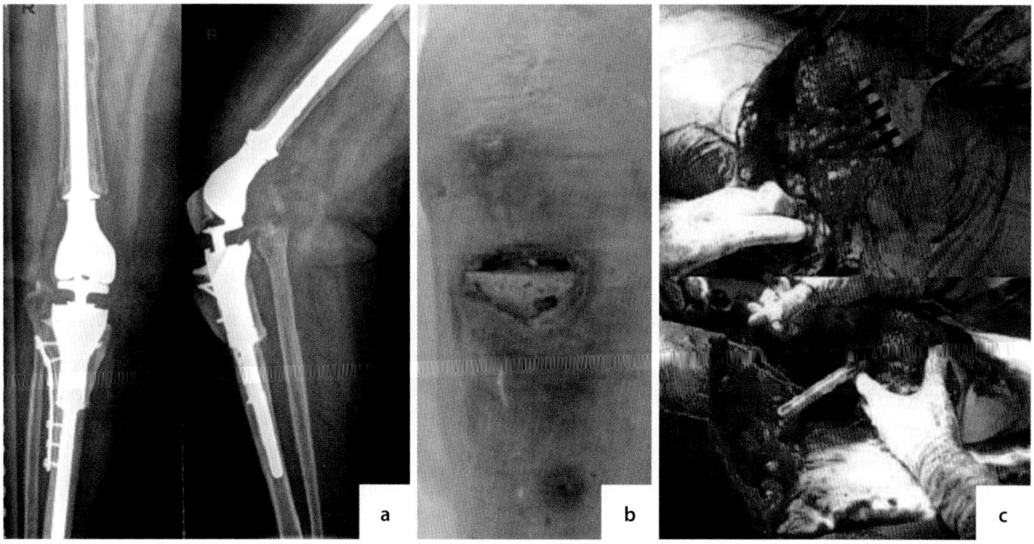

Fig. 6.14 Transfemoral amputation: A 76-year-old woman suffered from multiple infections after primary knee arthroplasty. The X-ray shows the right knee in anteroposterior and lateral view (**a**). Persistent chronic infection resulted in massive soft tissue damage and chronic draining infrapatellar sinus (**b**). A transfemoral amputation was performed successfully (**c**)

References

Amerstorfer F, Fischerauer S, Sadoghi P, Schwantzer G, Kühn KD, Leithner A, Glehr M (2016) Superficial Vancomycin Coating of Bone Cement in Orthopedic Revision Surgery: A Safe Technique to Enhance Local Antibiotic Concentrations. J Arthroplasty doi:10.1016/j.arth.2016.11.042

Atkins BL, Athanasou N, Deeks JJ, Crook DW, Simpson H, Peto TE, McLardy-Smith P, Berendt AR (1998) Prospective evaluation of criteria for microbiological diagnosis of prosthetic-joint infection at revision arthroplasty. The OSIRIS Collaborative Study Group. J Clin Microbiol 36(10):2932–2939

Goetz MB, Sayers J (1993) Nephrotoxicity of vancomycin and aminoglycoside therapy separately and in combination. J Antimicrob Chemother 32(2):325–334

Goldman RT, Scuderi GR, Insall JN (1996) 2-stage reimplantation for infected total knee replacement. Clin Orthop Relat Res 331:118–124

Insall JN, Thompson FM, Brause BD (1983) Two-stage reimplantation for the salvage of infected total knee arthroplasty. J Bone Joint Surg Ame 65(8):1087–1098

Kühn KD (2014) PMMA cements. Springer, Heidelberg ISBN-13 978-3-642-41535-7

MacDonald JH, Agarwal S, Lorei MP, Johanson NA, Freiberg AA (2006) Knee arthrodesis. J Am Acad Orthop Surg 14(3):154–163

Mahmud T, Lyons MC, Naudie DD, Macdonald SJ, McCalden RW (2012) Assessing the gold standard: a review of 253 two-stage revisions for infected TKA. Clin Orthop Relat Res 470(10):2730–2736

McPherson EJ, Woodson C, Holtom P, Roidis N, Shufelt C, Patzakis M (2002) Periprosthetic total hip infection: outcomes using a staging system. Clin Orthop Relat Res 403:8–15

Parvizi J, Zmistowski B, Berbari EF, Bauer TW, Springer BD, Della Valle CJ, Garvin KL, Mont MA, Wongworawat MD, Zalavras CG (2011) New definition for periprosthetic joint infection: from the Workgroup of the Musculoskeletal Infection Society. Clin Orthop Relat Res 469(11): 2992–2994

Tande AJ, Patel R (2014) Prosthetic joint infection. Clin Microbiol Rev 27(2):302–345

Trampuz A, Piper KE, Jacobson MJ, Hanssen AD, Unni KK, Osmon DR, Mandrekar JN, Cockerill FR, Steckelberg JM, Greenleaf JF, Patel R (2007) Sonication of removed hip and knee prostheses for diagnosis of infection. N Engl J Med 357(7):654–663

6.3 Treatment of Prosthetic Joint Infections

Hans J.G.E. Hendriks, Robin W.T.M. Van Kempen, and Laura van Dommelen

6.3.1 Introduction

In the 1970s, after almost two decades of optimizing mechanical issues related to prosthetic joint failure, safe revision of aseptic loosening of orthopaedic implants had become possible. The natural history of an infected total hip prosthesis (THP), however, still implied a 16% mortality after treatment, with only 13% of the survivors having a functioning prosthetic joint (Hunter and Dandy 1977). Prosthetic joint infections (PJI) remained a problem to be solved. In those years, Sir John Charnley focused on prevention rather than treatment of infection, since no effective treatment options for PJI were available (Charnley 1972). Nevertheless, centres of excellence in PJI treatment, such as the Endo Klinik in Hamburg, reported a 77% success rate for one-stage exchange arthroplasty in THP by the early 1980s (Buchholz et al. 1981).

6.3.2 Bacteria in a Biofilm

The description of the role of bacterial adherence to biomaterials and tissue in clinical sepsis by Gristina and Costerton in 1985 marked a paradigm shift in the understanding of the nature of PJI. The finding that the »biofilm« mode of bacterial growth is a natural situation, instead of the most often studied planktonic phase, changed laboratory research. Till then, the planktonic phase of bacterial growth had generally been studied. Studying biofilm subsequently changed diagnostic and therapeutic insights. Finding multiple strains of coagulase-negative staphylococci (CNS), small colony variants and anaerobic bacteria was once considered to be a contamination of the sample rather than infection (von Eiff et al. 1998). The success rate after one-stage exchange THP for infection concurrently went up to 87% (Hope et al. 1989).

6.3.3 Treatment

Antibiotics alone, although effective against many infections, generally fail to achieve cure in the case of PJI. The three main contributing factors are:

1. The implant itself gives rise to a so-called immuno-incompetent zone at its surface. In this zone the immune system is less effective (Gristina 1994).
2. Bacteria in biofilms produce extracellular matrix (slime) and have a limited metabolism making them less susceptible to antibiotics (Mah and O'Toole 2001).
3. The relatively poor tissue penetration of antibiotics at the site of infection (Winkelmann et al. 1978).

The first two factors suggest that antibiotic treatment can only be successful after removal of all foreign body material. After removal of the prosthesis, all treatment protocols recommend a thorough surgical debridement of the infected area. Surgical skills, particularly in dealing with soft tissue defects and available techniques for dealing with bone defects (requiring larger and often modular foreign body components or bone grafts), may limit the extent of debridement. Therefore, it is likely that the definition of what the surgeon considers as thorough varies widely and this may be why debridement is seldom described in detail. This makes it hard to compare therapeutic results that are reported for PJI in the literature.

To address the third factor, the use of local antibiotic therapy was developed. Although rinsing the wound with antibiotic solutions has not been shown to be successful, the use of gentamicin beads and collagen fleeces has been shown to yield higher antibiotic concentrations in the tissues involved in PJI than would be possible by systemic administration (Härle and Ritzerfeld 1979; Swieringa et al. 2008). Clinical research has yielded good results using gentamicin beads, even against gentamicin-resistant strains (Jannsen et al. 2016). Despite these reports on the results after clinical use, no randomized controlled trials have been published. Furthermore, there have been unproven concerns about developing antibiotic resistance, and nephrotoxicity has been found with use of gentamicin beads (De Klaver et al. 2012). As a result, the use of local antibiotic therapy has not been generally applied in the treatment of PJI. The use of antibiotic-loaded spacers was adopted with less reluctance, although the evidence base is not much better. Besides, persistence of contamination on their surface was shown (Schmolders et al. 2014). We do not regard the use of antibiotic-loaded spacers as a means of local antibiotic therapy.

Just like antibiotics alone, surgery alone – although effective against soft tissue abscesses – cannot cure PJI. It is obvious that treatment of PJI involves a combination of antibiotic and surgical management. The surgical strategy can be divided into one-stage and two-stage protocols. Treatment protocols for PJI that involve two operations have been investigated more thoroughly. With success rates of 92–95%, the two-stage protocols report better outcome than those relying on one-stage exchange (Haddad et al. 1995). Although the literature reports a tendency of the gap between published results from one-stage and two-stage strategies to be decreasing, two-stage remains the favoured strategy in general (Lange et al. 2012). In PJI of the knee, the evidence basis for two-stage treatment is also larger (Masters et al. 2013). Nevertheless, for knee PJI there is some evidence that a two-stage strategy may actually lead to poorer results than a one-stage procedure (Master et al. 2013). This appears to be particularly the case if a DAIR (debridement, antibiotics, irrigation, and retention of prosthesis) has preceded the revision surgery (Gardner et al. 2011; Sherrell et al. 2011).

6.3.4 One-Stage Protocol

A one-stage protocol involves a single operation in which the prosthesis is removed and the debridement is carried out, after which the new prosthesis is directly implanted. This has the advantage that the patient can start functional recovery without the delay caused by a prosthesis-free interval waiting for the second stage. Often, it is thought that surgical time and costs are reduced as well. This may not be the case, since provisional wound closure and re-prepping and re-draping the patient before continuing with the re-implantation with a fresh set of instruments (sometimes referred to as a three-step procedure) are mandatory from a hygiene point of view. Nevertheless, the overall costs of treatment with a one-stage protocol may be lower thanks to shorter hospitalization time and shorter antibiotic courses.

6.3.5 Two-Stage Protocol

A two-stage protocol has two basic advantages over a one-stage. Firstly, it leaves room for another debridement. Secondly, this debridement results in material that can be used to further diagnose the infection being treated. This is particularly interesting since biofilm infections have been found to be caused by multiple strains in almost 20% of cases (Holleyman et al. 2016). Having treated the strain(s) that was/were found in the first operation, taking cultures during the second operation makes it possible to find strains that went undetected after the first procedure. The reason for not finding them at first may lie in the relative ease of growth of common virulent strains versus small colony variants and other slow-growing micro-organisms. In addition, if the new strains were resistant to the treatment so far, redirecting treatment to cover these strains as well logically results in better outcome.

Finally, a two-stage protocol leaves room for adapting the initial treatment aim to clinical reality. Serious complications may preclude further antibiotic treatment or surgery. Failure to achieve infectious control may necessitate additional debridements. Discussing these circumstances with the patient may well lead to accepting a more certain outcome of a Girdlestone procedure or arthrodesis over a protracted and more hazardous course toward a functioning prosthetic joint.

A two-stage protocol obviously has drawbacks as well. The costs of treatment to society are perceived to be higher. With the outcomes of any infection treatment being dependent on more factors than just the one- or two-stage protocol, it can be argued that a one-stage protocol may be favourable (Kendoff and Gehrke 2014). Another drawback of the two-stage protocol directly involving the patient is the morbidity during the prosthesis-free interval, the second-stage surgical procedure and after the second operation. Also, antibiotic courses are generally more prolonged than with one-stage protocols, which could give rise to antibiotic-related complications.

To minimize functional impairment in the interval between the operations, a spacer made of antibiotic-loaded acrylic cement is commonly left in place. The spacer fills up the dead space created by removal of the prosthesis and prevents soft tissue contracture. Also, antibiotic-loaded bead chains can be used. The use of a spacer has been shown to contribute to an increase in antibiotic concentrations locally, but not to the same degree as antibiotic beads (Anagnostakos et al. 2009). The use of bead chains leaves the joint less functional, but can be appreciated as a means of providing the area of infection with a higher antibiotic concentration than can be achieved through treatment (intravenous or oral) alone.

We opt for gentamicin beads in difficult cases instead of a spacer, since the beads have more predictable elution characteristics related to the respective surface areas than spacers do (Holtom et al. 1998).

In order to be able to choose the optimal treatment and inform the patient in this respect, it is necessary to have insight into the factors that predict success or failure in each specific case. Most treatment protocols are based on the work of the Lausanne group or the Endo Klinik (Zimmerli et al. 2004; Kendoff and Gehrke 2014). Treatment is based on the duration of the PJI, the stability of the implant, the clinical situation of the patient as well as the (preoperative) identification of the micro-organism involved and the feasibility of antimicrobial treatment. Unfortunately, most of these issues require clinical judgement that is hard to describe scientifically. This results in a lack of objective data that could lead to an overestimation of the effect of treatment, or in statistical terms a type-1 error.

Furthermore, almost all clinical studies on PJI are hampered by serious limitations such as retrospective study design, small group sizes, heterogeneous groups mixing acute and chronic PJI and various joints involved. This leads to an increased probability of a type-2 error when comparing study groups. As a result it is all the more difficult to find a difference in the effect of various treatment protocols. The presence of such a difference may be cloaked by the large number of theoretically relevant factors that were not distributed evenly among the study groups and could not be corrected for.

6.3.6 Treatment Algorithm

One of the most important questions in prosthesis-related infection from a clinical point of view is which treatment method is optimal for this patient at this point. To answer this question, we have developed a treatment algorithm to guide our decisions on the one hand. On the other hand, we have constructed our own database of patients, not only including the types of bacteria involved and technical matters like bone stock but also comprising many patient factors that are correlated to treatment outcome.

Our treatment algorithm identifies five treatment scenarios:

- DAIR
- Failure to respond to DAIR
- Two-stage protocol
- Inadvertent one-stage protocol
- No wish for operation/inoperable patients

Debridement, Antibiotics, Irrigation, and Retention

When confronted with an acute PJI with a well-fixed prosthesis, DAIR is the treatment of choice. Our protocol makes no difference between cases that present in the early postoperative period or those that present late and may or may not have a haematogenous infection. As long as patients have symptoms for less than 4 weeks, we advocate DAIR. In the emergency room, no antibiotics are given to patients if they have a possible PJI. Soft tissue debridement is performed until bleeding surfaces are achieved and a set of five cultures is taken. A sample is also sent for histological examination. If during the surgical procedure loose components are found, they are removed, but not re-implanted at the same time. The wound is instilled with 0.37% solution of povidone–iodine for 3 min. Irrigation is performed with at least 6 l of saline using pulsatile lavage. Dead space can be managed with gentamicin beads or gentamicin collagen fleeces. To reduce wound leakage, these are left only underneath the deep fascia. Wounds are closed in customary fashion without any wound drains. After the last culture has been taken, intravenous flucloxacillin (8 g/24 h, continuous infusion) is started. Treatment is redirected based on the outcome of cultures. Rifampicin is started in the case of staphylococcal infection and if proven susceptible to prevent mono-treatment, which has been shown to lead to rifampicin resistance.

Removal of all foreign body material may offer better chance of infection control, but results of DAIR indicate that this is not necessary in the majority of cases. Furthermore, it exposes the patient to greater surgical risks (increase in blood loss, operating time and perioperative fracture), which is all the more threatening in a patient with an acute infection and a septic profile. Renewing exchangeable parts has shown to have good results in the literature. It also makes sense, bearing in mind that the biofilm on those parts that are exchanged no longer needs to be eradicated. Furthermore, it allows for a more radical debridement of the joint lining. However, not all prostheses used in our hospitals have parts that can be removed without sacrificing soft tissue balance and some parts are no longer available off the shelf. For this reason, we have chosen only to remove parts that can *easily* be exchanged. This lowers the threshold for starting the treatment protocol as soon as possible, since none of our staff members has to wait for a hip, knee or shoulder specialist to be present. Although there will always be discussion on the time limit until when DAIR can be started (particularly if measured in weeks), we feel that a delay in the start of treatment of a couple of days does matter in the majority of acute PJI presentations.

Failure to Respond to DAIR

Treatment effect is monitored by clinical observation, C-reactive protein (CRP) level and leukocyte counts. Kidney function is also monitored, which is particularly important when gentamicin has been used as local antibiotic treatment. If there is insufficient improvement after 2 weeks or if there is a secondary rise in CRP or wound leakage, a second DAIR procedure is performed. We have arrangements with surrounding hospitals to refer patients to our PJI unit. If gentamicin beads have been used, the second stage is planned in all cases. This is done by one of the colleagues dealing with PJI. If *easily* exchangeable parts have not been replaced, we plan to do so at the second DAIR.

This process can be repeated again, but should there be no response after the third DAIR we normally proceed to removing all the foreign body material. The prosthesis is sent to the laboratory for sonication and culture if no probable micro-organism was found.

Two-Stage Protocol

When facing a chronic PJI, we perform the procedure as in DAIR, up to the point that the prosthesis is removed with all foreign material. Antibiotics are again withheld up to the point of having taken all the cultures. When no positive culture is available from the work-up or from prior operations, we generally use a spacer as dead space management. The spacer is made from gentamicin- and clindamycin-loaded cement. In the case of overt pus, use of gentamicin beads is an option. When an infecting agent is known preoperatively we will do the same, unless the infection is deemed to be »difficult to treat«. In that case, in hips a Girdlestone procedure is performed without any interposing flaps and in knees an external fixator is applied. Since we make our spacers during the procedure, we have the option of adding additional antibiotics to the bone cement. However, this is only seldom necessary.

Treatment effect is monitored as described previously. Should the need for an extra stage arise, the spacer is replaced with a new one. If the response to treatment is satisfactory, the second stage is planned after a minimum of 6 weeks. Antibiotic treatment is continued up to the point of the re-implantation stage. Rifampicin treatment is withheld in the interval, since evidence to support this is lacking and mono-treatment of a possibly not yet discovered staphylococcal strain would risk developing resistance. The procedure is basically the same as the DAIR, only now, a new prosthesis is placed again after taking five cultures. For hips, antibiotic therapy is continued for 3 months, for knees, 6 months.

Again, treatment effect is monitored, although interventions are not described in detail. Should the need arise it is discussed in the PJI team.

Inadvertent One-Stage Protocol

In all revision procedures we take cultures. Despite a high index of suspicion for PJI, sometimes only after extensive perioperative culturing will a PJI be found. Although we do not perform a revision for a non-suspected PJI as a three-step procedure (as described earlier), we do start with a pre-emptive antibiotic treatment. This means giving at least 2 days of cefazolin 1,000 mg three times daily. After 2 days, the cultures are inspected for the first time. Virulent bacteria will have usually grown by then, meaning we continue treatment. If there is some doubt as to whether there might be an infectious cause after all, the pre-emptive treatment will be extended up to 1 or even 2 weeks. At these points the cultures are inspected again. After 2 weeks the cultures are discontinued. We feel that the results reported for missed »low-grade« infections justify this approach (Boot et al. 2015).

No Wish for Operation/Inoperable Patients

There is a small group of older patients who show signs of failure of their prosthetic joint with a PJI that does not cause sepsis. Unfortunately, this may be the outcome of a prior treatment as described under the first four points. These patients may be very reluctant to undergo further surgery, or in some cases may be inoperable because of comorbidity. A risk that threatens these patients is that bone resorption can lead to periprosthetic fracture. This could lead to catastrophic failure and severe impairment of mobility. The challenge to find proper management in this group is even greater than for a »simple« PJI, since there is a lack of evidence for any treatment. It is impossible to use the combination of antibiotic and surgical treatment as described, and thus no predictable results can be expected. We resort to either using suppressive antibiotic treatment or in rare cases to drain the infection by surgically creating a fistula.

Antibiotic treatment is an option if there is a known causative bacteria that can be treated by an oral regimen, which has little chance of complications. This carries a risk of antibiotic resistance developing in the PJI. It has been suggested to change the antibiotic of choice every couple of weeks in order to limit this risk.

Creating a fistula is an option if there is a large amount of fluid that causes pain and discomfort. We create the fistula by decompressing the fluid collection and suturing a modified 20-ml syringe into the skin. The point of the syringe is cut off to make a hollow tube. The plunger is removed and the wings are trimmed to a few millimetres. This end is inserted into the wall of the abscess, and the other end is perforated and sutured into the skin with non-resorbable material. This is covered by a pouch such as used in stomas. After about 4–6 weeks, the tract is sufficiently epithelialized to remove the syringe. This can lead to retention of an infected prosthesis for months or a few years.

6.3.7 Conclusion

In conclusion, not all PJIs are alike, but all share the biofilm mode of growth. This makes PJI hard to treat, but results reported in the literature have shown improvement over time up to a cure rate of 95%. Using a two-stage protocol generally gives better outcome than a one-stage procedure, although inadvertent one-stage treatment in »low-grade« PJI still yields acceptable results. We treat PJI using accurate microbiological diagnosis and treatment, debridement, local antiseptic and antibiotic treatment, monitoring the effect of treatment and re-debridement to eradicate the biofilm infection. Having defined the various PJI treatment scenarios helps us to rapidly start optimal treatment, without having to wait for an exact definition of type of infection and, in time, causative organism or grade.

We have used this approach for the past 5 years and have started to prospectively collect patient, infection and technical details in a revision cohort. This cohort is followed up using clinical as well as patient-reported outcome measures. The data we collect can be used to inform patients about their options when faced with PJI and to help us to refine our protocol and as such PJI treatment outcome.

Take-Home Message

- Antibiotics alone, although effective against many infections, generally fail to achieve cure in the case of PJI, because of the immuno-incompetent zone at the implant surface, lack of biofilm accessibility and poor tissue penetration of antibiotics at the site of infection.
- Successful treatment of PJI involves a combination of antibiotic and surgical management. The use of treatment algorithms improves the discussion of patients in a multidisciplinary setting. Algorithm-based treatment results can be used to inform patients on their expected outcome.

References

Anagnostakos K, Wilmes P, Schmitt E, Kelm J (2009) Elution of gentamicin and vancomycin from polymethylmethacrylate beads and hip spacers in vivo. Acta Orthop 80(2): 193–197

Boot W, Moojen DJ, Visser E, Lehr AM, De Windt TS, Van Hellemondt G, Geurts J, Tulp NJ, Schreurs BW, Burger BJ, Dhert WJ, Gawlitta D, Vogely HC (2015) Missed low-grade infection in suspected aseptic loosening has no consequences for the survival of total hip arthroplasty. Acta Orthop 86(6):678–683

Buchholz HW, Elson RA, Engelbrecht E, Lodenkamper H, Rottger J, Siegel A (1981) Management of deep infection of total hip replacement. J Bone Joint Surg Br 63:342–353

Charnley J (1972) Postoperative infection after total hip replacement with special reference to air contamination in the operating room. Clin Orthop 87:167–187

De Klaver PA, Hendriks JG, van Onzenoort HA, Schreurs BW, Touw DJ, Derijks LJ (2012) Gentamicin serum concentrations in patients with gentamicin-PMMA beads for infected hip joints: a prospective observational cohort study. Ther Drug Monit 34(1):67–71

Gardner J, Gioe TJ, Tatman P (2011) Can this prosthesis be saved?: implant salvage attempts in infected primary TKA. Clin Orthop Relat Res 469:970–976

Gristina AG (1994) Implant failure and the immuno-incompetent fibro-inflammatory zone. Clin Orthop 298:106–118

Gristina AG, Costerton JW (1985) Bacterial adherence to biomaterials and tissue. The significance of its role in clinical sepsis. J Bone Joint Surg Am 67:264–273

Haddad FS, Muirhead-Allwood SK, Manktelow AR, Bacarese-Hamilton I (2000) Two-stage uncemented revision hip arthroplasty for infection. J Bone Joint Surg Br 82:689–694

Härle A, Ritzerfeld W (1979) The release of gentamycin into the wound secretions from polymethylmethacrylate beads. A study with reference to the animal experiment. Arch Orthop Trauma Surg 95(1–2):65–70

Holleyman RJ, Baker PN, Charlett A, Gould K, Deehan DJ (2016) Analysis of causative microorganism in 248 primary hip arthroplasties revised for infection: a study using the NJR dataset. Hip Int 26(1):82–89

Hope PG, Kristinsson KG, Norman P, Elson RA (1989) Deep infection of cemented total hip arthroplasties caused by coagulase-negative staphylococci. J Bone Joint Surg Br 71:851–855

Holtom PD, Warren CA, Greene NW, Bravos PD, Ressler RL, Shepherd L, McPherson EJ, Patzakis MJ (1998) Relation of surface area to in vitro elution characteristics of vancomycin-impregnated polymethylmethacrylate spacers. Am J Orthop 27(3):207–210

Hunter G, Dandy D (1977) The natural history of the patient with an infected total hip replacement. J Bone Joint Surg Br 59:293–297

Janssen DM, Geurts JA, Jütten LM, Walenkamp GH (2016) 2-stage revision of 120 deep infected hip and knee prostheses using gentamicin-PMMA beads. Acta Orthop 28:1–9

Kendall RW, Duncan CP, Beauchamp CP (1995) Bacterial growth on antibiotic-loaded acrylic cement. A prospective in vivo retrieval study. J Arthroplasty 10: 817–822

Kendoff D, Gehrke T (2014) Surgical management of periprosthetic joint infection: one-stage exchange. J Knee Surg 27(4):273–278

Lange J, Troelsen A, Thomsen RW, Søballe K (2012) Chronic infections in hip arthroplasties: comparing risk of reinfection following one-stage and two-stage revision: a systematic review and meta-analysis. Clinical Epidemiology 4:57–73

Mah TF, O'Toole GA (2001) Mechanisms of biofilm resistance to antibicrobial agents. Trends Microbiol 9:34–39

Masters JP, Smith NA, Foguet P, Reed M, Parsons H, Sprowson AP (2013) A systematic review of the evidence for single stage and two stage revision of infected knee replacement. BMC Musculoskelet Disord 14:222

Schmolders J, Hischebeth GT, Friedrich MJ, Randau TM, Wimmer MD, Kohlhof H, Molitor E, Gravius S (2014) Evidence of MRSE on a gentamicin and vancomycin impregnated polymethyl-methacrylate (PMMA) bone cement spacer after two-stage exchange arthroplasty due to periprosthetic joint infection of the knee. BMC Infect Dis 14:144

Sherrell JC, Fehring TK, Odum S, Hansen E, Zmistowski B, Dennos A, Kalore N (2011) The Chitranjan Ranawat Award: fate of two-stage reimplantation after failed irrigation and débridement for periprosthetic knee infection. Clin Orthop Relat Res 469:18–25

Swieringa AJ, Goosen JH, Jansman FG, Tulp NJ (2008) In vivo pharmacokinetics of a gentamicin-loaded collagen sponge in acute periprosthetic infection: serum values in 19 patients. Acta Orthop 79(5):637–642

Von Eiff C, Lindner N, Proctor RA, Winkelmann W, Peters G (1998) Auftreten von Gentamicin-resistenten small colony variants von S. aureus nach Einsetzen von Gentamicin-Ketten bei Osteomyelitis als mögliche Ursache für Rezidive. Z Orthop Ihre Grenzgebiete 136:268–271
Winkelmann W, Schulitz KP, Knothe H, Schoening B (1978) Knochen- und Hämatomspiegel des Aminogylkosid-Antibiotkums Tobramycin. Infection 6:277–282
Zimmerli W, Trampuz A, Ochsner PE (2004) Prosthetic-joint infections. N Engl J Med 351(16):1645–1654

6.4 The University Hospitals of Louvain Experience and Care Pathways for PJIs: How We Do It

Jeroen Neyt

6.4.1 The Diagnostic Stage

A proper referral of the patient to our centre is required, including information on the following:

- Reason for referral (second opinion or transfer of care)
- History of sequence of events with problem prosthesis including original indication for index surgery
- Past diagnostic work-up (Peersman et al. 2001)
- Results and sensitivity of cultured germs, details of the aspirate, swab, tissue culture/biopsy
- Proper medical and surgical history
- Present medication including antibiotics (last time and length of period taken for whatever indication)
- Family history, social history, and professional occupation
- Allergies and specific evaluation of possible immuno-incompetencies (Jamsen et al. 2009), e.g. diabetes mellitus (Adams et al. 2013), rheumatoid arthritis (RA; Schrama et al. 2010), past oncological history ((chemotherapy/radiation), chronic steroid use (Berbari et al. 2012), co-morbidities and solid organ transplant (Vergidis et al. 2012), smoking, skin diseases (e.g. psoriasis, history of vascular surgery, kidney function, nutritional status (overweight, underweight, unexplained weight loss, body mass index), substance abuse, chronic pain syndrome, psychological/psychiatric status, post-trauma management, disease insight
- Past or present enrolment in other treatment protocols/studies (e.g. new disease-modifying anti-rheumatic drugs [DMARDS])
- Evaluation of aspiration results (Berbari et al. 2010)
- Recent blood samples, investigations and imaging studies including plain radiographs, computed tomography (CT) scans, magnetic resonance imaging (MRI) scans, nuclear scans including white blood cell-labelled scans, single-photon emission CT (SPECT) etc. via Pacs on Web or DVD loaded on the Clinical Workstation Software by the reception desk staff at patient arrival

At our institute, a thorough clinical examination (according to PJI location) is performed of both limbs, which are fully exposed, and an evaluation of the axial musculoskeletal system if required. The examiner should look, feel, check and test for the presence of swelling, redness, and fistulae; the amount of leakage should be examined by checking gauzes and inquiring about the frequency of changes and also about increased temperature; further, the quality of the skin and soft tissue envelope should be assessed. The range of motion (ROM) of the affected and adjacent joints is checked before performing a thorough neurovascular examination, in particular testing the capillary refill time and distal pulses.

We recommend taking several clinical photos of the patient in standing and supine position after drawing all scars with indelible marking (unfortunately crossed train line rail appearance not unusual). Subsequently, the care pathway is explained to the patient and consent is obtained. As a next step, imaging studies are ordered, i.e. at least up-to-date plain radiographs of the involved joint in weight-bearing position but also of any suspect areas of symptomatic metalwork (disc replacement, other arthroplasties). Nuclear scintigraphy scans or other scans can be considered in uncertain cases (Chryssikos et al. 2008)

Blood samples are then taken to assess the following: ionogram, erythrocyte sedimentation rate (first timers), C-reactive protein (CRP), coagulation studies (sickle cell), HbA1C for hidden diabetes (Jamsen et al. 2012), iron, calcium, and phosphate, alkaline phosphatase, hepatic function, albumin, transferring saturation, and vitamin D for the patient's nutritional status (Gherini et al. 1993; Fletcher and Fairfield 2002; Jaberi et al. 2008).

It is advised to plan at least one or two joint aspirations not only of the troubled joint but possibly also of the other (possibly symptomatic) prosthetic replacements (perform first!) in sterile conditions (proper surgical gown and theatre set-up) after an antibiotic-free interval of at least 2 weeks (Parvizi et al. 2011; Zmistowski et al. 2012; Dinneen et al. 2013).

The patient should be alerted to possible acute relapses of the infection within 2 weeks of stopping antibiotics, and a 24-h helpline number should be provided. Also, PCR or next generation sequencing studies of the aspiration sample could be performed if the antibiotic-free period is too short for a particular reason. If appropriate, broad-spectrum oral antibiotics can be restarted until the follow-up visit (Della et al. 2010).

6.4.2 Before Hospital Admission

Before the patient is admitted to hospital, the examination results should be discussed with the patient and their family, outlining the treatment plan, i.e. single-stage versus two-stage exchange procedure.

The clinical status of the patient should be optimal before embarking on infection control or eradication. If ankle–brachial index studies, transcutaneous oxygenation, angio-CT, angio-MRI, or any balloon or bypass procedures are required, these should be carried out first. Proper advice should be sought from plastic and reconstructive surgeons so as to allow the team to plan ahead. Both teams should be kept on standby when performing exchange surgery. Internists should review the medication so as to start treating hitherto hidden diabetes, to correct anaemia, and to plan the pathway to suspend DMARDS etc. and evaluate and correct any malnutrition.

The next step is to get a detailed anaesthesiology opinion (Spahn 2010) and plan for pre-, peri- and post-operative care including pain control and PCA pumps.

The admission office must be informed about the planned treatment and the requirement to stop antibiotics 2 weeks before admission. Patients can call the 24-h helpline if symptoms such as fever (appropriately measured by thermometer, >38°C), night sweats and tremor, or significantly increased redness and painful swelling around affected prosthesis develop, warranting earlier admission and aspiration unless the patient is scheduled for a first-stage revision.

Communication is maintained with the patient and the family physician about any unexpected events in the run-up to the procedure such as initiation of antibiotic treatment for an unrelated condition, e.g. bronchopneumonia, which would obviously delay the planned surgical procedure. The 2-week antibiotic-free period starts again after the end of the antibiotic course.

Plan to meet your patient at admission (your personally or a properly instructed member of surgical team). An anamnestic checklist should be completed again for any recent developments or changes of treatment plans, e.g. after rheumatology or nephrology clinic visits. With both of the patient's limbs fully exposed, we draw dotted lines over all scars in the proximity of the infected prosthesis with a permanent marker as well as a large double arrow to prevent surgery of the wrong site. After obtaining confirmation and informed consent from patient, an anaesthetist re-evaluates the status of patient and his/her wishes as to the anaesthetic modality including the setting up of a deep venous catheter and patient-controlled anaesthesia pump. If not already completed, the nursing staff completes the patient questionnaire to record the patient's home medication and status of their network or family support if not already. We then discuss the risk stratification process with the surgical team to classify the patient's status according to the Cierny–Mader, the McPherson (McPherson et al. 2002), and the Haddad scoring systems. We confirm via telephone and e-mail the methicillin-resistant *Staphylococcus aureus* (MRSA), carbapenamase-producing enterobacteriaceae (CPE), vancomycin-resistant enterococci (VRE), human immunodeficiency virus (HIV), hepatitis B/C (Orozco et al. 2013), and tuberculosis (TBC) status of the patient so as to determine the biohazard status and risks for the operating theatre staff. This information also helps to establish the requirements for (a) surgical instrumentation and materials (usually ordered and planned weeks beforehand), (b) the presence of industrial representatives, (c) fluoroscopy, (d) the set-up for cultures/biopsies, (e) irrigation schemes, (f) a clean phase or suite, and (g) tourniquet, packed cells, and tranexamic acid. We ascertain that our patient has had preoperative showering, has no surgical site/limb skin ulcers and has had the hair on the surgical site removed with electrical clippers (on the morning of the surgery; Mangram et al. 1999; Tanner et al. 2011).

6.4.3 The Day of Surgery

The Preoperative Stage

The theatre suite should be heated (Melling et al. 2001) and the entire team of surgical, anaesthetic and nursing staff should stay inside the operating theatre to reduce OR traffic in and out (McPherson and Peters 2011). The operating theatre traffic is reduced by logging/monitoring all traffic (Stocks et al. 2010) aided by door-opening counters and a small (pass on item slide) window built in the main door. A separate nurse outside the OR room is responsible for completing the paperwork and preparing the surgical and anaesthetic equipment for the procedure to follow. The nurse also passes on any additionally required items, e.g. cement, prefabricated spacers, local and systemic antibiotics and certifies the WHO check-list and time-out procedure (de Vries et al. 2010). Anaesthetic induction is performed in a septic suite with two peripheral intravenous access lines, at least one arterial line and one deep venous catheter. Recent appropriate radiographs are used on electronic screens with permanent markings showing. The theatre scrub nursing and surgical team wear impermeable gowns and Charnley helmets (for protection) with a fan and light focus for the two main surgeons. The running nurse, visitor, and anaesthetic staff wear add-on yellow gowns to remind them not to simply walk out for a chat. In the time period from incision to wound closure or the moment the dressing over an open existing wound is taken off, only authorized staff can walk out or in and with valid reasons. If there are no contra-indications or thrombo-embolic events in the past, the anaesthetist is instructed to instil tranexamic acid (Exacyl®) in a weight-adjusted dose (Zhou et al. 2013) as we do later in situ (Wong et al. 2010).

We plan to abandon the routine use of urinary catheters (except for first-stage revision hip replacements) with post-operative bladder scans and single catheterization. In the case of MRSA-, CPE-, or VRE-colonized patients, the set-up with internal and external nursing staff is organized the moment the patient is rolled into the theatre suite, not only when dressings are removed.

The sequence of prepping in the OR room is as follows: Charnley helmets are covered and only then is the battery-charged head ventilation unit switched on, immediately followed by pulling on a sterile gown. The instrumenting nurse or OR technician helps the surgeon with green gloves first, with white gloves on top secondly, and if desired (sharp objects hazard) a third pair of linen gloves. The sequence of prepping and draping of the patient is as follows: on the ward in the morning before the procedure, the patient is transferred to the OR, hair in and around the incision zone is trimmed with a battery-charged clipper. In the OR, the operating zone is surrounded or blocked off from either the perineal area in hip surgery, from the upper thigh zone in knee surgery or from the axillary pit in shoulder surgery by plastic U-shaped sticky sheets. Disinfection of the operating zone is carried out with iodine alcohol or chlorhexidine. The patient is covered and isolated from the anaesthetic team by several triple water-impermeable sheets or drapes. A large Ioban sticky plastic foil (or none if iodine allergy) is attached to the operating zone (Fairclough et al. 1986) before amenities or utilities are deployed such as monopolar electro-cautery 50/50, suction, a Zimmer irrigation pulse lavage gun (or from other companies) and a second suction system.

The Intraoperative Stage

At this stage, we obtain permission to start from the anaesthetist and scrub nurse. An »all in place check« is made to reduce operating time. We use double gloving, changing every 90 min as well as before and after cementation (Beldame et al. 2012). The next step is to excise any scar, wound edges, and fistulae (if required, contrast dye or methylene blue is injected). Once the skin and subcutaneous tissues have been incised, we proceed with aspiration (this method prevents skin bacteria contamination) and arrange for fluids to be collected in (adult or paediatric [richer broth]) an aerobic haemoculture, anaerobic haemoculture (HC) bottle, and cytology tube for further testing including leukocyte esterase, alpha-defensin, and other desired markers. On the side table – called the Oxford table at our institution – there are 12 vials in six pairs with each pair allocated a disposable knife, a forceps, and a bone nibbler (Mikkelsen et al. 2006).

Once the joint capsule has been incised after careful haemostasis, biofilm samples are obtained by means of separate Oxford table instruments and they are geographically defined and logged, e.g. biofilm behind the cup or inside the tibia channel aiming to reduce cross-contamination by use of the same instrument and to validate preoperative investigations – for instance, hot spot on a white blood cell scan corresponds to infection/biofilm in that particular location. Each biofilm sample is split up into a culture part and a pathology part, after which the three aforementioned instruments are discarded. A large and a small uterine curette are kept on the Oxford table to scrape off biofilm from inside the canals or cup.

Once six samples have been collected, logged, described and split, the anaesthesia team is informed to give the patient antibiotics according to the bacteriological results obtained by aspiration some weeks before or according to microbiological advice or blindly (usually vancomycin 1 g twice a day with subsequent therapeutic drug monitoring on the ward and piperacillin tazobactam is involved) and anti-mycotics if desired and planned beforehand.

Subsequently, the prosthetic components are carefully removed with the controlled and combined use of the following (in knee surgery): fine long osteotomes, oscillating saw, component extractors, Gigli saw carefully preserving as much bone stock as possible. If a Whiteside osteotomy for the tibia or a limited distal femoral osteotomy is required to either remove a long stem or cement, an Ultra-Drive or Midas dental bur system can help. Continuous irrigation is required to prevent thermal osteonecrosis. If required, an extended trochanteric osteotomy (ETO) (Morshed et al. 2005), a tibial Whiteside osteotomy, or a femoral gutter osteotomy is created and followed by the use of saline-cooled high-speed dental burs. Once metal components have been removed, the cement mantle – if present – is taken out piecemeal with special cement osteotomes and curettes as well as canal reamers (carefully increasing in size and with fluoroscopy guidance if required). We make sure the trunnion is not damaged if the stem remains stuck and Wagner or similar extended trochanter osteotomies are not carried through. The cement plastic plugs are usually drilled through and taken out by long hooks. We prefer to remove a hip prosthesis through the posterior approach (identifying the location and course of the sciatic nerve). Care is taken to scrape off the biofilm in its entirety from the cup and medullary cavity checking for cortical breakthroughs and hidden fistulae. Prosthetic components are handed out preferably with a no-touch technique in specially designed bags for sonication, especially useful for urgent DAIR procedures or in cases of an antibiotic-free interval of less than 14 days (Trampuz et al. 2007). One should explore in particular the posterior aspects of the proximal/distal femur (THA/TKA) and proximal aspect of the tibia (TKA). We then perform a thorough open synovectomy with the cutting electro-stick in a systematic round-the-clock manner as well as a debridement of suspicious or devitalized tissues. We use the saw to trim bony surfaces removing hitherto unreachable pockets. We always use cooling fluid to reduce thermal osteonecrosis.

We change the suction tip every 60 min (Givissis et al. 2008; Insull and Hudson 2012). Next, the planned irrigation scheme is started (Draeger and Dahners 2006) but it should be noted that between fluid bag sessions further debridement might be necessary. Usually we start with 3 l of warm saline with an intermittent pressure pump (Munoz-Mahamud et al. 2011) and splash sheet to prevent spreading of microscopic air droplets followed by a short soaking of diluted hydrogen peroxide (without pressure to prevent embolism and only if the site is pus loaded for additional mechanical debridement). Otherwise, we do not use hydrogen peroxide because of the increased potential for stiffness presumably because of cytotoxicity even when diluted. Again, 3 l of warm saline with a splash sheet and engine-driven femoral and acetabular brush are used. If there is a known infection with Pseudomonas, we apply a short soaking with 1% acetic acid followed by the third 3-l volume bag. At this stage a second instrument nurse prepares the »clean table«. We do not mix dilution fluids with antibiotics. Subsequently, a mixture of 500 ml with two ocular vials of iso-betadine in H_2O prepared in a glass jar is poured on the site and allowed to soak for 10–15 min (minimum dose to prevent cytotoxicity but still efficient; Brown et al. 2012) whilst all but one of the scrubbed surgical team pull back from the »dirty table« and are given a new water-impermeable gown on top of the old one and new gloves. This is the »Economy« option.

The upgrade to »Business« option entails temporary closure of the wound and dressing application and whilst the patient remains anaesthetized all contaminated trays, drapes and instruments are discarded; the surgical team takes a coffee break and then starts scrubbing and prepping again with new instrument trays and set-up.

The »First Class« option is wound and dressing application as described above followed by transport of the anaesthetized patient to an adjacent clean theatre suite with a new set-up. In the Economy model the last member holds the limb elevated whilst the »clean-phase team« prepares and drapes the patient's limb again on top of the »dirty« drapes applying a new Ioban and putting down a new electrocautery set, suction line and wide-bore-diameter infusion line allowing the last and final bag of warm normal saline to run in. Two new clean-phase cultures are then taken to qualify the previous cleaning efforts.

The dirty-phase tables in the meantime are put aside and taken out. On the clean-phase table the prefabricated spacers (sized by measuring with templates in situ or with a ruler) are ordered and tested in situ for stability, correct sizing, extension and flexion gap – the preferred option if time runs short (tourniquet or fragile patient; Anderson et al. 2009; Fleck et al. 2011).

If required, Tecres plastic malls can be used to inject either cement loaded with vancomycin and gentamicin (we started inserting pieces of Spongostan® attempting to increase spacer porosity and to increase future antibiotic elution duration) or cement, mixed with the desired heat-stable antibiotics or anti-mycotics (Parvizi et al. 2008). Currently, we are testing a vast array of »canal fillers« to optimize our dead space management such as OsteoSet®, Osteofill® or Herafill®, Cerament® V and G and BonAlive®. The hip spacer stem (with a steel core) is sized appropriately. To prevent a mismatch between stem and ball size, we aim to go modular in the near future (Biomet). Congruency and stability without undue constraint are key to preventing undue spacer dislocation, maintaining a proper wide soft tissue volume and optimizing function for the mobile spacers. For the knee spacers, a match between flexion and extension gap can be obtained by sizing additional cement waffle augmentation and a possible short intramedullary cone or stub. Once we are satisfied with the test results, the spacers (hip stem calcar, the femoral and tibial component) and the surfaces are smeared with doughy cement and inserted. We position a laminar spreader or haemostat clamp in-between the femoral and tibial component to prevent them becoming stuck together and remove any unwanted cement pressurized out. We wait for the cement to cure fully before reducing the hip spacer after cleaning the cup area of any undesired cement debris. If the »banana peel technique« is used for the knee to explore pus pockets and hidden fistulae resulting in significant ligamentous instability, a static spacer is used with antibiotic-cemented steel pins or a cheap small Isola rod inserted into the femoral channel and a second one into the tibial channel partially sliding over and along each other with preservation of an acceptable extension gap. Subsequently, a doughnut with newly mixed doughy cement is created in situ around the cement nails. A piece of hard plastic cut out of a plastic bowl is used between the femur and tibia to prevent thermal damage and undesired warm waxing away of the curing cement. The plastic is pulled out once the cement is cured (Masri et al. 1998; Kühn 2007; Fink et al. 2011).

If indicated we use and additionally insert vancomycin sandwiches into the canals (vancomycin up to 8 g powder prepared with some normal saline as a cottage cheese spread onto Spongostans; O'Neill et al. 2011; Kuiper et al. 2013).

We reserve the so-called Girdlestone hip procedures, leaving no spacer in place, only as a last resort in those patients not able to go through a two-stage procedure or after several failed one- or two-stage attempts. The mobility and stability of the reduced spacer positions are tested and recorded. Two deep-drain plastic tubes (without suction but only gravity) are inserted and secured to the skin.

We then carry out careful and meticulous closure with separate Vicryl® 1plus sutures of the knee extensor mechanism or of the fascial and muscular soft tissue envelope of the hip.

Once properly sealed off, we use a local infiltration anaesthesia scheme with a syringe of 20 ml of Naropin® at a dosage of 5 mg/ml and three vials of tranexamic acid (500 mg/5 ml) in two 50-ml syringes topped up with normal saline. Subsequently, two subcutaneous drains (on suction) are inserted and secured.

Further subcutaneous stitching with Vicryl® 1plus is performed followed by stapling of the skin. Absorbing gauzes are secured by an elastic roll dressing, Mefix® sticky sheets and a simple extra-large cricket bat splint are used for the knee and an abduction pillow or anti-rotation splint for the hip. After waking up, the patient is turned from lateral to supine position for extubating if indicated and carefully transferred from the operation table to his/her bed via a long double-sliding plastic sheet cushion to prevent undesired bruises and discomfort and to ease transfer.

The patient is then rolled out of the septic theatre into the septic recovery suite with one-to-one care.

The Post-operative Stage

In the immediate post-operative phase the principle of a separate septic recovery room with a dedicated nurse in yellow attire is critical so as to isolate the patient from patients who have had clean orthopaedic procedures. The systemic and neurovascular status of the patient is regularly checked and recorded. Wound drains with or without vacuum suction are unlocked and the involved limb is elevated if indicated.

The two superficial drains are subjected to vacuum only after a 30–60-min post-operative delay. Requests are made for cultures, biopsies, post-operative X-ray of the chest (deep venous catheter check) and hip or knee. Post-operative care sheets are completed as well as sonication sheets. A thorough neurovascular examination of the motor and sensory function of the lower limb in particular active ankle/toe pulling is carried out and recorded. The awake patient is briefly talked to and reassured.

After the busy operating day (in the evening) an efficient post-operative ward round is run with short explanations to the patient and any immediate family members present. Thrombo-prophylaxis – e.g. Clexane® 40 mg s.c. – is usually given at 8 p.m. Post-operative radiographs are inspected and the surgical technique used is evaluated for feedback.

The antibiotic scheme is adjusted once culture results are available and antibiograms or antibiotic sensitivities are discussed with the attending microbiologist.

A physiotherapist team is recruited 48 h post-operatively and bed-to-chair transfers are started followed by careful ambulation efforts supported by assistive devices such as crutches, quadruped or rollator frames.

As soon as possible, the deep venous catheter positioned in the jugular vein is replaced with a peripherally inserted central catheter (so-called PICC line), which is reportedly less prone to catheter sepsis and more patient friendly.

We prefer to suture the wound meticulously in layers with Vicryl® 1plus and with mostly two deep (no suction) and two subcutaneous (vacuum suction) drains in place to reduce any post-operative haematomata and to »suck dead space dry«. In contrast to clean joint replacement procedures in which we preferably do not use any drains, the rationale is obviously entirely different in a septic setting.

We tend to use skin staples because we believe skin edges/margins heal in between the sutures and a classic through-stitching technique could potentially render skin and subcutaneous zones hypoxic leading to skin-edge necrosis, wound-edge dehiscence and ultimately wound breakdown.

Occlusive absorptive dressing is applied with the appropriate tension as well as an extension knee brace if required.

6.4.4 Comments on Different Treatment Options

At our institution we believe preoperative optimization of the patient's status and of all systems as well as risk stratification are critical in selecting the best surgical treatment and care plan so as to obtain the best possible outcome for the patient –i.e. single-stage (healthy patient, primary replacement, known sensitive germ) versus two- or three-stage procedures (high-risk immunocompromised patient, multiple procedures, excessive germs) with static spacers or none at all.

In the case of *Pseudomonas* or mycotic infection of knee replacements, we tend not to use articulating spacers but a bridging external fixator with an absent or short antibiotic-free interval between the first and second stage (Kotwal et al. 2012). A double or triple spacer exchange regimen might also be required (Azzam et al. 2009).

We have also noticed that some of our elderly, frail or severely immunocompromised patients appear to function well enough with spacers (merely limited ambulation or no perceived limitations) and they decline further surgery. The middle- to long-term fate of these spacers remains to be assessed and is monitored.

We do not rule out the concept of partial exchange of components especially for revision hip or knee replacements. If indeed the cup appears loose and there is ample biofilm found behind and, for instance, a fully coated long femoral stem appears completely ingrown and sealed off, meaning no entry sleeves at all at the calcar level, we consider a partial exchange in the elderly frail patient in whom an extended Wagner or Whiteside osteotomy or extended osteotomy (ETO) might be a bridge too far. Loose components are removed and exchanged with new ones after thorough debridement, cleaning and temporary closure with the new set-up in a clean theatre next door if possible. In infected hip replacements with a stem solidly stuck in the femoral canal, we use the technique of a bipolar head concept with an antibiotic smooth head sized according to the acetabular reaming size and moulded into sterile steel bipolar shells of different sizes filled with a layer of paraffin and antibiotic cement. Just above and inside the top layers, a cheap, small metal ball is kept from sinking with a 5-ml syringe inserted into the ball. Once cured, the bipolar head is gently hammered onto the trunnion and reduction is performed. The depth of the central position of the metal ball into the curing larger head requires a learning curve. A stable configuration can be achieved. Trunnion damage by inappropriately positioned gripping femoral stem extractor instruments is of significant concern if the stem is left in situ because of a failed extraction despite numerous attempts and if the surgeon then decides not to proceed with an extended trochanteric osteotomy for further removal attempts.

We believe there is a place for so-called DAIR procedures (Byren et al. 2009) with thorough incision and drainage, synovectomy, debridement (Romano et al. 2012) and exchange of modular prosthetic components performed for early infections or late haematogenous infections. These have a higher success rate in healthier patients, in infections with low-virulence organisms, and in optimized patients with a short period of symptoms and in absence of a sinus tract. If incision and drainage are to be attempted, it is imperative to ensure that the prosthesis is well fixed and well positioned and there is a good soft tissue envelope to cover the prosthesis (Zimmerli et al. 2004; Sukeik et al. 2012).

◘ Tab. 6.5 presents the list of available antibiotics and anti-fungals that can be used in spacers. The dose ranges reveal only the reported doses in the analysed studies and are not recommendations. The type of antibiotic and the dose need to be individualized for each patient based on the organism profile and antibiogram (if available) as well as on the patient's renal function and allergy profile.

6.4.5 Conclusion

The successful treatment of a patient with PJI requires a thorough recognition of the status of the patient (systemic, immune, socio-economic and familial circumstances), his/her wishes, technical feasibilities, realistic target setting and expectations, the surgeon's expertise or perhaps lack of it, the availability of resources and a multi-disciplinary and dedicated team. Although no PJI patient resembles another, some experience-based rules of thumbs are helpful for the best treatment approach.

Tab. 6.5 Spacers and antibiotics (from Parvizi and Gehrke 2013)

Antibiotic group	Type of antibiotic	Activity against	Dose per 40-g cement (in grams)
Aminoglycoside	Tobramycin	Gram-negative bacteria such as *Pseudomonas*	1–4.8
Aminoglycoside	Gentamicin	Gram-negative bacteria, *Escherichia coli, Klebsiella* and particularly *Pseudomonas aeruginosa* . Also aerobic bacteria (not obligate/facultative anaerobes)	0.25–4.8
Cephalosporin, first generation	Cefazolin	Gram-positive infections, limited Gram-negative coverage	1–2
Cephalosporin, second generation	Cefuroxime	Reduced gram-positive coverage, improved Gram-negative coverage	1.5–2
Cephalosporin, third generation	Ceftazidime	Gram-negative bacteria, particularly Pseudomonas	2
Cephalosporin, fourth generation	Cefotaxime	Gram-negative bacteria, no activity against Pseudomonas	2
Cephalosporin, fifth generation	Ceftaroline	Gram-negative bacteria, no activity against Pseudomonas	2–4
Fluoroquinolone	Ciprofloxacin	Gram-negative organisms including activity against *Enterobacteriacaea*	0.2–3
Glycopeptide	Vancomycin	Gram-positive bacteria, including methicillin-resistant organisms	0.5–4
Lincosamide	Clindamycin	Gram-positive cocci, anaerobes	1–2
Macrolide	Erythromycin	Aerobic Gram-positive cocci and bacilli	0.5–1
Polymyxin	Colistin	Gram-negative	0.24
β-Lactam	Piperacillin not available piptazobactam	Gram-negative bacteria (particularly *Pseudomonas*), Enterobacteria and anaerobes	4–8
β-Lactam	Aztreonam	Only Gram-negative bacteria	4
β-Lactamase inhibitor	Tazobactam	Gram-negative bacteria (particularly *Pseudomonas*), Enterobacteria, and anaerobes in combination with piperacillin	0.5
Oxazolidinones	Linezolid	Multidrug-resistant Gram-positive cocci such as MRSA	1.2
Carbapenem	Meropenem	Gram-positive and gram-negative bacteria, anaerobes, *Pseudomonas*	0.5–4
Lipopeptide	Daptomycin	Only Gram-positive organisms	2
Antifungals	Amphotericin	Most fungi	200
Antifungal	Voriconazole	Most fungi	300–600 mg

The type of antibiotic and the dose need to be individualized for each patient based on the organism profile and antibiogram (if available) as well as the patient's renal function and allergy profile. However, most infections can be treated with a spacer with vancomycin (1–4 g per 40-g package of cement) and gentamicin or tobramycin (2.4–4.8 g per 40-g package of cement)

Take-Home Message

- Preoperatively, optimization of the patient's status and all systems as well as risk stratification are critical for selecting the best surgical treatment and care plan so as to obtain the best possible outcome for the patient.
- Orthopaedic surgeons who might not be treating PJIs on a full-time basis require some guidance.
- Special medical services or expert opinions should be sought from competent professionals who are dedicated to complex PJI cases.
- The patient and his or her relatives should be involved in the decision-making process about the treatment pathway.
- OR team communication is essential for a successful surgery.
- Patients with complex PJI should be treated in special centres where a standard of care can be provided.
- Best outcomes are achieved with a comprehensive therapy consisting of surgical, systemic and local infection management.

References

Adams AL, Paxton EW, Wang JQ, et al (2013) Surgical outcomes of total knee replacement according to diabetes status and glycemic control, 2001 to 2009. J Bone Joint Surg Am 95(6):481–487

Anderson JA, Sculco PK, Heitkemper S, Mayman DJ, Bostrom MP, Sculco TP (2009) An articulating spacer to treat and mobilize patients with infected total knee arthroplasty. J Arthroplasty 24(4):631–635

Azzam K, Parvizi J, Jungkind D, et al (2009) Microbiological, clinical, and surgical features of fungal prosthetic joint infections: a multi-institutional experience. J Bone Joint Surg Am 91[Suppl 6]:142–149

Beldame J, Lagrave B, Lievain L, Lefebvre B, Frebourg N, Dujardin F (2012) Surgical glove bacterial contamination and perforation during total hip arthroplasty implantation: when gloves should be changed. Orthop Traumatol Surg Res 98(4):432–440

Berbari E, Mabry T, Tsaras G, et al (2010) Inflammatory blood laboratory levels as markers of prosthetic joint infection: a systematic review and meta-analysis. J Bone Joint Surg Am 92(11):2102–2109

Berbari EF, Osmon DR, Lahr B, et al (2012) The Mayo prosthetic joint infection risk score: implication for surgical site infection reporting and risk stratification. Infect Control Hosp Epidemiol 33(8):774–781

Brown NM, Cipriano CA, Moric M, Sporer SM, Della Valle CJ (2012) Dilute betadine lavage before closure for the prevention of acute postoperative deep periprosthetic joint infection. J Arthroplasty 27(1):27–30

Byren I, Bejon P, Atkins BL, et al (2009) One hundred and twelve infected arthroplasties treated with 'DAIR' (debridement, antibiotics and implant retention): antibiotic duration and outcome. J Antimicrob Chemother 63(6):1264-1271

Chryssikos T, Parvizi J, Ghanem E, Newberg A, Zhuang H, Alavi A (2008) FDG-PET imaging can diagnose periprosthetic infection of the hip. Clin Orthop Relat Res 466(6): 1338–1342

Della Valle C, Parvizi J, Bauer TW, et al (2010) Diagnosis of periprosthetic joint infections of the hip and knee. J Am Acad Orthop Surg 18(12):760–770

de Vries EN, Prins HA, Crolla RM, et al (2010) Effect of a comprehensive surgical safety system on patient outcomes. N Engl J Med 363(20):1928–1937

Dinneen A, Guyot A, Clements J, Bradley N (2013) Synovial fluid white cell and differential count in the diagnosis or exclusion of prosthetic joint infection. Bone Joint J 95B(4):554–557

Draeger RW, Dahners LE (2006) Traumatic wound debridement: a comparison of irrigation methods. J Orthop Trauma 20(2):83–88

Fairclough JA, Johnson D, Mackie I (1986) The prevention of wound contamination by skin organisms by the preoperative application of an iodophor impregnated plastic adhesive drape. J Int Med Res 14(2):105–109

Fink B, Vogt S, Reinsch M, Buchner H (2011) Sufficient release of antibiotic by a spacer 6 weeks after implantation in two-stage revision of infected hip prostheses. Clin Orthop Relat Res 469(11):3141–3147

Fleck EE, Spangehl MJ, Rapuri VR, Beauchamp CP (2011) An articulating antibiotic spacer controls infection and improves pain and function in a degenerative septic hip. Clin Orthop Relat Res 469(11):3055–3064

Fletcher RH, Fairfield KM (2002) Vitamins for chronic disease prevention in adults: clinical applications. JAMA 287(23):3127–3129

Gherini S, Vaughn BK, Lombardi AV, Jr., Mallory TH (1993) Delayed wound healing and nutritional deficiencies after total hip arthroplasty. Clin Orthop Relat Res 293:188–195

Givissis P, Karataglis D, Antonarakos P, Symeonidis PD, Christodoulou A (2008) Suction during orthopaedic surgery. How safe is the suction tip? Acta Orthop Belg 74(4): 531–533

Insull PJ, Hudson J (2012) Suction tip: a potential source of infection in clean orthopaedic procedures. ANZ J Surg 82(3):185–186

Jaberi FM, Parvizi J, Haytmanek CT, Joshi A, Purtill J (2008) Procrastination of wound drainage and malnutrition affect the outcome of joint arthroplasty. Clin Orthop Relat Res 466(6):1368–1371

Jamsen E, Huhtala H, Puolakka T, Moilanen T (2009) Risk factors for infection after knee arthroplasty. A register-based analysis of 43,149 cases. J Bone Joint Surg Am 91(1):3847

Jamsen E, Nevalainen P, Eskelinen A, Huotari K, Kalliovalkama J, Moilanen T (2012) Obesity, diabetes, and preoperative hyperglycemia as predictors of periprosthetic joint infection: a single-center analysis of 7181 primary hip and knee replacements for osteoarthritis. J Bone Joint Surg Am 94(14):e101

Kotwal SY, Farid YR, Patil SS, Alden KJ, Finn HA (2012) Intramedullary rod and cement static spacer construct in chronically infected total knee arthroplasty. J Arthroplasty 27(2):253–259 e254

Kuiper JW, Brohet RM, Wassink S, van den Bekerom MP, Nolte PA, Vergroesen DA (2013) Implantation of resorbable gentamicin sponges in addition to irrigation and debridement in 34 patients with infection complicating total hip arthroplasty. Hip Int 23(2):173–180

Kühn KD (2007) Antibiotic loaded bone cements- antibiotic release and influence on mechanical properties. In Walenkamp G (ed) Local antibiotics in arthroplasty. Thieme, p. 125

Mangram AJ, Horan TC, Pearson ML, Silver LC, Jarvis WR (1999) Guideline for Prevention of Surgical Site Infection, 1999. Centers for Disease Control and Prevention (CDC) Hospital Infection Control Practices Advisory Committee. Am J Infect Control 27(2):97–132

Masri BA, Duncan CP, Beauchamp CP (1997) The modified two staged exchange arthroplasty in the treatment of infected total knee replacement: The Prostalac system and other articulated spacers. In Engh GA, Rorabeck CH (eds) Revision total knee arthroplasty, vol. 13. Willams & Wilkins, Baltimore, pp. 394–424

McPherson EJ, Peters CL (2011) Chapter 20: musculoskeletal infection. Orthopedic Knowledge Update 10:239–258

McPherson EJ, Woodson C, Holtom P, Roidis N, Shufelt C, Patzakis M (2002) Periprosthetic total hip infection: outcomes using a staging system. Clin Orthop Relat Res 403:8–15

Melling AC, Ali B, Scott EM, Leaper DJ (2001) Effects of preoperative warming on the incidence of wound infection after clean surgery: a randomised controlled trial. Lancet 358(9285):876–880

Mikkelsen DB, Pedersen C, Hojbjerg T, Schonheyder HC (2016) Culture of multiple peroperative biopsies and diagnosis of infected knee arthroplasties. APMIS 114(6): 449–452

Morshed S, Huffman GR, Ries MD (2005) Extended trochanteric osteotomy for 2-stage revision of infected total hip arthroplasty. J Arthroplasty 20(3):294–301

Munoz-Mahamud E, Garcia S, Bori G, et al (2011) Comparison of a low-pressure and a high pressure pulsatile lavage during debridement for orthopaedic implant infection. Arch Orthop Trauma Surg 131(9):1233–1238

O'Neill KR, Smith JG, Abtahi AM, et al (2011) Reduced surgical site infections in patients undergoing posterior spinal stabilization of traumatic injuries using vancomycin powder. Spine J 11(7):641–646

Orozco F, Post ZD, Baxi O, Miller A, Ong A (2013) Fibrosis in hepatitis C patients predicts complications after elective total joint arthroplasty. J Arthroplasty 29:7–10

Parvizi J, Saleh KJ, Ragland PS, Pour AE, Mont MA (2008) Efficacy of antibiotic-impregnated cement in total hip replacement. Acta Orthop 79(3):335–341

Parvizi J, Jacovides C, Zmistowski B, Jung KA (2011) Definition of periprosthetic joint infection: is there a consensus? Clin Orthop Relat Res 469(11):3022–3030

Parvizi J, Gehrke T (2013) Proceedings of the international consensus meeting on periprosthetic joint infection. Data Trace Publishing Company, pp. 226–227

Peersman G, Laskin R, Davis J, Peterson M (2001) Infection in total knee replacement: a retrospective review of 6489 total knee replacements. Clin Orthop Relat Res 392: 15–23

Romano CL, Manzi G, Logoluso N, Romano D (2012) Value of debridement and irrigation for the treatment of peri-prosthetic infections. A systematic review. Hip Int 22 [Suppl 8]:S1924

Schrama JC, Espehaug B, Hallan G, et al (2010) Risk of revision for infection in primary total hip and knee arthroplasty in patients with rheumatoid arthritis compared with osteoarthritis: a prospective, population-based study on 108,786 hip and knee joint arthroplasties from the Norwegian Arthroplasty Register. Arthritis Care Res (Hoboken) 62(4):473–479

Sorensen LT (2012) Wound healing and infection in surgery. The clinical impact of smoking and smoking cessation: a systematic review and meta-analysis. Arch Surg 147(4):373–383

Spahn DR (2010) Anemia and patient blood management in hip and knee surgery: a systematic review of the literature. Anesthesiology 113(2):482–495

Stocks GW, Self SD, Thompson B, Adame XA, O'Connor DP (2010) Predicting bacterial populations based on airborne particulates: a study performed in nonlaminar flow operating rooms during joint arthroplasty surgery. Am J Infect Control 38(3):199–204

Sukeik M, Patel S, Haddad FS (2012) Aggressive early debridement for treatment of acutely infected cemented total hip arthroplasty. Clin Orthop Relat Res 470(11):3164–3170

Tanner J, Norrie P, Melen K (2011) Preoperative hair removal to reduce surgical site infection. Cochrane Database Syst Rev 11:CD004122

Trampuz A, Piper KE, Jacobson MJ, et al (2007) Sonication of removed hip and knee prostheses for diagnosis of infection. N Engl J Med 357(7):654–663

Vergidis P, Lesnick TG, Kremers WK, Razonable RR (2012) Prosthetic joint infection in solid organ transplant recipients: a retrospective case-control study. Transpl Infect Dis 14(4):380–386

Wong J, Abrishami A, El Beheiry H, et al (2010) Topical application of tranexamic acid reduces postoperative blood loss in total knee arthroplasty: a randomized, controlled trial. J Bone Joint Surg Am 92(15):2503–2513
Zhou XD, Tao LJ, Li J, Wu LD (2013) Do we really need tranexamic acid in total hip arthroplasty? A meta-analysis of nineteen randomized controlled trials. Arch Orthop Trauma Surg 133(7):1017–1027
Zimmerli W, Trampuz A, Ochsner PE (2004) Prosthetic-joint infections. N Engl J Med 351(16):1645–1654
Zmistowski B, Restrepo C, Huang R, Hozack WJ, Parvizi J (2012) Periprosthetic joint infection diagnosis: a complete understanding of white blood cell count and differential. J Arthroplasty 27(9):1589–1593

6.5 Treatment of Prosthetic Joint Infections

Olivier Borens and John McManus

6.5.1 Introduction

Owing to the increasing number of implanted prosthetic joints, the number of infected total joint arthroplasty (TJA) cases is expected to rise in the near future (Widmer 2001; Campoccia et al. 2006; Kurtz et al. 2007). The goal of the treatment is to achieve a pain-free and functional joint, and whenever possible free of infection (Buller et al. 2012). Yet, treatment of an infected TJA is difficult owing to various aspects related to the infection and to the patient. The challenge in treating an infected TJA begins with making the correct diagnosis. It is essential to differentiate infections from aseptic loosening of TJA because of the difference in clinical consequences (Zimmerli et al. 2004). Once the diagnosis of infection has been confirmed, a specifically tailored treatment for each patient should be chosen and initiated. Treatment options for infected TJA include antibiotic suppression (systematically and locally), debridement and retention combined with exchange of the mobile parts, one-stage or two-stage exchange, arthrodesis and amputation, or Girdlestone procedure (Zimmerli et al. 2004).

To achieve a positive outcome in treating patient with TJA infection, a treatment concept is needed that takes into account different important aspects. The concept is based on five major pillars:

1. Teamwork
2. Understanding the »biofilm« problem
3. Diagnostics
4. Definition and classification
5. Patient-tailored treatment

6.5.2 Teamwork

Infection after TJA presents an important problem for the patient, the general practitioner and the orthopaedic surgeon who has implanted the artificial joint. When the TJA is evidently infected, for example, when a sinus tract is present (Zimmerli et al. 2004), the diagnosis of a TJA infection cannot be missed and is made very easily. On the other hand, when the signs of infection of the TJA are subtle, expertise from other medical specialists may be needed. Radiological evaluation can be important but close teamwork with an infectious disease (ID) specialist is paramount. The ID specialist needs to cooperate with a clinical or medical microbiologist to obtain more information on the involved pathogen and its susceptibility, as well as on other laboratory results.

This multidisciplinary approach is needed in treating TJA infections since the combination of good diagnosis, surgery and antibiotic treatment has been shown to have the highest success rate in eradication of infection (Zimmerli et al. 2004). Non-surgical treatment alone with suppressive antibiotics will not be able to eradicate infection (Zimmerli et al. 2004). The surgeon will choose the best of the possible surgical options and the ID specialist together with the microbiologist will decide on the best option among the antibiotic arsenal. The multidisciplinary team for treating TJA infection can be reinforced further by a plastic surgeon, a vascular surgeon or an internal medicine specialist.

6.5.3 Understanding »Biofilm«

TJA, like other foreign bodies (Elek and Conen 1957), are prone to colonization by micro-organisms. Micro-organisms that colonized foreign bodies form biofilms (Trampuz and Zimmerli 2005).

Biofilms can be defined as communities of bacteria attached to surface (O'Toole et al. 2000). Unlike their free-living (planktonic) counterparts, bacteria in biofilms live in an organized structure (Davies 2003). The formation of biofilms is a rapid process, which Gristina described as »the race for the surface« (Gristina 1987). Within minutes to hours, bacteria attach to the surface of an implant. In the following stages, these bacteria become embedded in a matrix (glycocalyx) and they enter a stationary growth phase (Davies 2003).

Problems associated with biofilm in TJA result from the characteristics of the biofilm. Firstly, biofilms are difficult to clear by immune killing or by treatment with antibiotics. Bacteria in biofilm are difficult to attack because of the compact structure of biofilm and because they enter the stationary phase (Stewart and Costerton 2001; Davies 2003). Secondly, biofilms might be capable of shedding individual bacterial and sloughed pieces of biofilm into surrounding tissues that cause infection. Therefore, local antibiotics would play a significant role.

Tab. 6.6 Criteria to define prosthetic joint infection proposed by the American Academy of Orthopaedic Surgeons (AAOS)

1.	A sinus tract communicating with the prosthesis; or
2.	A pathogen is isolated by culture from two separate tissue or fluid samples obtained from the affected prosthetic joint; or
3.	Four out of the following six criteria: – Elevated serum erythrocyte sedimentation rate (ESR) or C-reactive protein (CRP) concentration (CRP can be normal in low-grade infections!) – Elevated synovial white blood cell (WBC) count – Elevated synovial neutrophil percentage (PMN%) – Presence of purulence in the affected joint – Isolation of a micro-organism in one culture of periprosthetic tissue or fluid – Greater than five neutrophils per high-power field in five high-power fields observed from histological analysis of periprosthetic tissue at 400× magnification

6.5.4 Diagnostics

To date, there is no single set of accepted criteria for prosthetic joint infection (PJI) that can be considered as gold standard (Parvizi et al. 2011). Recently, the American Academy of Orthopaedic Surgeons (AAOS) published their proposed criteria to define PJI (Parvizi et al. 2011). In this proposal, diagnosis can be made based on signs only, or microbiological culture of tissue only, or a combination of laboratory and pathological findings. According to this proposal, a definite diagnosis of PJI can be made when several conditions are met (Tab. 6.6). Several of these diagnostic criteria included in this proposal are worth discussing. While in this proposal isolating a pathogen from two separate intraoperative tissue samples is enough to make the diagnosis, several other authors request at least three positive samples (Atkins et al. 1998). It is important to bear in mind not to perform culture of the superficial swab because of a low sensitivity (68%) (Font-Vizcarra et al. 2010). Recent evidence recommends prolonged aerobic and anaerobic culture of up to 14 days in order to find slow-growing micro-organisms such as *Propionibacterium* and *Peptostreptococcus* species (Schafer et al. 2008; Butler-Wu et al. 2011). Since antibiotics can prevent isolation of intraoperative organisms (Trampuz et al. 2007), it is advisable to stop antibiotics 14 days before taking a tissue biopsy.

Besides ESR and CRP, a systematic review performed in 2010 showed that interleukin-6 is another promising molecule to be used in diagnosing PJI (Berbari et al. 2010). The cut-offs of WBC count and PMN% differ in the hip and knee joints. For the knee joint, a WBC count of $>1.7\times10^9$/l showed a sensitivity of 94% and specificity of 88%. When this WBC count was combined with PMN >65%, the sensitivity and specificity become 97% and 98%, respectively (Trampuz et al. 2004). For the hip the WBC count is >4.2×109/l and the percentage of PMN is >80% (Schinsky et al. 2008).

Several novel diagnostic methods are not included in the proposal, such as sonication and polymerase chain reaction (PCR), but are worth mentioning. Sonication is a method used in the microbiology laboratory to dislodge micro-organisms from the biofilm formed on the surface of the prosthesis (Trampuz et al. 2007). This technique has been shown to have higher sensitivity for the microbiological diagnosis of PJI than tissue culture. Sonication is particularly helpful in detecting bacteria in patients who have been recently treated with antibiotics. It is also useful for detecting micro-organisms that cause low-grade infections that would otherwise go undetected using periprosthetic tissue cultures, such as *Propionibacterium acnes* (Borens et al. 2012). PCR is a molecular technique that amplifies the 16s rRNA gene of bacteria (Achermann et al. 2010). Multiplex PCR (meaning that multiple primers are used to amplify the 16s rRNA gene in order to detect multiple bacteria types) has been developed and was shown to increase the sensitivity and specificity of PJI detection. The increase in diagnostic performance is even more compelling when multiplex PCR is performed on the sonication fluid (Achermann et al. 2010).

6.5.5 Definition and Classification

PJI can be classified as: early, delayed and late (◘ Tab. 6.7; Zimmerli et al. 2004). Early infections occur within 3 months of implantation. The germs causing early infections are usually acquired during the implantation of the TJA. Delayed infections occur between 3 and 24 months after implantation. The germs responsible for delayed infections are also acquired during surgery but they are usually less virulent like *Propionibacterium acnes* or *Staphylococcus epidermidis*. Late infections are generally haematogenous and occur later than 24 months after implantation surgery. *Staphylococcus aureus* is the most frequent cause of haematogenous TJA infection (Uckay et al. 2009). Yet, in the majority of the cases, no primary focus of infection can be found.

After the classification, the next step is to differentiate whether the infection of TJA is acute or chronic. This differentiation is important for the choice of the treatment option. In acute infection the beginning of the symptoms should be less than 3 weeks before the diagnosis. Infection is considered to be chronic when the beginning of the symptoms is longer than 3 weeks. Acute infection can occur in the early postoperative phase, and is usually due to highly virulent germs like *Staphylococcus aureus* (Zimmerli et al. 2004). Acute infection can also occur after years. The symptoms start without warning, after infection of the prosthetic joint by haematogenous seeding of the micro-organisms from a distant infectious focus into a previously healthy and asymptomatic prosthesis. Chronic infection can be present early (1–3 months postoperatively), delayed or late (more than 24 months postoperatively). The patients have typically persistent pain.

6.5.6 Patient-Tailored Treatment

Once the diagnosis has been made and the type of infection has been determined, the orthopaedic surgeon together with the ID specialist must make a treatment plan to achieve their goal of a painless, functional and infection-free TJA. Solely medical treatment will not lead to eradication of the infection (Bengston and Knutson 1991). Therefore, it

◘ Tab. 6.7 Types of infected TJA according to when the symptoms start after implantation

Classification	Beginning of the infection after implantation	Pathogenesis	Typical germs
Early infection	< 3 months	During surgery	Highly virulent germs, e.g. *S. aureus* or Gram-negative bacilli
Delayed infection	3–24 months	During surgery	Less virulent germs, e.g. *S. epidermidis* or *P. acnes*
Late infection	>24 months	Mainly haematogenous	Typically highly virulent germs, e.g. *S. aureus*, streptococci or Gram-negative bacilli

should be only used in patients with multiple co-morbidities (e.g. patients too sick to endure surgery), in patients who refuse surgery or when surgery is technically too challenging (Zimmerli et al. 2004; Moran et al 2010). In all other situations, surgery in combination with appropriate antibiotics (systemically and locally) is the best if not the only way to reach the treatment goal. The choice of surgical treatment is determined by several factors: The type of infection (acute vs chronic), the state of the soft tissue, the type of pathogens and their susceptibility to antibiotics, and the patient's expectation. There five surgical options are the following:

1. Debridement and retention with exchange of mobile parts
2. One-stage exchange
3. Two-stage exchange
   - Short interval (2–4 weeks)
   - Long interval (6 weeks and more)
4. Arthrodesis
5. Amputation/Girdlestone

Debridement and Retention with Exchange of Mobile Parts

Initially it was thought that debridement and retention of the implant was a surgical procedure to be done by arthroscopy. Today it has been shown that adequate debridement and retention with good results can only be done through an open procedure (Waldmann et al. 2000). It consists of arthrotomy, extensive synovectomy, irrigation with at least 9 l of saline and debridement of all infected soft tissue followed by exchange of the mobile parts (◻ Tab. 6.8) (Bengston and Knutson 1991). The removal and exchange of the mobile parts in the knee, for instance, is important to facilitate synovectomy in the posterior parts of the total knee arthroplasty (TKA) and because there is a higher concentration of biofilm on the polyethylene than on the metal of the prosthesis. Intraoperative cultures are taken and mobile parts are sent for sonication. The patients are further treated with antibiotics for 3 months.

Compared with one- or two-stage exchange, there are several potential advantages of this method. Firstly, many patients can return to full activity quickly as the surgery is less invasive with reduced blood loss

◻ **Tab. 6.8** Key points in the treatment of infected TJA using debridement and retention

1.	Open and wide debridement of all infected tissue
2.	Removal of mobile parts
3.	Extensive synovectomy
4.	Cultures and sonication
5.	Low-pressure pulsed lavage
6.	New and sterile mobile parts
7.	Antibiotics (systemic) for 3 months

compared with exchange procedures (Waldmann et al. 2000). Secondly, surgical time and costs (only one surgery is performed and only mobile parts are exchanged) are lower. Thirdly, the risk of intraoperative fracture of the surrounding bone is low since the bone stock is left intact, unlike removal of a well-fixed prosthesis where bone loss occurs. Lastly, there will be no soft tissue distension or retraction unlike in two-stage exchange where spacers are implanted. These possible advantages should be weighed against the lower chance of a successful outcome. The percentage chance of a successful outcome for this procedure is commonly reported just below 50% (Waldmann et al. 2000; Deirmengian et al. 2003; Marculescu et al. 2006; Buller et al. 2012). Where debridement and retention fail, there are also consequences concerning further surgical treatment. Sherrell and co-workers showed that two-stage revision replacement in patients who had previous debridement and implant retention had a high risk of failure (34%; Sherrell et al. 2011).

There are several requirements for a successful outcome when debridement and retention are performed (Zimmerli et al. 2004; Sendi and Zimmerli 2011; Buller et al. 2012). Firstly, the implant should be stable. Secondly, the infection should be acute (i.e. less than 3 weeks). Thirdly, the soft tissue should be intact. Lastly, the pathogens should be sensitive to biofilm active antibiotics (i.e. rifampin, ciprofloxacin, fosfomycin).

One-Stage Revision

This surgical option consists of removal of the prosthesis, debridement of infected soft tissue, re-implantation of the prosthesis (Zimmerli et al. 2004). Intraoperative cultures are taken and the removed prosthesis is sent for sonication. The patients are further treated with antibiotics for 3 months.

The most important theoretical advantage of this procedure compared with two-stage exchange is the elimination of the demanding second surgery that could result in complications (Jenny et al. 2012), prolonged hospital stay and increased patient morbidity related to the spacer. A disadvantage is the need to do more aggressive debridement and often the need for more constrained implants, especially in infected TKA.

There are several requirements in performing one-stage exchange. Firstly, the soft tissue condition should be satisfactory. If soft tissues are not sound, the risk of wound breakdown and persistence of infection or super-infection is increased. Secondly, like in debridement and retention, the pathogens should be sensitive to biofilm active antibiotics (i.e. rifampin, ciprofloxacin, fosfomycin; Zimmerli et al. 2004). The success rate of one-stage exchange is high. A recent study by Jenny and co-workers showed that 87% of the patients treated with one-stage exchange were free of any infection during a 3-year follow-up (Jenny et al. 2012).

Two-Stage Revision

This procedure has become the gold standard treatment in the United States (Freeman et al. 2007; Sherrell et al. 2011) and appears to be the most effective surgical management for PJI with a success rate of 88–96% (Zimmerli et al. 2004) if debridement and retention are not possible.

In the first stage, the prosthesis is removed. Intraoperative cultures are taken and the removed prosthesis is sent for sonication. After wide debridement, a cement spacer can be implanted. Among the general benefits of cement spacers are: prevention of abundant scar tissue formation, maintenance of joint space, prevention of contraction of the joint, facilitation of exposure and revision, and improvement of patient comfort between the stages (Booth and Lotke 1989; Calton et al. 1997). In current practice, cement spacers for two-stage exchange are impregnated with antibiotics since they can deliver local antibiotics in much higher doses than using intravenous administration (Hanssen and Spangehl 2004; Hsu et al. 2007). There are two types of cement spacers: non-articulating (fixed) (Ferhing et al. 2000; Johnson et al. 2012) and articulating (dynamic) spacers (Ferhing et al. 2000; Hsu et al. 2007; Johnson et al. 2012). Fixed spacers have some shortcomings such as: inability of the patient to bend the knee, potential increase of bone loss, and quadriceps scarring and arthrofibrosis (Cui et al. 2007). By contrast, dynamic spacers allow for joint motion. Moreover, due to less bone loss and decrease in scar formation, dynamic spacers facilitate exposure during re-implantation (Calton et al. 1997; Ferhing et al. 2000; Meek et al. 2004; Cui et al. 2007). Owing to these characteristics, dynamic spacers also improve patient satisfaction (Calton et al. 1997; Meek et al. 2004; Johnson et al. 2012), but come with an increased risk of dislocation or other mechanical failures. Grossly, there are two types of articulating spacer: one that is made completely of antibiotic-impregnated cement using performed moulds and the other is made of metal and plastic coated with antibiotic-impregnated cement (Calton et al. 1997; Ferhing et al. 2000; Hofmann et al. 2005; Cui et al. 2007). Antibiotic concentration in the cement spacer is higher (>1 g per unit of 40 g cement) when it is used to treat infection than when it is used as prophylaxis (≤1 g per unit of 40 g cement; Hanssen and Spangehl 2004). In two-stage exchange, 2 g of vancomycin and 4 g of tobramycin/gentamicin should be added to the 40-g pack of bone cement (Masri et al. 1998; Koo et al. 2001). If the surgeon chooses not to create the spacer themselves, preformed off-the-shelf spacers can be used as well. After the first stage, intravenous antibiotics are also given to the patient.

In general, we can differentiate the time of re-implantation into short and long intervals. The short interval is when the re-implantation is performed 2–3 weeks after the first stage. In the long interval, the re-implantation is performed at 6–8 weeks after the first stage or even later. A short interval is preferred over long intervals in situations where the soft tissues are in good state and the pathogens are not difficult to treat (i.e. sensitive to rifampin or ciprofloxacin). Among the benefit of short- over long-intervals are: less scarring or contracture and shorter intravenous antibiotic therapy needed and subsequently less cost for monitoring this therapy (Burnett et al. 2007).

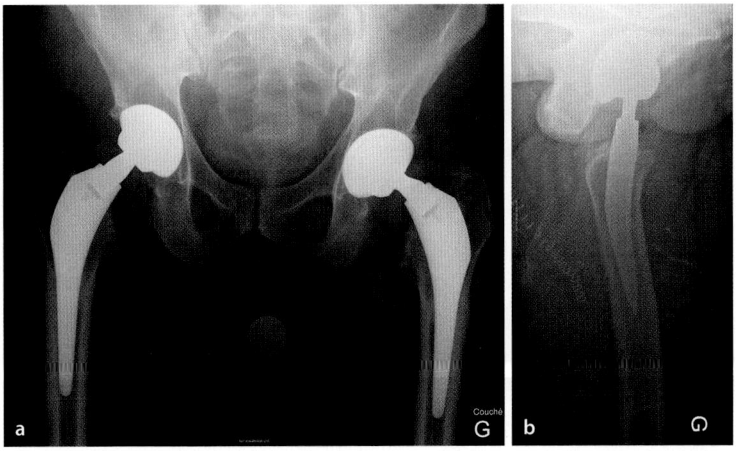

Fig. 6.15 **a** Bilateral total hip arthroplasty with modular stem, acute haematogenous infection on the left side. **b** Axial view with drain after revision

The question of when is the best time for re-implantation is not easy to answer. As rule of thumb, re-implantation should be conducted when no clinical, radiographic and laboratory findings of persisting infection are present (Huang et al. 2006). It is worth mentioning that progressively decreasing markers (e.g. ESR, CRP) are more practical and favourable for use than to wait until these markers become normal before re-implantation (Ghanem et al. 2009).

In the second stage, the spacer is removed and the prosthesis is re-implanted. The spacer should be sent for sonication and tissue cultures should be taken for microbiological examination. If after the re-implantation the cultures are negative, intravenous antibiotics can be converted to oral antibiotics for a period of 3 months in all. If the cultures are positive, intravenous antibiotics have to be continued for 2 weeks followed by 10 weeks of oral treatment (like in a one-stage exchange). These decisions and the choice of antibiotics should be based on the recommendations of the ID specialists.

In summary, the optimal surgical procedure is closely related to the type of infection, the soft tissue situation and the possible antibiotic treatment. The less aggressive the surgical choice is, the better the functional outcome will be; the shorter the interval between explantation and re-implantation is, the better the outcome will be. Offering only one stereotypical surgical procedure, e.g. only one-stage exchange or only two-stage exchange, is no longer regarded as sufficient or adequate for our patients. Each of our patients deserves personalized treatment as every single one of them presents with his or her own special situation of a PJI.

Case Studies

In the following, we describe five different cases from our hospital.

Case 1: Debridement and Retention with Exchange of the Mobile Parts

A 48-year-old man, with a history of alcohol abuse, underwent bilateral total hip arthroplasty 5 years earlier for aseptic necrosis of the femoral head related to his alcoholism. The post-operative recovery was uncomplicated.

The patient presented to our department with a fever of 39.1 °C with shivering and increasing pain in his left hip over the preceding 24 h. Laboratory testing revealed an elevated leukocyte count of 25 g/l and an elevated CRP of 148 mg/l. Radiologically, the prosthesis did not show signs of loosening (Fig. 6.15a and b). Joint aspiration was cloudy and the patient was commenced on an empirical treatment with Co-amoxiclav (3×2.2 g i.v.).

The short delay between presentation and surgery allowed us to carry out, the following morning, a wide debridement, lavage and retention procedure with exchange of the mobile parts (insert, head and neck).

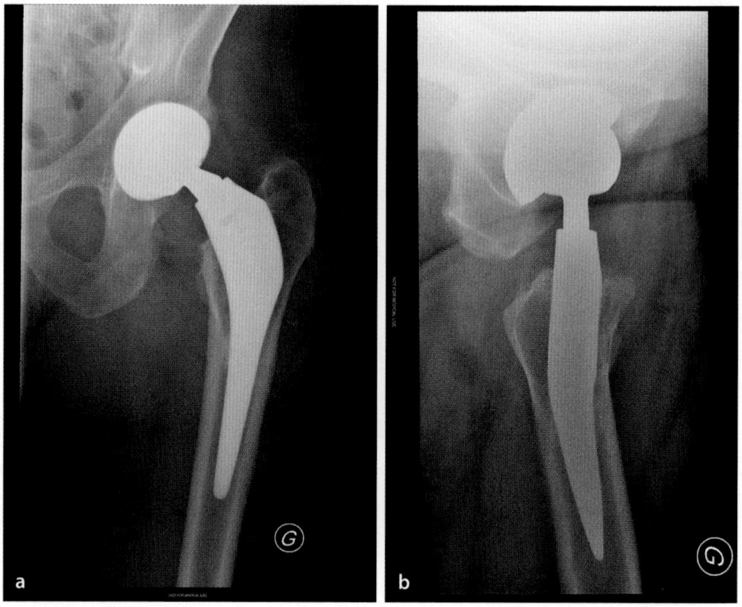

Fig. 6.16 **a** Anteroposterior view of left hip 1 year post-operatively, no lysis around stem or acetabular cup in asymptomatic patient. **b** Axial view 1 year post-operatively

The microbiological cultures of the tissue biopsies and sonication revealed the pathogen to be methicillin-sensitive *Staphylococcus aureus* (MSSA). The antibiotic therapy was changed to flucloxacillin (4×2 g i.v.) for a total of 2 weeks, followed by levofloxacin (2×500 mg p.o.) and rifampin (2×450 mg p.o.) for a total of 3 months of antibiotic therapy. Close follow-up of the patient's liver function tests was indicated during the rifampin therapy because of the patient's known alcohol abuse. The patient progressed well postoperatively (Fig. 6.16a and b).

Case 2: One-Stage Exchange

A 73-year-old man presented with painful joint effusions on multiple occasions in the years following a primary TKA. Each time the patient was afebrile, while the CRP and leukocyte counts were within normal limits. Multiple joint aspirations were carried out, and each time the cultures were sterile and did not show any evidence of a crystalline arthropathy. No cytological examination was carried out. The patient was even assessed by a dermatologist to rule out the possibility of an allergic reaction to the prosthesis, with negative results.

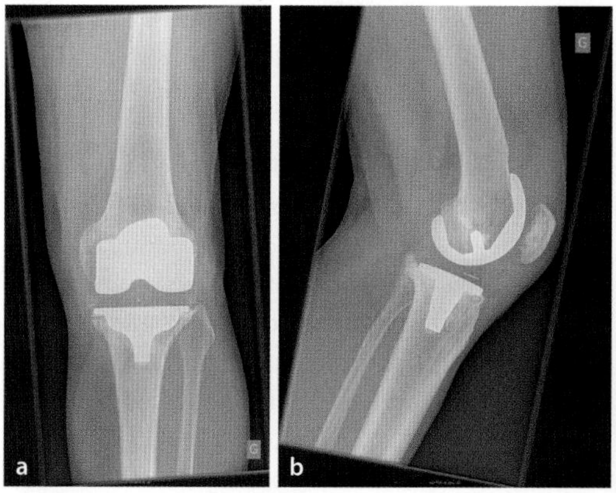

Fig. 6.17 **a** Chronic infection 2 years after total knee arthroplasty with *S. epidermidis*, anteroposterior view, signs of loosening medial plateau. **b** Lateral view

The patient presented to our department with a further episode of painful joint effusion. He remained afebrile with unremarkable blood tests. Radiologically, there were signs of osteolysis around the tibial implant (Fig. 6.17a and b). Joint aspiration showed increased cellularity 35 g/l with 80% neutrophils. Microbiological cultures of the joint aspirate confirmed the presence of *S. epidermidis*.

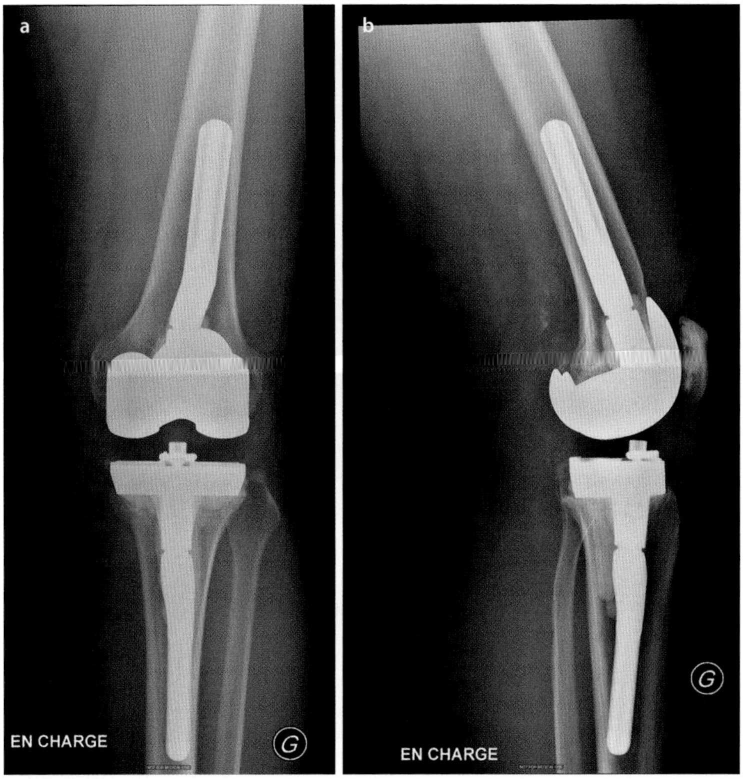

■ **Fig. 6.18** **a** Postoperative anteroposterior view 3 months after one-step exchange. **b** Lateral view

Owing to the long delay from the onset of symptoms, a biofilm had clearly formed on the surface of the prosthesis rendering retention of the implants impossible. However, because the germ was easy to treat and sensitive to multiple antibiotics, we chose to undertake a one-stage exchange with extensive debridement (■ Fig. 6.18a and b). The patient was treated with flucloxacillin (4×2 g i.v. for 2 weeks). Sonication of the implant confirmed the diagnosis of *S. epidermidis* infection. The patient was then treated with oral levofloxacin (2×500 mg p.o.) and rifampin (2×450 mg p.o.) for a total period of 3 months postoperatively. Apart from postoperative anaemia, the patient's recovery was unremarkable.

Case 3: Two-Stage Exchange (Short Interval)

A 54-year-old female patient, in good general health, presented with medial knee pain of the right knee with a history of prior trauma (■ Fig. 6.19a and b). After unsuccessful conservative treatment with non-steroidal anti-inflammatory drugs (NSAIDS) and physiotherapy, it was decided to proceed with a unicompartmental knee prosthesis (■ Fig. 6.20 b). The postoperative period was uncomplicated with good return of function. Two years following the primary surgery, the patient developed significant pain with loosening of the femoral component.

The inflammatory markers were within normal limits. No joint aspiration was performed. The patient underwent conversion to a TKA (■ Fig. 6.21a and b).

Biopsies and sonication of the prosthesis showed infection with *S. epidermidis*, but only after enrichment of the samples. Antibiotic therapy with oral levofloxacin and rifampicin was commenced only 3 weeks following the surgery.

Ongoing pain led to referral of the patient to our institution. Loosening of the tibial plateau was confirmed with standard radiographs (■ Fig. 6.22a and b).

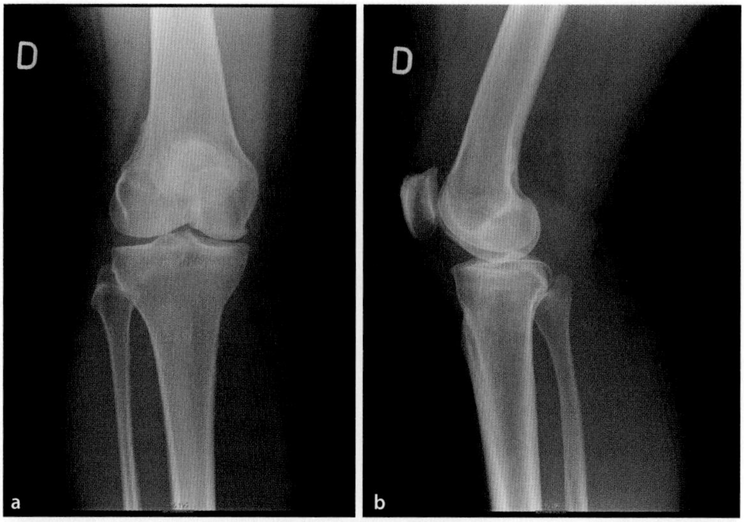

■ **Fig. 6.19** **a** Preoperative anteroposterior view. **b** Preoperative lateral view

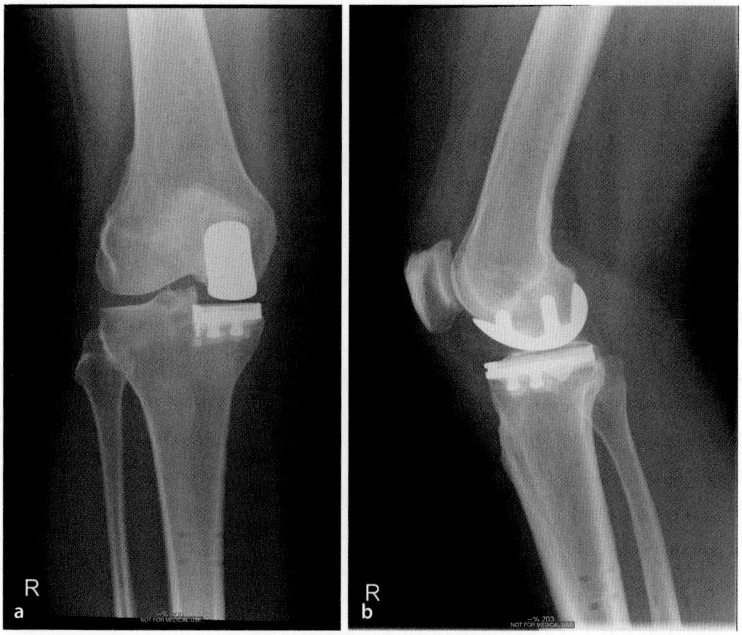

■ **Fig. 6.20** **a** Post-operative anteroposterior view after unicompartmental knee prosthesis. **b** Lateral view

We suspected persistence of chronic infection with *S. epidermidis* and decided to undertake a two-step exchange with a short interval to allow confirmation of the pathogenic organism.

A two-component cement spacer loaded with additional antibiotics was hand-made (■ Fig. 6.23a–f). Each component of the spacer was made with 40 g of Palacos® with 1.2 g of tobramycin and 2 g of vancomycin added. A dynamic spacer was chosen because of the good soft tissue status and so as to allow for mobilization of the knee with physiotherapy during the interval. The patient was also allowed weight-bearing as tolerated with protection of a splint.

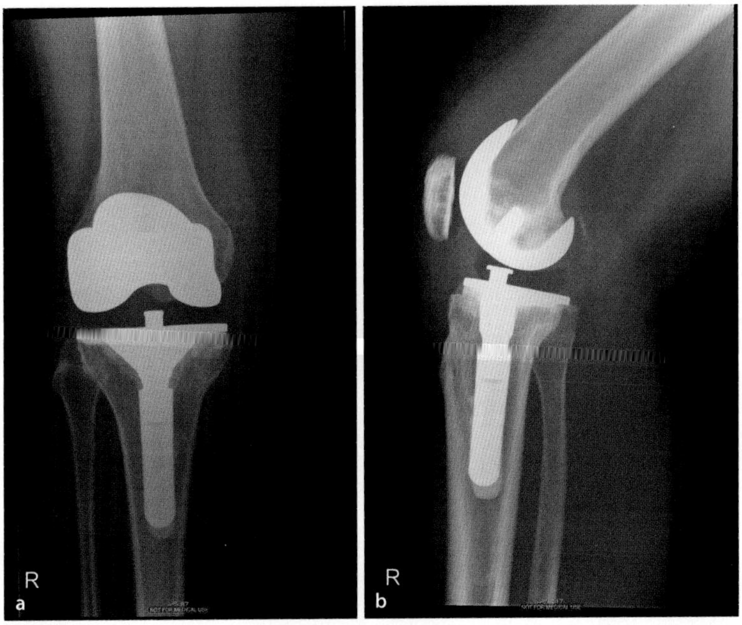

Fig. 6.21 **a** Anteroposterior view after conversion to total knee arthroplasty. **b** Lateral view

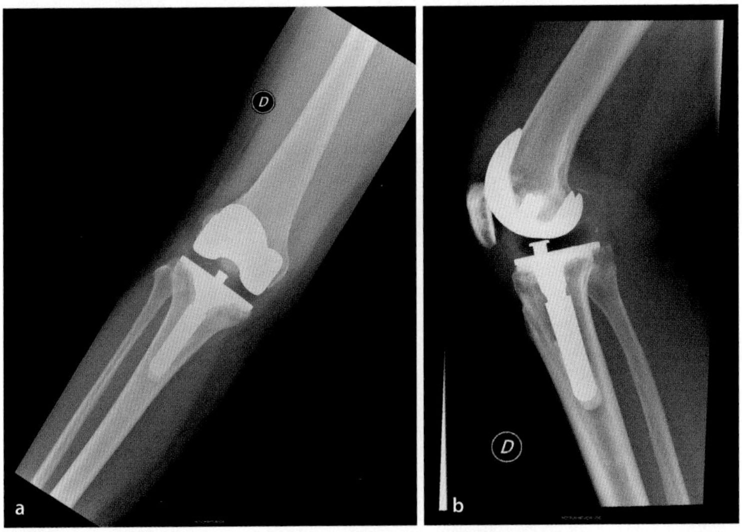

Fig. 6.22 **a** Signs of early loosening around tibial plateau on anteroposterior view. **b** Lateral viewateral view

Sonication and cultures confirmed our suspicion of *S. epidermidis* infection and the germ was sensitive to rifampin allowing us to re-implant after a short interval of only 2 weeks. In the interval, the patient received flucloxacillin (4×2 g i.v.) and under ongoing antibiotic treatment the patient underwent re-implantation of an LCCK (NexGen Legacy® Constrained Condylar Knee, Zimmer Biomet) (Fig. 6.24a and b). Sonication of the spacer and tissue cultures were negative. The patient was started on oral levofloxacin (2×500 mg p.o.) and rifampin (2×450 mg p.o.) to complete a total of 3 months of

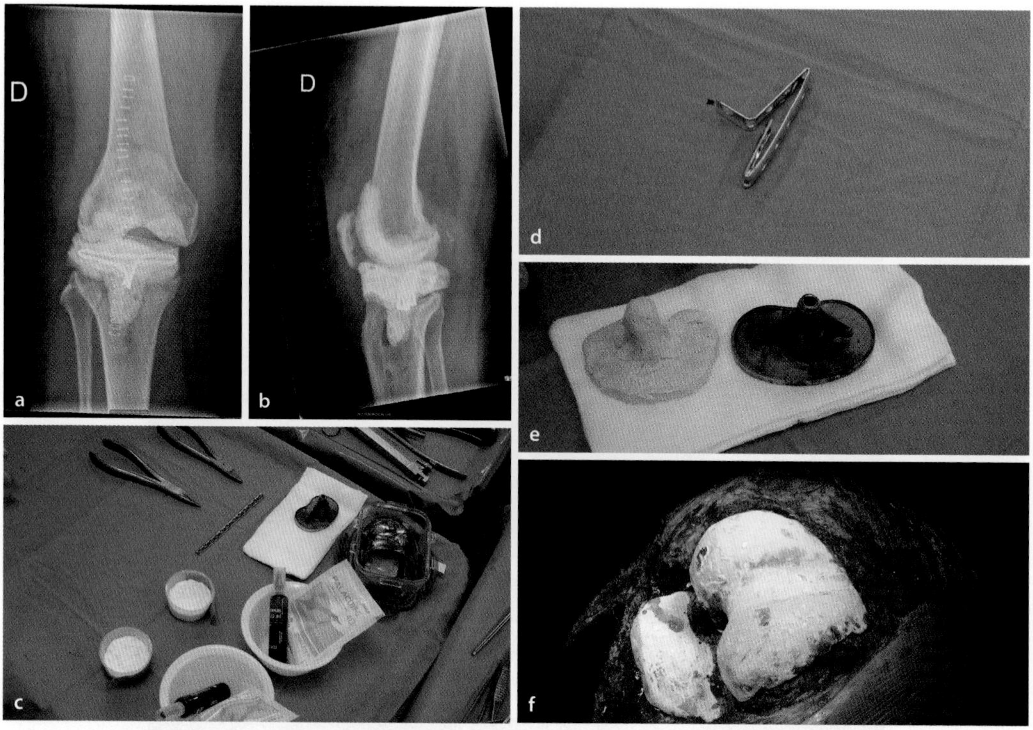

Fig. 6.23 **a** Anteroposterior view after removal of TKA and implantation of mobile handmade spacer. **b** Lateral view. **c** Material for producing handmade knee spacer. **d** One third tubular plate for tibial part of spacer. **e** Handmade tibial spacer before implantation. **f** Intraoperative view and testing of flexion

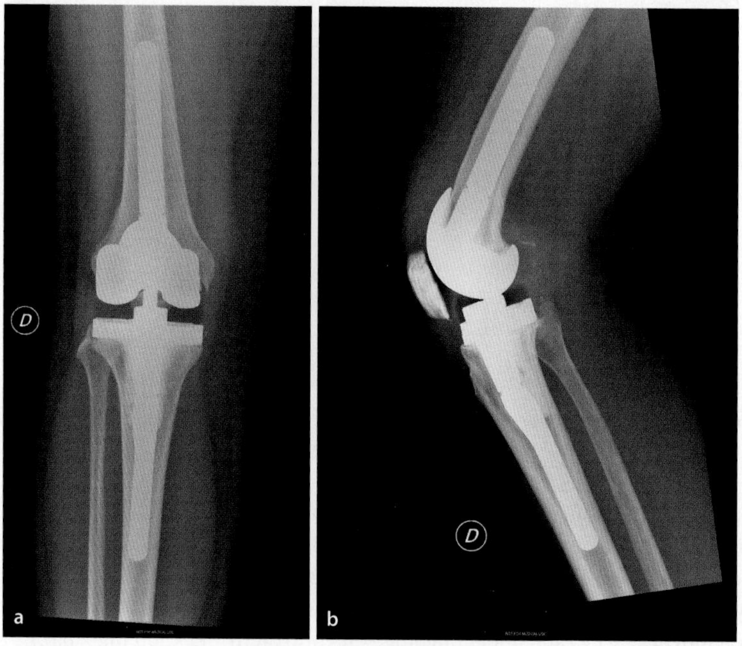

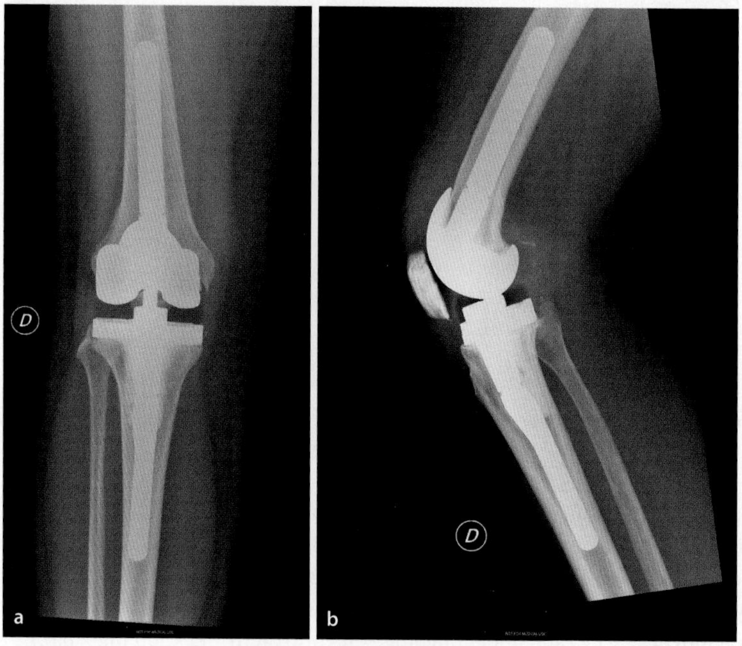

Fig. 6.24 **a** Anteroposterior view of Legacy® Constrained Condylar Knee 2 years after implantation. **b** Lateral view

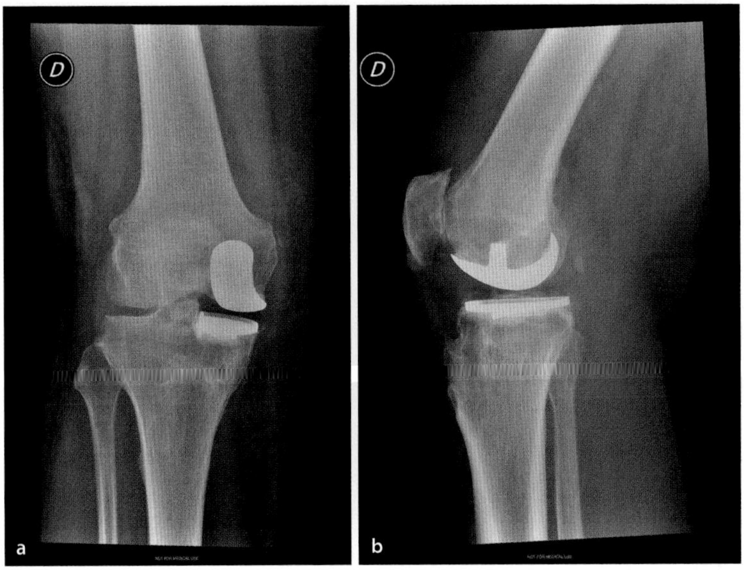

Fig. 6.25 **a** Anteroposterior view of chronically infected unicompartmental knee prosthesis. **b** Lateral view

antibiotic therapy. The postoperative follow-up at 2 years was uneventful.

Case 4: Two-Stage Exchange (Long Interval)

A 66-year-old male patient, with a history of obesity and type II diabetes, underwent implantation of a medial hemi-prosthesis of the right knee 3 years previously in another hospital. The post-operative period was uncomplicated and the patient progressed well (Fig. 6.25a and b). Two years following the surgery, the patient developed severe pain and was found to have an infection with *Campylobacter fetus*.

He underwent debridement, lavage and exchange of the removable parts of the prosthesis. The initial post-operative evolution was favourable; however, the patient presented to our department 6 months after his initial diagnosis of infection. He complained of a painful joint effusion, which was aspirated revealing a purulent liquid that later grew *Streptococcus agalactiae*.

The patient was treated empirically with Co-amoxiclav (3×2.2 g) and underwent removal of the prosthesis, resection of the remaining joint surfaces and implantation of a made-to-measure two-component dynamic cement spacer with additional antibiotics (Fig. 6.26a and b).

The tissue biopsies and sonication of the prosthesis confirmed the presence of *S. agalactiae*. The antibiotic therapy was modified to penicillin and gentamicin followed by ceftriaxone until the re-implantation.

The clinical evolution was good with normalization of the inflammatory markers, allowing us to re-implant a revision knee prosthesis 6 weeks after implantation of the spacer (Fig. 6.27a and b). Tissue biopsies and sonication of the spacer were sterile. The antibiotic therapy was continued with amoxicillin (3×1 g) for 6 weeks, thus completing 3 months of antibiotics.

The post-operative period was uncomplicated apart from moderate post-operative anaemia treated with iron supplementation.

Case 5: Two-Stage Exchange with Arthrodesis

A 66-year-old male patient underwent TKA in 2005 for post-traumatic osteoarthritis of the right knee following a patellar fracture in the 1960s. Six months after implantation, he developed an infection with *Beta haemolytic streptococci*, and underwent a two-stage exchange of the TKA with re-implantation after a 2-month interval. Initially the recovery seemed favourable; however, the symptoms re-

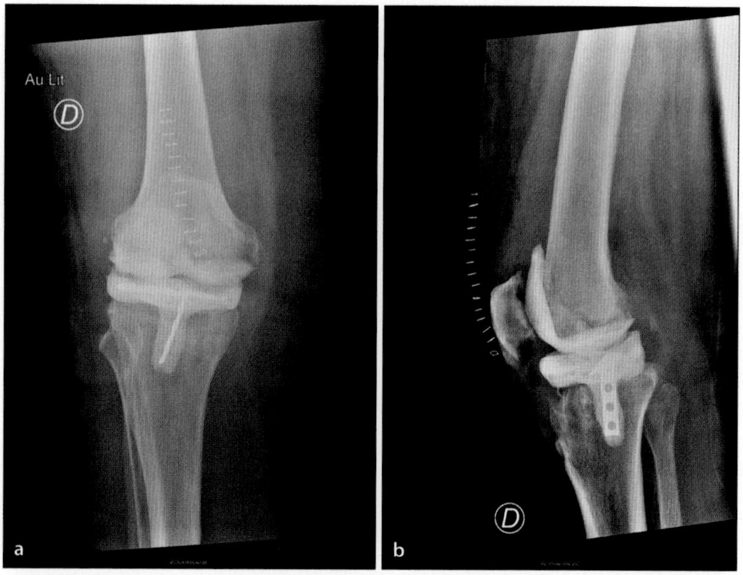

Fig. 6.26 **a** Anteroposterior view with spacer. **b** Lateral view

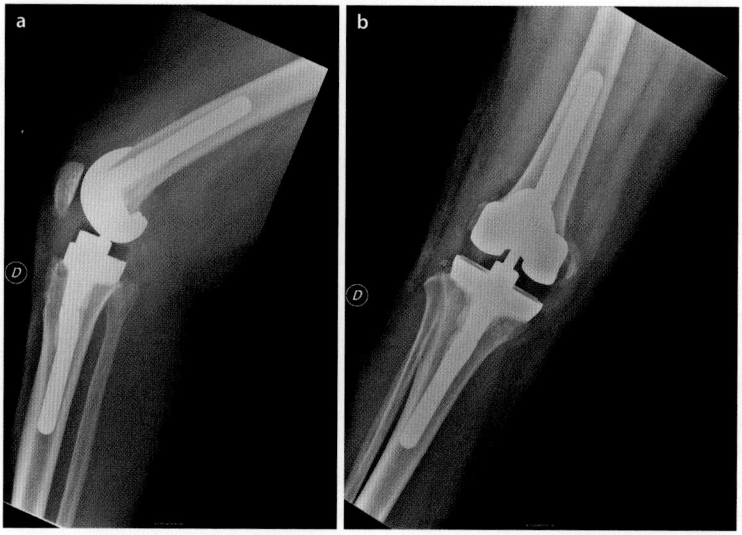

Fig. 6.27 **a** Anteroposterior view of Legacy® Constrained Condylar Knee. **b** Lateral view

turned. The patient underwent multiple surgeries and revisions over several years at another hospital but without eradication of the infection.

He presented to our hospital with a long-standing discharging sinus and significant pain (Fig. 6.28a and b). The patient underwent removal of the prosthesis with implantation of a non-articulating spacer with added antibiotics Fig. 6.29a–c). The patient was started on a treatment with i.v. Co-amoxiclav. Microbiological cultures and sonication of the prosthesis confirmed the presence of *S. epidermidis* and *Candida albicans*. Fluconazole was added to the treatment. Despite antibiotic and anti-mycotic treatment, the situation did not settle and the wound reopened. Multiple tissue samples revealed the presence of *Achromobacter xylosoxidans*

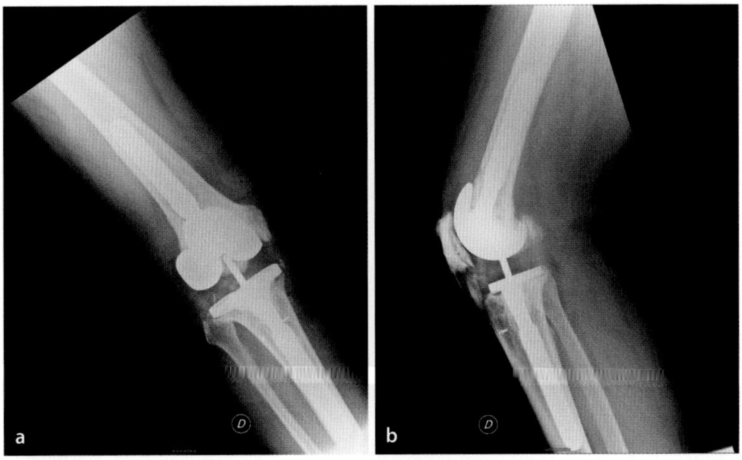

■ **Fig. 6.28** **a** Anteroposterior view of chronically infected rotating hinged knee. **b** Lateral view

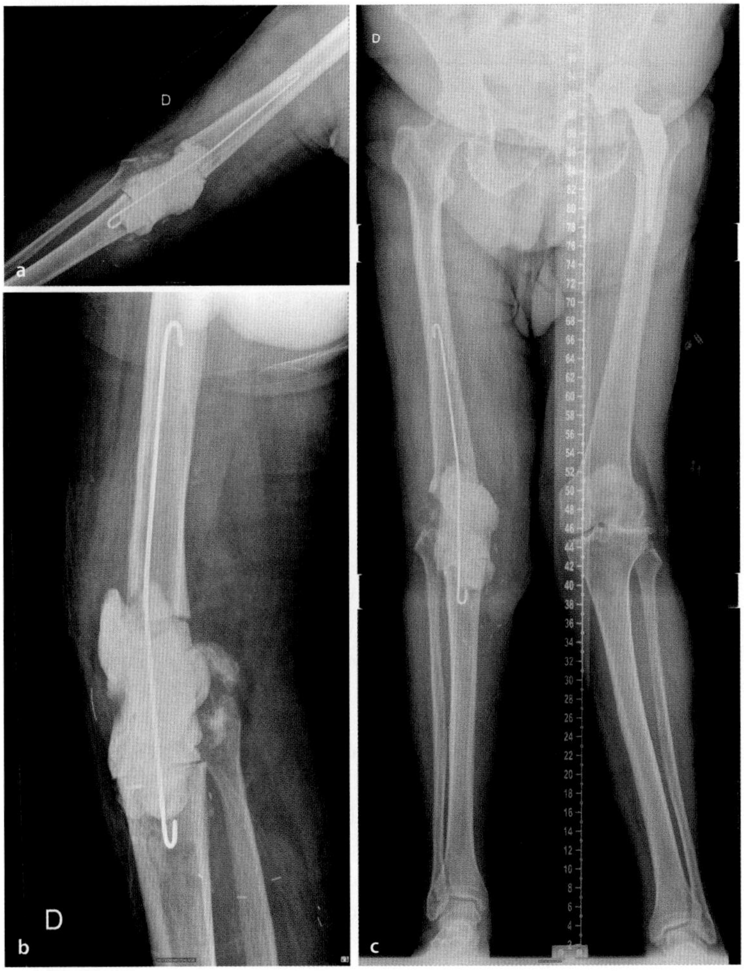

■ **Fig. 6.29** **a** Anteroposterior view of non-articulating knee spacer. **b** Lateral view, resected patella. **c** Long axis with non-articulating spacer Long axis with non-articulating spacer

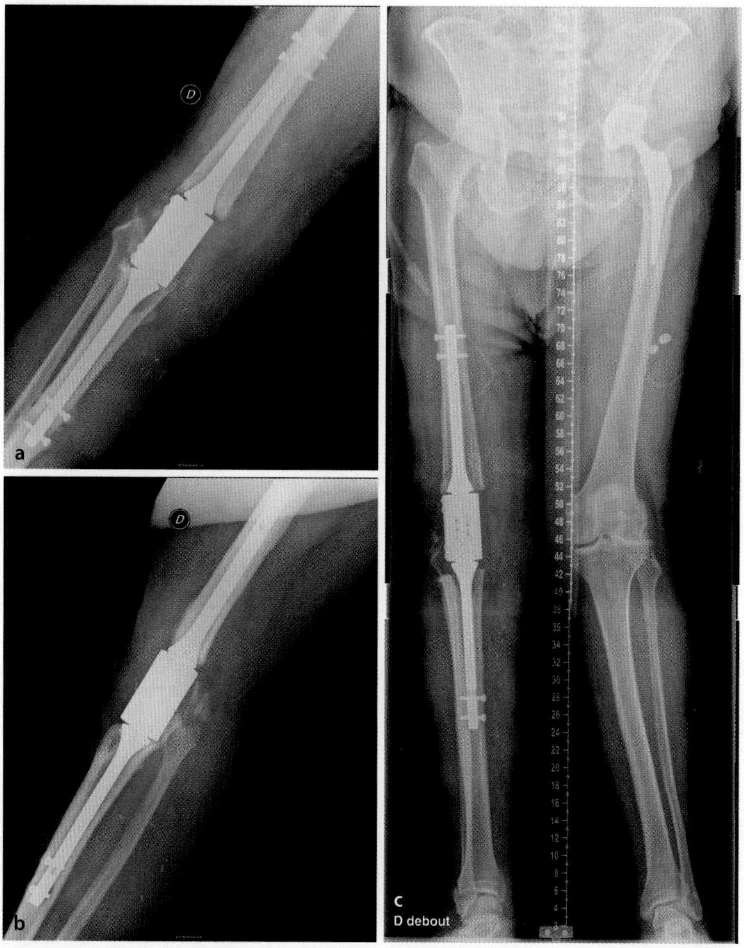

Fig. 6.30 **a** Anteroposterior view of arthrodesis nail. **b** Lateral view. **c** Long axis

infection. The *Achromobacter* was found to also be present after removal of a peripherally inserted central catheter line. The spacer was exchanged after significant local debridement and lavage. The treatment was adapted with i.v. vancomycin followed by i.v. teicoplanin, then oral clindamycin for a total of 3 months of antibiotics, with fluconazole therapy continuing for 6 months.

Owing to the catastrophic soft tissue situation and the incompetent extensor apparatus, a new revision TKA was deemed inappropriate. Two months after revision of the spacer, we opted for arthrodesis of the knee using an arthrodesis nail (Fig. 6.30a–c).

Post-operative recovery was good and the patient was happy and pain-free in the right knee. He was significantly more limited by his painful left knee.

6.5.7 Conclusion

If a patient-adapted treatment for infected total joints is applied, an overall success rate of above 90% can be obtained, even with difficult-to-diagnose or difficult-to-treat germs.

Take-Home Message

- The patient-adapted treatment concept in PJI is based on five pillars: teamwork, understanding biofilm, proper diagnostics, proper infection definition/classification and patient-tailored treatment.
- After classifying PJI into early, delayed and late, it is necessary to differentiate whether the infection is acute or chronic. These criteria are important for determining the best surgical and pharmaceutical treatment options.
- Possible advantages for each treatment option should be weighed against the chance of a successful outcome for the patient.
- Implant retention is only promising if the prosthesis is stable, the infection is acute, the soft tissues are intact, and the pathogens are sensitive to biofilm active antibiotics.
- The formation of biofilm is a rapid process starting with the »race for the surface«. Within minutes to hours, bacteria attach to the surface of an implant and enter a stationary growth phase. After 3 weeks, maturation of biofilms is established. Systemically and locally applied antibiotics play an important role to prevent biofilm formation.
- The cut-offs of WBC count and PMN% differ in the hip and knee joints at >4.2×109/l and PMN >80% and >1.7×109/l and PMN >65%, respectively.
- At least three positive samples and prolonged aerobic and anaerobic cultures for up to 14 days are recommended in order to find slow-growing microorganisms.
- Sonication is particularly helpful for detecting bacteria that cause low-grade infections or for patients who have been treated with antibiotics during the previous 14 days.

References

Achermann Y, Vogt M, Leunig M, Wust J, Trampuz A (2010) Improved diagnosis of periprosthetic joint infection by multiplex PCR of sonication fluid from removed implants. J Clin Microbiol 48:1208–14

Atkins BL, Athanasou N, Deeks JJ, Crook DW, Simpson H, Peto TE, et al (1998) Prospective evaluation of criteria for microbiological diagnosis of prosthetic-joint infection at revision arthroplasty. The OSIRIS Collaborative Study Group. J Clin Microbiol 36:2932–2939

Bengtson S1, Knutson K. (1991) The infected knee arthroplasty. A 6-year follow-up of 357 cases. Acta Orthop Scand 62:301–311

Berbari E, Mabry T, Tsaras G, Spangehl M, Erwin PJ, Murad MH, et al (2010) Inflammatory blood laboratory levels as markers of prosthetic joint infection: a systematic review and meta-analysis. J Bone Joint Surg Am 92:2102–2109

Booth RE, Jr., Lotke PA (1989) The results of spacer block technique in revision of infected total knee arthroplasty. Clin Orthop Relat Res 1989(248):57–60

Borens O, Corvec S, Trampuz A (2012) Diagnosis of periprosthetic joint infections. Hip Int 22:S9–14

-Buller LT, Sabry FY, Easton RW, Klika AK, Barsoum WK (2012) The preoperative prediction of success following irrigation and debridement with polyethylene exchange for hip and knee prosthetic joint infections. J Arthroplasty 27:857–864 e1-4

Burnett RS, Kelly MA, Hanssen AD, Barrack RL (2007) Technique and timing of two-stage exchange for infection in TKA. Clinical Orthop Relat Res 464:164–178

Butler-Wu SM, Burns EM, Pottinger PS, Magaret AS, Rakeman JL, Matsen FA, 3rd, et al. (2011) Optimization of periprosthetic culture for diagnosis of Propionibacterium acnes prosthetic joint infection. J Clin Microbiol 49:2490–2495

Calton TF, Fehring TK, Griffin WL (1997) Bone loss associated with the use of spacer blocks in infected total knee arthroplasty. Clin Orthop Relat Res 1997(345):148–154

-Campoccia D, Montanaro L, Arciola CR (2006) The significance of infection related to orthopedic devices and issues of antibiotic resistance. Biomaterials 27:2331–2339

Cui Q, Mihalko WM, Shields JS, Ries M, Saleh KJ (2007) Antibiotic-impregnated cement spacers for the treatment of infection associated with total hip or knee arthroplasty. J Bone Joint Surg Am 89:871–882

Davies D (2003) Understanding biofilm resistance to antibacterial agents. Nat Rev Drug Disc 2:114–122

Deirmengian C, Greenbaum J, Lotke PA, Booth RE, Jr., Lonner JH (2003) Limited success with open debridement and retention of components in the treatment of acute Staphylococcus aureus infections after total knee arthroplasty. J Arthroplasty 18:22–26

Elek SD, Conen PE (1957) The virulence of Staphylococcus pyogenes for man; a study of the problems of wound infection. Br J Exp Pathol 38:573–586

Fehring TK, Odum S, Calton TF, Mason JB (2000) Articulating versus static spacers in revision total knee arthroplasty for sepsis. The Ranawat Award. Clin Orthop Relat Res 380:9–16

Font-Vizcarra L, Garcia S, Martinez-Pastor JC, Sierra JM, Soriano A (2010) Blood culture flasks for culturing synovial fluid in prosthetic joint infections. Clin Orthop Relat Res 468:2238–2243

Freeman MG, Fehring TK, Odum SM, Fehring K, Griffin WL, Mason JB (2007) Functional advantage of articulating

versus static spacers in 2-stage revision for total knee arthroplasty infection. J Arthroplasty 22:1116–1121
Ghanem E, Azzam K, Seeley M, Joshi A, Parvizi J (2009) Staged revision for knee arthroplasty infection: what is the role of serologic tests before reimplantation? Clin Orthop Relat Res 467:1699–1705
Gristina AG (1987) Biomaterial-centered infection: microbial adhesion versus tissue integration. Science 237:1588--95
Hanssen AD, Spangehl MJ (2004) Practical applications of antibiotic-loaded bone cement for treatment of infected joint replacements. Clin Orthop Relat Res 427:79–85
Hofmann AA, Goldberg T, Tanner AM, Kurtin SM (2005) Treatment of infected total knee arthroplasty using an articulating spacer: 2- to 12-year experience Clin Orthop Relat Res 430:125–131
Hsu YC, Cheng HC, Ng TP, Chiu KY (2007) Antibiotic-loaded cement articulating spacer for 2-stage reimplantation in infected total knee arthroplasty: a simple and economic method. J Arthroplasty 22:1060–1066
Huang HT, Su JY, Chen SK (2006) The results of articulating spacer technique for infected total knee arthroplasty. The J Arthroplasty 21:1163–1168
Jenny JY, Barbe B, Gaudias J, Boeri C, Argenson JN (2012) High infection control rate and function after routine one-stage exchange for chronically infected TKA. Clin Orthop Relat Res 471:238--243
Johnson AJ, Sayeed SA, Naziri Q, Khanuja HS, Mont MA (2012) Minimizing dynamic knee spacer complications in infected revision arthroplasty. Clin Orthop Relat Res 470:220–227
Koo KH, Yang JW, Cho SH, Song HR, Park HB, Ha YC, et al (2001) Impregnation of vancomycin, gentamicin, and cefotaxime in a cement spacer for two-stage cementless reconstruction in infected total hip arthroplasty. J Arthroplasty 16:882–892
Kurtz S, Ong K, Lau E, Mowat F, Halpern M (2007) Projections of primary and revision hip and knee arthroplasty in the United States from 2005 to 2030. J Bone Joint Surg Am 89:780–785
Marculescu CE, Berbari EF, Hanssen AD, Steckelberg JM, Harmsen SW, Mandrekar JN, et al (2006) Outcome of prosthetic joint infections treated with debridement and retention of components. Clin Infect Dis 42:471–478
Masri BA, Duncan CP, Beauchamp CP (1998) Long-term elution of antibiotics from bone-cement: an in vivo study using the prosthesis of antibiotic-loaded acrylic cement (PROSTALAC) system. J Arthroplasty 13:331–338
Meek RM, Dunlop D, Garbuz DS, McGraw R, Greidanus NV, Masri BA (2004) Patient satisfaction and functional status after aseptic versus septic revision total knee arthroplasty using the PROSTALAC articulating spacer. J Arthroplasty 19:874–879
Moran E, Byren I, Atkins BL (2010) The diagnosis and management of prosthetic joint infections. J Antimicrob Chemother 65:45–54
O'Toole G, Kaplan HB, Kolter R (2000) Biofilm formation as microbial development. Ann Rev Microbiol 54:49–79
Parvizi J, Jacovides C, Zmistowski B, Jung KA (2011) Definition of periprosthetic joint infection: is there a consensus? Clin Orthop Relat Res 469(11):3022–3030
Schafer P, Fink B, Sandow D, Margull A, Berger I, Frommelt L (2008) Prolonged bacterial culture to identify late periprosthetic joint infection: a promising strategy. Clin Infect Dis 47:1403–1409
Schinsky MF, Della Valle CJ, Sporer SM, Paprosky WG (2008) Perioperative testing for joint infection in patients undergoing revision total hip arthroplasty. J Bone Joint Surg Am 90:1869-1875
Sendi P, Zimmerli W (2011) Challenges in periprosthetic knee-joint infection. Int J Artif Organs 34:947–956
Sherrell JC, Fehring TK, Odum S, Hansen E, Zmistowski B, Dennos A, et al (2011)The Chitranjan Ranawat Award: fate of two-stage reimplantation after failed irrigation and debridement for periprosthetic knee infection. Clin Orthop Relat Res 469:18–25
Stewart PS, Costerton JW (2001) Antibiotic resistance of bacteria in biofilms. Lancet 358:135–138
Trampuz A, Hanssen AD, Osmon DR, Mandrekar J, Steckelberg JM, Patel R (2004) Synovial fluid leukocyte count and differential for the diagnosis of prosthetic knee infection. Am J Med 117:556–562
Trampuz A, Zimmerli W (2005) Prosthetic joint infections: update in diagnosis and treatment. Swiss Med Wkly 135:243–251
Trampuz A, Piper KE, Jacobson MJ, Hanssen AD, Unni KK, Osmon DR, et al (2007) Sonication of removed hip and knee prostheses for diagnosis of infection. New Engl J Med 357:654–663
Uckay I, Lubbeke A, Emonet S, Tovmirzaeva L, Stern R, Ferry T, et al (2009) Low incidence of haematogenous seeding to total hip and knee prostheses in patients with remote infections. J Infection 59:337–345
Waldman BJ, Hostin E, Mont MA, Hungerford DS (2000) Infected total knee arthroplasty treated by arthroscopic irrigation and debridement. J Arthroplasty 15:430–436
Widmer AF (2001) New developments in diagnosis and treatment of infection in orthopedic implants. Clin Infect Dis 33:S94–106
Zimmerli W, Trampuz A, Ochsner PE (2004) Prosthetic-joint infections. New Engl J Med 351:1645–1654

6.6 Prosthetic Joint Infection: Treatment

James R. Berstock and Jason C.J. Webb

6.6.1 Background

The overall rate of revision for prosthetic hip joint infection is 0.078% (95% CI: 0.075–0.081) per patient per year during the first 11.75 years (National

Joint Registry for England 2015). Additional data from the 2015 report of the National Joint Registry for England, Wales, Northern Ireland and the Isle of Man show the patient-time incidence rate (PTIR) for revision of a prosthetic hip joint infection decreases with time from the primary procedure (see ◻ Tab. 6.9).

Other analyses of the incidence of prosthetic joint infection (PJI) have suggested an annual incidence of approximately 2% of all primaries performed in the United States (Kurtz et al. 2012), and a 5-year revision rate of 0.71% in the Nordic Arthroplasty Register (Dale et al. 2012). Difficulty identifying the true population at risk of PJI may account somewhat for the varying incidence rates reported. Likewise, whilst the absolute number of PJIs may be rising, concerns regarding a genuine upward trend in the incidence of PJI need careful appraisal. Finally, registry data regarding the incidence of PJI may not detect infections treated medically or by debridement or excision arthroplasty.

The human cost of PJI is significant (Zimmerli et al. 2004), with a 4% 90-day mortality associated with the first-stage procedure alone (Berend et al. 2013). The median Oxford Hip Score following two-stage exchange revision arthroplasty has been reported as 27 out of 48, equating to a »fair« outcome; however, less than 27 would equate to a »poor« outcome based on categories adopted from the Harris Hip Score (Bejon et al. 2010). Meta-analyses of studies reporting persistent infection following revision demonstrate re-infection rates of 8.2% (95% CI: 6.0–10.8) following one-stage surgery, and 7.9% (95% CI: 6.2–9.7) following two-stage revision (Kunutsor et al. 2015). In addition, a European cost-analysis study reported that the treatment of PJI was over €32,000 per patient, twice the cost of revision surgery for other causes (Klouche et al. 2010).

In our unit we aim to treat PJI in accordance with modern practice put forward by Zimmerli et al. (2004). The central tenet of this approach is to base the treatment upon the clinical features of the infection and the medical status of the patient. We provide the regional prosthetic joint service and work in a multidisciplinary team including microbiologists, radiologists, nurses, physiotherapists and occupational therapists.

◻ Tab. 6.9 Revision rates for infection following index procedure.

Time from primary	Number of revisions per 1,000 patient-years (95% CI)
<1 year	1.39 (1.30–1.48)
1–3 years	0.81 (0.76–0.87)
3–5 years	0.53 (0.48–0.59)
5–7 years	0.44 (0.38–0.50)
>7 years[a]	0.38 (0.32–0.47)
Overall	0.78 (0.75–0.81)

[a] Maximum observed follow-up, 11.75 years

6.6.2 Case 1: Debridement and Implant Retention

Case 1 is a 65-year-old woman with chronic obstructive pulmonary disease who underwent primary left total hip replacement which suddenly became painful (◻ Fig. 6.31). She was promptly investigated with an aspiration of the hip joint which revealed a methicillin-sensitive *Staphylococcus aureus*. The diagnosis of PJI was made within 3 weeks of the initial symptoms, and subsequently the patient underwent a radical debridement, exchange of modular components followed by intravenous oral antibiotic therapy with Co-trimoxazole and rifampicin. Her C-reactive protein (CRP) level was monitored weekly and then monthly in the community with follow-up arranged in the multidisciplinary PJI clinic. Antibiotics were subsequently withheld with no recurrence of infection for 3 years. A recent radiograph did not reveal any evidence of component loosening (◻ Fig. 6.32).

Learning point

DAIR indicated in view of early diagnosis of PJI with a sensitive organism.

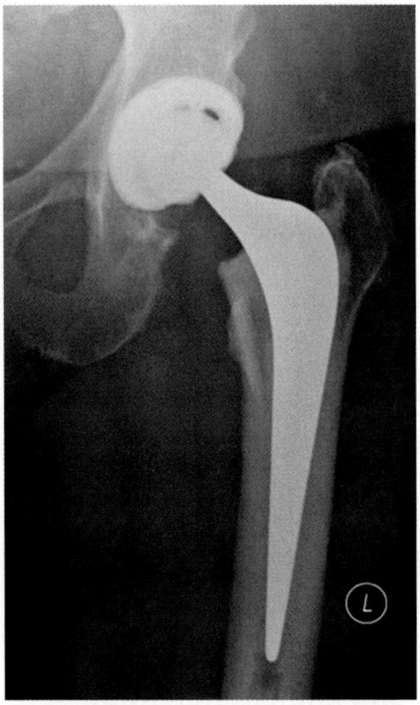

■ **Fig. 6.31** Imaging prior to debridement and implant retention (DAIR)

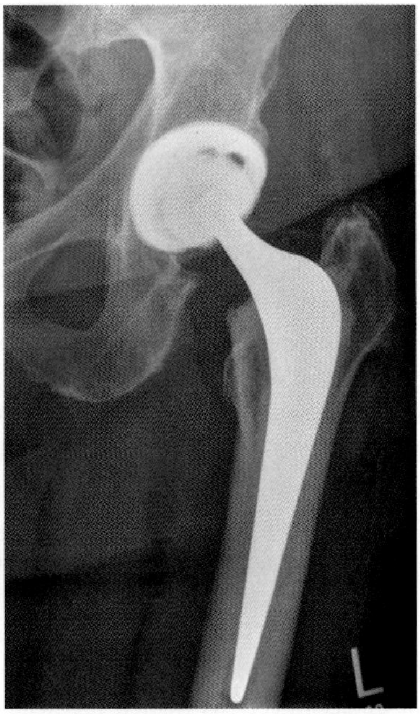

■ **Fig. 6.32** Image of most recent follow-up

6

6.6.3 Case 2: Single-Stage Exchange Arthroplasty

Case 2 is an 89-year-old man who underwent primary right-sided Exeter®/Duraloc® total hip replacement 13 years earlier with good function for over 10 years before he developed some swelling and erythema over the lateral aspect of the hip. This was treated as suspected cellulitis with oral antibiotics by his general practitioner but failed to resolve. He was therefore referred for a specialist opinion. His co-morbidities include immunosuppression secondary to polymyalgia rheumatica, oral steroid therapy, myelodysplasia and chronic renal failure. However, he enjoyed a good quality of life and walked unaided. Once referred, his CRP was noted to be 38 mg/l, having been off antibiotics for 1 week, and an ultrasound scan of the right hip showed a superficial collection communicating with the joint itself. An aspiration at the time of the ultrasound was sent for microbiological analysis and *Bacillus licheniformis*, a Gram-positive organism commonly found in soil, was cultured. The patient remained off antibiotics and was promptly taken to the operating theatre for a debridement and exchange of modular components. Following surgery he was treated with intravenous vancomycin and rifampicin, and deep tissue specimens isolated coagulase-negative *Staphylococcus epidermidis* on microbiological culture. Once his CRP level had fallen below 50 mg/l, treatment was converted to oral antibiotics, following the advice of the microbiologist, for a period of 6 weeks. He was followed up in the PJI clinic where his clinical condition and CRP were monitored following the discontinuation of oral antibiotics.

The wound remained quiet and his CRP below 10 mg/l for 1 year before a recurrence of the swelling and erythema in association with a sinus discharging purulent material that led to his second presentation. An ultrasound-guided aspiration of the hip joint confirmed coagulase-negative staphylococci once again, and following a discussion about potential treatment options the patient was happy to be randomized to either a one- or two-staged procedure as part of the INFORM trial. He received a single-stage exchange of components to a Stryker Trident Tritanium® revision cup and long-stem Exeter® femoral component with Modular Dual Mobility® bearings (Stryker)

Learning point

Note the history of previous debridement and implant retention (DAIR). One-stage revision appropriate option for frail elderly patient with sensitive organism. It is the practice of our unit to use proprietary antibiotic laden bone cement in the femoral reconstruction of elderly patients. We ensure that the antibiotics contained within the cement match the antibiogram of the cultured organisms. If this is not the case, then we add the appropriate antibiotics to the cement in theatre.

(◘ Fig. 6.33, ◘ Fig. 6.34). Intraoperatively, the Orthosonics® OSCAR 3 ultrasonic arthroplasty revision instrument was used to remove all cement from the femoral canal. Following removal of the primary implants and a thorough debridement, the patient was re-draped, new sterile instruments opened and the surgical team re-scrubbed prior to re-implantation. He received intravenous rifampicin and vancomycin in the post-operative period whilst cultures were awaited. Coagulase-negative *Staphylococcus epidermidis* were confirmed on all deep tissue specimens. Owing to an adverse haematological reaction caused by ciprofloxacin, he is currently completing a course of oral minocycline and rifampicin, and is being reviewed regularly in the PJI clinic.

6.6.4 Case 3: Two-Stage Exchange Arthroplasty

The patient of case 3 underwent a primary right-sided Exeter® total hip replacement at the age of 72 years (◘ Fig. 6.35), which became infected in the early post-operative period but was treated with a

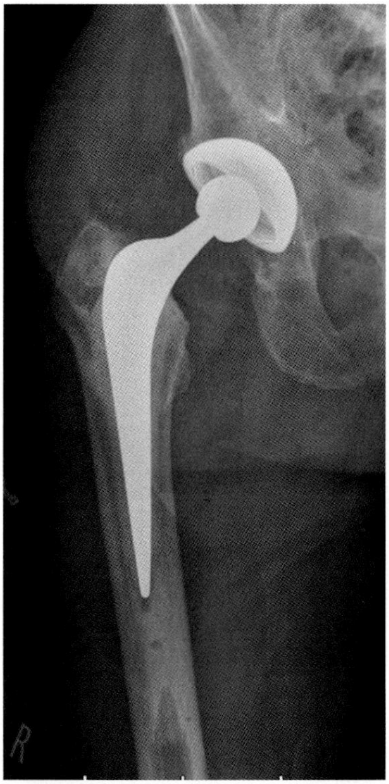

◘ **Fig. 6.33** Primary Exeter®/Duraloc® following DAIR

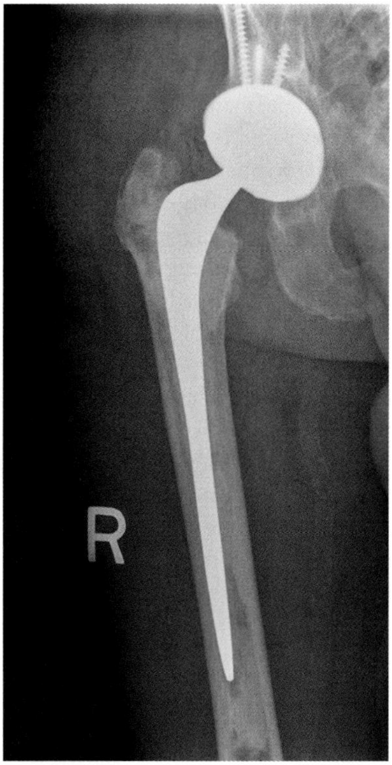

◘ **Fig. 6.34** Single-stage revision to Tritanium®/long-stem Exeter®

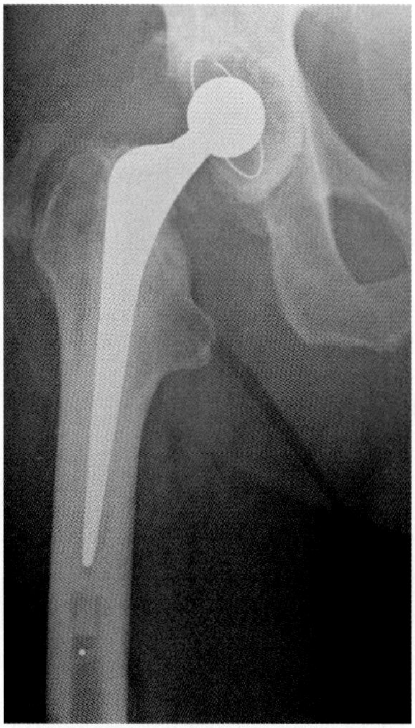

Fig. 6.35 Primary total hip replacement

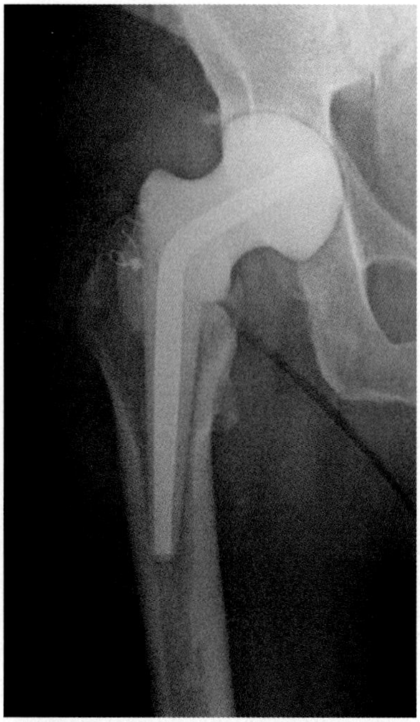

Fig. 6.36 Tecres® spacer following first-stage procedure

3-week course of oral antibiotics rather than further surgery. The wound then healed but the patient continued to suffer pain. He did not receive any further treatment at his original hospital. At 1 year after surgery, his general practitioner referred him to our unit. His past medical history included thrombocytopoenia and prostate cancer treated with hormone therapy. His CRP was raised at 27 mg/l and he underwent aspiration of the right hip replacement under fluoroscopy. This sample grew a coagulase-negative Staphylococcus species. In view of the delay in presentation and the incomplete previous treatment, the patient was offered exchange arthroplasty surgery and opted for a two-stage approach.

The first-stage operation comprised removal of implants, radical debridement and insertion of a proprietary gentamicin-loaded Tecres® cement spacer (Fig. 6.36). The same coagulase-negative Staphylococcus species was identified on deep tissue culture. Following a 2-week period of intravenous antibiotics, treatment was converted to oral therapy and 3 months later underwent a second-stage revision where a Tritanium® revision cup was inserted with an Exeter® stem (Fig. 6.37). He

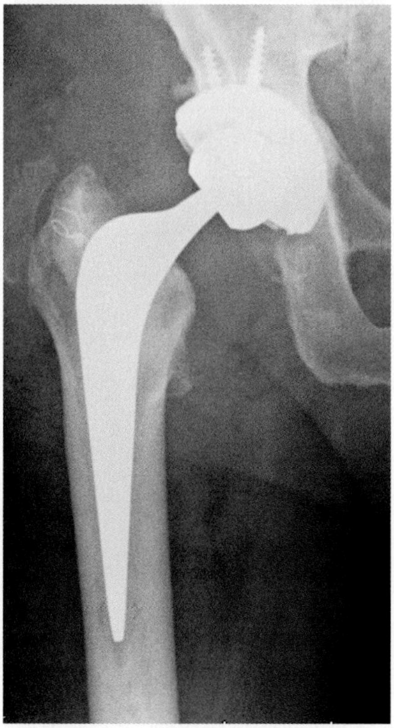

Fig. 6.37 Revision to Exeter®/Tritanium®

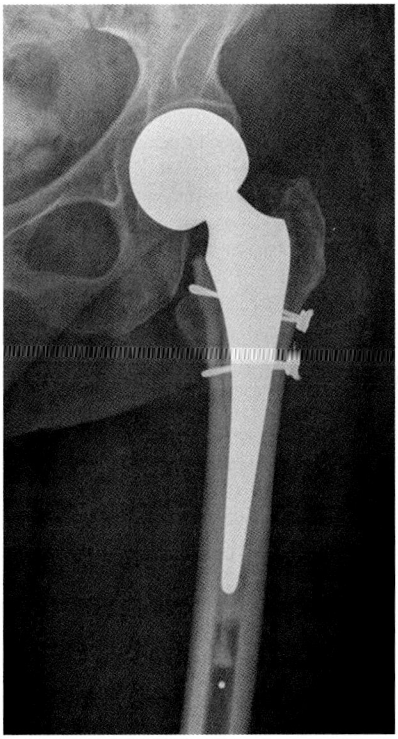

Fig. 6.38 Furlong® hemiarthroplasty

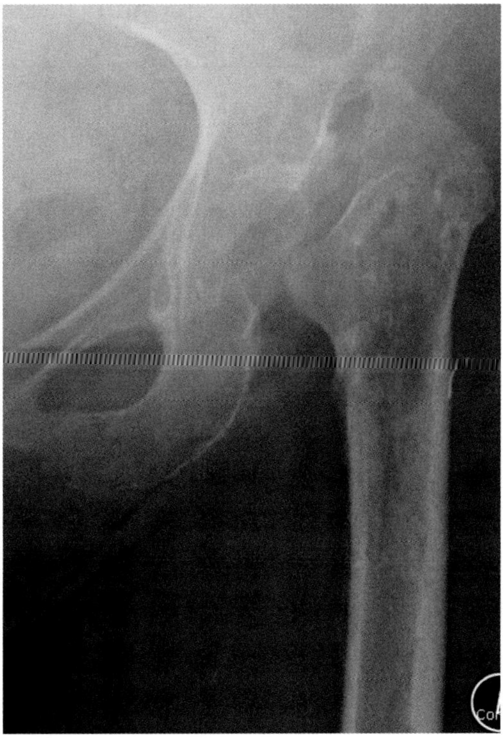

Fig. 6.39 Girdlestone excision arthroplasty

stopped antibiotics after 2 weeks, when delayed cultures showed no growth. Three months later he experienced a single dislocation, which was treated by a closed reduction. He remains clinically free of infection and off antibiotics without further complications for 5 years.

Learning point

Appropriate option for frail elderly patient with sensitive organism.

6.6.5 Case 4: Excision Arthroplasty

Case 4 is of a frail 72-year-old woman with multiple medical comorbidities, who fell and sustained a hip fracture which was treated with a hemiarthroplasty (Fig. 6.38). Post-operatively, the wound continued to discharge haemoserous fluid for 7 days before settling; however, at the 2-week mark it started to leak again and she was taken for a radical debridement and closure of the wound. Tissue specimens cultured *Staphylococcus epidermidis* and a vancomycin-resistant enterococcus. The wound continued to discharge fluid despite the cessation of chemical thromboprophylaxis and the use of a negative pressure dressing. To control the infection, the patient underwent a repeat surgical debridement and this was combined with an excision arthroplasty (Fig. 6.39). The wound then went on to heal. She was monitored in the PJI clinic where the CRP level settled and antibiotic therapy was discontinued. She remained clear of infection for 1 year following excision arthroplasty and declined reconstructive surgery despite an Oxford Hip Score of 6 out of 48, with 0 representing the worst possible score.

Learning point

Excision arthroplasty used to treat a medically unfit patient with early infection following hip fracture surgery who was cured of infection but suffered poor functional recovery.

6.6.6 Case 5: Lifelong Antibiotic Suppression

Case 5 is of an 89-year-old woman with a history of a cerebral vascular accident and subsequent right-sided hemiparesis, who presented with a discharging sinus over a right total hip replacement. The hip replacement had been in situ for many years but there was a history of recurrent urinary tract infections. Significant osteomyelitis was evident from her radiographs and aspiration revealed *E. coli* organisms. The PJI team had a frank discussion of her treatment options with the patient. She had been well throughout the clinical episode and taking her medical co-morbidities and age into account, she elected for lifelong antibiotic suppression. She was prescribed Co-trimoxazole and stoma bag dressings for the discharging sinus. The sinus subsequently healed on antibiotics negating the requirement for stoma bag dressings. She is closely monitored in our PJI clinic for signs of worsening infection and antibiotic side effects.

> **Learning point**
> A significant proportion of elderly patients choose antibiotic suppression if their PJI is pain free and they remain well.

6.6.7 Summary

We have used these case scenarios and the many options for treatment of PJI in a modern regional clinic. Although surgery offers the only hope for cure, we offer patients all treatment options with descriptions of the likely clinical course. We maintain close follow-up of all the patients and change strategies based on clinical progress and the patient's wishes.

> **Take-Home Message**
> - The management of prosthetic joint infection (PJI) requires a collaboration within a truly multidisciplinary specialist team
> - The treatment categories include:
>   - DAIR (debridement and implant retention) indicated if early diagnosis of PJI with a sensitive pathogen
>   - One-stage exchange with antibiotic-loaded bone cement as appropriate option with sensitive organisms
>   - Two-stage exchange with PMMA spacer
>   - Excision arthroplasty
>   - Lifelong antibiotic suppression

References

Bejon P, Berendt A, Atkins BL, Green N, Parry H, Masters S, et al (2010) Two-stage revision for prosthetic joint infection: predictors of outcome and the role of reimplantation microbiology. J Antimicrob Chemother 65(3):569–575

Berend KR, Lombardi AV Jr, Morris MJ, Bergeson AG, Adams JB, Sneller MA (2013) Two-stage treatment of hip periprosthetic joint infection is associated with a high rate of infection control but high mortality. Clin Orthop Relat Res 471(2):510–518

Dale H, Fenstad A M, Hallan G, Havelin L I, Furnes O, Overgaard S, et al (2012) Increasing risk of prosthetic joint infection after total hip arthroplasty. Acta Orthop 83(5):449–458

Klouche S, Sariali E, Mamoudy P (2010) Total hip arthroplasty revision due to infection: a cost analysis approach. Orthop Traumatol Surg Res 96(2):124–132

Kunutsor SK, Whitehouse MR, Blom AW, Beswick AD, Team I (2015) Re-infection outcomes following one- and two-stage surgical revision of infected hip prosthesis: a systematic review and meta-analysis. PLoS One 10(9):e0139166

Kurtz S M, Lau E, Watson H, Schmier JK, Parvizi J (2012) Economic burden of periprosthetic joint infection in the United States. J Arthroplasty 27[8 Suppl]: 61–65e1

No authors listed (2015) National Joint Registry for England, Wales, Northern Ireland, and the Isle of Man: 12th Annual Report

Zimmerli W, Trampuz A, Ochsner PE (2004) Prosthetic-joint infections. N Engl J Med 351(16):1645–1654

6.7 Dutch Protocol for Treatment of PJIs with Illustrative Clinical Cases

René H.M. ten Broeke

6.7.1 Introduction

Recently in the Dutch Orthopaedic Society, a consensus was proposed by the Working Group on Orthopaedic Infections on how to diagnose, treat and follow up prosthetic joint infections (PJIs) (www.orthopeden.org). Six treatment strategies were determined that could cover all possible patient categories. The strategies for treating possible or confirmed PJIs are:

- Debridement, antibiotics and implant retention (DAIR with prosthesis still in situ)
- Revision of the prosthesis in one stage
- Revision in two stages with or without the use of local antibiotics during the interval
- Definitive explantation, arthrodesis or amputation
- Suppressive antibiotic treatment
- »Supervised neglect«

6.7.2 Debridement, Antibiotics, and Implant Retention

DAIR (Hartman et al. 1991) is the treatment of choice for cases of early infection (within 3 months of the index operation) or when symptoms have presented only recently in cases of haematogenous infection (until 4–6 weeks, although there is evidence from our group that retaining the prosthesis can be successful in more than 50 % of cases until 8 weeks after the onset of symptoms) (Geurts et al. 2013). This protocol should only be considered when the prosthesis is well fixed and soft tissues are of good quality.

The rate of success for a debridement in situ depends on several factors. The results are worse with longer intervals between primary implantation and onset of symptoms (4 weeks, 90%; 8 weeks 80%; >8 weeks, 50%) (Geurts et al. 2013). Implant retention also has a higher failure rate in cases of inferior soft tissues and a micro-organism that is difficult to treat (high minimum inhibitory concentration [MIC] or resistance against several antibiotics; Deirmengian et al. 2003; Azzam et al. 2010; Koyonos et al. 2011; Odum et al. 2011).

In the case of DAIR, it is advised not to administer the antibiotics before cultures have been taken. At least five to six cultures have to be taken from joint fluid and tissues with separate, clean instruments. Excision of the infected tissues should be extensive (complete synovectomy and excision of the surrounding tissue of the abscess). Abundant irrigation with 0.9% NaCl or Ringer's lactate solution with pulse lavage (6 l or more) and exchange of all mobile components is advised (total hip replacement [THP]: modular head and liner; total knee prosthesis [TKP]: tibial insert), in order to be able to debride the posterior part of the knee joint and the femoral taper and inner side of the acetabular shell. The use of local antibiotic carriers (beads, fleeces) can be considered (NB: for non-dissolvable carriers, a re-operation has to be performed).

In the case of a persistent infection after two to three debridements, in the case of micro-organisms that are difficult to treat, and in cases with suboptimal patient and local circumstances, extraction of the prosthesis is usually necessary (Azzam et al. 2010).

The aim of the antibiotic therapy must also be focussed on the treatment of the biofilm. The working spectrum is aimed at the cultured bacteria: It should be broad until the results of deep cultures are known, and should be narrow as soon as the sensitivity of the causal micro-organism is known. If the prosthesis is to be retained, antibiotics should be continued for 3 months, at least 2 weeks intravenously and orally thereafter.

6.7.3 One-Stage Revision

Indications

One stage revisions may be performed if the following criteria are met (Gehrke et al. 2013):

- Infection can no longer be treated with debridement and implant retention because of the duration of the infection and/or a prosthesis which is no longer well fixed.
- The patient is not septic (no systemic signs of infection).

- The causal micro-organism is known (by preoperative cultures of synovial fluid or periprosthetic tissues), and is sensitive to available antibiotics.
- Soft tissues are of good quality (vital and giving good coverage of the prosthesis).

The preoperative identification of the causal micro-organism from synovial cultures is a prerequisite for the admission of adequate antibiotics, both locally in the cement as well as systemically through intravenous or oral treatment. The micro-organism needs to be highly sensitive for the chosen antibiotics, culturing must be continued for at least 14 days (preferably 21 days), and the patient must have had an antibiotic-free break of at least 14 days (Ure et al. 1998; Callaghan et al. 1999; Hanssen and Osmon 2000; Oussedik et al. 2010; Gehrke et al. 2013).

6

Contra-indications

Absolute contra-indications (Hanssen and Osmon 2000; Oussedik et al. 2010) for a one-stage septic procedure are:

- A septic patient with systemic signs of infection
- Failure of an earlier one-stage procedure
- Preoperatively unidentified or unclear micro-organism
- No adequate antibiotics available (locally or systemically)
- Sinus tract with unclear specification of the causal micro-organism

Relative Contra-indications

The relative contra-indications for a one-stage septic procedure are:

- Serious soft tissue involvement with inadequate coverage (particularly around the knee) requiring plastic surgery
- Complete loss of extensor mechanism of the knee in combination with serious PJI (strong indication for arthrodesis with external fixator or intramedullary nail in a one- or two-stage procedure)
- Extensive bony defects in need of reconstruction with allograft, or associated osteomyelitis (requiring resection and reconstruction which may be technically too complicated)
- Seriously immunocompromised patients (i.e. due to chemotherapy).

Conditions for a Successful One-Stage Septic Revision

Important conditions for a successful one-stage septic revision are (Singer et al. 2012):

- Radical debridement until healthy bleeding tissues (bone and soft tissue), including total radical synovectomy
- Special revision instruments for removal of the implant(s) and cement
- Cultures of relevant tissues (fluid, interface, and capsule) for microbiological and histopathological analysis, at least five to six specimens, no swabs
- Low pulse lavage (at least 6 l with saline)
- New sterile instruments as well as new sterile operating room (OR) clothes before the re-implantation phase
- Repeated dose of antibiotics in the case of OR time of > 2× $T_{1/2}$ of the antibiotics or of blood loss/ fluid resuscitation > 1–2.2 l
- Preferably cemented implants (release of antibiotics supports local antibiotic-therapy), and in the case of a TKP, a hinged design is advised because of the extensive amount of debridement, as a result of which condylar prostheses do not provide sufficient stability.

Antibiotic Treatment

Convincing evidence for the ideal length of antibiotic treatment is not available. International consensus advises the administration of 2–6 weeks of (micro-organism specific) intravenous therapy, with the recommendation of a supplementary oral period (Parvizi and Gehrke 2013).

The Infectious Diseases Society of America (IDSA) protocol suggests for Staphylococcus species a 2–6-week period of micro-organism-specific intravenous therapy combined with rifampicin. This should be followed by 3 months of additional oral treatment (rifampicin and ciprofloxacin or levofloxacin). If rifampicin treatment is not possible (because of allergic reactions in the past, for example) 4–6 weeks of intravenous therapy is advised (Osmon et al. 2013).

For the other pathogens, 4–6 weeks of pathogen-specific intravenous or high »bioavailability oral antibiotic treatment is recommended (Osmon et al. 2013).

6.7.4 Revision in Two or More Stages with or Without Application of Local Antibiotic Carriers During the Interval Period

Indications

- The infection is no longer eligible for debridement with implant retention after two attempts have been made. It can be considered with causative agents both easy or difficult to treat (high MIC or resistance against antibiotic).
- Another reason for this policy can be poor soft tissue quality (fistula or abscess; Parvizi et al. 2010).

Steps of Implant Removal

The steps to be followed during removal of the implant are:

- Taking at least five to six (preferably an uneven number) cultures of joint fluid, capsule, and interface tissue with separate instruments; sonification of the explants is also advised.
- Starting broad-spectrum antibiotics following the taking of cultures, or narrow-spectrum antibiotics in the case of an identified micro-organism.
- Extensive excision and radical debridement of all infected tissue.
- Pulsatile lavage with 0.9% NaCl or Ringer's lactate solution.
- Depending on the bone and soft tissue quality and on the causative micro-organism, a temporary spacer can be introduced with specifically added antibiotics. Other local carriers like beads can also be chosen. In the case of a spacer, (partial) weight-bearing is allowed, but this should not be advised if beads are used. In the knee, extra stability should be provided with an external fixator or a splint.
- It may be necessary to repeat the debridement and exchange of the local antibiotic carrier based on the clinical picture and the laboratory results (erythrocyte sedimentation rate [ESR] and C-reactive protein [CRP]).

The Interval Period

- Depending on the micro-organism and the tendency of wound healing, the interval period (Tsukayama et al. 1996; Segawa et al. 1999; Hanssen and Spangehl 2004; Pitto and Spika 2004) can be adapted.
- The sensitivity of the micro-organism is of great importance for the choice of the cement and the specific antibiotics that can further be added to the cement; for this, close collaboration with the microbiologist is crucial.
- In the case of local antimicrobial therapy (antibiotic-loaded spacer/PMMA beads) the length of treatment can be short or long. After a short interval (2–6 weeks), the delivery of antibiotics will be insufficient, making the spacer become a foreign body with the risk of renewed biofilm formation. When a decision for a short interval has been made, the administration of antibiotics can be interrupted for at least 2 weeks before performing re-implantation. Because theoretically during these 2 weeks a biofilm may develop, the antibiotic break may be skipped and re-implantation executed under an antibiotic umbrella for 6 weeks. If, however, during the placement of the prosthesis new cultures still show bacteria, the antibiotics will have to be continued for (at least) 3 months.
- In infections that are difficult to treat, the spacer therapy can be prolonged and the new prosthesis postponed (long-term interval). The patient can then be discharged from hospital with the spacer in situ. It is not advised to leave beads for such a long time in the hip or knee joint. After this period, it is advisable to include a reliable antibiotic-free interval again of at least 2 weeks, before re-implantation is performed.
- When soft tissues are inadequate for good coverage, consultation of a plastic surgeon is advised for additional surgical treatment during the prosthetic implantation.

The Re-implantation

- It is preferred not to start antibiotics before taking renewed deep cultures.
- Once again, at least five to six cultures (preferably an uneven number) are advised with separate clean instruments.
- After cultures are taken, antibiotic therapy should be started aimed at the already known micro-organism(s), or otherwise once again a broad-spectrum antibiotic is chosen.
- Debridement of necrotic or potentially infectious tissue should again be executed before prosthetic re-implantation.
- Thorough lavage is then performed with 3–6 l 0.9% NaCl or Ringer's lactate solution, with or without povidone-iodine as an aqueous solution.
- In the case of preoperative or intraoperative doubt about the status of the infection, a new interval with antibiotic treatment can be chosen.
- Both a cemented or an uncemented prosthesis can be considered; in the case of a cemented implant, the active antibiotic can be applied to the cement, and if chosen it should also be used in a bone graft (Witsø et al. 1999).
- Plastic surgery may be necessary during the re-implantation for an additional soft tissue procedure.

After the Re-implantation

- If the patient has been treated with antibiotics, and the cultures taken at re-implantation and following a drug-free interval of at least 2 weeks are negative, then antibiotic treatment can be stopped.
- However, if a local antibiotic carrier is used during the interval, and there is re-implantation without a drug-free interval, the cultures are less reliable and it is advised to continue the antibiotic medication for 6 weeks.
- If new bacteria are found in the intraoperative cultures, the antibiotic regimen should be adapted and the newly implanted prosthesis has to be protected for 12 weeks again.
- During this period and afterwards, the patient must be followed up by checking infection parameters such as the ESR, CRP and white blood cell count until they are normal again. In the case of potentially nephrotoxic and hepatotoxic medication, liver and kidney functions should also be checked regularly.

6.7.5 Definitive Explantation, Arthrodesis, and Amputation

Depending on the condition of the bone and soft tissues, as well as on the status of the patient and on any existing co-morbidities, the best choice may be a definitive extraction of the prosthesis creating a persistent Girdlestone of the hip. In the case of a failed knee prosthesis, the exarticulation may result in an arthrodesis or an exarticulation or amputation. Obviously the patient's wish and the doctor's advice will have to match in these difficult cases.

Arthrodesis/Exarticulation of the Knee

- This may be necessary in the case of insufficient viable bone stock and/or deficient extensor mechanism.
- In the initial stage, external fixation is preferred with the fixator pins as far away from the joint as possible without compromising stability.
- If the infection has settled, further treatment may be optimized with plate fixation or intramedullary fixation.

Upper Leg Amputation

- If no adequate soft tissue coverage can be anticipated, an upper leg amputation may have to be chosen. The level of amputation should be as far as possible from the infected area; however, the necessity of the patient having to rely on an orthesis should be taken into account. Therefore close consultation with the rehabilitation specialist is obligatory.
- In the case of an amputation through infected tissue, it may be indicated to treat the patient with antibiotics for 6 weeks.

Definitive Girdlestone of the hip is indicated in the following cases

- Extensive bone and peri-articular muscular damage (particularly of the abductor mecha-

nism) when bad hip function may be anticipated after renewed prosthetic implantation.
- When recurrent infections have led to repeated failure of the THP.

6.7.6 Antibiotic Suppression of the Infection (Lifelong)

Indications for this Treatment

- Inoperable patients
- Patients refusing surgical interventions.
- Availability of oral antibiotics with no or few side effects.
- For this group, a permanent fistula without prosthetic complaints is in itself not an indication for antibiotic suppression therapy. However, when a fistula closes under antimicrobial medication, interrupting the antibiotics may result in accumulation of wound secretion and in infection symptoms, even sepsis (Goulet et al. 1988; Segreti et al. 1998; Rao et al. 2003; Zimmerli et al. 2004).

6.7.7 Supervised Neglect

In the case of mild complaints and symptoms, the patient and doctor may agree to wait and see and abstain from any (surgical and drug) treatment at all. Serious co-morbidities and resistance against many antibiotics can motivate this decision. Nevertheless, it is advised to perform clinical and radiological evaluations on regular basis in this patient group.

6.7.8 Case 1

This case describes a 50-year-old female patient who underwent total hip replacement (THR) of the left hip in 1995 at another hospital, which was revised in 1997 and eventually extracted in 1999 for a PJI. Cultures showed *Staphylococcus epidermidis*, and it was decided after several debridements not to perform a re-implantation because of persistent positive cultures and insufficient bone stock (▪ Fig. 6.40).

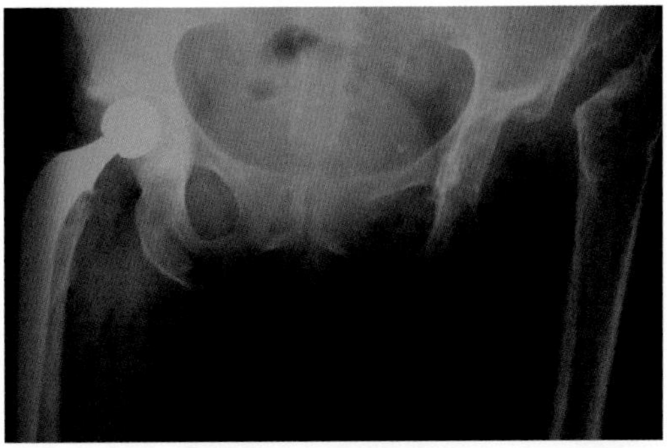

▪ **Fig. 6.40** Girdlestone situation of the left hip after total hip removal and several unsuccessful debridements

We saw the patient for a second opinion in 2002 and on computed tomography (CT) analysis we confirmed an extensive bone loss with large segmental defects in the dome and in both the anterior and posterior acetabular wall (▪ Fig. 6.41).

Because the patient had been free of symptoms for 2 years, it was decided to take deep cultures again followed by a renewed debridement. Gentamicin PMMA beads were implanted and she was treated intravenously with vancomycin (▪ Fig. 6.42). Because the cultures remained negative and because the patient had a strong wish to regain her mobility, we agreed to restore the bone stock and re-implant a THP. A strut graft for the cranio-posterior segmental defect and impaction bone grafting for the central cavitary defect was followed by the implantation of an anti-protrusio cage and a cemented cup on the acetabular side, and a fully hydroxyapatite (HA)-coated revision stem with prophylactic wiring on the femoral side (▪ Fig. 6.43).

During the following years the patient had no pain, normal laboratory test results, and was able to walk long distances even in the alpine mountains without any complaints. Nevertheless, there was a gradual migration of the ring cage with femoral osteolysis (see ▪ Fig. 6.44).

In 2013 she returned with complaints about her left hip. At that time an infection of the hip was suspected on the basis of laboratory test results and a positron emission tomography (PET)-CT scan. In 2014 she was treated for a fistula with DAIR and a fistulectomy at the hospital where she had originally presented. Furthermore, she received i.v. ri-

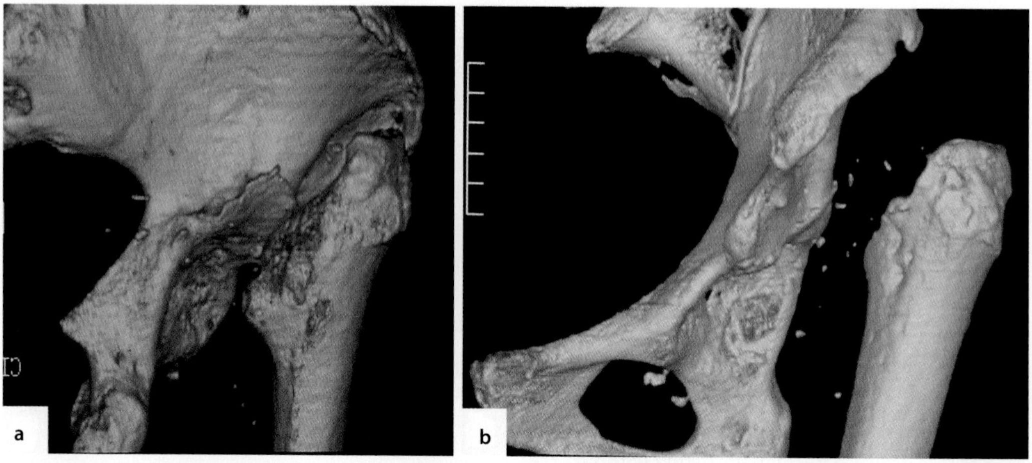

■ Fig. 6.41 Computed tomography scan showing bone loss of acetabular dome, anterior (a) and posterior (b) acetabularwall

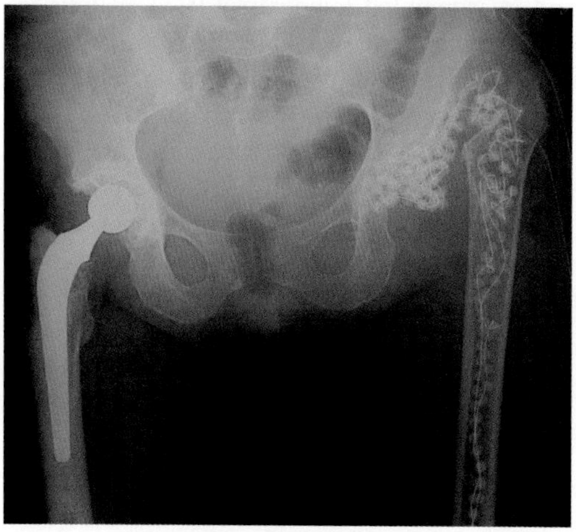

■ Fig. 6.42 Gentamicin PMMA beads in situ

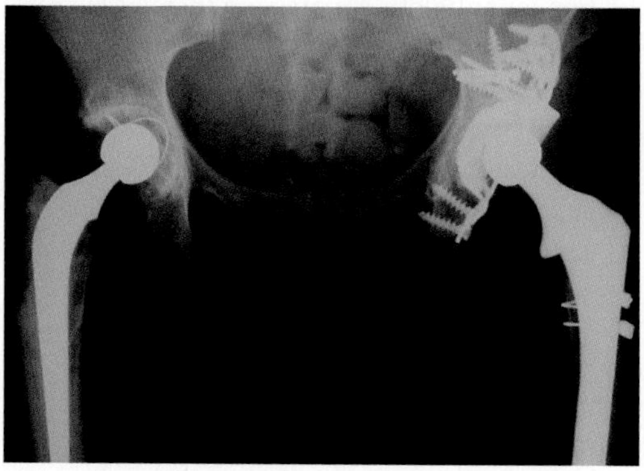

■ Fig. 6.43 Radiographic results after extensive bone reconstruction, anti-protrusio cage and reversed hybrid total hip replacement of the left hip

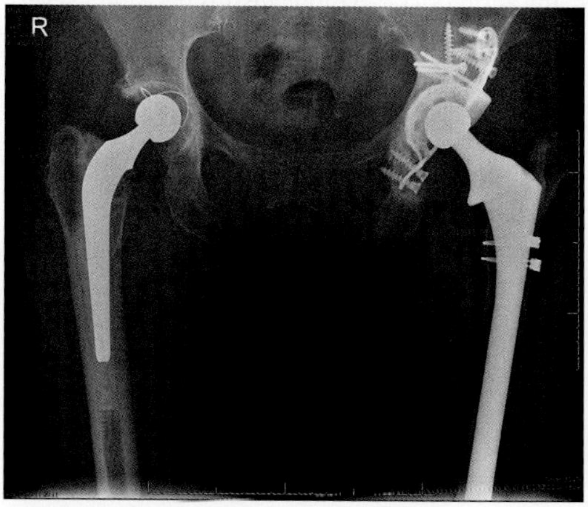

■ Fig. 6.44 Bone loss of the ischial bone with migration of the cage. Note remarkable stress shielding of the proximal femur

fampicin and Fucidin. Although there was a progressive protrusion, no action was taken and the patient once again returned to our hospital for a renewed second opinion.

At that time new X-rays showed a complete protrusion of the cage into the small pelvis (■ Fig. 6.45). She was re-admitted and soon afterwards underwent re-operation. Several deep cultures were taken and the cage and cup were extracted. Because the femoral stem on the PET-CT did not show an elevated uptake and particularly because of the extensive stress shielding, it was decided to leave the stem in situ and put a cement spacer loaded with gentamicin and vancomycin on top of the cone (■ Fig. 6.46).

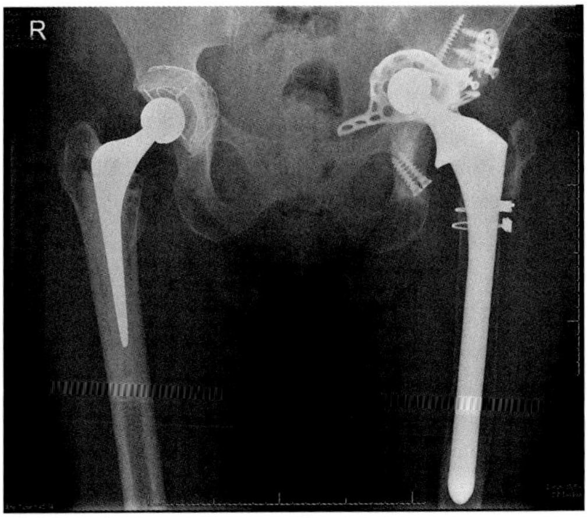

■ **Fig. 6.45** Central protrusion and fracture of the cage

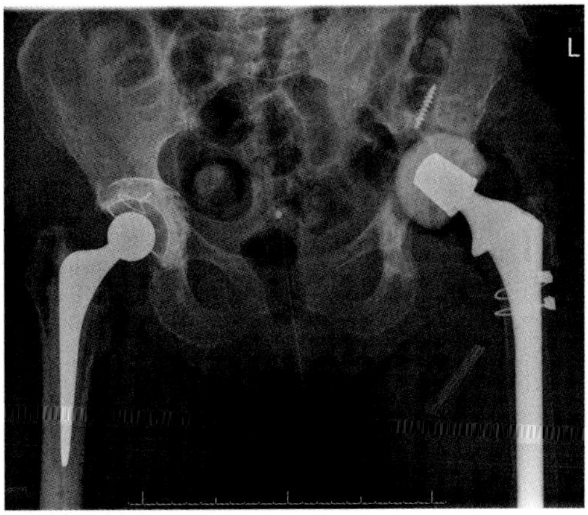

■ **Fig. 6.46** Antibiotic-loaded cement spacer in the acetabulum after removal of the dislocated cage

Two months after the operation, the patient had a fever with a high CRP level (211 mg/l) and underwent debridement again with exchange of the spacer and adaptation of the antibiotics based on cultures showing *Pseudomonas aeruginosa*. Antibiotics were continued for 3 months. After that she was free of complaints, had normal laboratory test results (ESR, 20 mm/h; CRP, 9 mg/l; leukocytes, 7.8 10^3/µg/l), and requested again to have a THP.

It was decided to wait for another 3 months without antibiotics. Because she remained symptom-free with normal laboratory results, we agreed to perform another re-implantation with restoration of the acetabular bone defects using medial wall and segmental rim meshes with bone impaction grafting (■ Fig. 6.47, ■ Fig. 6.48, ■ Fig. 6.49, ■ Fig. 6.50).

Since then (6-month follow-up at the time of writing) the patient has been doing well and has no complaints or signs of infection.

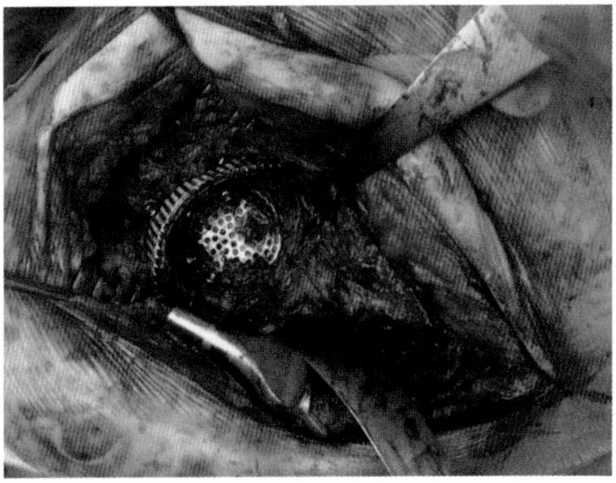

■ **Fig. 6.47** Medial wall and rim mesh

6.7.9 Case 2

A 59-year-old male patient was referred to our hospital in July 2015 for persistent PJI of a total knee arthroplasty (TKA) of the right knee. The prosthesis had been implanted 4 years earlier. The patient's medical history noted diabetes. His current complaints started after a recent episode of urosepsis with kidney failure.

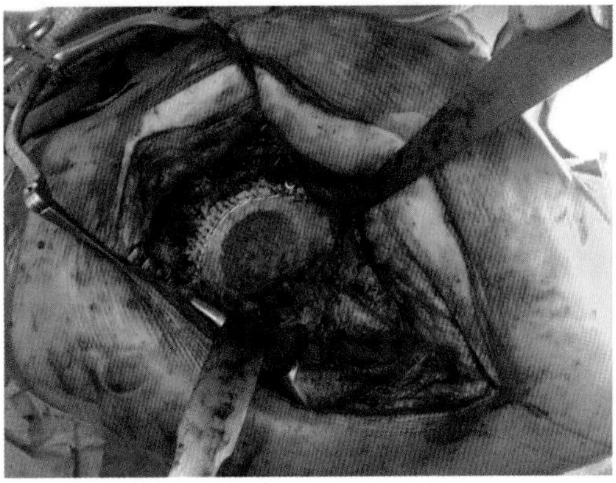

■ **Fig. 6.48** After impaction of morcellized bone graft

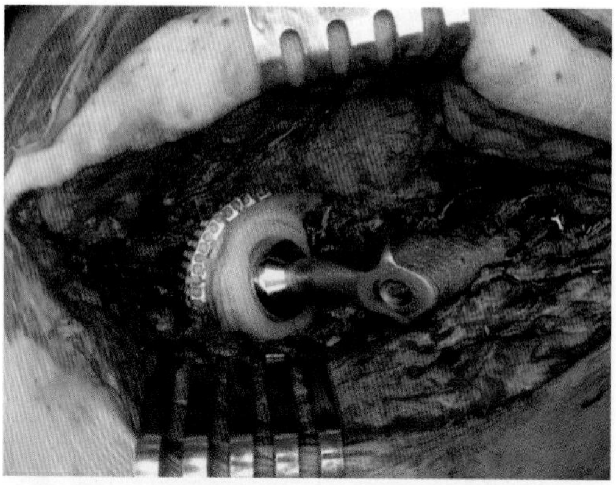

Fig. 6.49 Cemented cup and reduced stem

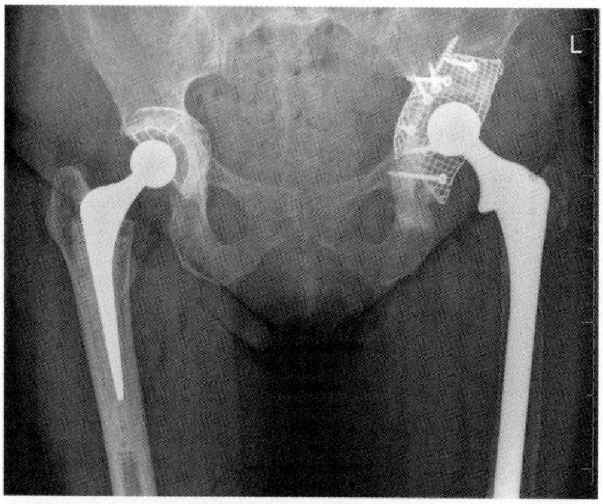

Fig. 6.50 Post-operative X-ray

On physical examination of the right knee swelling, redness and tenderness were seen with a limited and painful range of motion. Laboratory results showed a CRP level of 82 mg/l and an ESR of 33 mm/h. An X-ray displayed bone loss under the tibial tray (Fig. 6.51), while a single-photon emission (SPECT)-CT suggested loosening of the tibial component. A leukocyte scan showed clear elevated uptake of the right TKA (Fig. 6.52).

Arthrocentesis was performed and Gram-negative rods were cultured from the aspirated synovial fluid. A late haematogenous infection of the right TKP was concluded, for which a two-stage revision was planned with extraction of the prosthesis, 6 weeks of antibiotics, and early re-implantation after a short interval with a spacer.

Operation 1 (August 2015) consisted of removal of the prosthesis, deep cultures of the synovial fluid, the synovial tissue/capsule and the interface of femur and tibia, as well as sonication of the explants. The joint was rinsed with 6 l of fluid and a spacer of gentamicin and clindamycin cement was left in situ together with gentamicin PMMA beads in the large osteolytic tibial defect, for optimal local antibiotic treatment (Fig. 6.53).

In all cultures as well as in the sonicated material, *Proteus mirabilis* was identified, for which i.v. ciprofloxacin with co-trimoxazole was started.

Operation II was performed 2 weeks later (August 31) with removal of the beads, renewed exten-

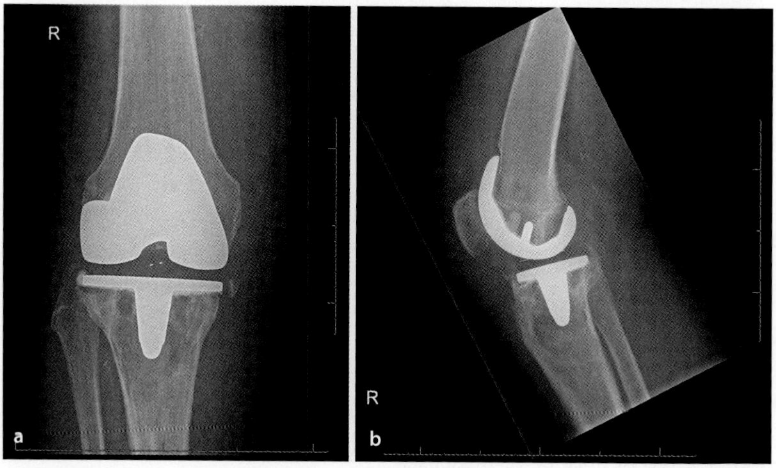

Fig. 6.51 X-rays showing extensive periprosthetic bone loss of the proximal tibia (**a**) and distal femur (**b**)

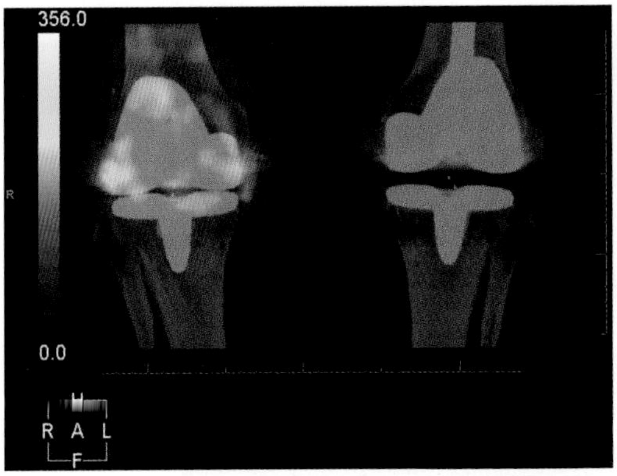

Fig. 6.52 Leukocyte scan showing elevated uptake of right total knee arthroplasty

sive debridement, and renewal of the spacer. After 3 weeks, antibiotics were orally continued (ciprofloxacin) and the patient was discharged from hospital (Fig. 6.54).

Six weeks after the first surgery, operation III was performed, during which a revision prosthesis was placed with augments and a tibial sleeve for the bone defects. Gentamicin and clindamycin cement was used for fixating the components (Fig. 6.55). One week later the patient could be discharged from hospital.

However, 6 months later (April 2016), the patient presented again with sudden knee pain, which felt warm and tender. Although he had not experienced fever, his temperature was 38.6°C and the laboratory tests showed a CRP level of 154 mg/l with 14.3 $10^3/\mu g/l$ leukocytes. Therefore, he was operated on again (operation IV) on the same day. DAIR was performed and mobile parts (tibial insert) were replaced also for better access to the popliteal fossa during lavage. Gentamicin PMMA beads were left in the joint. It was considered to be a delayed infection, but because there was a short duration of symptoms, a stable implant which was already a revision type of implant, no fistulas, no severe soft tissue damage, and good susceptibility to antibiotics, the prosthesis was left in situ (Fig. 6.56).

Cultures taken during this last operation now showed *Staphylococcus aureus* and cefazolin was started i.v. and after 3 days rifampicin was added and continued for 3 months.

Two weeks later (operation V; May 2016) the beads were removed again, and the tibial insert was once again replaced. All cultures and the sonicated material were negative. Laboratory results normalized and therefore antibiotics were switched to clindamycin with rifampicin, which was continued orally for 3 months.

At the most recent follow-up more than 3 months after the fifth operation, there were no complaints, a CRP level of 1 mg/l and an ESR of 5 mm/h, and a good radiological result (Fig. 6.57).

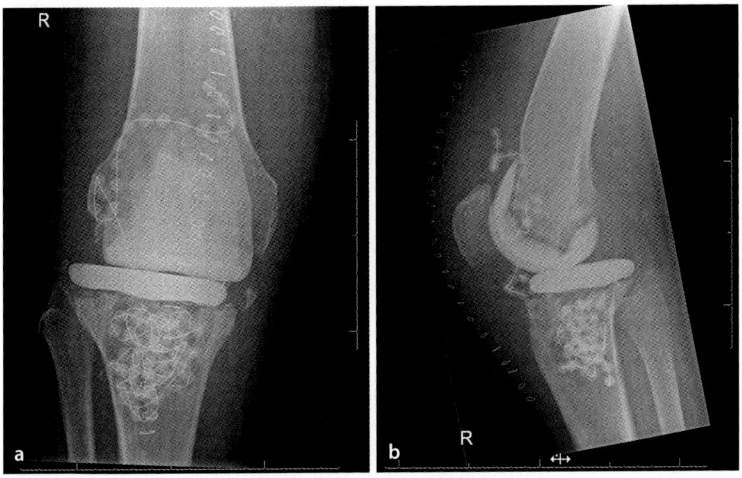

Fig. 6.53 **a, b** Spacer and gentamicin PMMA beads for local antibiotic treatment

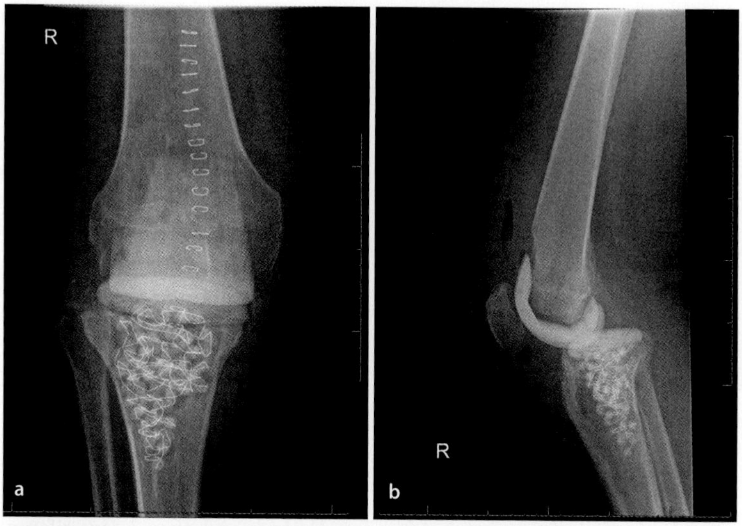

Fig. 6.54 a, b Situation after renewal of both the spacer and the gentamicin PMMA beads

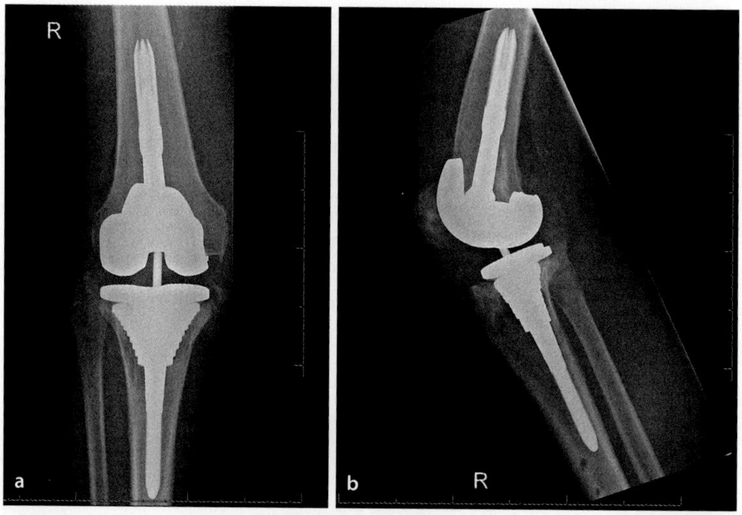

Fig. 6.55 a, b X-ray showing TKP with stem extensions and augments

6.7.10 Case 3

In 2012, a 71-year-old male patient was referred to our department with a persistent PJI of the TKA in his left knee, which was implanted in 2010. Furthermore, he had psoriasis and was morbidly obese. After his index operation in 2010 there had been no problems with wound healing (Fig. 6.58).

In August 2012, he presented with a red, tender, and swollen knee which was treated with only i.v. antibiotics at his initial hospital. This resulted in only short-term improvement, with aggravated symptoms soon after the antibiotics were stopped, leading to pulmonary insufficiency and admission to the IC unit. Laboratory tests showed an ESR of 86 mm/h, leukocytes of 8.1 10^3/µg/l and a CRP level of 37 mg/l. *Proteus mirabilis*, *Escherichia coli* and *Enterococcus faecalis* were identified via an arthrocentesis. A bone scan showed signs of loosening or infection. In October

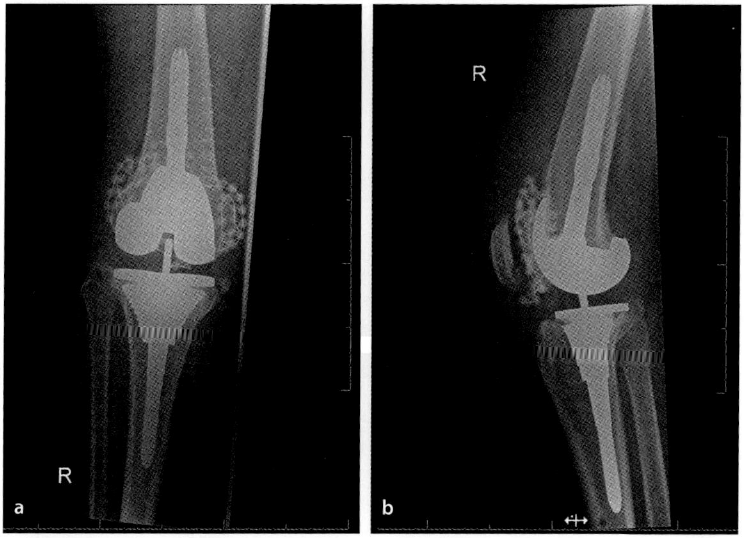

Fig. 6.56 a, b Renewed DAIR with retained revision TKP

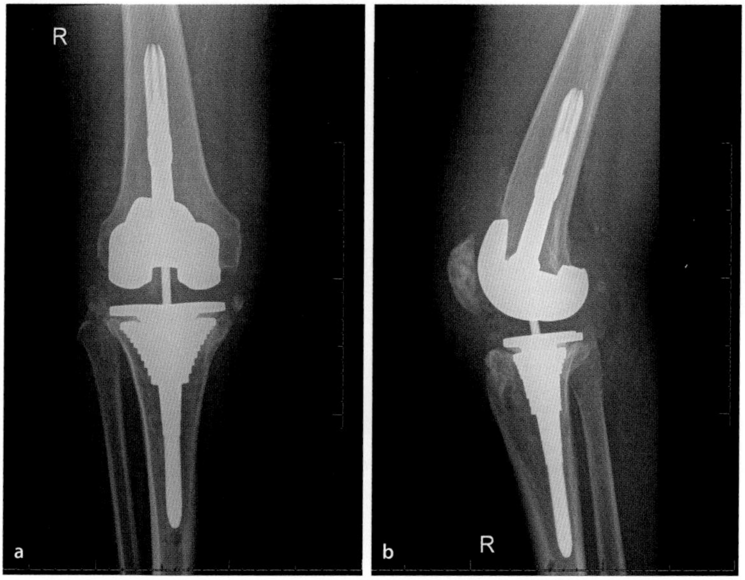

Fig. 6.57 a, b No signs of infection, no osteolysis, no periosteal reaction

2012 he was referred to our hospital and underwent surgery.

The operation (no. I) consisted of extraction of the knee prosthesis, taking of deep cultures, thorough debridement with 6 l NaCl 0.9%, and leaving gentamicin PMMA beads intra-articularly (Fig. 6.59). Treatment with i.v. flucloxacillin was started.

The gentamicin PMMA beads were removed 2 weeks later and a Palacos® R+G spacer was introduced (operation II). Flucloxacillin was continued for 6 weeks i.v. followed by clindamycin given orally for 6 weeks. Laboratory results improved dramatically (ESR, 24 mm/h; CRP, 11 mg/l; leukocytes, 7.8 $10^3/\mu g/l$; Fig. 6.60).

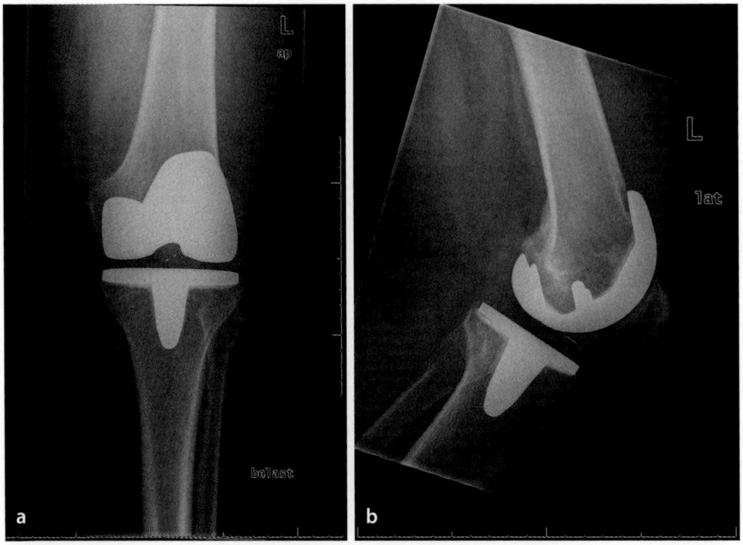

■ **Fig. 6.58 a, b** X-rays showing situation following initial total knee replacement

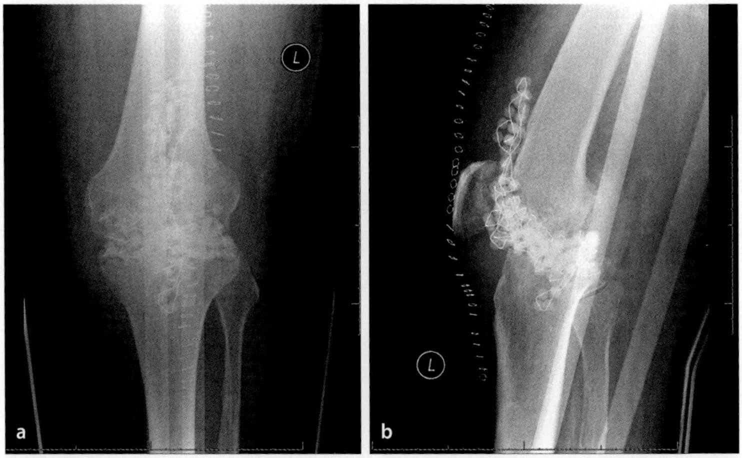

■ **Fig. 6.59 a, b** X-rays after extraction of TKP, debridement and gentamicin PMMA beads for optimal local antibiotic treatment

Because of other health problems and after an antibiotic-free interval, a revision TKA was implanted in May 2013, with the normal 24-h antibiotic prophylaxis (operation III). Wound healing was uneventfull (■ Fig. 6.61).

However, in November 2013 he had to be re-admitted to hospital for clinical deterioration with elevated infection parameters; ESR, 68 mm/h, CRP, 106 mg/l; leukocytes, 11.4 10^3/µg/l. Because earlier cultures had shown coagulase-negative staphylococci (CNS), the patient was treated with vancomycin i.v., and after a few days rifampicin was added. This last antibiotic had to be interrupted because of liver failure, but vancomycin could be continued for 6 weeks. CRP levels improved to 16 mg/l.

In June 2014, the patient had to be admitted again for 1 week owing to worsening of symptoms. Because of his personal wish, it was agreed to leave the implant in situ and only treat him with antibiotics again. Flucloxacillin i.v. was started and was continued ambulatory for 6 weeks again.

Nevertheless, the patient was unable to become symptom free and pain free, and because of recur-

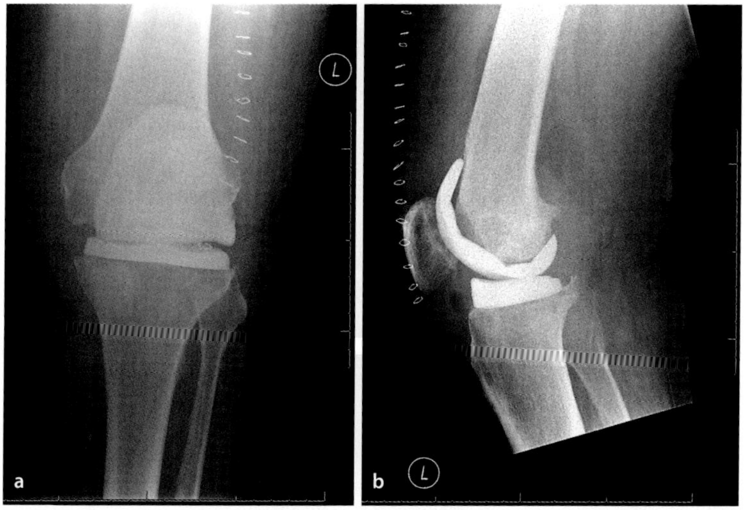

Fig. 6.60 a, b After 2 weeks the gentamicin PMMA beads were replaced by an antibiotic spacer

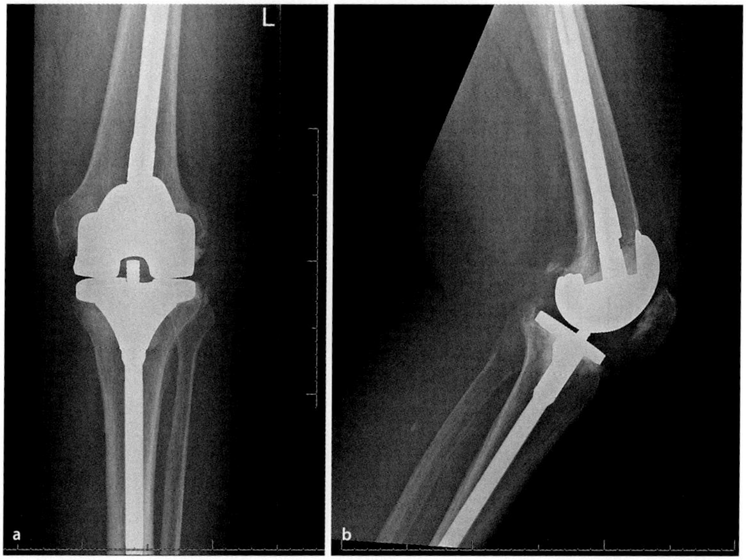

Fig. 6.61 a, b Situation after re-implantation of a revision TKP

rent infections which were resistant to several debridements, to an earlier extraction and to i.v. antibiotic treatments, and because of several disabling comorbidities, it was decided to extract the TKA and perform an arthrodesis (operation IV, October 2014; Fig. 6.62).

Cultures taken during the surgery showed CNS and *Proteus mirabilis* infection, and i.v. treatment consisted of vancomycin and amoxicillin, which was continued orally after 2 weeks.

In March 2015 a delayed union was diagnosed with severe bone defect on CT (Fig. 6.63).

Therefore, a conversion to intramedullary fixation was done with treatment of the bone defect with bone graft harvested from the contralateral femur using RIA (reaming with irrigation and aspiration) combined with bioglass (operation V; Fig. 6.64).

Post-operatively, vancomycin and rifampicin were continued intravenously for 6 weeks. ESR

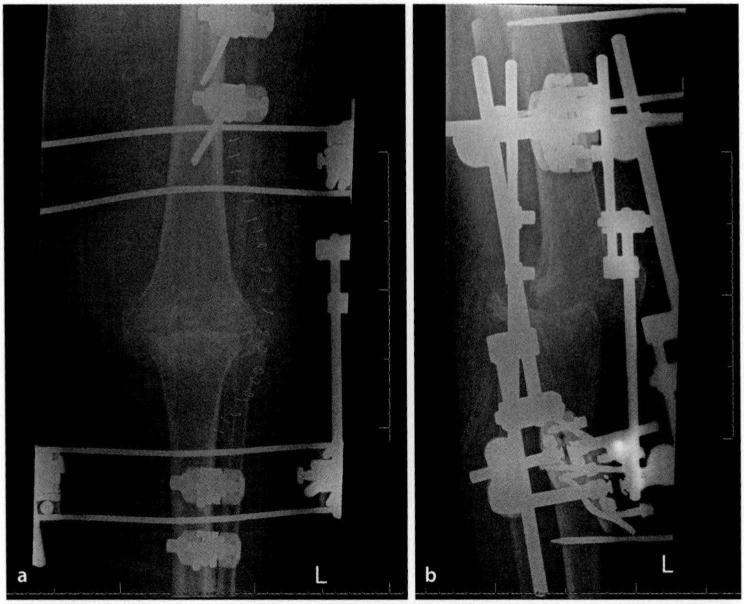

■ **Fig. 6.62 a, b** X-ray after extraction of the TKP and conversion to arthrodesis of the knee using an external fixator

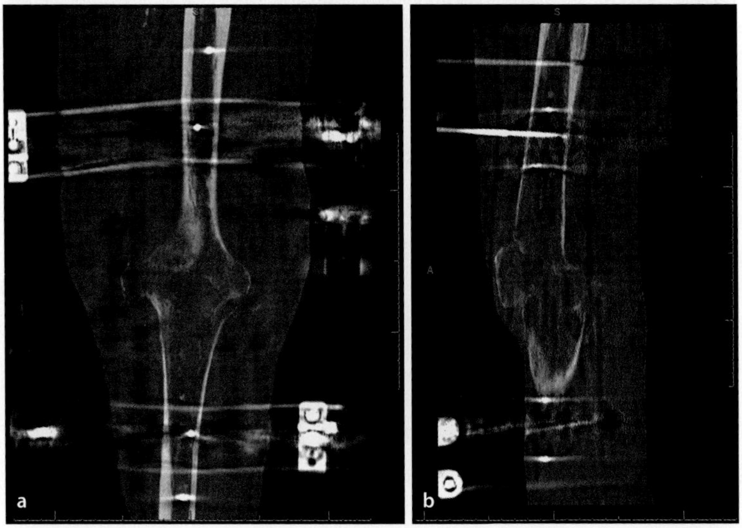

■ **Fig. 6.63 a, b** X-rays showing bone loss and delayed union of the knee arthrodesis

(36 mm/h) and CRP levels (1 mg/l) normalized almost entirely and radiographically a good fusion was accomplished. No further signs of infection were seen during further follow-up. Nevertheless, the patient kept complaining of pain on weight-bearing, which is a common result after so many surgical interventions.

6.7.11 Case 4

During the past 10 years, we have gradually adapted our policy for cases of PJIs from performing a three-stage procedure (using initially gentamicin or vancomycin beads, followed by an antibiotic-loaded spacer and subsequently prosthesis

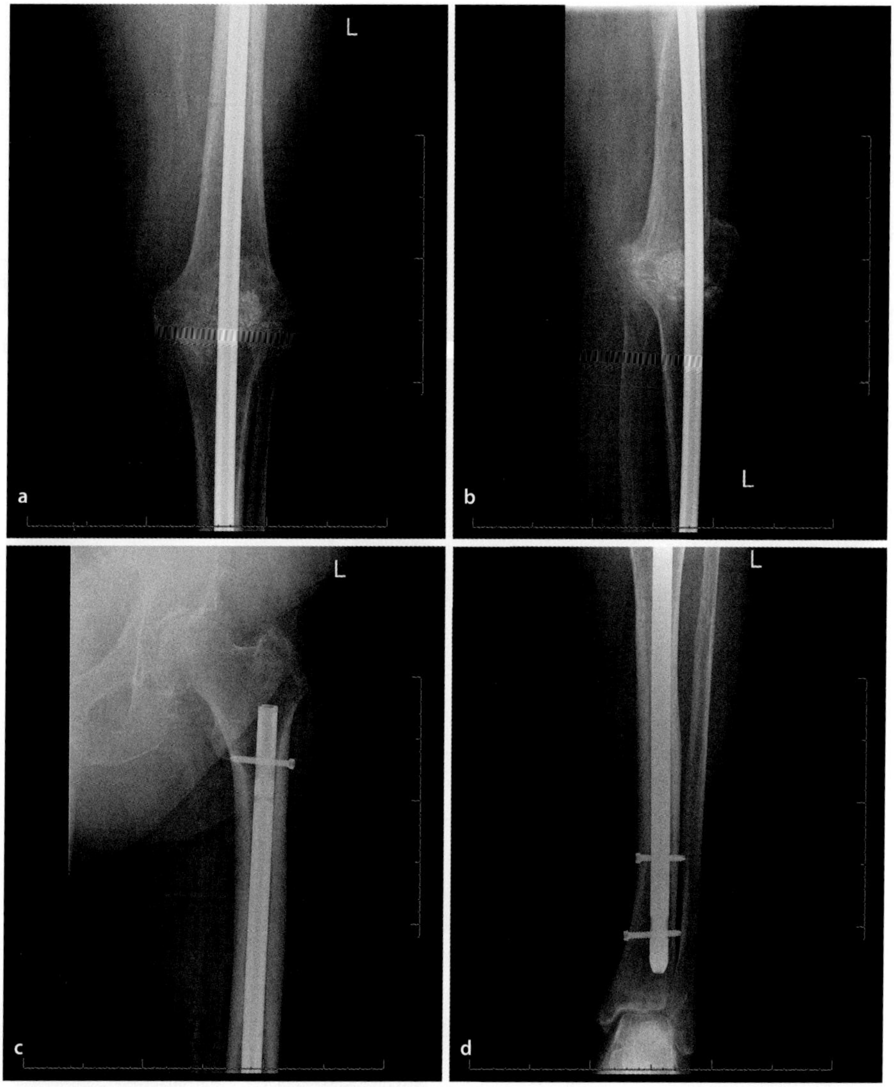

■ **Fig. 6.64 a–d** Union of the knee arthrodesis after bone grafting and compression intramedullary nailing

re-implantation) to a two-stage procedure using either beads or a spacer as the first step to final re-implantation. For bridging the period without a THP with a spacer, we choose a short interval (6–8 weeks) or a long one (several months). Depending on the case (first infection or recurrent infection), an antibiotic-free interval is preferred or antibiotics are continued until re-implantation. Here, we offer a few examples to illustrate the steps and underlying motivation of these procedures.

The first example is a 72-year-old woman who had undergone surgery of her left hip at a different hospital, and which had been revised a few years later because of »aseptic loosening of the cup«. At that time, no cultures were taken and the acetabular bone loss was filled with Tutoplast (■ Fig. 6.65). Soon afterwards, however, this cup also migrated and renewed arthrocentesis did not reveal any micro-organism (■ Fig. 6.66).

At that stage the patient was referred to our hospital and it was decided to extract both components

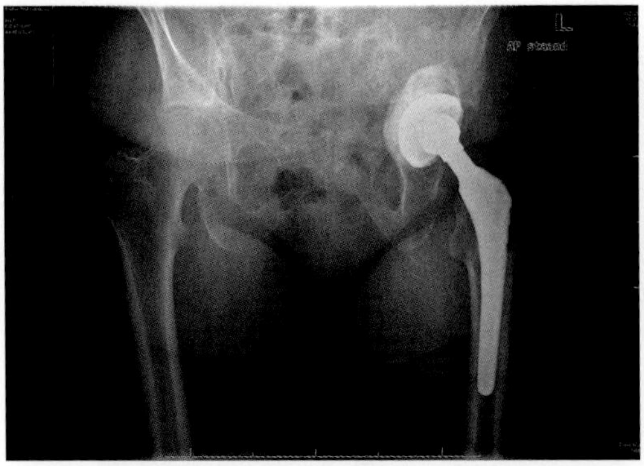

Fig. 6.65 Revised cup and acetabular bone loss filled with Tutoplast

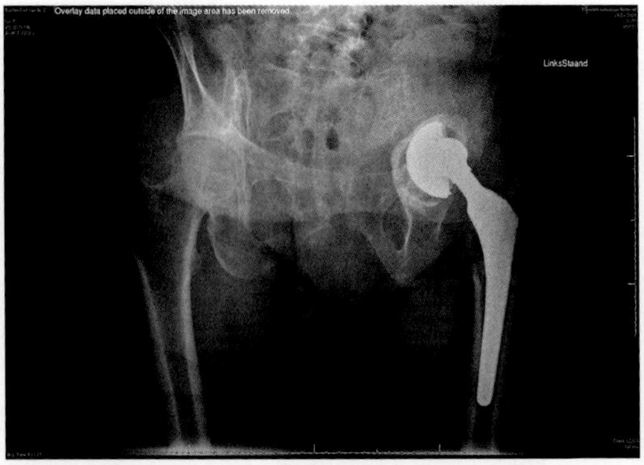

Fig. 6.66 Renewed cup loosening with migration of the implant

6

of the prosthesis as well as the Tutoplast. This was done in January 2009. Intraoperative cultures of the interface and soft tissues all showed *Proprionibacterium acnes* for which treatment with intravenous penicillin was started (6×1 g) in combination with local antibiotics in the form of gentamicin PMMA beads (Fig. 6.67). Our second operation (February 2009) consisted of removing the beads and leaving a vancomycin-loaded cement ball in the acetabulum (Fig. 6.68), because the medial wall was initially considered too vulnerable and prone to central protrusion of a conventional spacer. The third operation followed 2 weeks later during which the cement ball was, nevertheless, replaced by a second-generation vancomycin-loaded spacer (high sensitivity of the bacteria to vancomycin) for a longer interval (Fig. 6.69). She was discharged from hospital on oral clindamycin for 6 weeks (4×600 mg).

In July 2009 after an antibiotic-free interval of almost 3 months her laboratory test results had returned to almost normal values (ESR, 33 mm/h, CRP, 3 mg/l, leukocytes, 6.3 $10^3/\mu g/l$) and cultures of joint aspirates were negative. In August we therefore re-implanted a THP with bone impaction grafting of the central cavitary acetabular defect and a cemented cup. An uncemented HA-coated revision stem was used on the femoral side (Fig. 6.70). She healed without further signs of infection and the most recent X-ray at the 7-year follow-up showed a nice remodelling of the graft and no signs of recurrent infection (Fig. 6.71).

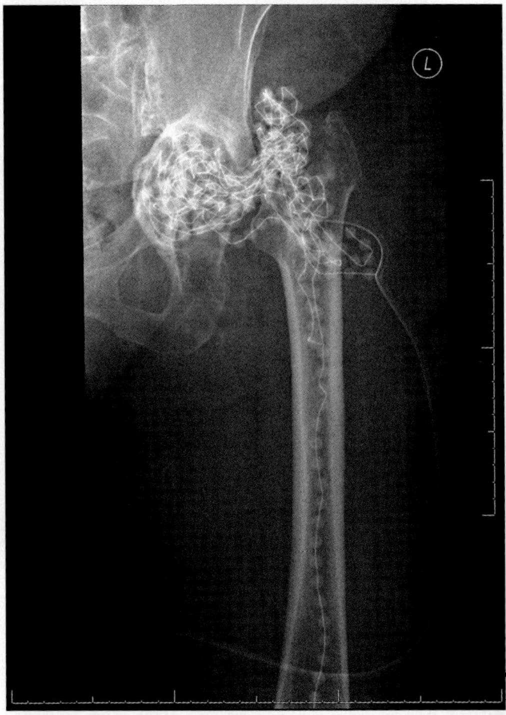

Fig. 6.67 After removal of the cup and Tutoplast and local antibiotic treatment with beads

6.7.12 Case 5

Another example of a three-stage solution is the case of a 50-year-old male patient who was treated with three cannulated screws for an intracapsular fracture of the right hip (operation I, 2006;

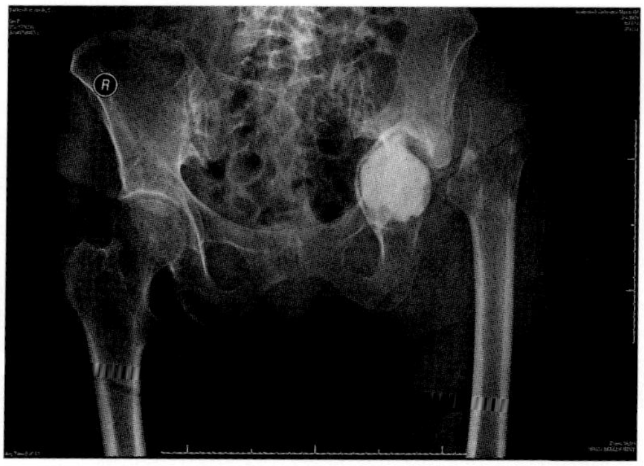

Fig. 6.68 Situation after placement of temporary antibiotic-loaded cement ball

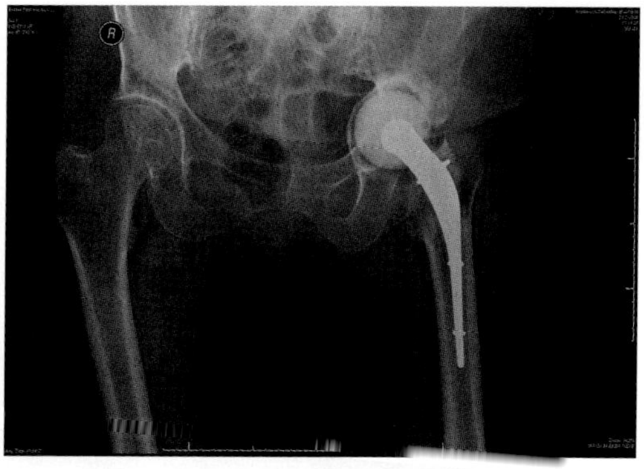

Fig. 6.69 Situation after placement of spacer

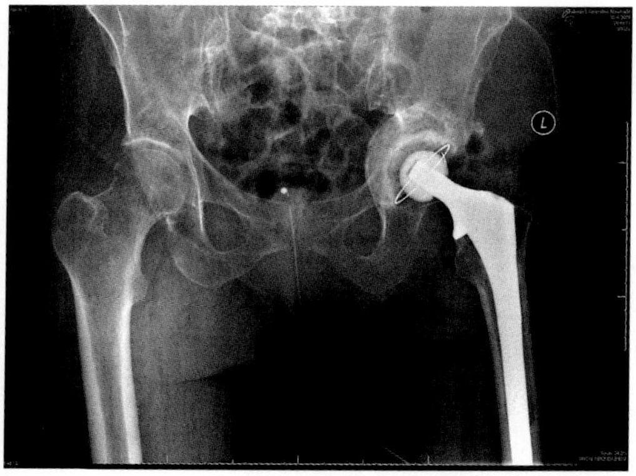

Fig. 6.70 After extensive acetabular antibiotic-loaded bone grafting and cemented cup with uncemented revision stem

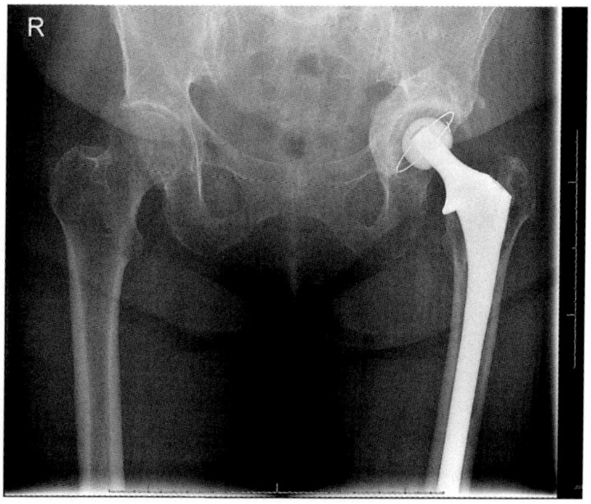

Fig. 6.71 X-ray at the 7-year follow-up

Fig. 6.72). Possibly due to an incorrect indication (Pauwels III) and reduction, combined with a non-compliant patient with alcohol abuse, an early collapse of the fracture followed (Fig. 6.73), and was succeeded by a conversion to a cemented THA (operation II, September 2006; Fig. 6.74). Cultures taken during this surgery later showed *Pseudomonas aeruginosa*, which was treated with piperacillin.

The patient showed persistent wound drainage post-operatively beyond 10 days. Therefore, a debridement was performed (operation III, Oct 2006) during which the femoral component appeared to be loose and was removed, including the cement mantle and cup. Cultures were again taken and gentamicin PMMA beads were inserted. These cultures showed *Enterobacter cloacae* and a *Stenotrophomas (Xanthomonas) maltophilia*, for which co-trimoxazole was given (Fig. 6.75).

Because of persistent high infection parameters, we exchanged the beads every 2 weeks, in order to apply renewed levels of local antibiotics until clinical parameters showed clear improvement. In this case this was done twice (operations IV and V), further followed by the introduction of a spacer (operation VI, November 2006; Fig. 6.76). Cultures still showed *Pseudomonas aeruginosa* and Corynebacterium, only sensitive to vancomycin. This was administered intravenously for 2 weeks. When the clinical situation improved with progressive

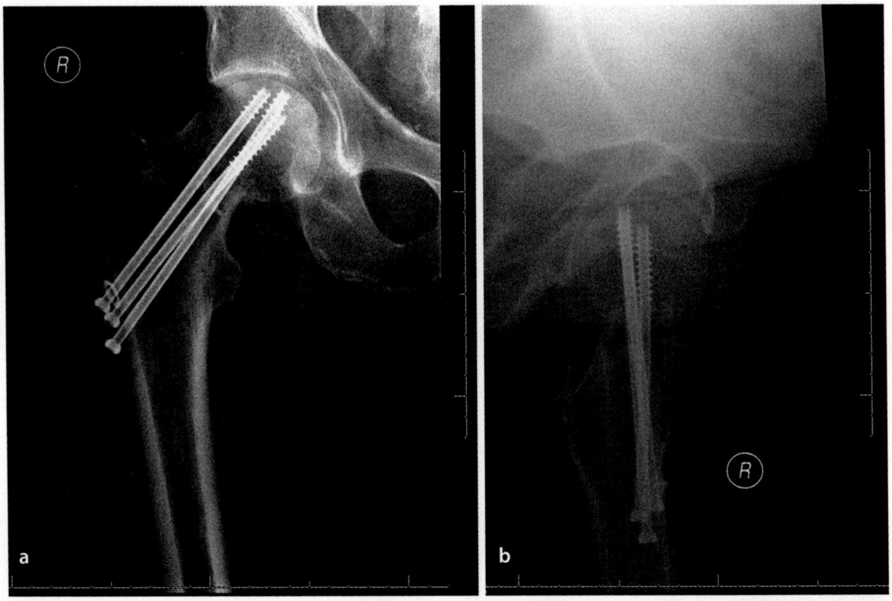

■ **Fig. 6.72 a, b** Three cannulated screws for an intracapsular hip fracture in a young male patient

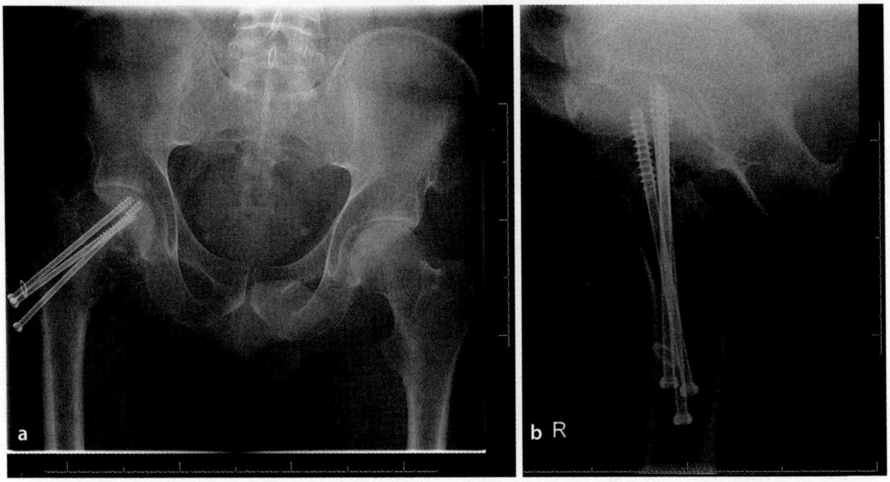

■ **Fig. 6.73 a, b** Pressive collapse of the fracture with non-union

wound healing and normalization of the laboratory parameters, antibiotics could be continued orally with doxycycline. After 3 months, the spacer appeared to be broken (a frequent occurrence with first-generation spacers; ■ Fig. 6.77). Antibiotics, which in those days were still given for 3 months also after removal of all implants, were stopped and subsequent cultures after arthrocentesis were negative. Laboratory tests now showed an ESR of 3 mm/h and a CRP level of 2 mg/l. In April 2007 the broken spacer was removed and re-implantation of a non-cemented THA was performed (operation VII; ■ Fig. 6.78).

Cultures from this last operation now showed CNS, sensitive to only vancomycin and rifampicin. Because the patient again suffered from compro-

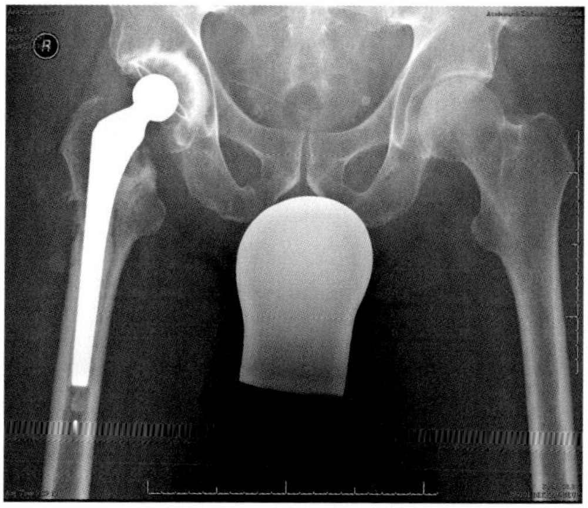

Fig. 6.74 X-ray after conversion to a cemented THP

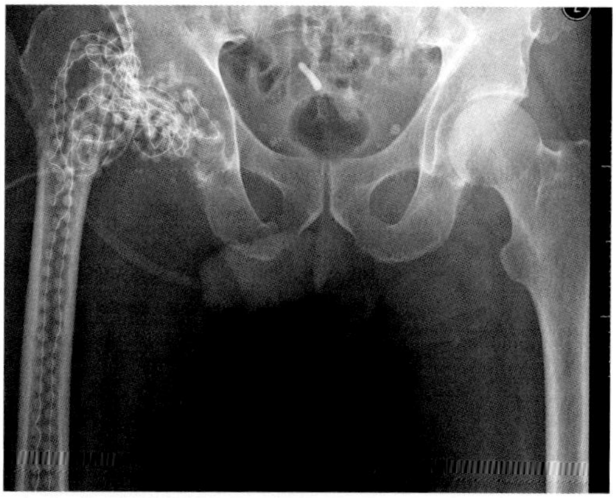

Fig. 6.75 Early removal of the THP and cement leaving beads for local antibiotic treatment

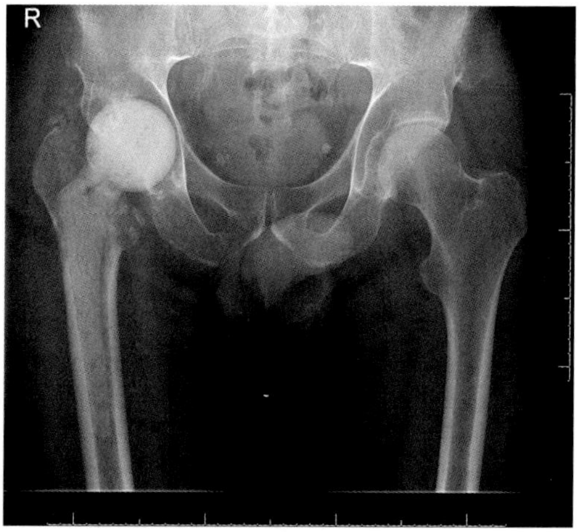

Fig. 6.76 First-generation spacer implanted after two 2-week periods of beads

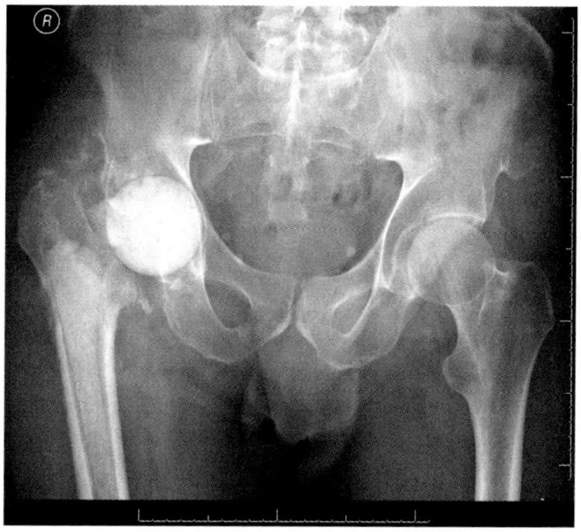

Fig. 6.77 Broken spacer

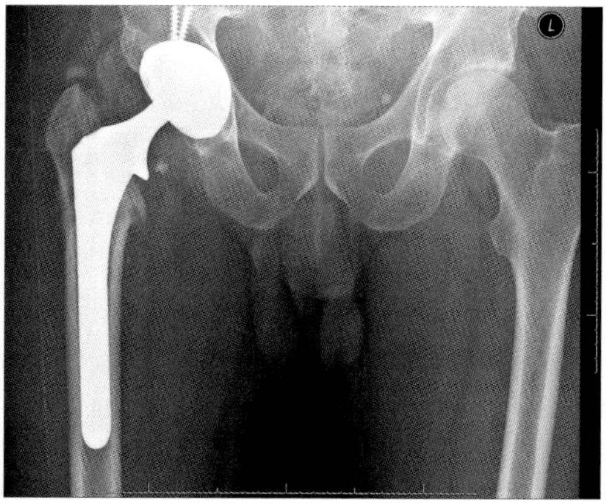

Fig. 6.78 Re-implantation of an uncemented THP after healing of the infection

mised wound healing with dehiscence, another DAIR had to be performed after 10 days (operation VIII). Systematic antibiotics were once more repeated intravenously for 2 weeks (vancomycin + rifampicin), and continued orally for another 4 weeks (linezolid and rifampicin). After that, wound healing ensued without further complications. Since this protracted history, no further infection of the hip occurred, although the mobility of the patient remained limited because of persistent muscular inefficiency.

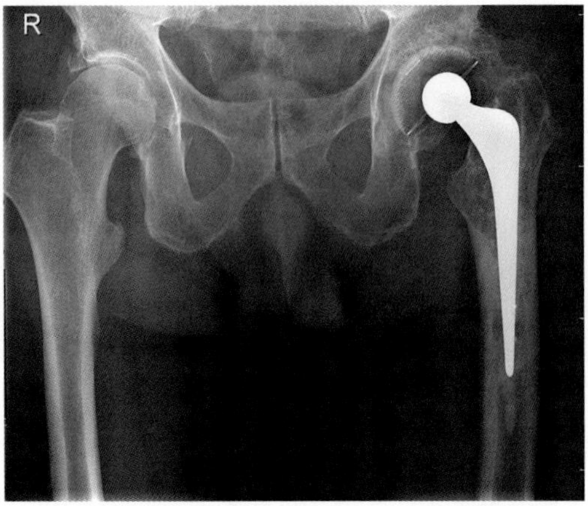

Fig. 6.79 Femoral bone showing endosteal cavitation and periosteal reactions

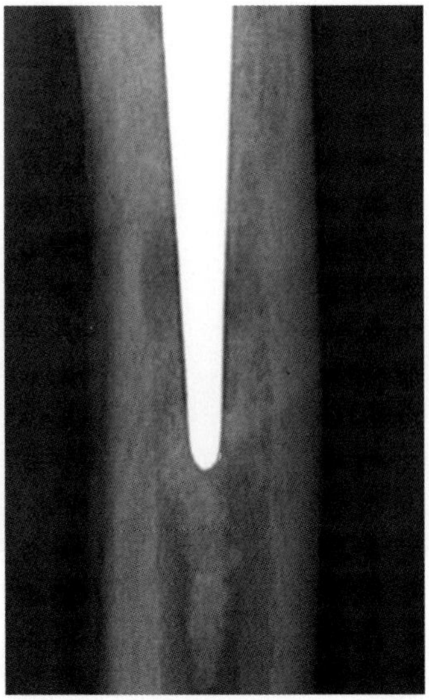

Fig. 6.80 Detail of Fig. 6.79

6.7.13 Case 6

Case 6 is an example of a two-stage revision, with a short interval, of a 75-year-old male patient who was seen in our hospital in 2006 with lateral hip pain on the left side. He had a THP in 1998 at a nearby hospital, which had to be revised in 2000 because of loosening of the stem. There was no information on the possible micro-organisms involved. After the revision in 2000, there was compromised wound healing with dehiscence and early deep infection which had to be treated with two debridements. Once again, there were no results of the cultures available.

In 2006 the patients complained of pain with limited range of motion but without any fever, shivers, general illness or other signs of infection. X-rays showed osteolysis both proximally and distally, with radiolucent endosteal cavitation and periosteal reactions (Fig. 6.79 and Fig. 6.80).

CRP levels and ESR were high, but cultures taken from hip aspirates were negative. Arthrography did not show contrast medium at the implant–cement or cement–bone interfaces. Therefore, scintigraphy was performed, which showed elevated uptake at the osteolytic area around the distal stem (Fig. 6.81). Although there was no conclusive evidence of sepsis we decided to remove the prosthesis because of high suspicion for a low grade infection.

In June 2007 we extracted the THP, took several cultures of the synovial fluid, the capsule and the interfaces and introduced gentamicin PMMA beads (Fig. 6.82). Results showed one positive (of six) cultures for CNS, indicating probable contamination.

Because there was uneventful wound healing and laboratory results returned to normal within 2 weeks, it was considered safe to re-implant a THP after 3 weeks with normal perioperative antibiotic prophylaxis (Fig. 6.83). After 8 years of follow-up, the hip functions well and there have not been any signs of recurrent infection (Fig. 6.84).

6.7.14 Case 7

This final case is an example of a two-stage revision with a short interval using a third-generation spacer, which allows for independent sizing of both the stem and head component, and the possibility to use sleeves for adaptation of the neck length. The patient was a 70-year-old man with a history of low back pain and spinal surgery. In 2014 he had undergone THA of the right hip in another hospital. After 6 weeks, pain in the hip recurred, particularly in the groin. Analysis in the initial hospital consisted of laboratory investigations (normal results), conven-

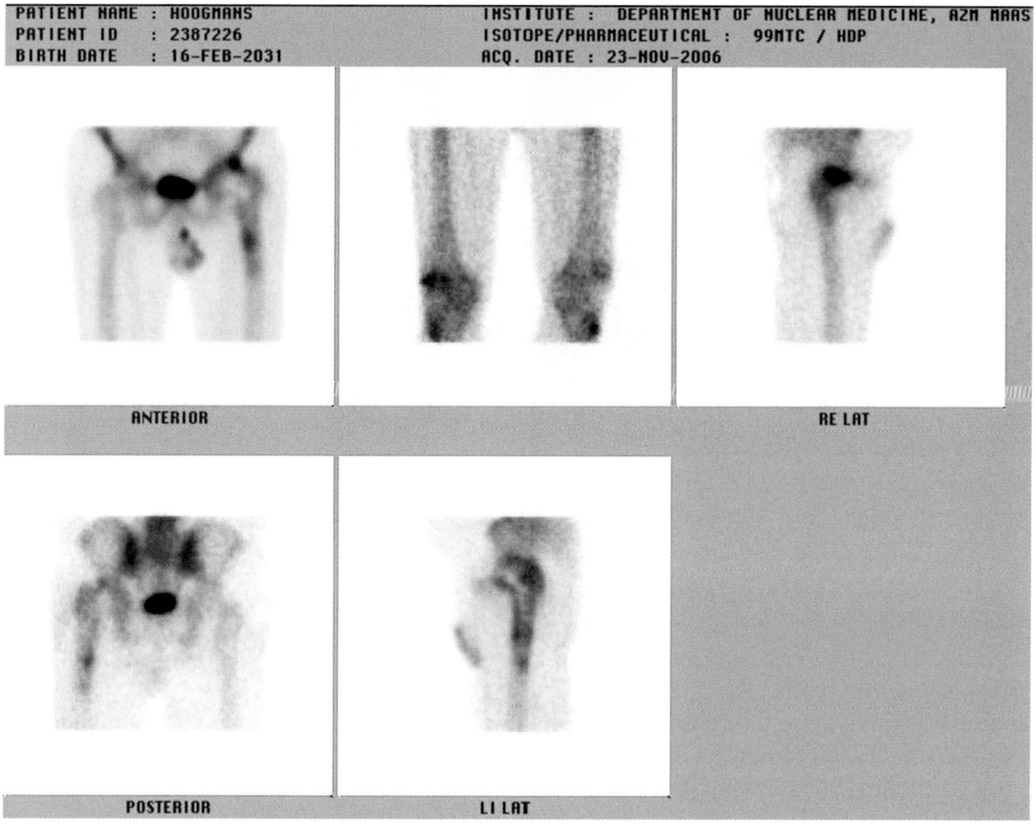

Fig. 6.81 Elevated femoral tracer uptake suggestive of infection

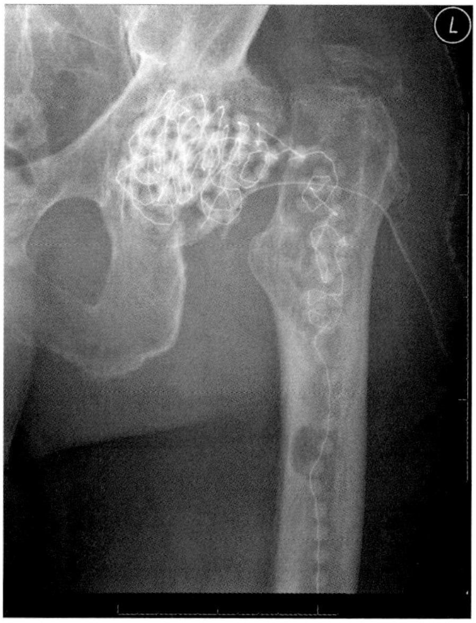

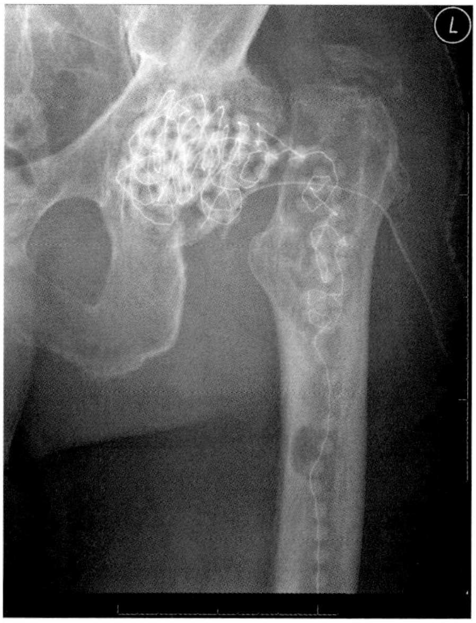

Fig. 6.82 After removal of the THP and cement, with debridement, leaving gentamicin PMMA beads

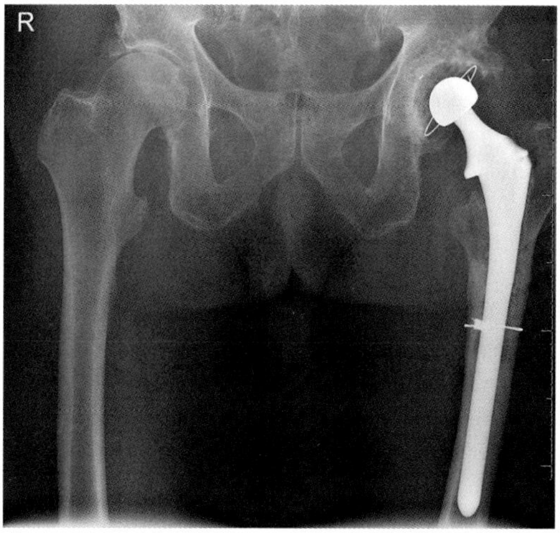

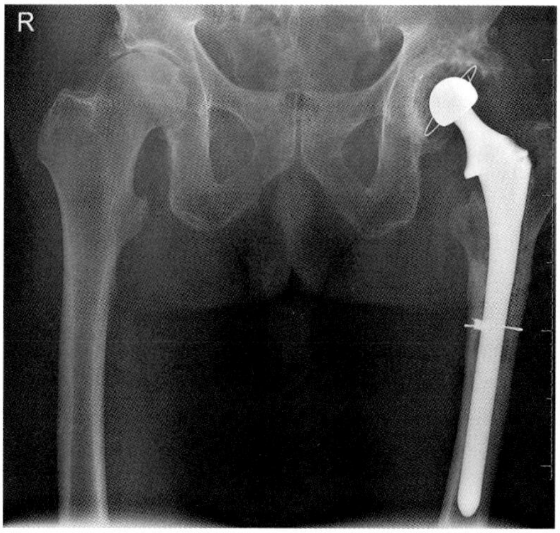

Fig. 6.83 X-rays after early re-implantation

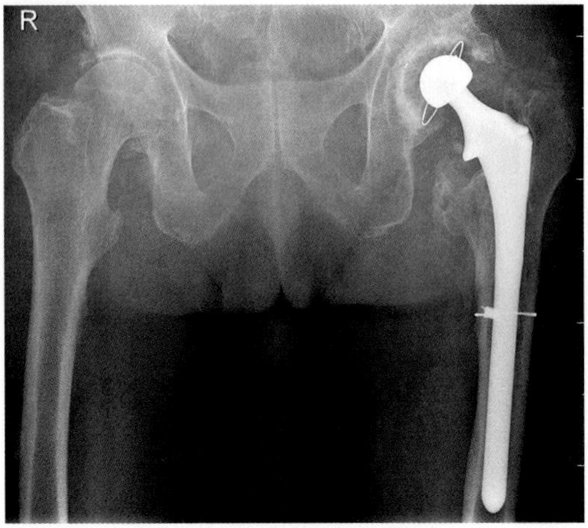

■ **Fig. 6.84** After 8-year follow-up

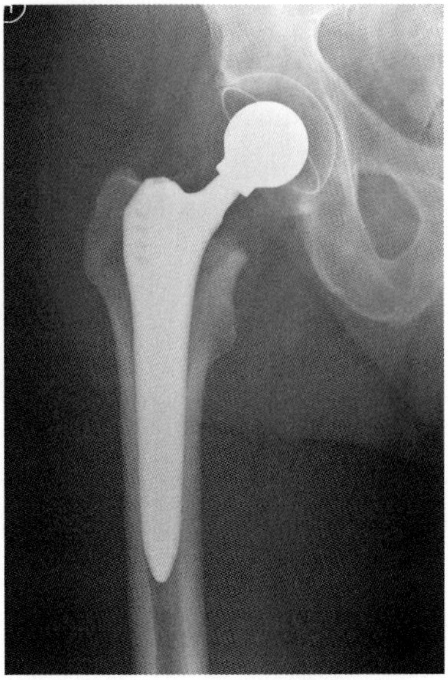

■ **Fig. 6.85** X-rays showing no signs of periprosthetic infection

tional radiography (normal findings), sonography (no inguinal hernia and no psoas impingement) and CT (no abnormalities). Pain treatment by the anaesthetist had no effect. The patient received second and third opinions in other hospitals, which did not result in new insights or treatment options.

In December 2015 he visited our department. X-rays (■ Fig. 6.85) and laboratory test results were normal but an FDG-PET scan showed elevated uptake of the FDG tracer around the femoral component.

On the basis of these findings, we performed an arthrocentesis and took cultures that showed *Pseudomonas aeruginosa*. Late results of these cultures also revealed *Enterobacter cloacae*.

The case was therefore handled as a late infection and the patient was treated with a two-stage revision using a spacer. In January 2015, the THP was removed through an extended trochanteric osteotomy and after cultures and thorough debridement, a spacer was inserted (■ Fig. 6.86). The patient was treated systemically with piperacillin + tazobactam.

Subsequently, laboratory results normalized within 2 weeks. Intraoperative cultures now revealed CNS which, however, was considered contamination by the microbiology department (one of six cultures positive). After 3 weeks, the patient was operated on again and a non-cemented THP was inserted (■ Fig. 6.87). Cultures taken during this intervention were all negative and laboratory parameters all returned to normal values within a short interval (CRP from 165 to 6 mg/l, ESR from 74 to 5 mm/h and leukocytes from 11.1 to 7.2 $10^3/\mu g/l$). Nevertheless, the patient kept complaining of severe pains in spite of a considerable amount of pain medication.

6.7.15 Conclusion

During the past decade, the protocol for the treatment of PJIs in the Netherlands has changed considerably. The reports in this chapter and the clinical cases presented here are a reflection of this evolution. Although the use of gentamicin or vancomycin beads has not been abolished, there is a trend toward earlier use of spacers even though their antibiotic effect is not considered as effective as that of beads. There still remain several other controversies as well in this field of orthopaedics, for example the choice of cemented versus uncemented reconstructions, even in cases of one-stage exchange. Furthermore the way how to mix additional antibiotics in the cement with the goal to enhance antibiotic release is to be established from future release studies. Also the choice and length of a antibiotic holiday

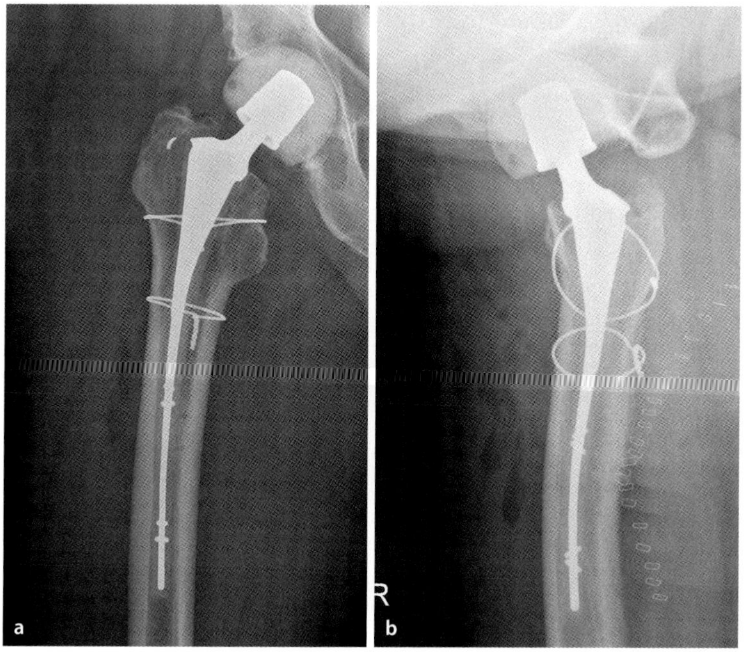

Fig. 6.86 a, b Modular spacer in situ with cerclage wiring for closure of the extended trochanteric osteotomy

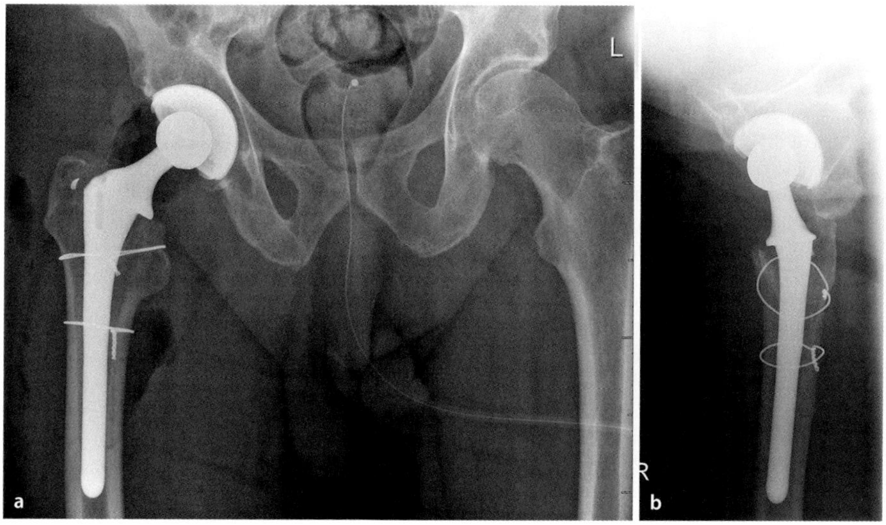

Fig. 6.87 a, b X-rays after two-stage revision with early re-implantation of an uncemented THP

before prosthesis re-implantation in a two-stage setting has to be determined. Finally the choice and length of antibiotic suppressive treatment is also still under debate.

In recent meetings of the European Bone and Joint Infection Society (EBJIS) and in the current literature, it has become clear that this is an ongoing process that has not yet come to an end. Particularly new tools and biomarkers for early and better diagnosis will further influence decision-making in this complex area of orthopaedics.

Take-Home Message

- The strategies for treating PJI are: DAIR, one-stage revision, two-stage revision with (or without) local antibiotics, definitive explantation, arthrodesis or amputation, suppressive antibiotic treatment (lifelong).
- The antibiotic therapy must also be focussed on treatment of the biofilm (one-stage).
- The preoperative identification of the causal micro-organism is a prerequisite for administration of adequate antibiotics, both locally in the bone cement as well as systemically (two-stage).
- Dependent on the condition of the bone and soft tissues, as well as on the status of the patient and existing co-morbidities, in particular circumstances the best choice may be a definitive extraction of the prosthesis creating a persistent Girdlestone of the hip. In the case of a failed knee prosthesis the exarticulation may result in an arthrodesis or an exarticulation or amputation.
- The indications for the different treatment protocols of PJIs provide a rational and effective algorithm for dealing with infections of orthopaedic implants.

References

Azzam KA, Seeley M, Ghanem E, Austin MS, Purtill JJ, Parvizi J (2010) Irrigation and debridement in the manegement of prosthetic joint infection: traditional indications revisited. J Arthroplasty 25:1022–1027

Callaghan JJ, Katz RP, Johnston RC (1999) One-stage revision surgery of the infected hip. A minimum 10-year followup study. Clin Orthop Relat Res 369:139–143

Deirmengian C, Greenbaum J, Lotke PA, Booth Re, Lonner JH (2003) Limited success with open debridement and retention of components in the treatment of acute Staphylococcus Aureus infections after Total knee arthroplasty. J Arthroplasty 18:22–26

Gehrke T, Zahar A, Kendoff D (2013) One-stage exchange. It all began here. BJJ 95B[Suppl A]:77–83

Geurts JA, Janssen DM, Kessels AG, Walenkamp GH (2013) Good results in postoperative and hematogenous deep infections of 89 stable total hip and knee replacements with retention of prosthesis and local antibiotics. Acta Orthop 84(6):509–516

Goulet JA, et al (1988) Prolonged suppressionof infection in total hip arthroplasty. J Arthroplasty 3(2):109–116

Hanssen AD, Osmon DR (2000) Assessment of patient selection criteria for treatment of the infected hip arthroplasty. Clin Orthop Relat Res 381:91–100

Hanssen AD, Spangehl MJ (2004) Practical applications of antibiotic-loaded bone cement for treatment of infected joint replacements. Clin Orthop Relat Res 427:79–85

Hartman MB, Fehring TK, Jordan L, Norton HJ (1991) Periprosthetic knee sepsis. The role of irrigation and debridement. Clin Orthop Relat Res 273:113–118

Koo KH, Yang JW, Cho SH, et al (2001) Impregnation of vancomycin, gentamicin, and cefotaxime in a cement spacer for two-stage cementless reconstruction in infected total hip arthroplasty. J Arthroplasty 16(7):882–892

Koyonos L, Zmistowski B, Della Valle CJ, Parvizi J (2011) Infection control of irrigation and debridement for periprosthetic joint infection. Clin Orthop Relat Res 469:3043–3048

Odum SM, Fehring TK, Lombardi AV, et al (2011) Irrigation and debridement for periprosthetic infections: does the organism matter? J Arthroplasty 26: 114–118

Osmon DR, et al (2013) Diagnosis and management of prosthetic joint infection: clinical practice guidelines by the infectious diseases society of America. Clin Inf Dis 56(1):e1–25

Oussedik SI, Dodd MB, Haddad FS (2010) Outcomes of revision Total hip replacement for infection after grading according to a standard protocol. J Bone Joint Surg (Br) 92(9):1222–1226

Parvizi J, Zmistowski B, Adeli B (2010) Periprosthetic joint infection: tretament options. Orthopedics 33(9):659

Parvizi J, Gehrke T (2013) Proceedings of the international consensus meeting on periprosthetic joint infection. ISBN 978-1-57400-147-1

Pitto RP, Spika IA (2004) Antibiotic-loaded bone cement spacers in two-stage management of infected total knee arthroplasty. Int Orthop 28(3):129–133

Rao N, Crossett LS, Sinha RK. Le Frock JL (2003) Long-term suppression of infection in total joint arthroplasty. Clin Orthop Relat Res 414:55–60

Segawa H, Tsukatama DT, Kyle RF, Becker DA, Gustillo RB (1999) Infection after total knee arthroplasty. A retrospective study of the treatment of eightly-one infections. J Bone Joint Surg [Am] 81(10):1434–1445

Segreti J, Nelson JA, Trenholme GM (1998) Prolonged suppressive antibiotic therapy for infected orthopedic prosthesis. Clin Infct Dis 27:711–713

Singer J, Merz A, Frommelt L, Fink B (2012) High rates of infection control with one-stage revision of septic knee protheses excluding MRSA and MRSE. Clin Orthop Relat Res 470(5):1461–1471

Ure KJ, Amstutz HC, Nasser S, Schmalzried TP (1998) Direct-exchange arthroplasty for the treatment of infection after total hip replacement. An average ten-year follow-up. J Bone Joint Surg [Am] 80(7):961–968

Tsukayama DT, Estrada R, Gustillo RB (1996) Infection after total hip arthroplasty. A study of the treatment of one

hubdred and six infections. J Bone Joint Surg [Am] 78(4):512–523
Witsø E, Persen L, Løseth K, Bergh K (1999) Adsorption and release of antibiotics from morselized cancellous bone. In vitro studies of 8 antibiotics. Acta Orthop Scand 70(3):298–304
Working Group Orthopedic Infections of the Dutch Orthopedic Society (2015) Aanbeveling werkwijze behandeling prothese infecties orthopedie. Retrieved from www.ortrhopeden.org
Zimmerli W, Trampuz A, Ochsner P (2004) Prosthetic joint infections. N Engl J Med 351(16):1645–1654

Antibiotic-Loaded Bone Cement

K.-D. Kühn (Ed.), *Management of Periprosthetic Joint Infection*
DOI 10.1007/978-3-662-54469-3_7

7.1 Benefit and Risks of Antibiotic-Loaded Bone Cements

Pablo Sanz-Ruiz, Manuel Villanueva-Martínez, and Christoph Berberich

7.1.1 Introduction

Since the past mid-century, surgeons have started to look at the advantages of a local application of anti-infective substances aiming at a better infection prophylaxis and/or eradication of an already established infection in organs or tissues which are generally »difficult to access« for systemic antibiotics (AB). The bone and joint compartments belong to such restricted body compartments because of poor blood vascularization. In 1970, the German surgeon Buchholz (Buchholz and Engelbrecht 1970) first introduced the concept of antibiotic-loaded bone cement (ALBC) as prophylaxis and later for treatment of prosthetic joint infections. This is also reflected by the sharp increase in the number of corresponding scientific and clinical publications as well as patents regarding antibiotic-loaded polymethylmethacrylate (PMMA) over the time period 1970–2015 (see ◘ Fig. 7.1 and ◘ Fig. 7.2)

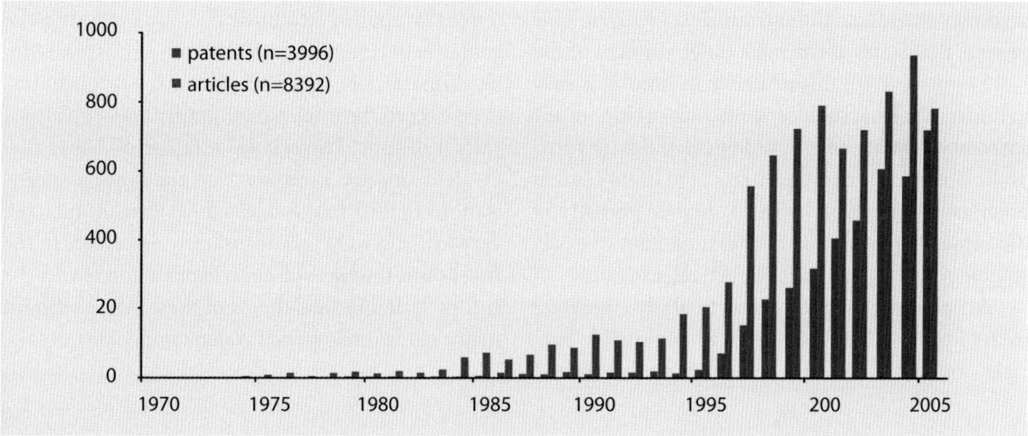

◘ **Fig. 7.1** Publications and patents on local anti-infective delivery systems since 1970 (Walenkamp 2007)

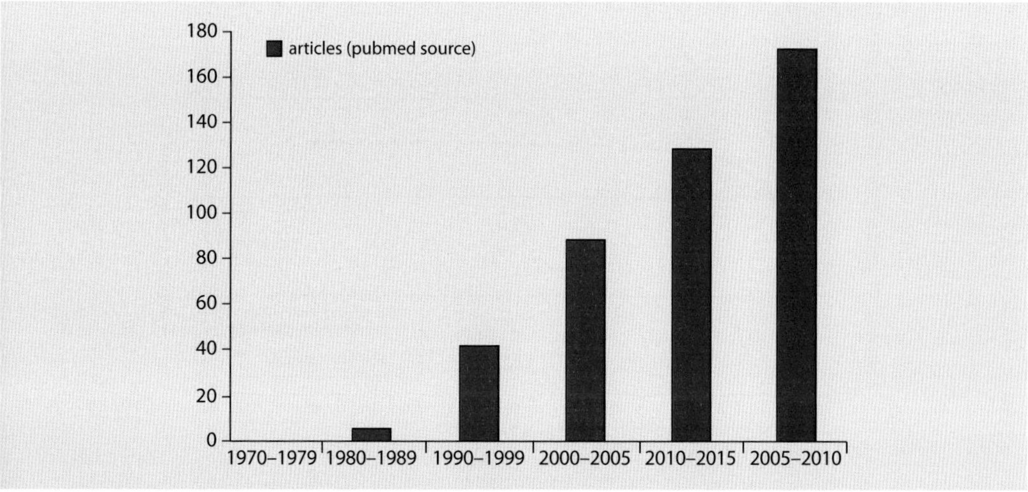

◘ **Fig. 7.2** Number of articles published in PubMed using the keywords »antibiotic loaded bone cement«

7.1.2 Mechanisms of Action of Antibiotic-Loaded Bone Cement

With our increasing knowledge on the pathomechanisms of implant-related bone and joint infections, it has become clear that the understanding of the elution mechanisms of AB out of PMMA is fundamental for the best patient- and germ-adapted use of ABLC.

The liberation process of the AB which is enclosed in the cured bone cement mantle follows essentially the law of reciprocal diffusion: In the same way in which body fluid (water) penetrates into the outer surfaces of the bone cement leading to a dissolution of the AB molecules, the AB are gradually eluted into the surrounding medium. This process first starts at the most outer surfaces of the bone cement. With this principle in mind it is easy to understand that such cements with (a) higher absorption capacity of physiological fluids (hydrophilic index) as a consequence of the bone cement polymer composition, with (b) higher porosity of the cement mantle and with (c) a content of easily soluble AB will show superior AB release rates.

A high elution capacity is particularly important in the first 24–72 h (◘ Fig. 7.3), when possible bacterial contaminants, host-derived granulocytes and fibroblasts compete to colonize the implant in the so-called race for the surface (Gristina 1987). As a general rule it can be stated that the higher the local concentration of a bactericidal AB, such as the aminoglycoside gentamicin, the better its decontaminating efficacy in case bacteria have seeded at the surgical site. After this initial peak release, AB elution continues over the following weeks and – at very low levels – even for years. The latter observation has prompted concerns that these very low AB concentrations may then favour the emergence of AB resistance if the bacteria have not been killed during the »high elution phase«.

As evidenced by studies comparing bone tissue concentrations of gentamicin from locally and systemically applied gentamicin or by analysing the gentamicin release from PMMA in a prosthesis-related interfacial gap model, the local AB concentrations exceed the minimal inhibitory concentrations (MIC) of most bacteria by a factor of 100–1,000 (Walenkamp 1983). By contrast, the serum concentrations of the PMMA-derived AB were found to be very low and were only transiently detectable in the first hours, thus providing an explanation of why the risk of systemic side effects of these AB is without major clinical relevance (Walenkamp 1983).

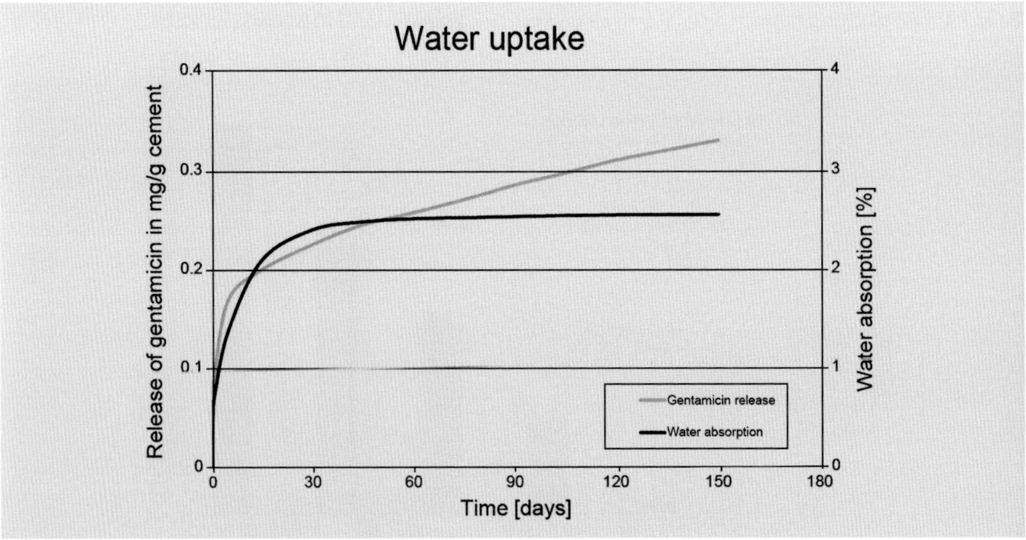

◘ **Fig. 7.3** Release of gentamicin from a high-viscous bone cement into phosphate buffer solution (mixture containing 0.5 g gentamicin per 40 g cement powder) (Kühn 2014)

Tab. 7.1 Overview of the basic physical, chemical and microbiological properties of AB required for their use in PMMA (Frommelt and Kühn 2005)

Physicochemical properties	Microbiological properties
Water solubility	Broad spectrum against Gram-negative and Gram-positive bacteria
Sterilizability via γ/EtO	Bactericidal
Thermostability	Low primary resistance rates
No chemical interference with PMMA	Low resistance induction rates (secondary resistance)
High elution from PMMA	Low interaction with proteins
Storage stability	Low allergic potential

7.1.3 Choice of Antibiotic

As important as the selection of the best bone cement matrix is the choice of the appropriate AB for successful clinical use of ALBC (Kühn et al. 2016). If adding an AB to PMMA, it must fulfil a series of basic physiochemical and microbiological requirements (see Tab. 7.1). As some of these necessary properties are often not predictable, recommendations have been issued on which AB can be added at which concentration to PMMA in line with its antimicrobial spectrum. These recommendations are also based on clinical experience derived from the analysis of arthroplasty registry data, clinical trials or case report studies (Hendrich and Frommelt 2005; Parvizi et al. 2013).

With these principles in mind it becomes apparent that the choice of an inappropriate AB may not only lead to failure of the local antibacterial strategy, but may also drastically affect the mechanical properties of the bone cement. In extreme cases, the AB–PMMA mixture may no longer be suitable for fixation of implants in orthopaedic surgery.

Another controversial issue is the concentration of AB which can be added to PMMA without affecting the mechanical strength of the mixture. When referring to the AB content, the percentage of AB is typically calculated for one pack of 40 g PMMA powder. Since the release of the AB is also positively correlated with the quantity added to cement, many surgeons argue in the case of acute or chronic infections to use a high-dose cement in order to further prolong the antimicrobial efficacy. From a mechanical point of view, the following statements can be made:

- In vitro study results cannot always be extrapolated to the in vivo situation, as the physiological medium additionally influences the mechanical properties (Sanz-Ruiz et al. 2014).
- Any additional ingredient leads in principle to a deterioration of the mechanical properties of PMMA. Therefore, the more of an antibiotic powder is added, the more pronounced the effect. Apart from the concentration, the type and chemical nature of the added AB also exert an important effect on the mixture (Sanz-Ruiz et al. 2014). As a general rule of thumb, only a limited or no clinically relevant effect on the mechanical properties below the American Society for Testing and Materials (ASTM) and the International Organization for Standardization (ISO) minimal technical standards for acrylic cements should be expected at a »threshold« of 2.5% AB load for most of the common AB used with ALBC (van de Belt et al. 2001; Hendriks et al. 2004).

A summary of the typical AB concentrations in PMMA in agreement with the aim of the clinical application is provided in Tab. 7.3.

The kinetics of elution of two or more AB from bone cement has also been extensively studied. The idea to add more than a single AB arose after the emergence of resistant bacteria and after the findings of a synergistic action of two or more AB broadening the anti-bacterial spectrum and often increasing the mutual elution from the cement matrix (Kühn 2014). As shown in Tab. 7.2, AB combinations in PMMA have become an increasingly common practice in septic revision surgery.

Tab. 7.2 Examples for options of AB combinations for preparation of ALBC in agreement with the pathogen susceptibility pattern (Frommelt and Kühn 2005)

Amount of AB per 40 g of cement powder	Bacteria
1 g Clindamycin + 1 g Gentamicin	*S. aureus/S. epidermidis*, Streptococci and Propionibacteria
3 g Cefuroxime + 1 g Gentamicin	*S. aureus/S. epidermidis*, Streptococci and Propionibacteria
2 g Vancomycin + 1 g Ofloxacin + 1 g Gentamicin	MRSA MRSE
2 g Vancomycin + 1 g Ampicillin+ 1 g Gentamicin	Enterococci
2 g Cefoperazone + 1 g Amikacin	*Pseudomonas aeruginosa*
2 g Ofloxacin + 1 g Gentamicin	*Pseudomonas aeruginosa*

AB antibiotics, *ALBC* antibiotic-loaded bone cement, *MRSA* methicillin-resistant *Staphylococcus aureus*, *MRSE* methicillin-resistant *Staphylococcus epidermidis*

Tab. 7.3 Recommendations on how much AB to use in ALBC in agreement with the clinical application objective

Quantity of antibiotic (percentage in 40 g PMMA)	Surgical application
Low doses: <2.5%	Prevention of PJI – prophylaxis
High doses: 2.5–7.5%	Combined indications: Fixation of (revision) implants, filling of bone and joint cavities and spacer management (if fixation purpose is predominant, do not exceed 5%)
Very high doses: 10% (in some cases even more)	Exclusive use for bone–cement spacer

AB antibiotics, *ALBC* antibiotic-loaded bone cement, *PJI* prosthetic joint infection, *PMMA* polymethylmethacrylate

7.1.4 How Can the Use of ALBC Be Justified?

Fortunately, prosthetic joint infection (PJI) is a rare pathology with an incidence rate of 1% or less in specialized arthroplasty centres (Willis-Owen et al. 2010). However, the absolute infection numbers are on the rise owing to population ageing and the higher demands for joint replacement procedures, as well as the increasing number of operations on patients with comorbidities putting them at higher risks for infections. To fully understand the epidemiological burden of PJI now and in the future, Kurtz et al. compared the number and percentage of septic revision cases in 2005 (8.4%) and in 2030 (47.5%) on the basis of the expected growth of primary and revision joint replacement procedures (100% growth of hip arthroplasty and 600% growth for knee arthroplasty) in the United States (Kurtz et al. 2007).

Treatment of a periprosthetic joint infection is often complex and also increasingly challenging as a consequence of the growing prevalence of difficult-to-treat multi-resistant pathogens. Apart from the surgical problem and the suffering of the patient, there is also a high cost involved in PJI treatment, which is often twice as high as (or even higher) the costs of an aseptic joint replacement (Kontekakis et al. 2013).

The high »vulnerability« of any implant for bacterial colonization and the increasing demand for knee and hip replacement serves to emphasize the importance of implementing strategies to minimize the risk of infections (Bistolfi et al. 2011). However, as long as there is yet nothing commercially available to meet the aim of reducing the adhesion and subsequent bacterial colonization risk of implants, surgeons still have to rely on »old« strategies for infection prevention, which includes strict theatre hygiene, quick operation times and appropriate systemic and local antibiotics.

7.1.5 Treatment

Despite a growing interest in PJI treatment concepts without use of any acrylic cement (almost exclusively in septic hip replacement), there is still a wide consensus that the available clinical data and the therapeutical success rates favour a concept in which AB-eluting bone cements play a pivotal role in the fixation of the revision implant in one-stage procedures (Rudelli et al. 2008; Winkler et al. 2008; Singer et al. 2012) and/or as interim spacer in two-stage revision procedures (Villanueva et al. 2006; Toulson et al. 2009; Silvestre et al. 2013). Infection treatment success rates do not differ much between the two techniques and were often reported to be around 90% or more. ◘ Fig. 7.4 provides two examples of articulating PMMA spacers implanted in the hip or knee joint cavity after removal of the primary implant and surgical debridement of the infected bone and soft tissue.

7.1.6 Prophylaxis

Although the cementation with ALBC is widespread practice in most Scandinavian countries, the UK and Germany, its routine use in arthroplasty is still controversially discussed in other regions, such as Southern Europe or the United States. Among the arguments against routine application of ALBC are concerns of AB resistance development and the added costs of the surgeries. In addition, the regulatory approval status differs among regions. In the United States, for example, ALBC is only approved for local prophylactic purpose in revision arthroplasty.

> The rationale of combining systemic AB prophylaxis and local AB via PMMA as a delivery system follows two principles: First, from a pharmacokinetic point of view, both administration routes complement each other – systemic AB provide high concentrations in serum and parenchymatous organs, while local AB released from PMMA provide high concentrations in the poorly vascularized and therefore difficult-to-access compartments, such as bone tissue and joint spaces. Second, from an antimicrobial efficacy point of view, the mode and target of action of the systemic AB (often a cephalosporin for prophylactic purpose) is complemented by the action of the aminoglycoside gentamicin or combinations of it with other AB.

This does not only widen the antimicrobial spectrum, but represents »two independent security levels«, in case the systemic AB prophylaxis has not been given at the correct time and/or in the correct dose prior to incision. The local AB barrier may also be effective in cases of primary resistance of bacterial contaminants to the systemic AB.

The data from several arthroplasty registers can be considered as proof of concept that the combination of both systemic and local AB prophylaxis »works« best. Engesaeter and co-workers (Engesaeter et al. 2003) analysed the data from 22,170 total hip arthroplasty procedures recorded in the Norwegian hip register and found that the revision risk for any reason as well as the revision risk for septic reasons was lowest when systemic and local AB prophylaxis had been combined. Similar results were also obtained from the Finnish knee register

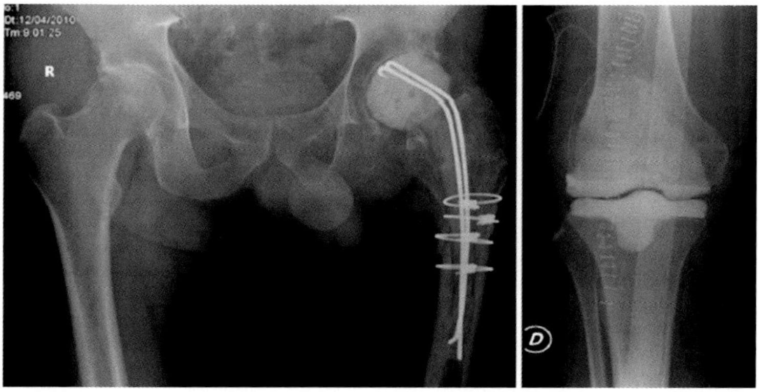

◘ **Fig. 7.4** Articulating PMMA spacers for the treatment of PJI in two-stage revision protocols: *left*, hip spacer; *right*, knee spacer

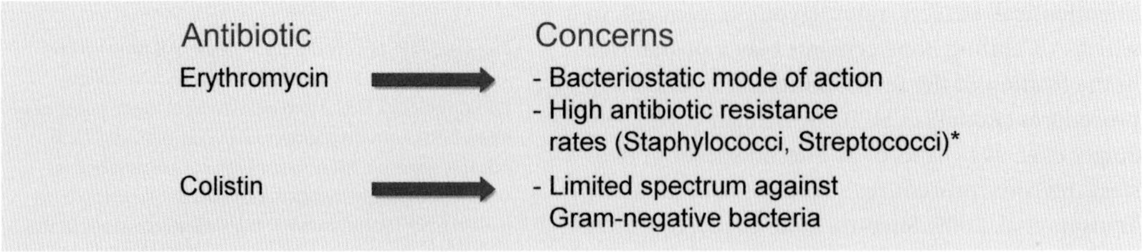

Fig. 7.5 Features and concerns of the AB erythromycin and colistin used in Simplex® P bone cement for the local AB prophylaxis of knee replacement procedures (Hinarejos et al. 2013). *According to European antimicrobial resistance surveillance data 2012 (EARRS network)

(Jamsen et al. 2009). The author of this study even concluded that no or inappropriate local AB prophylaxis with bone cement was a higher risk factor for infections than putting aside the systemic AB prophylaxis. The most recent patient cohort data are derived from a French study with 100,200 patient data suggesting a clear association between the use of bone cement and the survivorship of total hip prostheses. It was found that cemented hip arthroplasty not only showed a lower revision risk in general compared with uncemented hip replacement procedures, but that the use of ALBC added a significant survival benefit to the cemented hip implants (Colas et al. 2015). In an attempt to summarize all the clinical evidence available until then from arthroplasty registries, clinical trials and prospective cohort studies, Parvizi concluded in 2008 in his meta-analysis that the routine use of ALBC as an additional local prophylactic measure to systemic AB reduced the number of implant infections in total hip replacement by approximately 50%.

Based on these reports one might argue that the picture is clear. But it is also part of a differentiated judgement to mention some recent publications which have questioned the additional benefit of ALBC. Among these the prospective study of Hinarejos et al. may be highlighted in which no reduction of PJI risk was observed in 3,000 knee arthroplasties analysed, if cementation of the knee implants was done with ALBC instead of plain cement (Hinarejos et al. 2013). The standard systemic prophylaxis was comparable in both groups. However, this study is also a good example of how quick results with a particular bone cement brand and a particular AB combination (in this study Simplex® P bone cement with erythromycin and colistin) are extrapolated to any other ALBC brand. In fact, it has not only been shown that the AB elution capacity of Simplex® P is inferior to the comparator cement Palacos® R (Stevens et al. 2005), but that the AB combination analysed in this study can be problematic because of the mode of action and the relatively high AB resistance level of erythromycin (see Fig. 7.5).

7.1.7 Concerns with ALBC

Toxicity

The attractiveness of the local AB concept is also based on observations that high local AB concentrations can be achieved without clinically relevant cytotoxic effects on osteoblasts combined with a very low systemic burden (AB concentrations are 100- to 1,000-fold lower in serum and parenchymatous organs). This principle has already been shown by Walenkamp (1983) (see Fig. 7.6).

So far, no reports of a systemic toxicity related to the use of low-dose ALBC for infection prophylaxis purposes have been published. However, a few reports are available which describe some clinical cases of systemic toxicity, in particular renal failure. These severe side effects were always associated with the implementation of high-dose AB-loaded cement spacers in two-stage revision arthroplasty. In a recent meta-analysis, Luu and colleagues (Luu et al. 2013) analysed the reported incidence of acute kidney injury (AKI) and infection recurrence in a period of 13 years, in order to assess the risk–benefit ratio of ALBC spacers. Ten observational studies (n=544 patients) with clinical outcomes showed an average incidence of AKI of 4.8% and a treatment success rate of 89%. Although these severe side ef-

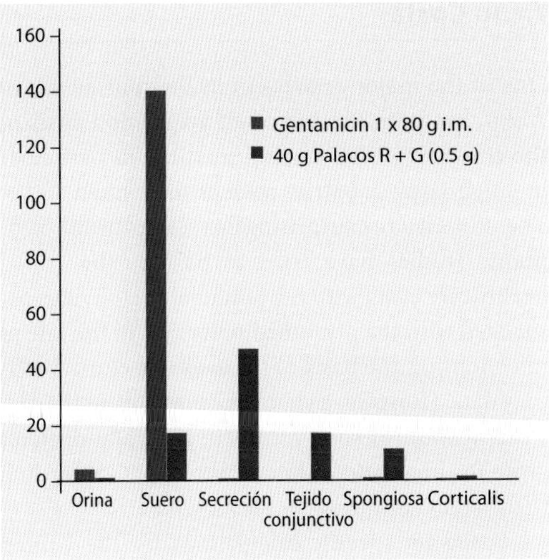

Fig. 7.6 Gentamicin concentrations in cortical (*corticalis*) and spongy (*spongiosa*) bony tissue, the surrounding soft tissue (*tejido conjunctivo*), in drainage fluid (*secreción*) from operated joints, in serum (*suero*) and in urine (*orina*) as a function of the application route (*purple bars*, gentamicin applied i.m.; *red bars*, gentamicin applied via ALBC; adapted from Walenkamp 1983)

fects appear higher than previously reported, it must be noted that the doses of local AB (often vancomycin) differed widely, with AB concentrations frequently exceeding 20% (8 g AB per 40 g cement) (Hsieh et al. 2009). A study by Springer et al., on the other hand, did not report any systemic toxicity and allergic reactions at huge local AB doses (in addition to different systemic AB), as high as 10.5 g vancomycin and 12.5 g of gentamicin loaded into PMMA. In light of these data, it can be concluded that systemic toxicity does not appear to be an issue of major clinical relevance, but clinicians should always be aware of the potential side effect on kidney function if using high-dose ALBC spacer in high-risk patients (Springer et al. 2004).

7.1.8 Influence on the Mechanical Properties of PMMA

Another argument often posed by opponents of prophylactic ALBC use is the concern of an increase in the fatigue properties of bone cement leading to a higher risk of mechanical implant failure and subsequent prosthesis loosening. There is a large body of evidence, however, that does not support this point of view. In 1999 Klekamp (Klekamp et al. 1999) published a study in which he did not find a significant difference in the mechanical parameters of the bone cements Palacos® R or Simplex® P compared with plain cement if the concentration of added vancomycin powder did not exceed 5%. In all cases, the ISO or ASTM norms were fulfilled. Based on Klekamp's studies, it was, however, recommended that vancomycin always be added in powder form to PMMA, as he observed a drastic negative effect on PMMA stress resolutions if the AB was mixed in liquid form into bone cement. Such concerns are generally of lower priority when high-dose ALBC is used for spacer management in two-stage revisions because of the limited implantation time of the spacer in the joint cavity. A few studies have also compared industrially produced ALBC and manually manufactured ALBC in the theatre with respect to mechanical strength and AB elution capacity. It was found that the manual addition of a generic tobramycin powder to the bone cement Simplex® P decreased the mechanical strength by 38% (DeLuise and Scott 2004) and that the elution of equal amounts of manually added gentamicin to the bone cement Palacos® R was inferior to the elution of the antibiotic Palacos® R with gentamicin (Schering; Neut et al. 2003).

The data from the Scandinavian arthroplasty registries can also be considered as clinical proof of concept that low-dose AB in bone cement does not negatively influence the survival of implants: Implants cemented with ALBC did not lead to higher »aseptic« revision rates (because of prosthesis loosening) in the observation periods of many years. On the contrary, such implants showed a lower incidence of septic revision cases, which might be explained by the additional infection prophylaxis effect (Jämsen et al. 2009).

7.1.9 Resistance

A recurrent controversy is the concern that the routine use of ALBC in arthroplasty might promote the development of bacterial resistance in the orthopaedic ward as a consequence of the prolonged exposure to the AB at sub-inhibitory levels after the initial burst of elution from the cement mantle. Using an animal infection model, Thomes et al. (2002) found a lower incidence of infections in those animals receiving gentamicin-loaded bone cement instead of plain cement (41% vs 73%), but this was at the expense of a significantly higher rate of gentamicin-resistant Staphylococci in the ALBC group (78% vs 19%). These findings corresponded to earlier clinical observations made by Hope et al. (1989), that gentamicin-resistant germs could be found with higher frequency in PJI patients in whom ALBC had been initially used for the primary joint replacement procedure compared with plain cement (88% vs 16%). On the other hand, it is reported that the shift from plain cement (Simplex® P) to ALBC (Simplex® P with Tobramycin) at their institution in 2003 did not cause notable changes in the AB resistance profile of *S. aureus* or coagulase-negative Staphylococci in PJI cases. It was even observed that the prevalence of methicillin-resistant *Staphylococcus aureus*/methicillin-resistant *Staphylococcus epidermidis* (MRSA/MRSE)-infections tended to decrease in the observation period as well as the cross-resistance level to tetracyclines (from 20% to 5%) and erythromycin (from 70% to 50%), possibly reflecting a more careful consumption of these antibiotics in the hospital wards (Hansen et al. 2014). In view of these conflicting results, it may be concluded that the clinical relevance of this important issue is not fully clear yet. It should be also noted in this context that concentration-dependant strictly bactericidal AB, such as gentamicin, are not prone to induce resistance, but rather lead to a selection of primary resistance if present. This principle would also explain why the antibiotic resistance rates in the Scandinavian countries continue to be low despite the widespread use of ALBC for decades. To obviate this serious concern it has been proposed to carefully weigh the pros and cons according to the patient's individual infection risk and the type of operation. Another strategy to minimize the risk of resistance selection is the combination of two antibiotics with different modes of action in special situations, such as for spacer management in septic revision cases or for joint replacement procedures in patients with a particular high-risk profile (Stefánsdóttir et al. 2013).

7.1.10 Costs

One of the major drawbacks in the routine use of ALBC has been the increased acquisition costs of the commercial AB-cement mixture, in particular in »high-cost« countries such as the United States. Therefore, it is not surprising that several health-economic studies have tried to balance the added health-care costs with the potential cost savings associated with the presumed reduction in the rate of infections on the basis of the available clinical efficacy data. However, it should be pointed out that the extrapolation of such results is generally difficult given the huge price differences of ALBC according to different countries.

Based on specific calculations for the United States, Jiranek et al. (2006) suggested that the routine use of ALBC in primary arthroplasty procedures was not justified despite the prophylactic effect against PJI (Jiranek et al. 2006). The cost–benefit analysis was done on the basis of the following assumptions: (1) ALBC would be applied in 50% of the estimated 500,000 primary arthroplasties performed annually in the United States at an added cost of $600 for two 40-g packs of ALBC used on average in each procedure; (2) an average treatment cost for each PJI case of $50,000. To recover the costs associated with the routine use of ALBC, it was concluded that the PJI incidence rate would have to fall from the calculated 1.5% to 0.3%, thus exceeding the most optimistic efficacy calculations of approximately 50% PJI risk reduction. A more recent US study has specifically calculated the economics of using prophylactic ALBC in total knee replacement procedures assuming, however, a more realistic average cost per PJI case of $109,805 (Lavernia et al. 2006). The authors concluded that depending on the type of AB-loaded cement used, its cost in all primary total knee replacements ranges between $2,112.72 and $112,606.67 per case of infection that is prevented (Gutowski et al. 2014).

In an attempt to adjust the calculation basis of such health-economic evaluations to the »European situation«, we performed an independent cost-efficacy analysis in our own institution. The study was based on our observations in a 2-year period before and after the switch from plain cement to the ALBC Palacos® R + G (Heraeus Medical, Germany) in

2011 for any cemented primary knee or hip replacement (including hemiarthroplasties after femoral neck fractures). We observed a drastic reduction in the PJI incidence rate from 4.3% before to 1.8% after switching to ALBC. Since such observational studies always bear the risk of a significant bias, we used a group of uncemented implants as internal control. Interestingly, no reduction in the infection rate could be observed in this comparator group before and after 2011. If we balance this effect on the PJI rate against the added costs of routine ALBC use (basis for this calculation is a cost difference of approximately €10 per 40-g pack in Spain) assuming similar treatment costs per PJI case as calculated by Jiranek et al., we calculated a net saving of €1,123,846 in this period, which would correspond to €992 per patient (Sanz-ruiz et al. 2016).

The aforementioned evaluations are good examples of the »transatlantic paradox« showing that the conclusions of such cost-efficacy studies largely depend on the economic parameters used for the statistical analysis. Because of their large variations, conclusions for one country may often not be extrapolated to another country. It is mandatory that each country performs such cost-efficacy calculations independently.

7.1.11 Our Institutional Experience with ALBC

In 2011 it was decided in our institution to perform any cemented arthroplasty procedure for total knee and hip replacements including hemiarthroplasties after femoral neck fractures routinely with gentamicin-loaded bone cements. We chose the commercial brand Palacos® R+G (Heraeus Medical GmbH, Wehrheim, Germany) including 0.5 g gentamicin per 40-g pack as the preferred bone cement basing our decision on its excellent outcome data with respect to revision rates and AB elution capacity.

In order to assess whether this change of clinical practice had an impact on the infection rates in our institution we compared the number of PJI cases in a 2-year period before and after the introduction of routine use of ALBC in primary arthroplasty on the basis of 2,500 procedures performed in these two periods. As internal control we used the PJI rate of

Tab. 7.4 PJI incidence before and after the introduction of the routine use of Palacos® R+G in primary cemented joint replacement procedures

Period	Total joint infection risk	Total knee infection risk	Hip arthroplasty infection risk								
			Total			Total hip infection risk			Hemiarthroplasty hip infection risk		
			Global	Non-cemented	Cemented	Global	Non-cemented	Cemented	Global	Non-cemented	Cemented
Before ALBC use	4.3%	3.3%	5.4%	3.5%	8.4%	1.6%	1.3%	7.1%	8.5%	8.7%	8.5%
After ALBC use	1.88%	1.3%	2.4%	2.8%	2.3%	2.4%	2.3%	2,8%	2.4%	4.4%	2.3%
% Reduction infection risk/ RR	57%/ RR 0.42 *	60.6%/ RR 0.37 *	65.6%/ RR 0.45 *	20%/ RR 0.35	72.6%/ RR 0.27 *	>44%/ RR 1.9	>176%/ RR 1.8	60.6%/ RR 0.3	31.8%/ RR 0.26 *	59.5%/ RR 0.48	73%/ RR 0.25 *

*Statistically significant differences at $p<0.001$
RR relative risk

Tab. 7.5 Calculation of the added costs of using ALBC vs the cost savings as a result of the reduction of the incidence of PJI at our institution

	Total joints	Total knees	Hip arthroplasty
Added cost per use ALBC	€11,330	€5,550	€2,570
Cost per all infection prevented	€1,135,176	€445,962	€689,214
Total net saving Net saving per patient	€1,123,846 €992	€440,412/ €801	€686,644 €2,672

uncemented arthroplasties in the same observation periods, which would allow us to monitor the influence of other factors leading to a possible bias in our retrospective analysis. As shown in Tab. 7.4, it was found that the overall infection rate was significantly reduced from 4.3% to 1.8% resulting in a reduction of the infection risk of 57% for all cemented total joint replacements (60% for TKR; 73% for hemiarthroplasty procedures; 44% for THR).

The higher than usually reported infection rates at our institution in the period before the switch to ALBC may be explained by the high-risk profile of our patients, often transferred from smaller hospitals to our more specialized University General Hospital, treating more complicated cases, patients with comorbidities and also emergencies and polytrauma patients.

In a further study, these remarkable results were then used to balance the added costs of using ALBC in primary cemented arthroplasty instead of plain cement against the potential cost savings per prevented PJI case. We calculated a net saving of €1,123,846 for all prevented infections in the 2-year period following the change in our clinical practice toward using ALBC (see Tab. 7.5). This corresponds to a net saving per patient of €992. It should also be emphasized that we did not observe changes in the pattern of PJI causing pathogens, nor a significant variation in the AB resistance profile of the micro-organisms.

7.1.12 Summary

PJI is a devastating complication after total joint replacement. Its incidence is predicted to grow further as a consequence of the increasing number of arthroplasty procedures, the trend to operate on comorbid patients with higher infection risks and the expanding AB resistance of PJI-causing micro-organisms. Therefore, optimization of infection prevention strategies is mandatory. In the opinion of the authors, the clinical evidence is sufficient to support the recommendation of using ALBC as an additional prophylactic measure to systemic preoperative AB. The positive effects should outweigh the concerns that a reduction of the mechanical strength of ALBC may lead to a higher risk of prosthesis loosening, that systemic toxic side effects affect the patient's health status and that AB resistance may increase. It is, however, necessary to choose the appropriate bone cement matrix with high initial AB elution capacities and the appropriate AB.

The cost–benefit analysis of the routine use of ALBC should always consider the added costs and the »real« infection rates in the institution. Our own experience has shown that this calculation can be positive.

Take-Home Message

- The choice of bone cement and the added AB has a big impact on the outcome.
- The goal of all surgeons is to prevent the difficult-to-treat and expensive complication PJI.
- Local AB in addition to systemic AB provide high concentrations (of AB) in difficult-to-access areas. They also provide an additional security level when systemic AB is not given correctly.
- There is a proven connection between ABLC and the survival of prostheses.
- The rise of mechanical failure of the bone cement comes with high doses and manually added AB.

- Some cases of systemic toxicity were reported when high-dose ALBC spacers were used.
- The general concern of creating AB resistance when using ALBC cannot be proven nor disproven with certainty.
- Depending on the individual situation (country + hospital) the use of ALBC may or may not be cost efficient. Therefore individual evaluations are recommended.

References

Bistolfi AG, Massazza E, Verne A, Masse D, Deledda S, Ferraris M, Miola F, Galetto F, Crova M (2011) Antibiotic-loaded cement in orthopedic surgery: a review. ISRN Orthop http://dx.doi.org/10.5402/2011/290851

Buchholz HW, Engelbrecht H (1970) [Depot effects of various antibiotics mixed with Palacos resins]. Chirurg 41(11): 511–515

Colas SC, Collin P, Piriou P, Zureik M (2015) Association Between Total Hip Replacement Characteristics and 3-Year Prosthetic Survivorship: A Population-Based Study. JAMA Surg 150(10): 979–988

DeLuise M, Scott CP (2004) Addition of hand-blended generic tobramycin in bone cement: effect on mechanical strength. Orthopedics 27(12):1289–1291

Engesaeter LB, Lie SA, Espehaug B, Furnes O, Vollset SE, Havelin LI (2003) Antibiotic prophylaxis in total hip arthroplasty: effects of antibiotic prophylaxis systemically and in bone cement on the revision rate of 22,170 primary hip replacements followed 0-14 years in the Norwegian Arthroplasty Register. Acta Orthop Scand 74(6): 644–651

Frommelt L, Kühn KD (2005) Properties of bone cement: Antibiotic-loaded cement. In: Breusch S, Malchau H (eds) The well-cemented total hip arthroplasty. Springer, Heidelberg, p 86–92

Gristina AG (1987) Biomaterial-centered infection: microbial adhesion versus tissue integration. Science 237(4822):1588–1595

Gutowski CJ, Zmistowski BM, Clyde CT and Parvizi J (2014) The economics of using prophylactic antibiotic-loaded bone cement in total knee replacement. Bone Joint J 96-B(1): 65–69

Hansen EN, Adeli B, Kenyon R and Parvizi J (2014) Routine use of antibiotic laden bone cement for primary total knee arthroplasty: impact on infecting microbial patterns and resistance profiles. J Arthroplasty 29(6):1123–1127

Hendriks JG, van Horn JR, van der Mei HC, Busscher HJ (2004) Backgrounds of antibiotic-loaded bone cement and prosthesis-related infection. Biomaterials 25(3):545–556

Hinarejos P, Guirro P, Leal J, Montserrat F, Pelfort X, Sorli ML, Horcajada JP, Puig L (2013) The use of erythromycin and colistin-loaded cement in total knee arthroplasty does not reduce the incidence of infection: a prospective randomized study in 3000 knees. J Bone Joint Surg Am 95(9):769–774

Hope PG, Kristinsson KG, Norman P and Elson RA (1989) Deep infection of cemented total hip arthroplasties caused by coagulase-negative staphylococci. J Bone Joint Surg Br 71(5):851–855

Hsieh PH, Tai CL, Lee PC and Chang YH (2009) Liquid gentamicin and vancomycin in bone cement: a potentially more cost-effective regimen. J Arthroplasty 24(1): 125–130

Jaemsen E, Huhtala H, Puolakka T, Moilanen T (2009). Risk factors for infection after knee arthroplasty. A register based analysis of 43,149 cases. J Bone Joint Surg Am 91(1):38–47

Jiranek WA, Hanssen AD, Greenwald AS (2006) Antibiotic-loaded bone cement for infection prophylaxis in total joint replacement. J Bone Joint Surg Am 88(11): 2487–2500

Klekamp J, Dawson JM, Haas DW, DeBoer D, Christie M (1999) The use of vancomycin and tobramycin in acrylic bone cement: biomechanical effects and elution kinetics for use in joint arthroplasty. J Arthroplasty 14(3):339–346

Kontekakis A, Berghaus M, Gaiser S, Kühn KD (2013) Evidence generation for medical devices- the case of cemented joint replacement sugery in arthroplasty registries. In: Scholz M (ed) Biofunctional Surface Engineering 13, Pan Stanford, Singapore, p 291–314

Kühn KD (2014) PMMA cements Springer, Heidelberg, doi 10.1007/978-3-642-41536-4

Kühn KD, Lieb E, Berberich C (2016) PMMA bone cement: what is the role of local antibiotics. Maîtrise Orthopédique 255:12–18

Kurtz SM, Ong KL, Schmier J, Mowat F, Saleh K, Dybvik E, Karrholm J, Garellick G, Havelin LI, Furnes O, Malchau H, Lau E (2007) Future clinical and economic impact of revision total hip and knee arthroplasty. J Bone Joint Surg Am 89(Suppl3):144–151

Lavernia C, Lee DJ, Hernandez VH (2006) The increasing financial burden of knee revision surgery in the United States. Clin Orthop Relat Res 446:221–226

Luu A, Syed F, Raman G, Bhalla A, Muldoon E, Hadley S, Smith E and Rao M (2013) Two-stage arthroplasty for prosthetic joint infection: a systematic review of acute kidney injury, systemic toxicity and infection control. J Arthroplasty 28(9):1490–1498

Neut D, van de Belt H, van Horn JR, van der Mei HC and Busscher HJ (2003) The effect of mixing on gentamicin release from polymethylmethacrylate bone cements. Acta Orthop Scand 74(6):670–676

Parvizi J, Gehrke T and Chen AF (2013) Proceedings of the International Consensus on Periprosthetic Joint Infection. Bone Joint J 95-B(11):1450–1452

Rudelli S, Uip D, Honda E, Lima AL (2008) One-stage revision of infected total hip arthroplasty with bone graft. J Arthroplasty 23(8):1165–1177

Sanz-Ruiz P, Paz E, Abenojar J, Carlos del Real J, Vaquero J, Forriol F (2014) Effects of vancomycin, cefazolin and test conditions on the wear behavior of bone cement. J Arthroplasty 29(1):16–22

Sanz-Ruiz P,Matas-Diez JA, Sanchez-Somolinos M, Villanueva-Martínez M, Vaquero-Martín J. (2016) Is the Commercial Antibiotic-Loaded Bone Cement Useful in Prophylactic and Cost Saving After Knee and Hip Joint Arthroplasty? The Transatlantic Paradox. J Arthroplasty. Nov 15. pii: S0883-5403(16)30812-9. doi: 10.1016/j.arth.2016.11.012. [Epub ahead of print]

Silvestre A, Almeida F, Renovell P, Morante E, Lopez R (2013) Revision of infected total knee arthroplasty: two-stage reimplantation using an antibiotic-impregnated static spacer. Clin Orthop Surg 5(3):180–187

Singer J, Merz A, Frommelt L, Fink B (2012) High rate of infection control with one-stage revision of septic knee prostheses excluding MRSA and MRSE. Clin Orthop Relat Res 470(5):1461–1471

Springer BD, Lee GC, Osmon D, Haidukewych GJ, Hanssen AD, Jacofsky DJ (2004) Systemic safety of high-dose antibiotic-loaded cement spacers after resection of an infected total knee arthroplasty. Clin Orthop Relat Res(427):47–51

Stefánsdóttir A, Johansson A, Lidgren L, Wagner P, W-Dahl A (2013) Bacterial colonization and resistance patterns in 133 patients undergoing a primary hip- or knee replacement in Southern Sweden. Acta Orthopaedica 84(1): 87–91

Stevens CM, KD Tetsworth, Calhoun JH and Mader JT (2005) An articulated antibiotic spacer used for infected total knee arthroplasty: a comparative in vitro elution study of Simplex and Palacos bone cements. J Orthop Res 23(1):27–33

Thomes B, Murray P, Bouchier-Hayes D (2002) Development of resistant strains of Staphylococcus epidermidis on gentamicin-loaded bone cement in vivo. J Bone Joint Surg Br 84(5):758–760

Toulson C, Walcott-Sapp S, Hur J, Salvati E, Bostrom M, Brause B, Westrich GH (2009) Treatment of infected total hip arthroplasty with a 2-stage reimplantation protocol: update on »our institution's« experience from 1989 to 2003. J Arthroplasty 24(7):1051–1060

van de Belt H, Neut D, Schenk W, van Horn JR, van der Mei HC, Busscher HJ (2001) Infection of orthopedic implants and the use of antibiotic-loaded bone cements. A review. Acta Orthop Scand 72(6):557–571

Villanueva M, Rios A, Pereiro J, Chana F, Fahandez-Saddi H (2006) Hand-made articulating spacers for infected total knee arthroplasty: a technical note. Acta Orthop 77(2):329–332

Walenkamp GHIM (2007) Local antibiotics in Arthroplasty: State of the art from an interdisciplinary point of view. Thieme, Stuttgart

Walenkamp, G. (1983). Gentamicin PMMA BEads. A clinical, pharmacokinetic and toxicological study. Dissertation, Radboud University

Willis-Owen CA, Konyves A, Martin DK (2010) Factors affecting the incidence of infection in hip and knee replacement: an analysis of 5277 cases. J Bone Joint Surg Br 92(8):1128–1133

Winkler H, Stoiber A, Kaudela K, Winter F, Menschik F (2008) One stage uncemented revision of infected total hip replacement using cancellous allograft bone impregnated with antibiotics. J Bone Joint Surg Br 90(12): 1580–1584

7.2 Therapy Using Antibiotic-Loaded PMMA

Götz von Foerster, Lars Frommelt, and Thorsten Gehrke

7.2.1 Principles of Therapy in Periprosthetic Joint Infection

Periprosthetic joint infection (PJI) is an infection resulting from pathogens that are sessile on the surface of artificial joint replacements in biofilm. The infection, as an interaction between host and pathogen, takes place in the tissue adjacent to the artificial joint replacement (Gristina 987; Costerton et al. 1987; Frommelt 2000).

Bacteria in biofilm are protected from the activities of antimicrobial agents and the cellular host defence. Phagocytosis of mature biofilm is not possible and thus the bacterial pathogen cannot be eliminated. Therefore, antibiotic therapy alone is not able to terminate PJI by elimination of the causative agent, the pathogen. To control PJI, surgical revision with removal of the prosthesis and all foreign material, e.g. bone cement, screws and other hardware, is necessary. In addition, antibiotics are able to act on the remaining bacteria.

Antimicrobial agents can be administered systemically via the intravenous route or via oral application. Another route of application is possible by delivery systems that are placed directly at the site of infection: the application of PMMA bone cement known as ALAC (antibiotic-loaded acrylic cement) or ALBC (antibiotic-loaded bone cement) is widely used (Buchholz and Engelbrecht 1970).

7.2.2 ALBC as a Carrier for Local Antibiotics

The elution of antibiotics from PMMA depends on the type of bone cement, its ability uptake of water and the available surface. It starts in the very beginning with an extremely high concentration, which drops down within minutes to a lower concentration that will be eluted for a distinct period depending on the antimicrobial agents and the bone cement specialty (Kühn 2014; Lewis 2015; Mader et al. 1997).

ALAC may be used for prophylaxis (Espehaug et al. 1997; Dunbar 2009) and as antibiotic delivery device in fixation of the TJR in one-stage revision arthroplasty or as a spacer material in two-stage revision (Buchholz et al. 1979; Gehrke et al. 2013; Romanò et al. 2012).

One of the advantages is that ALAC offers the possibility of specific antimicrobial therapy to the surgeon if the pathogen is known before revision. This can be realized by using industrial specialties containing gentamicin alone or in combination with clindamycin or vancomycin. If no industrial preparation containing effective antimicrobial agents for the pathogen is found, effective antibiotics may be admixed to the PMMA bone cement by hand in the operating theatre (Chen and Parvizi 2014; McLaren et al. 2009).

Some antimicrobial agents are inactivated in PMMA, e.g. by the heat resulting during polymerization. The choice of antibiotics must respect the property of being eluted from acrylic bone cement (Frommelt 2007). Suitable antibiotics with proven elution properties for admixing are shown in ◘ Tab. 7.6. For admixing, only antibiotics that are certified

◘ **Tab. 7.6** Antimicrobial agents qualified for admixing in PMMA bone cement

	Antimicrobial agents (selection)	Remarks
Antimicrobial agents with well-known activity	Gentamicin	
	Tobramycin	Mostly used in the United States
	Clindamycin	
	Vancomycin	Good elution in the presence of gentamicin
	Erythromycin	Historical use in therapy, indicated in prophylaxis
	Colistin	For critical PJI due to multiresistant Gram-negative rods
	Cefazedone	No longer available
	Cefoperazone	No longer available
	Thiamphenicol	No longer available in human medicine owing to toxicity
	Streptomycin	For tuberculosis (TBC)
Antimicrobial agents with moderate activity	Ofloxacin	Only in combination with other antibiotics
	Cefazolin	Short-acting by hydrolysis
	Cefuroxim	Short-acting by hydrolysis
	Ampicillin	Short-acting by hydrolysis
	Mezlocillin	Short-acting by hydrolysis
Antimicrobial agents with poor in vivo studies	Meropenem	Gram-negative multiresis-tant pathogens *Pseudomonas aeruginosa*
	Teicoplanin	
	Daptomycin	Vancomycin-resistant enterococci (VRE) or staphylococci

for i.v. administration and are available as powder must be used.

7.2.3 How to Admix Antimicrobial Agents to PMMA Bone Cement

Well-trained members of staff must carry out the application of antimicrobial agents to PMMA bone cement under sterile conditions in the operating theatre. Here, we describe the procedure using a mixing system for PMMA bone cement (Zahar 2016):

- **Step 1**

The circulating nurse opens the vial containing sterile antibiotic powder and puts the powder in a sterile bowl which is positioned in sterile area.

- **Step 2**

The scrub nurse in the sterile area homogenizes the crystalline antibiotic powder with a proper device like a pestle.

- **Step 3**

The PMMA polymer powder and the homogenized antibiotic powder are filled in the mixing system.

- **Step 4**

The handle is mounted and closes the mixing system and a member of the scrub team mixes the two powders in order to obtain a homogeneous mixture.

- **Step 5**

The mixture of PMMA polymer powder and antibiotic powder is removed from the mixing system under sterile conditions.

- **Step 6 to End**

The manufacturer's instructions for mixing PMMA bone cement are followed with the exception that instead of the pure polymer powder the mixture of PMMA and antibiotic powder as prepared in steps 1–5 is used.

7.2.4 Periprosthetic Joint Infection: When to Use ALBC

Prophylaxis

When PMMA bone cement is used for the fixation of a prosthesis, ALBC should be used together with the appropriate systemic antibiotic prophylaxis. The use of gentamicin has been evaluated by the Norwegian registry (Espehaug et al. 1997). Whether the use of other agents is of benefit has not been evaluated to date and remains an unsolved challenge.

Retention of Prosthesis in the DAIR Procedure

In the DAIR procedure (debridement, antibiotics, irrigation, retention), ALBC is not necessary. The application of ALBC beads should not be used so as not to damage the articulating surfaces of the TJR that should be retained.

One-Stage Exchange Procedure

The use of local antibiotics is an essential part of the one-stage revision as introduced by Buchholz. Knowledge of the pathogen is one of the prerequisites to carrying out specific local antimicrobial therapy by admixing antibiotics, which are effective according to the susceptibility of the pathogen. Thus it is possible to limit the systemic antimicrobial therapy to a period of about 2 weeks depending on the patient's individual situation and the pathogen present.

As to the amount of antibiotics, not more than 10% of the weight of the PMMA should be used in adding antibiotics in order to obtain mechanical stable fixation of the TJR especially when mixing by hand (McLaren 2009; Frommelt 2007). Whenever possible, industrial preparations should be used because, thanks to the standardization of the manufacturing process, reliable mechanical properties of the PMMA bone cement are guaranteed.

Contraindications for this type of one-stage revision are failure to identify the pathogen preoperatively, lack of antimicrobial agents that can be eluted from PMMA, or the patient having an allergy to the antibiotics, without alternative antibiotic options.

Two-Stage Revision with ALBC as Spacer

Spacers are mostly prepared by using PMMA bone cement. If ALBC is used, the spacer becomes an antibiotic delivery system, which allows for a tailored local antibiotic therapy. The use of industrial produced devices is as crucial as in ALBC for fixation of TJR because the primary stability is not of crucial importance. This allows us to override the 10% limit and create high-dosage PMMA spacers especially when using PMMA preparations with lower elution properties.

7.2.5 Local Antibiotic Therapy and Case-Based Illustrations

Case 1: One-Stage Exchange Revision of the Hip

- **E.A., male, 75 years of age at the time of septic revision (Fig. 7.7, Fig. 7.8, Fig. 7.9)**

The patient suffered from coxarthrosis of the left hip. In August 2009, he was treated with total hip replacement (THR) with cement-free fixation in Papenburg, Germany. Post-operatively the patient was free of complaints but in December 2009 he developed sudden pain under load and in motion. The patient reported no unspecific signs of infection.

On 5 February 2010 the patient visited an outpatient clinic (ENDO-Klinik Hamburg) where joint aspiration of the left hip was performed. *Staphylococcus capitis* was isolated from the synovial fluid. Because the patient was treated with THR on the right side, aspiration of the right hip was performed: The synovial fluid was unremarkable and the culture remained sterile. The patient's C-reactive protein (CRP) level was not elevated.

The patient had undergone THR for the right hip in 2005; in 2008, revision was carried out with exchange of the socket owing to aseptic loosening. In September 2009, a urinary tract infection followed by a bacterial infection of the prostate due to *Escherichia coli* and *Enterococcus faecalis* was reported.

On 1 June 2010, a one-stage revision with exchange of the left side of the THR was performed with radical debridement, irrigation and fixation of the THR using hand-mixed ALBC.

Local therapy in PMMA bone cement comprised:
- 2 g vancomycin admixed to 40 g clindamycin-/gentamicin-PMMA bone cement (Revision Bone Cement, BIOMET, Sweden)

Systemic antibiotic therapy comprised:
- Levofloxacin 500 mg i.v. q12 h
- Rifampicin 600 mg i.v. q12 h
- (Post-operatively the antibiotic administration was changed to oral therapy using the same drugs and dosage)
- Duration of 10 days

From intraoperative biopsies, the same pathogen as before was found, *Staphylococcus capitis*.

The patient was free of complaints until recurrent dislocation of the left hip. In October 2011, revision with exchange of the socket and the prosthetic head was performed.

Preoperatively and from intraoperative biopsies, no bacteria were found.

In 2016, follow-up took place at the outpatient clinic: The patient was free of complaints and no sign of persistent infection could be found.

Case 2: One-Stage Exchange Revision of the Knee

- **D.G., female, 52 years of age at the time of septic revision (Fig. 7.10, Fig. 7.11)**

The patient underwent arthroscopic examination and operation of the right knee in July 2007, Febru-

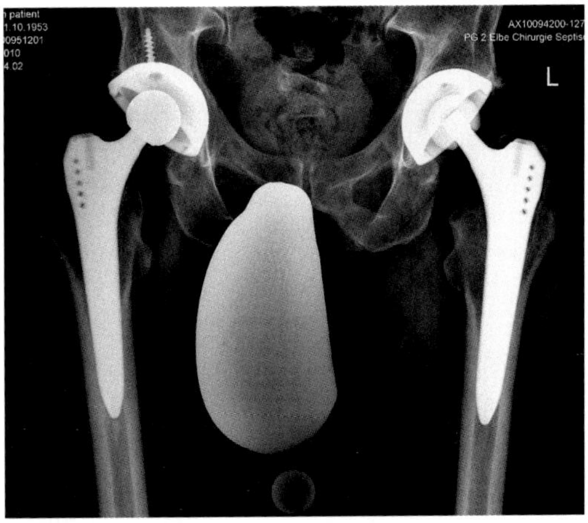

Fig. 7.7 Preoperative X-ray (31 May 2010)

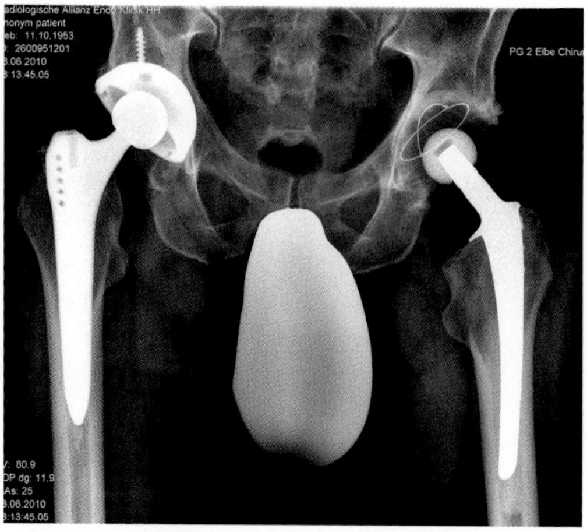

Fig. 7.8 Post-operative X-ray (8 June 2010)

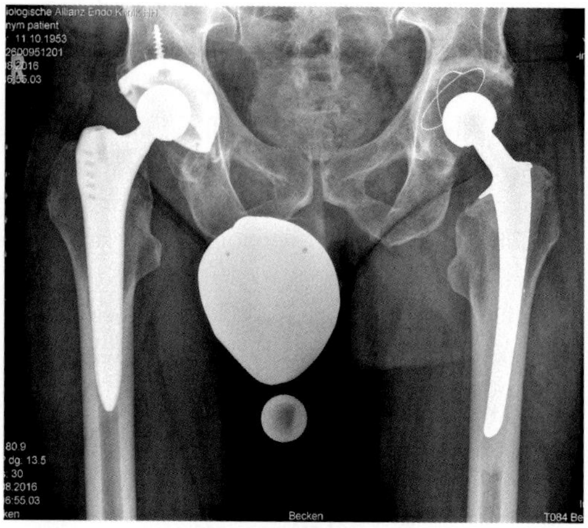

Fig. 7.9 Follow-up X-ray (18 August 2016)

ary 2008, and February 2009 in Sendenhorst and Gütersloh, Germany. In July 2009, prosthetic treatment in the right knee was performed by surface replacement. Post-operatively the patient's complaints became more intense and the range of motion was restricted.

In November 2009, aspiration of the right knee was done and *Staphylococcus epidermidis* was detected in the culture. The patient's family doctor prescribed antibiotic therapy with clindamycin. During antibiotic therapy, the patient reported deterioration of his general condition and increasing pain.

On 7 January 2010, the patient visited the outpatient clinic (ENDO-Klinik Hamburg). An aspiration of the right knee was performed while the patient was still on antibiotic therapy; the synovial fluid for cytology was suggestive of infection but no bacteria was detected in the culture.

After stopping the antibiotic therapy on 29 January 2010, another aspiration of the right knee was performed: The findings from cytology and microscopy were highly suggestive of infection, and in culture *S. epidermidis* was found again.

On admission to the ENDO-Klinik Hamburg on 22 February 2010, the right knee joint was swollen, hyperthermic and slightly reddened.

On 23 February 2010, a one-stage revision was performed with debridement, irrigation and exchange of the surface replacement knee prosthesis to a highly constrained total knee replacement (TKR) in the right knee. For fixation of the TKR, antibiotic-loaded PMMA bone cement (hand-mixed) was used:

Local therapy in PMMA bone cement comprised:
- 2 g vancomycin admixed to 40 g clindamycin-/gentamicin–PMMA bone cement (Revision Bone Cement, BIOMET, Sweden)

Systemic antibiotic therapy comprised:
- Vancomycin 1 g i.v. q12h
- Rifampicin 600 mg i.v. q12
- (Post-operatively, the antibiotic administration of rifampicin was changed to oral therapy using the same drug and dosage)
- Treatment was applied for 14 days

From intraoperative biopsies the same pathogen as before, *Staphylococcus epidermidis*, was found.

Post-operatively, there was wound healing disturbance and in June 2010 a superficial revision was done. Neither preoperatively nor from intraoperative biopsies were bacteria isolated. Wound healing was without any complications and the CRP level decreased with time.

In 2014, follow-up was done in the outpatient clinic: The patient was free of complaints and no signs of persistent infection were found.

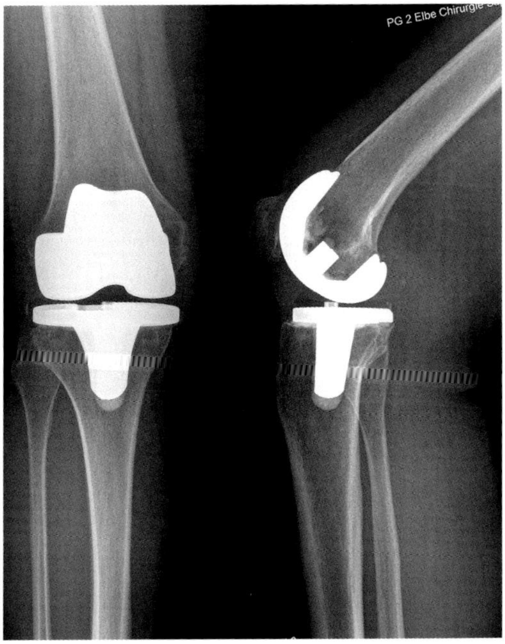

■ **Fig. 7.10** Preoperative X-ray (22 February 2010)

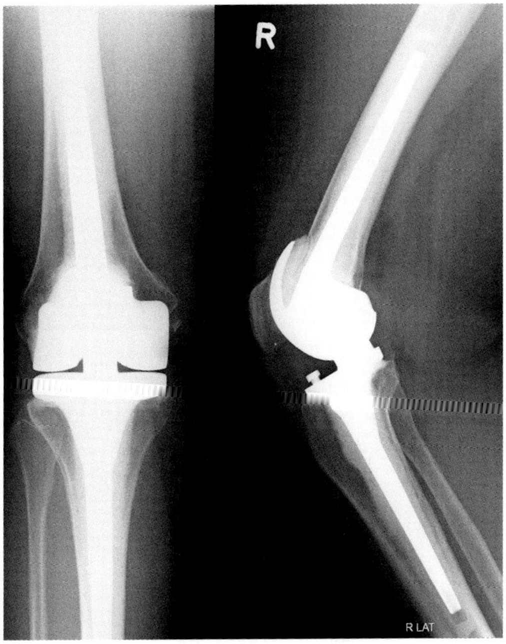

■ **Fig. 7.11** Post-operative X-ray (8 June 2010)

Case 3: One-Stage Exchange Revision of the Hip (E. coli)

- **S. V., female, 76 years of age at the time of septic revision (■ Fig. 7.12, ■ Fig. 7.13, ■ Fig. 7.14)**

In 1999, the patient was treated with THR on both hip joints because of necrosis of the femoral head on both sides.

In 2006, the patient developed pancreatic head carcinoma. Whipple's procedure was performed followed by poly-chemotherapy. Septicaemia originating from a port infection with *Escherichia coli* occurred in 2009. Aspiration of the right hip showed *E. coli* and a revision of the right hip was carried out with exchange of the cup and application of gentamicin-loaded PMMA beads/chains. This therapy was accompanied by systemic administration of ciprofloxacin until November 2009.

On 17 March 2010, a one-stage revision was performed with debridement, irrigation and replantation of the THR on the right side using hand-mixed antibiotic-loaded PMMA bone cement.

Local therapy in the PMMA bone cement comprised:
- 2 g ofloxacin[1] admixed to 40 g clindamycin-/gentamicin–PMMA bone cement (Revision Bone Cement, BIOMET, Sweden)

Systemic antibiotic therapy comprised:
- Meropenem 1 g i.v. q8h
- Levofloxacin 500 mg i.v. q12h
- Post-operatively, the antibiotic administration of levofloxacin was changed to oral therapy without changing the dosage
- Treatment continued for 14 days (meropenem and levofloxacin)
- Levofloxacin was given for another 7 days

No bacteria were isolated from intraoperative biopsies.

In 2011, follow-up was done in the outpatient clinic: The patient was free of complaints and no sign of persistent infection was found.

1 The use of ofloxacin in PMMA is obsolete and is replaced by meropenem (2 g/40 g PMMA bone cement).

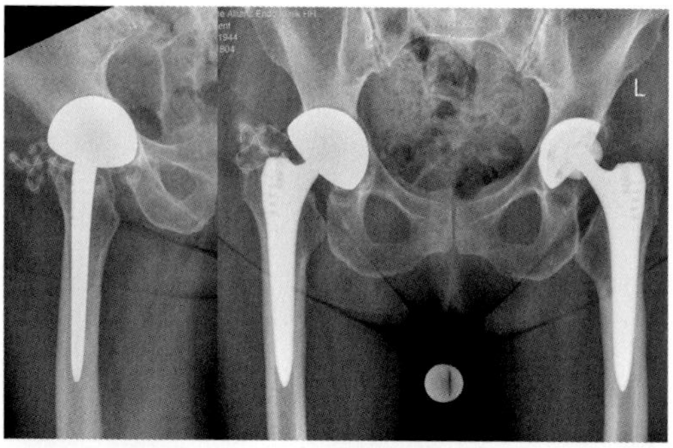

■ **Fig. 7.12** Preoperative X-ray (9 February 2010)

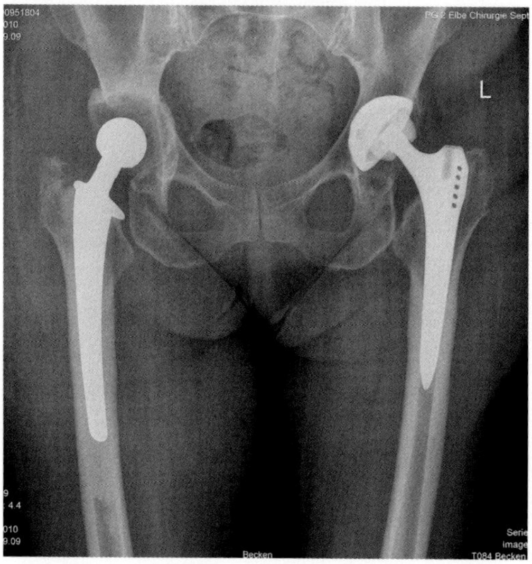

■ **Fig. 7.13** Post-operative X-ray (10 March 2010)

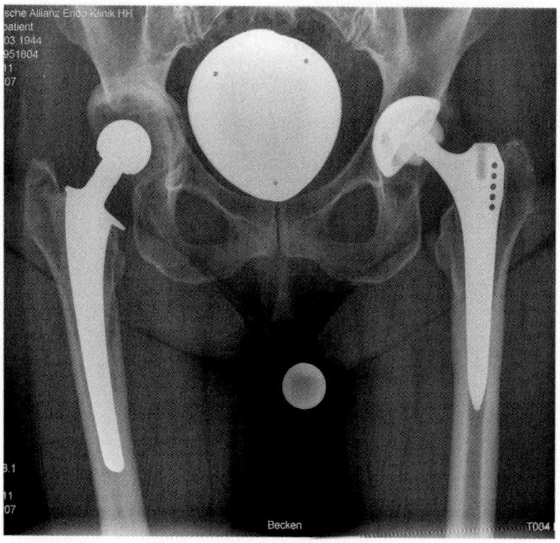

■ **Fig. 7.14** Follow-up X-ray (31 May 2011)

Case 4: Two-Stage Exchange Revision of the Knee

- **S.K.U.R., female, 75 years of age at the time of septic revision (■ Fig. 7.15, ■ Fig. 7.16, ■ Fig. 7.17) Pathogen Found by Sonication of the TKR and from the Periprosthetic Membrane**

The patient had undergone multiple arthroscopic procedures with surgical therapy of menisci and cruciate ligaments. In October 2012, treatment comprised open revision of the left knee and implantation of surface replacement TKR. Postoperatively, there was a persistent tendency for swelling with hyperthermia and restricted range of motion.

The patient first contacted the outpatient clinic of the ENDO-Klinik Hamburg on 15 December 2015. Aspiration of the left knee was done. The leukocyte esterase test of the synovial fluid yielded positive results with twofold higher values than normal, and the alpha-defensin level was definitely elevated whereas the culture remained sterile; these findings were reproduced when repeating the aspiration on 7 January 2016. Another aspiration was performed on 24 May 2016: The microbial culture

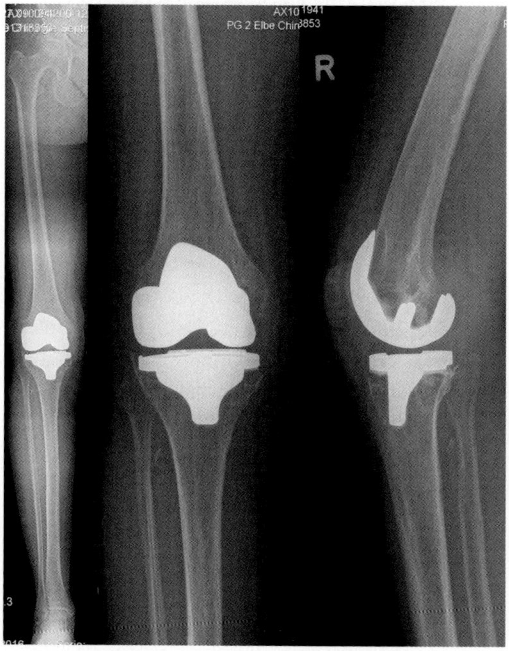

■ **Fig. 7.15** Preoperative X-ray (7 June 2016)

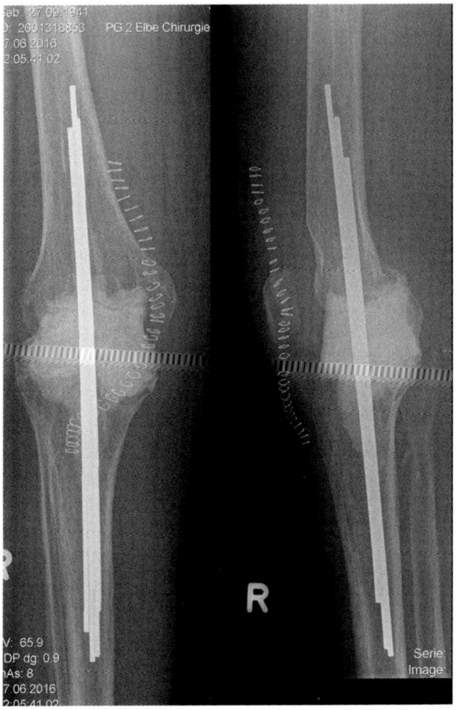

■ **Fig. 7.16** Post-operative X-ray with in-dwelling spacer after removal of TKR (17 June 2016)

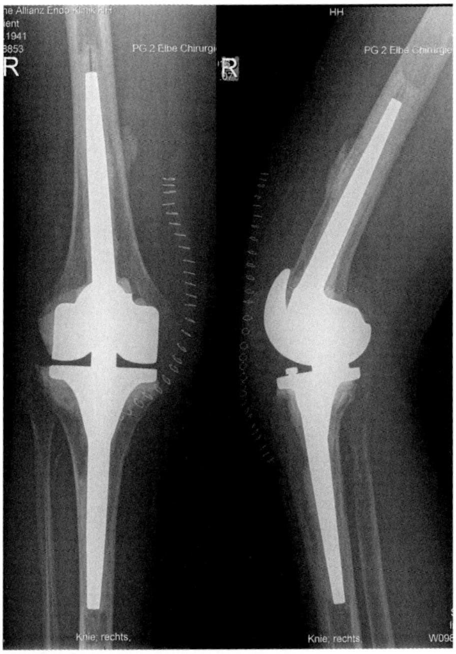

■ **Fig. 7.17** Post-operative X-ray after re-implantation of TKR (22 July 2016)

remained negative but at cytology 2,200 white blood cells/µl (80% polymorphonuclear leukocytes) were found.

Clinically there was no doubt that the patient suffered from PJI, which was supported by the leukocyte esterase test, the alpha-defensin and the cytology results, even though the latter does not serve the Musculoskeletal Infection Society (MSIS) criteria.

On 9 June 2016, in the context of a two-stage revision, the prosthesis was removed with debridement, irrigation and insertion of a static spacer of antibiotic-loaded PMMA bone cement reinforced by metal bars. For the local and systemic antibiotic therapy, broad-range empiric therapy was administered.

Local therapy in the PMMA bone cement comprised:

- 2 g meropenem admixed to 40 g vancomycin-gentamicin PMMA bone cement (Copal® G+V, Heraeus Medical, Germany)

Systemic antibiotic therapy comprised:

- Meropenem 1 g i.v. q8h
- Vancomycin 1.25 g i.v. q12h (drug monitoring! Goal: Trough 15–20 mcg/ml)
- Treatment continued for 14 days
- Treatment ended with doxycycline 200 mg p.o. q24h until re-implantation of TKR

In order to identify the true pathogen multiple biopsies were taken and the prosthesis was sent to a specialized laboratory for sonication.

From the sonicate fluid as well from two of the five biopsies, *Cellulosimicrobium cellulans* was isolated

Re-implantation was performed on 14 July 2016 using the same antibiotic regimen as when the prosthesis was removed.

Systemic antimicrobial therapy was carried out intravenously for 12 days and continued with oral sequential therapy with doxycycline until 24 August 2017.

Post-operatively, wound healing was uneventful and the CRP level dropped to the reference range.

7.2.6 Essentials in the Use of ALBC

Local antibiotics are of benefit in perioperative prophylaxis together with systemic antibiotic prophylaxis if PMMA bone cement is used.

Antibiotic-loaded PMMA bone cement allows us to create custom-made specific local antimicrobial agents for the pathogen. This may be realized by using commercially available bone cement preparations or by admixing suitable antibiotics by hand in the operation theatre.

In one-stage revisions of PJI, knowledge of the pathogen is a prerequisite for specific local antimicrobial therapy.

7

In two-stage revisions of PJI, knowledge of the pathogen is beneficial but it is possible to choose empirical antimicrobial agents. At the time of removal of the TJR, diagnostic efforts including sonication must be made in order to carry out specific antibiotic therapy at the time of re-implantation of a new TJR.

Take-Home Message

- Antibiotic-loaded PMMA bone cement (ALBC) is suitable as carrier for local antibiotics.
- The use of local antibiotics is well established for one-stage-revision procedures in periprosthetic joint infection.
- In two-stage revision procedures, the ALBC spacer becomes a local antibiotic-delivery device.
- Due to standardized mechanical properties, industrially produced ALBC should be used for fixation of total joint replacement whenever effective antibiotics are available in these preparations.

References

Buchholz HW, Engelbrecht H (1970) Über die Depotwirkung einiger Antibiotika bei Vermischung mit dem Kunstharz Palacos. Chirurg 41:511–515

Buchholz HW, Elson RA, Lodenkämper H (1979) The infected joint implant. In McKibbin B (ed) Recent advances in orthopaedics. Churchill Livingstone, New York, pp. 139–161

Chen AF, Parvizi J (2014) Antibiotic-loaded bone cement and periprosthetic joint infection. J Long Term Eff Med Implants 24(2-3):89–97

Costerton JW, Cheng KJ, Geesey GG, Ladd TI, Nickel JC, Dasgupta M, Marrie TJ (1987) Bacterial biofilms in nature and disease. Annu Rev Microbiol 41:435–64

Dunbar MJ (2009) Antibiotic bone cements: their use in routine primary total joint arthroplasty is justified. Orthopedics 32(9): doi: 10.3928/01477447-20090728-20

Espehaug B, Engesaeter LB, Vollset SE, Havelin LI, Langeland N (1997) Antibiotic prophylaxis in total hip arthroplasty. Review of 10,905 primary cemented total hip replacements reported to the Norwegian arthroplasty register, 1987 to 1995.J Bone Joint Surg Br 79(4):590–595

Gehrke T, Zahar A, Kendoff D (2013) One-stage exchange: it all began here. Bone Joint J 95-B[11 Suppl A]:77–83

Gristina AG (1987) Biomaterial-centered infection: microbial adhesion versus tissue integration. Science 237(4822): 1588–1595

Frommelt L (2000) Periprosthetic joint infection – bacteria and the interface between prosthesis and bone. In Learmonth ID (ed) Interfaces in total hip arthroplasty. Springer, London Berlin Heidelberg New York, pp. 153–161

Frommelt L (2007). Antibiotic choices in bone surgery – local therapy using antibiotic-loaded bone cement. In Walenkamp GHIM (ed) Local antibiotics in arthroplasty. State of the art from the interdisciplinary point of view. Georg Thieme Verlag, Stuttgart New York, pp. 59–64

Kühn KD (2014) PMMA cements. Springer, Berlin Heidelberg, ISBN 978-3-642-41535-7

Lewis G (2015) Not all approved antibiotic-loaded PMMA bone cement brands are the same: ranking using the utility materials selection concept. J Mater Sci Mater Med (2015) 26:48. doi:10.1007/s10856-015-5388-4

Mader JT, Calhoun J, Cobos J (1997) In vitro evaluation of antibiotic diffusion from antibiotic-impregnated biodegradable beads and polymethylmethacrylate beads. Antibmicrob Agents Chemother 41:415–418

McLaren ACI, Nugent M, Economopoulos K, Kaul H, Vernon BL, McLemore R (2009). Hand-mixed and premixed antibiotic-loaded bone cement have similar homogeneity. Clin Orthop Relat Res 467(7):1693–1698

Romanò CL, Gala L, Logoluso N, Romanò D, Drago L (2012) Two-stage revision of septic knee prosthesis with articulating knee spacers yields better infection eradication rate than one-stage or two-stage revision with static spacers. Knee Surg Sports Traumatol Arthrosc 20(12):2445–2453

Zahar A (2016) Local antibiotic therapy: Antibiotic loaded cement. In Kendoff D, Morgan-Jones R, Haddad FS (eds) Periprosthetic joint infections. Changing paradigms. Springer International Publishing, Switzerland, pp. 115–124

7.3 The Role of Antibiotic-Loaded Bone Cement in Periprosthetic Joint Infection

Yuhan Chang

7.3.1 Introduction

Total joint arthroplasty (TJA) is currently one of the most frequently performed and most successful surgical procedures in orthopaedics (Ethgen et al. 2004; Learmonth et al. 2007). Infection, however, remains the most common cause of failure of total knee arthroplasty (TKA; 25.2%) and the third most common indication for hip arthroplasty revision (14.7%; Bozic et al. 2009, 2010).

Antibiotic-loaded polymethyl methacrylate (PMMA) bone cements (ALBCs) have been widely used in the prevention and treatment of skeletal infection. The ability to deliver high local concentrations of antimicrobial agents has made ALBC into one of the standard measures for the treatment or prevention of skeletal infection, including periprosthetic joint infection (PJI; Hanssen 2005; Ueng et al. 2012).

7.3.2 Choice and Dose of Antibiotics in ALBCs

Several different antibiotics have been used in ALBCs, with aminoglycosides and vancomycin most commonly used. The dose of antibiotic in ALBCs can simply be divided into low and high dose (Jiranek et al. 2006). The use of ALBCs as a prophylactic measure requires the administration of low doses of antibiotics to avoid adverse mechanical effects on the cement used for the fixation of the prosthesis. In general, low-dose loading of antibiotic in the cement is defined as ≤1 g of powdered antibiotic per 40 g of PMMA bone cement (Jiranek et al. 2006). International industrial standards state that bone cement used for definitive fixation must have an ultimate compressive strength of at least 70 MPa. This standard was established to reduce the incidence of premature cement breakdown (Bridgens et al. 2008; Pelletier et al. 2009). The high-dose ALBCs are used for the treatment of PJI (Leone and Hanssen 2005; Jiranek et al. 2006; Jacofsky et al. 2010). High doses of antibiotics in bone cement have been shown to significantly reduce the cement's mechanical strength and cannot be used in prosthesis fixation (Jiranek et al. 2006). Thus, for therapeutic measures in infection, it has been suggested that the »minimum« dose of antibiotics should be 2 g of vancomycin and 2.4 g of tobramycin or gentamicin, whereas a »typical« dose should be 4 g of vancomycin and 4.8 g of an aminoglycoside.

Gram-positive pathogens including *Staphylococcus aureus* and coagulase-negative staphylococci (CoNS) are the most common organisms implicated in PJI (Tattevin et al. 1999; Zimmerli and Ochsner 2003). However, Gram-negative bacteria (although less commonly associated with PJI) constitute 6–23% of all cases of PJI (Tattevin et al. 1999; Hsieh et al. 2009a). *Pseudomonas aeruginosa* and *Escherichia coli* are the most common Gram-negative bacteria in PJIs (Hsieh et al. 2009a). When using ALBC to prevent or eradicate both Gram-positive and Gram-negative pathogens in PJIs, antibiotics with a broad spectrum of antibacterial activity are the most appropriate choice for ALBC (Chang et al. 2013).

However, the optimal combination of antibiotics in ALBCs is still unclear. Furthermore, the antibiotic release efficacy, antibacterial duration, and antibacterial spectrum of bone cement loaded with various combinations of antibiotics have not been well investigated. In order to provide a wide antibacterial spectrum and long antibacterial duration, ALBCs used as therapeutic measures commonly incorporate two different high-dose antibiotics.

In the author's laboratory, a study was carried out (Hsu et al. 2017) to determine the optimal formulation of ALBC for PJI using both in vitro and in vivo models incorporating various combinations of Gram-positive and Gram-negative antibiotics. The in vitro antibiotic release characteristics and antibacterial capacities of ALBCs loaded with either 4 g of vancomycin or teicoplanin and 4 g of ceftazidime, imipenem, or aztreonam were measured against methicillin-susceptible *S. aureus*, methicillin-resistant *S. aureus*, CoNS, *P. aeruginosa* and *E. coli*. ALBC spacers with superior in vitro antibacterial capacity were then implanted into patients with PJI. Antibiotic concentrations and antibacterial activities of joint fluid at the site of infection were measured during the initial period as well as several months following spacer implantation. Cement samples loaded with vancomycin/ceftazidime or teicoplanin/ceftazidime exhibited equal or longer antibacterial duration against test bacteria as compared with other ALBCs. Joint fluid samples exhibited antibacterial activity against the test micro-organisms including American Type Culture Collection (ATCC) strains and clinically isolated strains. Vancomycin/ceftazidime ALBC provided broad-spectrum antibacterial capacity both in vitro and in vivo and was shown to be a potentially effective therapeutic measure in the treatment of PJIs.

Iarikov et al. reviewed published studies evaluating the types and doses of antibiotics in spacers used in the interim stage of two-stage exchange arthroplasty. They conducted a PubMed search of all clinical study reports evaluating the use of ALBCs in a two-stage hip or knee arthroplasty for treatment of PJI (1988 through August 2011). The authors concluded that the published data are not sufficient to support recommendations on dosages. Prospective randomized trials comparing spacers with different loads of antibiotics are needed in further studies.

7.3.3 ALBC in the Prevention of PJI

Systemic prophylactic antibiotics have been widely accepted as effective agents for reducing the rate of deep infections in TJA (Walenkamp 2001). However, despite their use, a 1–2% prevalence of deep infection was noted in most of the large case series reporting on TJA (Hill et al. 1981; Norden 1985). The use of ALBC was shown to be effective in reducing the rate of early-to-intermediate deep infection after TJA of both the hip (Josefsson et al. 1990) and the knee (Chiu et al. 2002). ALBCs have been widely used in TJA, particularly for patients at high risk of infection (Chiu et al. 2001; Yang et al. 2001; Meding et al. 2003). On the basis of two prospective randomized trials, Chiu et al. reported that cefuroxime-impregnated bone cement was effective in reducing the rate of deep knee infection after TKA (Chiu et al. 2002), particularly in the case of diabetic patients (Chiu et al. 2001). The use of ALBC as a prophylactic measure requires the administration of low doses of antibiotics to avoid adverse mechanical effects on the cement used for the fixation of the prosthesis. In another study, bone cement loaded with low-dose oxacillin or vancomycin (1 g antibiotic in 40 g PMMA) released the antibiotic for up to 48 h, thereby retaining its antibacterial activity after implantation (Ueng et al. 2012). These results indicate that bone cement loaded with low-dose antibiotics could release the antibiotic effectively in an in vivo environment. The use of low-dose ALBC in TKA was able to prolong the antibacterial activity in the joint fluid after the discontinuation of intravenous prophylactic antibiotics. This longer duration of antibacterial activity in joint fluid may contribute to a lower infection rate in TKA performed using ALBC (Ueng et al. 2012).

Several commercial premixed ALBC products have been approved by the United States Food and Drug Administration (Jiranek et al. 2006). All of these commercial premixed ALBCs contain aminoglycoside combined with either tobramycin or gentamicin. Today, surgeons continue to mix antibiotics to PMMA by hand, if a specific antibiotic is not premixed commercially available. The primary drawback of using commercially premixed ALBC is that the antibiotic used is dictated by the bone cement chosen, and consequently surgeons are unable to tailor the antibiotic to a specific organism. Vendor marketing information claims commercial premixing saves operative time and that the antibiotic is more homogeneously mixed in the ALBC, leading to better drug delivery. We tested two commercial premixed ALBCs: Palacos® R+G, which contains 1 g gentamicin in 40 g PMMA, and Simplex® P, which contains 1 g tobramycin in 40 g PMMA (Chang et al. 2013). The premixed gentamicin-loaded ALBC showed a broad antibacterial spectrum against all of the tested bacteria, including Gram-positive and Gram-negative strains. Moreover, it provided the longest antibacterial duration against MSSA, CoNS, *P. aeruginosa* and *E. coli*. The premixed tobramycin ALBC also provided a broad antibacterial spectrum against all of the tested bacteria with the exception of MRSA. As compared with hand-mixed ALBCs, the commercial premixed gentamicin-loaded ALBC provided an equal or longer antibacterial duration against different bacteria in this study. However, this superiority in antibacterial activity was not observed in the premixed tobramycin ALBC as compared with hand-mixed ALBCs. The results indicated that not all available commercial premixed ALBCs always exhibit superior antibacterial activity over hand-mixed ALBCs (Chang et al. 2013).

7.3.4 ALBC in Two-Stage Exchange Arthroplasty of PJI

Two-stage exchange arthroplasty is currently considered the gold standard in the treatment of chronic PJI. The application of ALBC spacers has become a common approach in the management of patients between exchange arthroplasty stages (Hsieh et al. 2004, 2005). Although there are a number of studies on the efficacy of two-stage exchange arthroplasty, there is still ongoing debate as to the type of spacer that should be used between the stages. The traditional use of antibiotic-loaded cement beads or blocks works well to fill the dead space that is created at the time of resection arthroplasty and provides a high local concentration of antibiotics (Hovelius and Josefsson 1979; Duncan and Masri 1994).

The hip or knee joint is left in pseudo-arthrosis or static status with limited function. The second-stage procedure may be very complicated because of soft tissue contractures, distorted tissue planes, disuse osteopoenia and bone loss, especially when there is a long interval between resection and re-implantation (Younger et al 1998; Fehring et al. 2000). In the author's previous study, the results of hip PJI treated with antibiotic-impregnated cement beads or antibiotic-loaded cement prosthesis implantation after resection arthroplasty were compared (Hsieh et al. 2004). Antibiotic-impregnated cement beads or antibiotic-loaded cement prostheses both provided equal infection eradication rates. Hsieh et al. noted that the use of a spacer prosthesis was associated with: a higher hip functional score, a shorter hospital stay, and better walking capacity in the interim period; a decreased operative time, less blood loss, and a lower transfusion requirement at the time of re-implantation; and fewer postoperative dislocations (Hsieh et al. 2004). The use of a cement spacer prosthesis preserves soft tissue tension and planes, making the re-implantation procedure much easier to perform. Furthermore, the post-operative dislocation rate following re-implantation after resection arthroplasty was significantly reduced with the use of cement spacer prostheses. An ideal spacer should be durable, cost-effective, easily available, and effective in controlling infection while allowing for function during the interim periods. Traditionally, in knee PJI, static cement spacers have been used, but recent results indicate that articulating spacers may have some benefit such as interim functionality, preservation of bone stock, and improved final range of motion (Emerson et al. 2002; Park et al. 2010). Moreover, the static cement spacer is always associated with different degrees of bone loss (Fehring et al. 2000). The articulating cement spacer can maintain soft tissue tension with ligamentous stability, reduce the severity of disused muscle atrophy and disused osteoporosis, and conserve bone well enough to allow for less constrained types of prostheses thereby making the re-implantation procedure much easier to perform. However, prosthetic spacers invariably cost more than static cement spacers. Therefore, an articulating cement spacer prosthesis is a better choice in hip or knee PJI treatment after the resection arthroplasty as compared with antibiotic-loaded beads or static spacers.

7.3.5 Antibiotic Release Efficacy of ALBC

When antibiotics are used in cement, the release efficacy is the critical point determining the antibacterial activities. High porosity would be expected to increase the release of antibiotics from ALBC. The antibiotic-release kinetics of ALBCs depend on the penetration of dissolution fluids into the polymer matrix and subsequent diffusion of the dissolved drug from the ALBCs. To increase antibiotic release from ALBCs, soluble fillers such as glycine, xylitol, sucrose, or erythritol can be added into the bone cement to increase its porosity and consequently increase the penetration of dissolution fluids (McLaren et al. 2004; McLaren et al. 2006; McLaren et al 2007). Many powder antibiotics are effectively released from bone cement (Hsieh et al. 2004; Chang et al. 2011; Ueng et al. 2012). In con-

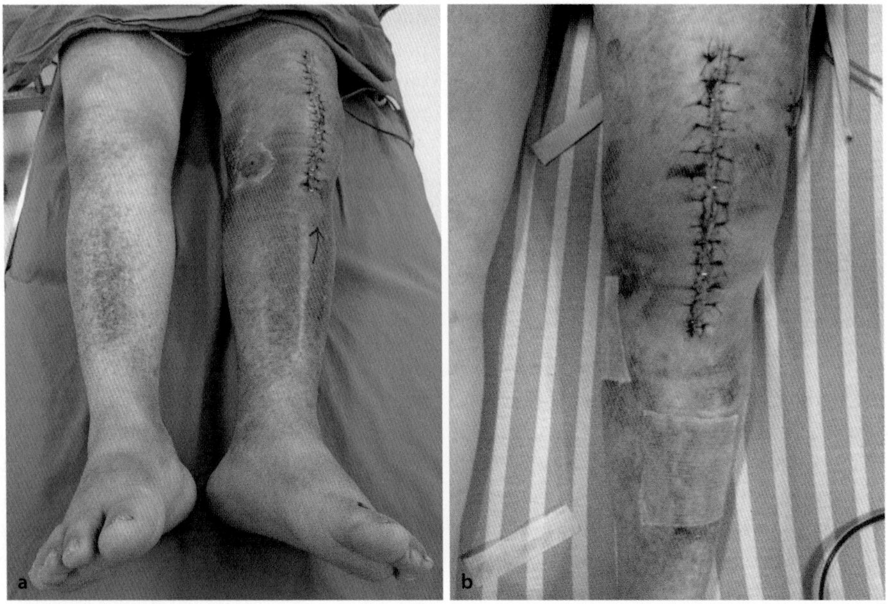

Fig. 7.18 **a** A 68-year-old female patient suffering from periprosthetic joint infection of the knee was treated with two-stage exchange arthroplasty. Two days after the implantation of an antibiotic-loaded bone cement spacer (vancomycin and ceftazidime), severe pruritus developed, initially localized to the operated knee but with subsequent spread. Erythematous, pruritic infiltrate extending from the knee to the whole body can be seen. **b** The pruritus and erythema receded 3 days after the removal of the antibiotic-loaded cement spacer

trast to the use of powder antibiotics, liquid antibiotics have not been widely used in bone cement because the mechanical integrity of the cement decreases by up to 50% when liquid antibiotics are added (Marks et al. 1976). Liquid gentamicin in bone cement has been reported to elute effectively and maintain its bactericidal activity (Seldes et al. 2005; Hsieh et al. 2009b), and liquid gentamicin combined with vancomycin in the same cement sample demonstrated a positive reciprocal effect on the elution of both antibiotics (Hsieh et al. 2009b). The positive effect on the elution of antibiotic by addition of liquid gentamicin to bone cement is caused by increased porosity of the cement. In a previous study, we showed that adding vancomycin or amphotericin B antibiotic powder in distilled water before mixing with bone cement can significantly improve the antibiotic-release efficacy compared to loading ALBC with the same dose of antibiotic powder (Chang et al. 2014).

7.3.6 Concerns and Complications

Although the use of ALBCs was shown to be effective in reducing the rate of deep infection after TJA (Chiu et al. 2001, 2002), the issue of whether to use ALBC routinely for prophylaxis against deep periprosthetic infection when performing primary or aseptic revision TJA is still controversial. The primary concerns regarding ALBC include the potential for detrimental effects on the mechanical structural characteristics of PMMA when antibiotics are admixed, systemic toxicity related to high antibiotic levels eluted from the cement, development of drug-resistant bacteria, allergic reactions to the specific antibiotic used, and the cost. Renal toxicity of vancomycin is notorious, and acute renal injury is attributable to the use of ALBCs in the treatment of PJI (van Raaij et al. 2002; Luu et al. 2013). From Hsieh's series of 46 patients with hip PJIs, however, no systemic side effects were noted after using high doses of vancomycin and aztreonam in bone cement (Hsieh ct al. 2006). Furthermore, in a series of 36 knee PJIs, Springer et al. reported no systemic adverse effects from the use of high-dose vancomycin and gentamicin in cement spacers (Springer et al. 2004).

There are some in vitro data suggesting that prolonged exposure of organisms to sub-inhibitory levels of antibiotics encourages mutational adaptations that confer resistance (Kendall et al. 1996; van de Belt et al. 2000). Hope et al. reported that a gentamicin-resistant infection developed in 88% of the patients who had gentamicin-loaded bone cement used in the primary arthroplasty compared with only 16% when plain cement was utilized (Hope et al. 1989). By contrast, Hansen et al. noted that the routine prophylactic use of ALBC for primary TKA did not lead to significant changes in the infecting pathogen profile (Hansen et al. 2014). The proportion of PJI cases caused by *S. aureus*, CoNS, or non-staphylococcal species did not change significantly following the introduction of ALBC. Hansen's report indicates that the routine prophylactic use of ALBC has not led to significant increases in antimicrobial resistance patterns of pathogens causing PJI. Therefore, this controversial issue needs further investigation.

Severe allergy reaction could be induced by ALBC, especially in high-dose ALBC (■ Fig. 7.18). If ALBC-induced severe allergic reaction is suspected, the ALBC spacer or beads should be removed as soon as possible.

7.3.7 Conclusion

Low-dose ALBC can be used for prosthesis fixation and they reduce the incidence of PJI significantly as compared with prostheses fixed with plain cement. High-dose ALBC has capacity for delivery of very high local antibiotic concentrations in the treatment of PJI.

Take-Home Message

- Infection remains the most common cause of failure in total knee arthroplasty (25.2%) and the third most common indication for hip arthroplasty revision (14.7%).
- When using ALBC to prevent or eradicate both Gram-positive and Gram-negative pathogens in PJIs, antibiotics with a broad spectrum of antibacterial activity are the most appropriate choice for ALBC loading.
- The use of low-dose ALBC in total knee arthroplasty (TKA) was able to prolong the antibacterial activity in the joint fluid after the discontinuation of intravenous prophylactic antibiotics. This longer duration of antibacterial activity in joint fluid may contribute to a lower infection rate in TKA performed using ALBC.
- An articulating cement spacer prosthesis is a better choice in hip or knee PJI treatment after the resection arthroplasty as compared with antibiotic-loaded beads or static spacers.

References

Bozic KJ, Kurtz SM, Lau E, Ong K, Vail TP, Berry DJ (2009) The epidemiology of revision total hip arthroplasty in the United States. J Bone Joint Surg Am 91:128–133

Bozic KJ, Kurtz SM, Lau E, Ong K, Chiu V, Vail TP, Rubash HE, Berry DJ (2010) The epidemiology of revision total knee arthroplasty in the United States. Clin Orthop Relat Res 468:45–51

Bridgens J, Davies S, Tilley L, Norman P, Stockley I (2008) Orthopaedic bone cement: do we know what we are using? J Bone Joint Surg Br 90:643–647

Chang Y, Chen WC, Hsieh PH, Chen DW, Lee MS, Shih HN, Ueng SW (2011) In vitro activities of daptomycin-, vancomycin-, and teicoplanin-loaded polymethylmethacrylate against methicillin-susceptible, methicillin-resistant, and vancomycin-intermediate strains of Staphylococcus aureus. Antimicrob Agents Chemother 55:5480–5484

Chang Y, Tai CL, Hsieh PH, Ueng SW (2013) Gentamicin in bone cement: A potentially more effective prophylactic measure of infectionin joint arthroplasty. Bone Joint Res 2:220–226

Chang YH, Tai CL, Hsu HY, Hsieh PH, Lee MS, Ueng SW (2014) Liquid antibiotics in bone cement: an effective way to improve the efficiency of antibiotic release in antibiotic loaded bone cement. Bone Joint Res 3:246–251

Chiu FY, Lin CF, Chen CM, Lo WH, Chaung TY (2001) Cefuroxime-impregnated cement at primary total knee arthroplasty in diabetes mellitus. A prospective, randomised study. J Bone Joint Surg Br 83:691–695

Chiu FY, Chen CM, Lin CF, Lo WH (2002) Cefuroxime-impregnated cement in primary total knee arthroplasty: a prospective, randomized study of three hundred and forty knees. J Bone Joint Surg Am 84-A:759–762

Duncan CP, Masri BA (1994) The role of antibiotic-loaded cement in the treatment of an infection after a hip replacement. J Bone Joint Surg Am 76:1742–1751

Emerson RH, Jr., Muncie M, Tarbox TR, Higgins LL (2002) Comparison of a static with a mobile spacer in total knee infection. Clin Orthop Relat Res:132–138

Ethgen O, Bruyere O, Richy F, Dardennes C, Reginster JY (2004) Health-related quality of life in total hip and total knee

arthroplasty. A qualitative and systematic review of the literature. J Bone Joint Surg Am 86-A:963–974
Fehring TK, Odum S, Calton TF, Mason JB (2000) Articulating versus static spacers in revision total knee arthroplasty for sepsis. The Ranawat Award. Clin Orthop Relat Res 9–16
Hansen EN, Adeli B, Kenyon R, Parvizi J (2014) Routine use of antibiotic laden bone cement for primary total knee arthroplasty: impact on infecting microbial patterns and resistance profiles. J Arthroplasty 29:1123–1127
Hanssen AD (2005) Local antibiotic delivery vehicles in the treatment of musculoskeletal infection. Clin Orthop Relat Res 91–96
Hill C, Flamant R, Mazas F, Evrard J (1981) Prophylactic cefazolin versus placebo in total hip replacement. Report of a multicentre double-blind randomised trial. Lancet 1:795–796
Hope PG, Kristinsson KG, Norman P, Elson RA (1989) Deep infection of cemented total hip arthroplasties caused by coagulase-negative staphylococci. J Bone Joint Surg Br 71:851–855
Hovelius L, Josefsson G (1979) An alternative method for exchange operation of infected arthroplasty. Acta Orthop Scand 50:93–96
Hsieh PH, Shih CH, Chang YH, Lee MS, Shih HN, Yang WE (2004) Two-stage revision hip arthroplasty for infection: comparison between the interim use of antibiotic-loaded cement beads and a spacer prosthesis. J Bone Joint Surg Am 86-A:1989–1997
Hsieh PH, Shih CH, Chang YH, Lee MS, Yang WE, Shih HN (2005) Treatment of deep infection of the hip associated with massive bone loss: two-stage revision with an antibiotic-loaded interim cement prosthesis followed by reconstruction with allograft. J Bone Joint Surg Br 87:770–775
Hsieh PH, Chang YH, Chen SH, Ueng SW, Shih CH (2006) High concentration and bioactivity of vancomycin and aztreonam eluted from Simplex cement spacers in two-stage revision of infected hip implants: a study of 46 patients at an average follow-up of 107 days. J Orthop Res 24:1615–1621
Hsieh PH, Lee MS, Hsu KY, Chang YH, Shih HN, Ueng SW (2009a) Gram-negative prosthetic joint infections: risk factors and outcome of treatment. Clin Infect Dis 49:1036–1043
Hsieh PH, Tai CL, Lee PC, Chang YH (2009b) Liquid gentamicin and vancomycin in bone cement: a potentially more cost-effective regimen. J Arthroplasty 24:125–130
Hsu Y-H, Hu C-C, Hsieh P-H, Shih H-N, Ueng SWN, Chang Y (2017) Vancomycin and ceftazidime in bone cement as a potentially effective treatment for knee periprosthetic joint infection. J Bone Joint Surg Am 99(3):223–231. DOI:10.2106/JBJS.16.00290
Jacofsky DJ, Della Valle CJ, Meneghini RM, Sporer SM, Cercek RM, American Academy of Orthopaedics (2010) Revision total knee arthroplasty: what the practicing orthopaedic surgeon needs to know. J Bone Joint Surg Am 92:1282–1292
Jiranek WA, Hanssen AD, Greenwald AS (2006) Antibiotic-loaded bone cement for infection prophylaxis in total joint replacement. J Bone Joint Surg Am 88:2487–2500
Josefsson G, Gudmundsson G, Kolmert L, Wijkstrom S (1990) Prophylaxis with systemic antibiotics versus gentamicin bone cement in total hip arthroplasty. A five-year survey of 1688 hips. Clin Orthop Relat Res:173–178
Kendall RW, Duncan CP, Smith JA, Ngui-Yen JH (1996) Persistence of bacteria on antibiotic loaded acrylic depots. A reason for caution. Clin Orthop Relat Res:273–280
Learmonth ID, Young C, Rorabeck C (2007) The operation of the century: total hip replacement. Lancet 370:1508–1519
Leone JM, Hanssen AD (2005) Management of infection at the site of a total knee arthroplasty. J Bone Joint Surg Am 87:2335–2348
Luu A, Syed F, Raman G, Bhalla A, Muldoon E, Hadley S, Smith E, Rao M (2013) Two-stage arthroplasty for prosthetic joint infection: a systematic review of acute kidney injury, systemic toxicity and infection control. J Arthroplasty 28:1490-1498 e1491
Marks KE, Nelson CL, Lautenschlager EP (1976) Antibiotic-impregnated acrylic bone cement. J Bone Joint Surg Am 58:358–364
McLaren AC, Nelson CL, McLaren SG, De CGR (2004) The effect of glycine filler on the elution rate of gentamicin from acrylic bone cement: a pilot study. Clin Orthop Relat Res 25–27
McLaren AC, McLaren SG, Smeltzer M (2006) Xylitol and glycine fillers increase permeability of PMMA to enhance elution of daptomycin. Clin Orthop Relat Res 451:25–28
McLaren AC, McLaren SG, Hickmon MK (2007) Sucrose, xylitol, and erythritol increase PMMA permeability for depot antibiotics. Clin Orthop Relat Res 461:60–63
Meding JB, Reddleman K, Keating ME, Klay A, Ritter MA, Faris PM, Berend ME (2003) Total knee replacement in patients with diabetes mellitus. Clin Orthop Relat Res doi:10.1097/01.blo.0000093002.90435.56:208–216
Norden CW (1985) Prevention of bone and joint infections. Am J Med 78:229–232
Park SJ, Song EK, Seon JK, Yoon TR, Park GH (2010) Comparison of static and mobile antibiotic-impregnated cement spacers for the treatment of infected total knee arthroplasty. Int Orthop 34:1181–1186
Pelletier MH, Malisano L, Smitham PJ, Okamoto K, Walsh WR (2009) The compressive properties of bone cements containing large doses of antibiotics. J Arthroplasty 24:454–460
Seldes RM, Winiarsky R, Jordan LC, Baldini T, Brause B, Zodda F, Sculco TP (2005) Liquid gentamicin in bone cement: a laboratory study of a potentially more cost-effective cement spacer. J Bone Joint Surg Am 87:268–272
Springer BD, Lee GC, Osmon D, Haidukewych GJ, Hanssen AD, Jacofsky DJ (2004) Systemic safety of high-dose antibiotic-loaded cement spacers after resection of an infected total knee arthroplasty. Clin Orthop Relat Res:47–51
Tattevin P, Cremieux AC, Pottier P, Huten D, Carbon C (1999) Prosthetic joint infection: when can prosthesis salvage be considered? Clin Infect Dis 29:292–295

Ueng SW, Hsieh PH, Shih HN, Chan YS, Lee MS, Chang Y (2012) Antibacterial activity of joint fluid in cemented total-knee arthroplasty: an in vivo comparative study of polymethylmethacrylate with and without antibiotic loading. Antimicrob Agents Chemother 56:5541–5546

van de Belt H, Neut D, Schenk W, van Horn JR, van der Mei HC, Busscher HJ (2000) Gentamicin release from polymethylmethacrylate bone cements and Staphylococcus aureus biofilm formation. Acta Orthop Scand 71:625–629

van Raaij TM, Visser LE, Vulto AG, Verhaar JA (2002) Acute renal failure after local gentamicin treatment in an infected total knee arthroplasty. J Arthroplasty 17:948-950

Walenkamp GH (2001) Gentamicin PMMA beads and other local antibiotic carriers in two-stage revision of total knee infection: a review. J Chemother 13 Spec No 1:66–72

Yang K, Yeo SJ, Lee BP, Lo NN (2001) Total knee arthroplasty in diabetic patients: a study of 109 consecutive cases. J Arthroplasty 16:102–106

Younger AS, Duncan CP, Masri BA (1998) Treatment of infection associated with segmental bone loss in the proximal part of the femur in two stages with use of an antibiotic-loaded interval prosthesis. J Bone Joint Surg Am 80: 60–69

Zimmerli W, Ochsner PE (2003) Management of infection associated with prosthetic joints. Infection 31:99–108

7.4 PMMA Cements in Revision Surgery

Ashutosh Malhotra, Elke Lieb, Christoph Berberich, and Klaus-Dieter Kühn

7.4.1 Introduction

Polymethyl methacrylate (PMMA), commonly known as bone cement, is the most frequently used material to fix a prosthesis to the bone. This special acrylic material has been shown to have a decisive role for the success of cemented total joint replacement by transferring the load between the bone and prosthesis (Breusch and Malchau 2005; Deb 2008). All cements are originally developed from dental acrylics and many clinical investigations have proven the non-toxicity of bone cements in joint replacement (Smith 2005; Kühn 2014a). Chemically, such cold curing two-component systems are Plexiglas® with special additives suitable for clinical use. Especially the addition of anti-infective agents to the PMMA powder and their release characteristics from the outer surface of the cement matrix allows antibiotic-loaded bone cements (ALBCs) to function as a local drug delivery system (DDS; Breusch and Kühn 2003). The efficacy of local antibiotics (AB) is based on the concept of providing a protecting antimicrobial drug film, which develops immediately after cement implantation.

PMMA cement continues to be one of the most enduring materials used in orthopaedic surgery. However, more and more brands and various types of cement have come on the market over the past years. For primary fixation, PMMA cement fills and levels off the implant–bone interface and stabilizes quickly the metallic implant in the bone tissue. Furthermore, the cement improves the even load distribution and gradually stiffens the cancellous bone around the prosthesis. ALBC has been successfully used for prophylactic purposes to prevent the bacterial colonization on metallic prostheses. In line with this function, usually a broad-spectrum antibiotic is added to the powder, e.g. aminoglycosides such as gentamicin or tobramycin in concentrations of 1.25–2.5% with respect to the powder fraction. The high initial release of gentamicin out of the cement matrix by diffusion leads to high local concentrations in the joint cavity and bactericidal efficacy against most of the germs (approximately 70%) responsible for periprosthetic joint infection (PJI), thereby reducing the risk of a deep infection (Parvizi et al. 2008). The high local antibiotic concentration provides an excellent colonization barrier for germs and prevents the subsequent formation of a biofilm on implant surfaces (Costerton et al. 1999).

Since any major surgical intervention poses an infection risk for patients, preventive actions are necessary. In this context, the efficacy of local AB that form a protective coat immediately after cement implantation plays a significant role. ALBCs have been shown to effectively reduce the risk of infections in primary arthroplasty.

The Role of ALBC in Arthroplasty

- ALBC = The PMMA cement surface acts locally as a barrier to bacterial colonization (Frommelt 2007), in particular at the implant site.
- ALBC = The use of ALBC is effective in preventing PJI with a favourable cost-efficiency profile using standardized cost and infection rates (Sanz-Ruiz et al. 2016).

For revision surgery, a single AB agent might not be sufficient. The prophylactic role of ALBCs is here even more important owing to the fact that often multiple revised patients were exposed to significantly higher infection risks. In addition, revision surgeries are typically of longer duration with the surrounding tissue being often less vascularized, which further compromises the immune defence. In addition, it must be taken into account that the implanted revision prosthesis is generally bigger and bone grafts are often necessary. Only a few cements are explicitly endorsed for use in revisions procedures (Tab. 7.7). In such revision cements, the powder component contains more than one antibiotic and the content of these drugs exceeds a volume proportion of 2.5%.

7.4.2 What Are Revision PMMA Cements?

Revision PMMA cements have specific functions compared with ALBC.

Revision Bone Cements
- Contains more than one AB or anti-infective substance
- Contains AB or drug concentrations higher than 2.5%
- AB combination results in a synergetic and synergistic (elution and/or efficacy) effect

Among currently marketed ALBCs, Stryker endorses the use of Antibiotic Simplex™ P with tobramycin (Simplex® T) bone cement for the fixation of prostheses to living bone in the second stage of a two-stage revision for total joint arthroplasty (Sterling et al. 2003). Simplex® T is offered as a revision bone cement on the market although there is no evident clinical rationale backing this claim (http://www.stryker.com/en-us/products/Orthopaedics/BoneCementSubstitutes/index.htm). Tobramycin as an AB is chemically similar to gentamicin, the spectrum is comparable and the amount of T within the Simplex® T cement is 1–40 g powder. All other revision cements contain two different ABs and the amount within the powder varies from 2.5% to 7.5%.

Antibiotic Simplex® with erythromycin and colistin (E+Col; Ruzaimi et al. 2006) was the first ALBC on the market that contained two AB (Rosenthal et al. 1976). However, the AB colistin and erythromycin do not cover the same pathogen spectrum as gentamicin. Further, it should also be pointed out that erythromycin acts bacteriostatically, but not bactericidally, the latter being a much preferred property of AB in joint infections. European and US resistance surveillance data show a relatively high degree of primary resistance of staphylococci and Enterobacteriaceae to erythromycin. The efficacy of erythromycin is limited in general to Gram-positive bacteria (pneumococci, *Clostridium* spp., *Corynebacteriae*, α-haemolytic streptococci of group A), which play only a minor role in PJI. Although colistin has experienced a revival in recent years because of its broad coverage of resistant Gram-negative bacteria (e.g. *Pseudomonas* spp.), this antibiotic is not ideal as it is more hydrophobic and less soluble in water leading to a rather low release of PMMA cement.

Mode of Action of E+Col Combination
- Erythromycin: inhibits protein synthesis on ribosomes
- Colistin: changes the permeability of the cytoplasmic membrane
- Erythromycin: acts bacteriostatically

Both Copal® G+C and Refobacin® Revision are gentamicin- (1 g) and clindamycin(1 g)-containing PMMA cements. This antibiotic combination acts synergistically with respect to the antimicrobial spectrum and mode of action. This combination targets even anaerobic bacteria, which are of growing importance as PJI pathogens, especially in low grade infections as well as streptococci, which are often found in late haematogenous infections and at low-grade infection sites. Another obvious advantage of this AB combination is its synergetic effect via a mutually increased elution from the PMMA matrix. Because of their high local diffusion, the concentration of gentamicin and clindamycin is significantly higher than the minimum inhibitory concentration (MIC) and the minimum bactericidal concentration (MBC) for several days and weeks at the surface of the cement. In addition, being a rath-

Tab. 7.7 Overall portfolio of commercially available revision ALBCs on the market

ALBC	Simplex® T	Antibiotic Simplex® E+Col	Copal® G+C	Copal® G+V	Refobacin® Revision	VancoGenx®
Polymer	PMMA with BPO + MA-styrene	PMMA with BPO + MA-styrene	MA/MMA 2x	MA/MMA 2x	MA/MMA 2x	PMMA+MA-styrene
Opacifier	Barium sulphate	Barium sulphate	Zirconium dioxide	Zirconium dioxide	Zirconium dioxide	Barium sulphate
BPO	BPO	BPO	BPO	BPO	BPO	BPO
Antibiotics	Tobramycin (1 g) –	Erythromycin (0.5 g) Colistin (0.25 g)	Gentamicin (1 g) Clindamycin (1 g)	Gentamicin (0.5 g) Vancomycin (2 g)	Gentamicin (1 g) Clindamycin (1 g)	Gentamicin (1 g) Vancomycin (1 g)
Colouring agent	–	–	E 141	E 141	–	–
Liquid	MMA+DmpT+HQ	MMA+DmpT+HQ	MMA+DmpT+HQ+ E 141	MMA+DmpT+HQ+ E 141	MMA+DmpT+HQ+ E 141	MMA+DmpT+HQ
Viscosity	medium	medium	high	high/medium	high/medium	medium/low
Handling at 23°C Sticky [min]	2.45	2.45	1.00	1.30	1.30	2.30
Working [min]	2.30	2.30	3.30	3.00	3.00	2.00
Setting [min]	10.30	10.30	7.00	9.00	9.00	10.00
Powder sterilization	Gamma	Gamma	Eto	Gamma	Eto	Gamma
P:L ratio	2:1	2:1	2:1	2:1	2:1	3:1
BPO:DmpT ratio	DmpT surplus (little)	DmpT surplus (little)	DmpT surplus (high)	DmpT surplus (high)	DmpT surplus (little)	BPO surplus (high)
Indication	Primary + revision	Primary + revision	Primary + revision	Revision	Primary + revision	Revision

MMA methylmethacrylate, *MA* methylacrylate, *BPO* benzoyl peroxide, *DmpT* dimethyl-para-toluidine, *HQ* hydroquinone, *P* powder, *L* liquid, *Eto* ethylene oxide er small molecule, clindamycin shows excellent bone and tissue penetration and exerts an intracellular bactericidal activity (Gehrke et al. 2001; Zimmerli et al. 2004; Fink et al. 2011; Kühn 2014a; Valour et al. 2015).

As proof of concept for the clinical benefit exhibited by addition of two AB to cement serves the observation that such cements are more protective against biofilm formation than cements containing only one antibiotic in a lower concentration (Ensing et al. 2008). Indeed, a recent clinical study has shown that the incidence of superficial and deep infections was significantly reduced in the presence of this double-loaded ALBC if applied in patients at high risk for infection (e.g. patients suffering from intracapsular neck fractures and treated with cemented hemiprostheses; Sprowson et al. 2013).

7

Consequently, in light of the clinical data, this AB combination can be recommended not only in septic revision cases where the antibiogram reveals sensitivity of the germ(s) to gentamicin and clindamycin, but also in high-risk patients where the risk of infection is higher than »normal«. Another indication for use could be those revision cases where the diagnosis is difficult and »uncertain« (e.g. culture-negative PJI cases) or in those situations where contaminations with anaerobic bacteria such as *Propionibacterium acnes* occur relatively frequently (e.g. shoulder arthroplasty).

Another hallmark of such AB combinations is the observation that the presence of two AB with different modes of action virtually rules out the risk of development of concomitant resistance to these two substances. Antibiotic combination therapies are a hallmark of all those chronic infections prone to resistance development, which require a prolonged antibiotic treatment including tuberculosis or eradication of *Helicobacter pylori* in peptic ulcers and gastritis.

Mode of Action of G+C Combination

- Gentamicin: disturbs the translation of mRNA on the 30s ribosomes
- Clindamycin: binds to 50s ribosomes and inhibits protein synthesis
- Clindamycin: usually acts bacteriostatically but locally in higher concentrations bactericidally

Despite the high local concentration of both ABs, systemic side effects are not a major clinical concern as evidenced by a safety study showing that gentamicin and clindamycin peak only transiently in serum and urine after local use and then quickly fall below detectable levels. Infection was resolved in all monitored patients during the observation period of 1 year (Gehrke et al 2001).

The choice of antibiotic added to ALBC is always dependent on the germ causing the infection. The idea of having different antibiotic combinations arose after the emergence of resistant bacteria. In particular, when it comes to MRSA resistances, vancomycin is the antibiotic of choice and is currently available with bone cements: Copal® G+V and VancoGenx® (Schmolders et al. 2014; Kühn et al. 2016). Both contain gentamicin and vancomycin in combination. Copal® G+V contains 0.5 g gentamicin and 2 g vancomycin, VancoGenx® contains 1 g gentamicin and 1 g vancomycin. Methicillin-resistant *S. aureus* (MRSA) is an important factor of hospital morbidity and mortality. However, of equal or even higher clinical concern are the growing rates of methicillin resistance *S. epidermidis* (MRSE). Current records indicate that MRSA/MRSE infections lead to significantly longer hospital stays, higher costs and an overall increase in mortality.

Mode of Action of G+V Combination

- Gentamicin: disturbs the translation of mRNA on the 30s ribosomes
- Vancomycin: inhibits the bacterial cell wall cross-link synthesis

In all those PJI cases in which a MRSA/MRSE pathogen has been identified, vancomycin-loaded PMMA cement is the AB of choice for local administration during revision arthroplasty. The highly synergistic effect of both AB gentamicin and vancomycin has been well known to the infectious disease specialist for many years (Mulazimoglu et al. 1996; Watanakunakorn 1982; Watanakunakorn and Tisone 1982a, b).

Again, it is highly recommended to combine vancomycin with gentamicin, as vancomycin alone diffuses very slowly out of the cement matrix because of its big size, structure and relative hydrophobicity. The synergetic elution effect with gentamicin ensures a far better diffusion of vancomycin (and gentamicin) leading to a strong antimicrobial effect against various MRSA strains (Bertazzoni Minelli et al. 2011; Kühn et al. 2016).

A reduction of the infection risk by a combined administration of systemic and local antibiotics is reported by several clinical studies and in arthroplasty registers (Balato et al. 2015; Colas et al. 2015; Jämsen et al. 2009; Bini et al. 2016). A comparison of the pharmacokinetics of systemic and local AB shows clear differences: Systemically applied AB build up quickly and are highly concentrated in serum and parenchymatous organs. By contrast, locally applied AB provide high concentrations in difficult-to-access body departments. Therefore, poorly vascularized areas such as bone tissue and joint spaces in total joint arthroplasty can successfully be reached by administration of local AB. Furthermore, the use of a combination of different antibiotic classes with different modes of actions often results in a synergistic and thus improved infection prophylaxis efficacy.

Taken together, it can be concluded that systemically given cephalosporins and locally applied aminoglycosides widen the antimicrobial spectrum and represent two independent security levels (Kühn et al 2016).

7.4.3 Role of Revision PMMA Cements in Surgery

Generally, it is important to have a clear treatment strategy (algorithm) for exchange revision procedures in PJI in mind. From a microbiological point of view, knowledge of the causative pathogen and its resistances, as well as the choice of the appropriate anti-infective agent(s), is mandatory for a successful eradication of the infection. As mentioned earlier, the combination of an aminoglycoside AB with a further drug component is often recommended.

As in the prophylactic situation, the administration of local AB to support treatment of an infection follows two rationales:

1. From a pharmacokinetic point of view, both administration routes should complement each other. Systemic AB provide high concentrations in serum and parenchymatous organs, while local AB released from PMMA provide high concentrations in the otherwise difficult-to-access departments, such as bone tissue and joint spaces, because of the poor vascularization of these tissues (Valour et al. 2015).
2. From an antimicrobial efficacy point of view, the mode and target of action of the systemic AB (often a cephalosporin for prophylactic purposes) are complemented by the action of the aminoglycoside gentamicin, or by its combination with other ABs. This does not only widen the antimicrobial spectrum, but represents »two independent security levels« in case the systemic AB prophylaxis has not been given at the correct time and/or in the correct dose prior to incision. The local AB barrier may also be effective in cases of primary resistance of bacterial contaminants to the systemic AB.

Use of ALBC has been common practice for a long time for the fixation of revision implants after two-stage revision procedures, as well as for the manufacture of interim spacers in the time interval between the first and second stage.

Claims for Revision PMMA Cements

- For fixation of revision implants
- For manufacturing of PMMA spacer (interim prostheses)
- Sometimes for fixation of primary implants in high-risk patients
- Containing more than one antibiotic of different antibiotic groups
- Containing more than 2 g of antibiotic powder to 40 g of PMMA powder

As already mentioned, AB locally released from cement matrix do not result in a significant systemic uptake of the active ingredient into organs and body compartments other than bone and joint tissue. This can be explained by the specific kinetics of release of the AB from the PMMA surface with a high initial elution rate, followed by constant release over several days. An absolute prerequisite of the antimicrobial effect of ALBC is a local AB concentration well above the minimal inhibitory concentration (MIC) and minimal bactericidal concentration (MBC) of those bacteria that may cause PJI after implantation of the prosthesis. Low-dose (0.5–1 g of AB) ALBC used in primary arthroplasty should in principle fulfil the requirement to act as a colonization barrier. However, according to several in vitro and clinical studies, the quantity of eluted AB and the duration of the AB release vary significantly among different commercial brands of ALBCs, thus suggesting careful selection of the ALBC brand (Anagnostakos et al 2006; Frommelt and Kühn 2005). It must be taken into account that the amount of antibiotics within PMMA powder does not correlate with the release. There are a lot of other important cement characteristics that significantly influence the elution properties (Kühn 2014a).

Being a strict concentration-dependent bactericidal AB, the absolute concentration of gentamicin is an important parameter of its efficacy to prevent biofilm formation of even intermediate resistant germs in the »race for the surface« (Gristina et al. 1988) together with the systemic AB prophylaxis. Once a biofilm has been formed, the MIC is increased by a factor of at least 1,000 because of the sessile bacterial phenotype (Kühn 2014b). Eradication of biofilm bacteria is therefore a great challenge requiring the complete explantation of the biofilm-contaminated implant components, followed by radical surgical debridement of neighbouring bone and soft tissue. To further support the eradication of the bacterial pathogens, the combination of anti-biofilm-active systemic AB, such as rifampicin (Fig. 9.1), and high-dose local AB are then required.

Rifampicin

- Rifampicin is the most common anti-biofilm-active AB against staphylococci

7.4.4 Registry Data and Clinical Outcome

A solid proof of concept that the combination of both systemic and local AB prophylaxis »works« best has come from the Scandinavian arthroplasty registries. It has been shown that no or inappropriate local AB prophylaxis is an even higher risk factor than no systemic AB prophylaxis at all (Jämsen 2009; Jämsen et al. 2010).

Recent results from the National Joint Registry (NJR) of England, Wales and Northern Ireland (the largest arthroplasty registry worldwide) add further evidence of the efficacy of ALBC in the prevention of revision surgery. The data, spanning the period 2004–2015, comprise 717,339 cemented total knee arthroplasty (TKA) and 421,604 cemented total hip arthroplasty (THA) procedures. Of these, 47% and 59% represent primary hip and knee arthroplasties, respectively. A statistically significant reduction in the number of both hip and knee arthroplasty revisions was reported in the data when ALBC was used. Furthermore, differences between different PMMA cement brands have also been detected (Implant Summary Report for Heraeus Medical Hips & Knees using Heraeus Palacos Antibiotic Cement, NJR Database extract, 12/02/2015.18:43, © 2014 Northgate Information Solutions Ltd.).

In a French cohort study, the data of 100,200 patients was analyzed by the French Ministry of Health. They found a clear association between total hip replacement characteristics and the survivorship of the implants. In general, cemented THA not only showed a lower revision risk compared with uncemented THA, but the use of ALBC added an additional survival benefit to the cemented hip implants (Colas et al. 2015).

Furthermore, the results from a recent (quasi) randomized clinical trial with 848 intracapsular neck fracture patients in the UK have added a strong argument about the extent to which a high-dose double AB-loaded cement is able to reduce the infection rate in high-risk patients. If Copal® G+C was used for cemented hemi-arthroplasty procedures instead of the low-dose Palacos® R+G cement, the incidence rate of superficial and deep infections was drastically reduced from 5.0% to 1.7% (Jensen et al 2013).

Also in revised TKAs, which are at higher risk of subsequent failure than THAs, the use of ALBC was associated with lower risk of further revision. A recent retrospective cohort study reported on 1,154 patients who underwent aseptic revision TKA between 2002 and 2013 that were followed up prospectively by a total joint replacement registry in the USA. Revision was defined as any operation in which an implanted component was replaced. ALBC was associated with half the risk of re-revision in this large patient cohort of aseptic revision total knee arthroplasties (Bini et al. 2016).

Because of the favourable clinical data for ALBCs, many associations and clinical guidelines, including the most recent guideline issued by the European Society of Clinical Microbiology and Infectious Diseases (ESCMID; Kontekakis et al. 2014; Høiby et al. 2015), recommend the use of ALBCs to reduce the incidence of prosthesis-associated biofilm infections.

7.4.5 Manual Addition of Drugs

The selection of local AB in bone cement should always be based on the expected or, even better, the confirmed aetiology of germs responsible for a PJI. The practice of manual admixing of AB to PMMA is currently widespread, as the commercially manufactured ALBCs do not cover all possible multi-resistant pathogens (combinations) causing PJI. Customized addition of AB according to the antibiogram makes it possible to select exactly those ABs that are effective (Zahar and Hannah 2016). However, the admixture of AB to bone cement is a science per se and several points must be taken into account (Parvizi and Gehrke 2013, Kühn 2014a):

- The distribution of the AB particles in the cement might not be uniform, resulting in non-reproducible release kinetics. The impact of the added AB on the working properties are often unknown and the mechanical long-term behaviour cannot be predicted.
- Any manual addition of AB in the OR is an off-label use. As a legal consequence, the surgeon becomes the responsible manufacturer and thus assumes liability for the product quality. Frommelt and Kühn (2005) and Ochsner et al. (2014) described instructions for adding and mixing cements to AB powder, in order to produce the best possible homogeneous mixture.
- High amounts of added AB to the PMMA powder influence the mechanical properties and may compromise the mechanical stability of the cement matrix. It is therefore critical not to exceed a certain amount of added AB (typically max. 10% of cement powder), if the cement is used for the fixation of the revision prosthesis. These mechanical aspects are not of high clinical concern if using high-dose ALBCs for the manufacturing of spacers.
- Some AB interfere strongly with the PMMA polymerization process. The addition of rifampicin to ALBC is highly problematic and prevents bone cement from curing because of the *p*-hydroquinone structure within the AB molecule (◘ Fig. 7.19). This structure has chemically the function of a radical catcher and reacts with the benzoyl radicals of the cement, which usually develop by the reduction oxidation process caused by the decomposition of the benzoyl peroxide (BPO) with dimethyl-para-toluidine (DmpT). A similar situation has been described for metronidazole.
- Risk of hydrolysis and inactivation by high temperatures: The manual admixture of carbapenems, in particular of imipenem, might be critical because of their weak β-lactam ring and the imine structure within the molecule, which is usually highly susceptible to hydrolysis. Especially water as well as BPO within the polymeric powder and a rising temperature during polymerization may cause a destroying potential of the imipenem molecules (◘ Fig. 7.20).

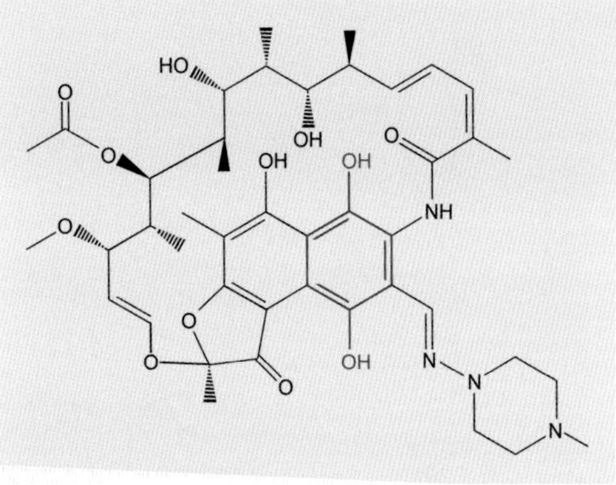

◘ **Fig. 7.19** Rifampicin molecule: The *p*-hydroquinone (*red*) structure acts as a radical catcher and inhibits the benzoyl peroxide-initiated radical polymerization

Usually hydrolytic reactions take place in solution. This argues against such a kind of interaction with PMMA cement. Meropenem, which is character-

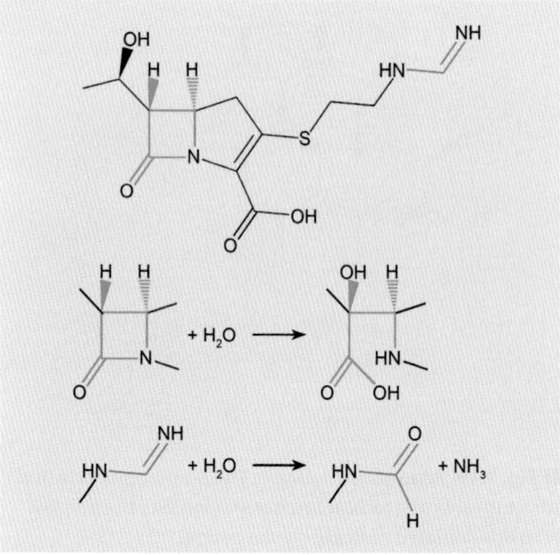

Fig. 7.20 Imipenem molecule containing one β-lactam ring (*green*) and an imine structure (*orange*)

ized by a similar molecule as imipenem, works well in combination with PMMA cement.

Liability of Manual Admixing

- Manual admixing of AB to PMMA = As a consequence, the surgeon becomes the responsible manufacturer especially because of an increasing risk of contaminations.

7.4.6 Antimycotics

The hydrophobic character of some anti-infective agents might be a problem preventing sufficient release out of the PMMA. This holds particularly true for most of the antimycotic (AM) substances such as amphotericin B (polyene-AM, consists of different formulation). Usually the concentration of added recommended AM is < 1 g/40 g polymer because of their strong side effects.

Mode of Action of Amphotericin B

- Binds with ergosterol (not a specific reaction) of the fungal cell wall
- Forms pores and increases cell permeability for ions
- Amphotericin B deoxycholate, liposomal formulation, and lipid complex formulations available

Therefore, synergistic or synergetic effects between ALBCs and antimycotic agents are not expected. The combination of a systemic and local antimycotic administration seems logical, whereas the systemic application is essential. In view of the limited penetration of antimycotic substances, a local rinsing with antimycotic substances might also be considered an option.

Mode of Action of Caspofungin

- Inhibits beta(1,3)-D-glucan synthesis
- Fungal cell wall becomes permeable
- Results in a cell lysis
- Beta(1,3)-D-glucan synthesis does not occur in human cells

Some more hydrophilic antimycotic substances – e.g. caspofungin (echinocandin AM), inhibits the beta(1,3)-D-glucan synthesis – have the tendency to stick on surfaces so that the release is significantly inhibited. Therefore, such substances are usually not suitable for a local application in PMMA spacer management.

7.4.7 Antiseptics

Antiseptic agents like octenidine (Weckbach et al. 2012) and chlorhexidine (Hiraishi et al. 2009) can be mixed with PMMA. The hydrophilic chlorhexidine diglyconate is especially suitable. Both antiseptics have a broad antimicrobial spectrum (bacterials, viruses and fungi) and are effective in low concentrations (<1 g/40 g). Antiseptics have a weak hypersensitivity or allergy potential.

During revision surgery of PJIs, the use of antiseptic agents or other anti-infective substances has been discussed if detected germs are resistant against AB added to PMMA.

7.4.8 Antimicrobial Resistances

As a consequence of growing antimicrobial resistances it is obvious that ALBC must sometimes be customized according to the specific germ profile. Multi-drug resistances do not only refer to MRSA/MRSE, but do also include the group of Gram-neg-

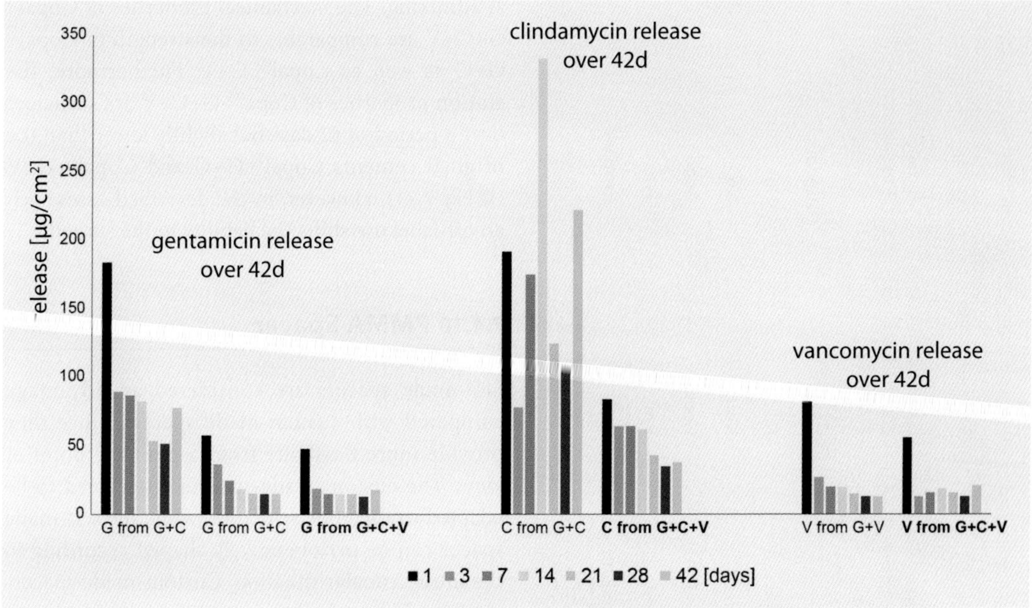

Fig. 7.21 Elution of Copal® G+C+V in comparison with Copal® G+C and Copal® G+C, *G* gentamicin, *C* clindamycin, *V* vancomycin, *d* days

ative bacteria and the heterogeneous mix of difficult-to-treat cases with polymicrobial aetiology, sometimes found in PJI.

As mentioned earlier, the identification of the causative organism and the assessment of possible AB resistances are of paramount importance for successful infection management. If it proves necessary to admix an AB to PMMA cement in septic revision surgery, it is recommended to contact a specialist to ensure that the chosen AB is sufficiently effective with PMMA. An inadequate quantity may compromise the stability of the prosthesis or a too-low elution out of the cement matrix may generate the emergence of resistant bacteria (Bistolfi et al. 2011).

Manual admixing of anti-infective agents into bone cement might prove necessary in septic revision situations, if no commercial revision bone cement is available that covers the germ(s) (Tab. 7.8).

7.4.9 Copal® G+C+V

From a clinical point of view, it is important that ALBC-eluted substances are measurable locally in the tissue around the cement matrix. Fink et al. (2011) demonstrated that the AB concentrations in the soft tissue surrounding a PMMA spacer (manufactured with Copal® G+C or Copal® G+C+manually added vancomycin) after 6 weeks of spacer implantation often exceed the minimal inhibitory concentrations (MIC) of susceptible germs.

Anti-infective combinations can be very effective by choosing the appropriate mode of application. The »correct« local combination of anti-infective substances in a PMMA spacer complements the choice of systemically applied AB.

One of the »best« local combinations in terms of germ spectrum and antimicrobial action might be the combination of gentamicin, clindamycin and vancomycin (Fink et al. 2011).

In clinical practice, vancomycin powder can be manually added to the commercial product Copal® G+C or clindamycin to the commercial product Copal® G+V. However, it should be pointed out that such a practice confers the risk of inhomogeneity of the product with negative consequence for the mechanical strength of the cement and the AB elution properties. Some surgeons have also reported their practice of mixing one unit of each Copal® cement (G+C plus G+V) together. This combination seems logical and the better option compared with manu-

Tab. 7.8 Efficacy of antibiotic combination: close the gap

Antibiotic(s)	Gram-positive					Gram-negative	
	Staphylococci methicillin S	Staphylococci methicillin R	Enterococci	Streptococci	Propionibacterium sp. *P. acnes*	Enterobacteriaceae *E. coli*, Proteus sp. *E. faecalis*	Pseudomonas sp. *P. aeruginosa*
Gentamicin (G)	Good	Poor	Good	Good	No	Good	Good
Vancomycin (V)	Good	Good	Good	Good	Good	No	No
Clindamycin (C)	Good	Good	No	Good	Good	No	No
G+C	Syn	Syn	Syn	Syn	Good	Good	Good
G+V	Syn	Syn	Syn	Good	Good	Syn	Syn
G+C+V	Excellent	Excellent	Excellent	Excellent	Excellent	Excellent	Excellent

Syn synergetic, *S* sensitive, *R* resistant

al admixing. The mechanical properties of Copal® G+C+V are comparable to the strength of Copal® G+C as well as Copal® G+V. Furthermore, the elution properties of Copal® G+C+V are sufficient over a period of 42 days but slightly lower than the original cements Copal® G+C and Copal® G+V (Fig. 7.21). However, in the described cases such an off-label use shifts the liability to the surgeon.

7.4.10 PMMA Spacer

Self-made spacers are considered an advantage compared with custom-made spacers, since they provide more flexibility from a practical point of view. The custom-made spacers often need to be adapted to the bone structure, while the self-made spacer can be perioperatively shaped according to the intra-articular situation. Custom-made spacers exhibit additional advantage with a nearly smooth cement surface, which results in a largely predictable release of agents under reproducible conditions. This reproducibility might be important from a microbiological view and in the case of legal disputes. Self-made spacers, on the other hand, have an irregular surface and a significantly higher rate of agent release. Fundamentally, spacers should be manufactured as flexibly and anatomically as possible, one piece for the hip, two pieces for the knee. Spacers in general can also have cement temperature peaks because of their bigger mass. This property must be taken into account when agents are added manually, since some anti-infective drugs are sensitive to temperature.

It is necessary to prevent spacers from getting into contact with liquids before implantation, in order to avoid premature elution of agents from the spacer surface. A hydrophilic and microporous spacer matrix can significantly improve and elongate the elution of agents nonetheless. Because of the restricted period of sufficient AB release out of the spacer surface, a too-long implantation interval should be avoided. The status of the soft tissue should allow for re-implantation, and subsequent systemic AB treatment should be long enough.

If articulating spacers are used, long implantation intervals may increase the risk of cement particle abrasion. In this case, it can be useful to utilize

Tab. 7.9 Mechanics of Copal mixed with different antibiotics

	Copal® G+C	Copal® G+V	Copal® G+C+V
ISO Bending	63.1	63	61.2
ISO Bending Modulus	2755	2926	2894
ISO Compression	87.3	84.9	88.2
DIN Bending	69.5	64	63.7
DIN Impact	3.1	3	3.1

spacers with low-abrasion surfaces. Special PMMA spacer cements with low-abrasive calcium carbonate/calcium sulphate as a contrast medium for radiology (Copal® spacem) may fulfil this expectation. The lower visibility of calcium carbonate on X-rays compared with conventional contrast agents such as zirconium dioxide and barium sulphate is not a major concern, since the lower visibility of calcium carbonate is compensated by the large size of the spacer. In addition, these spacers elute AB much better than »conventional« PMMA spacers because of the significantly higher hydrophilicity of the cement matrix (Kühn et al 2016). Therefore, Copal® spacem can also be considered as a revision PMMA cement matrix to which AB must be manually admixed.

Take-Home Message

- Periprosthetic joint infection is a devastating complication after total joint replacement. Prevention is mandatory and the use of anti biotic-loaded bone cement (ALBC) for the treatment of complex musculoskeletal infections is well established. Further addition of local antibiotics eluting from bone cement is also a possibility.
- Most commercially available premixed preparations contain 0.5–2 g of antibiotic per 40 g of polymethylmethacrylate (PMMA). An inadequate dose may be seen as the cause of failure of the prosthesis, as it may generate the emergence of resistant bacteria.
- The choice of antibiotic added to ALBC is always dependent on the germ causing the infection. The causative pathogen and its resistances, as well as the choice of the appropriate anti-infective agent(s), is mandatory for a successful eradication of the infection.
- The method of mixing is considered one of the most important factors affecting the release of the antibiotics and the mechanical properties of cement.
- Addition of two ABs to cement serves the observation that such cements are more protective against biofilm formation than cements containing only one antibiotic in lower concentration.
- ALBC for prophylaxis against infection has proven to be useful especially in high-risk patients. The use of ALBC during primary surgery in these patients is considered as a support strategy preventing the high-risk onset of infections.
- Cement spacers carrying high doses of antibiotic(s) are currently accepted during two-stage treatment of infected prosthetic joints.

References

Anagnostakos K, Fürst O, Kelm J (2006) Antibiotic-impregnated PMMA hip spacers: Current status. Acta Orthop 77(4):628–637

Balato G, Ascione T, Rosa D, Pagliano P, Solarino G, Moretti B, Mariconda M (2015) Release of Gentamicin from Cement Spacers in two-stage Procedures for Hip and Knee Prosthetic Infection: an in vivo pharmacokinetic study with clinical follow-up. J Biol Regul Homeost Agents 29(4):63–72

Bertazzoni Minelli E, Della Bora T, Benini A (2011) Different microbial biofilm formation on polymethylmethacrylate (PMMA) bone cement loaded with gentamicin and vancomycin. Anaerobe 17(6):380–383

Bini SA, Chan PH, Inacio MCS, Paxton EW, Khatod M (2016) Antibiotic cement was associated with half the risk of re-revision. Acta Orthopaedica 87(1):55–59

Bistolfi A, Massazza G, Verné E, Massè A, Deledda D, Ferraris S, Miola M, Galetto F, Crova M (2011) Antibiotic-loaded

cement in orthopedic surgery: a review. ISRN Orthop doi:10.5402/2011/290851
Breusch SJ, Kühn KD (2003) Bone cements based on polymethylmethacrylate. Orthopaede 32(1):41–50
Breusch S, Malchau H (2005) The Well-Cemented Total Hip Arthroplasty, Theory and Practice. Springer Verlag, Heidelberg
Colas S, Collin C, Piriou P, Zureik M (2015) Association Between Total Hip Replacement Characteristics and 3-Year Prosthetic Survivorship: A Population-Based Study. JAMA Surg 150(10):979–988
Costerton JW, Stewart PS, Greenberg EP (1999) Bacterial biofilms: a common cause of persistent infections. Science 284(5418):1318–1322
Deb S (2008) Orthopaedic bone cements King's College London. Woodhead Publishing, UK
Ensing GT, van Horn JR, van der Mei HC, Busscher HJ, Neut D (2008) Copal bone cement is more effective in preventing biofilm formation than Palacos R-G. Clin Orthop Relat Res 466(6):1492–1498
Fink B, Vogt S, Reinsch M, Büchner H (2011) Sufficient release of antibiotic by a spacer 6 weeks after implantation in two-stage revision of infected hip prostheses. Clin Orthop Relat Res 469(11):3141–3147
Frommelt L (2007) Antibiotic choices in bone surgery – local therapy using antibiotic-loaded bone cement. In: Walenkamp GHIM (ed) Local antibiotics in arthroplasty. State of the art from an interdisciplinary view. Thieme, Stuttgart New York, p59–64
Frommelt L, Kühn KD (2005) Properties of Bone Cement: Antibiotic-Loaded Cement. In: Breusch SJ, Malchau H (eds) The Well-Cemented Total Hip Arthroplasty: Theory and Practice. Springer Verlag, Heidelberg, p86–92
Gehrke T, Förster GV, Frommelt L (2001) Pharmacokinetic Study of a Gentamicin/Clindamicin Bone Cement Used in One-stage Revision Arthroplasty. In: Walenkamp GHIM, Murray DW (eds) Bone Cements and Cementing Technique, Springer, Berlin Heidelberg, p127–134
Gristina AG, Naylor P, Myrvik Q (1988) Infections from biomaterials and implants: a race for the surface. Med Prog Technol 14(3–4):205–224
Hiraishi N, Yiu CK, King NM, Tay FR (2009) Antibacterial Effect of Experimental Chlorhexidine-releasing Polymethymethacrylate based Root Canal Sealers. J Endod 35(9):1255–1258
Høiby N, Bjarnsholt T, Moser C, Bassi GL, Coenye T, Donelli G, Hall-Stoodley L, Holá V, Imbert C, Kirketerp-Møller K, Lebeaux D, Oliver A, Ullmann AJ, Williams C, ESCMID Study Group for Biofilms and Consulting External Expert Werner Zimmerli (2015) ESCMID guideline for the diagnosis and treatment of biofilm infections 2014. Clin Microbiol Infect 21(Suppl1):S1–25
Implant Summary Report for Heraeus Medical Hips & Knees using Heraeus Palacos Antibiotic Cement, NJR Database extract, 12/02/2015.18:43, © 2014 Northgate Information Solutions
Jämsen E, Stogiannidis I, Malmivaara A, Pajamäki J, Timo Puolakka T, Konttinen YT (2009) Outcome of prosthesis exchange for infected knee arthroplasty: the effect of treatment approach. Acta Orthop 80(1):67–77
Jämsen E, Furnes O, Engesæter LB, Konttinen YT, Odgaard A, Stefánsdóttir A, Lidgren L (2010) Prevention of deep infection in joint replacement surgery: A review. Acta Orthop 81(6):660–666
Jämsen E (2009) Risk Factors for Infection after Knee Arthroplasty: a register-based analysis of 43,149 cases. J Bone Joint Surg Am 91(1):38–47
Jensen C, Gupta S, Sprowson A, Chambers S, Inman D, Jones S, Aradhyula NM, Reed MR (2013) High dose, double antibiotic-impregnated cement reduces surgical site infection (SSI) in hip hemiarthropalsty: a randomized controlled trial of 848 patients with intracapsular neck of femur fractures. Orthopaedic Proceedings DOI:10.1186/1471-2474-14-356
Kontekakis A, Berghaus M, Gaiser S, Kühn KD (2014) Evidence generation for medical devices- the case of cemented joint replacement surgery in arthroplasty registries. In: Scholz M (ed) Biofunctional Surface Engineering 13. Pan Stanford Publishing, Singapore, ISBN 978-9814411-60-8, p291–314
Kühn KD, Lieb E, Berberich C (2016) PMMA bone cement: what is the role of local antibiotics**?** Matrise Orthopaedic**,** Proceeding of N°243, commission paritaire 1218T86410ISSN:1148 2362 12–18
Kühn KD (2014b) Antimicrobial coating. In: Scholz M (ed) Biofunctional surface engineering 6. Pan Stanford Publishing, Singapore, ISBN 978-9814411-60-8, p121–189
Kühn KD (2014a) PMMA Cements. Springer, Heidelberg, ISBN 978-3-642-41535-7
Mulazimoglu L, Drenning SD, Muder RR (1996) Vancomycin-gentamicin synergism revisited: effect of gentamicin susceptibility of methicillin-resistant Staphylococcus aureus. Antimicrob Agents Chemother 40(6): 1534–1535
Ochsner PE, Borens O, Bodler PM, Schweizerische Gesellschaft für Orthopädie und Traumatologie (2014) Infections of the musculoskeletal system. Published by Swiss Orthopaedics and the Swiss Society for Infectious Disease expert group »Infections of the musculoskeletal system«. 2. Edition
Parvizi J, Gehrke T (2013) Proceedings of the international consensus meeting on periprosthetic joint infection. Data Trace Publishing Company, Brooklandville, Maryland, ISBN 978-1-57400-147-1
Parvizi J, Saleh KJ, Ragland PS, Pour AE, Mont MA (2008) Efficacy of antibiotic-impregnated cement in total hip replacement. Acta Orthop 79(3):335–342
Rosenthal AL, Rovell JM, Girard AE (1976) [Polyacrylic bone cement with added erythromycin and colistin. In vitro studies on bacteriologic activity and diffusion properties]. MMW Munch Med Wochenschr 118(31):987–990
Ruzaimi MY, Shahril Y, Masbah O, Salasawati H (2006) Antimicrobial properties of erythromycin and colistin impreg-

nated bone cement. An in vitro analysis. Med J Malaysia 61(SupplA):21–26

Sanz-Ruiz P, Matas-Diez JA, Sanchez-Somolinos M, Villanueva-Martinez M, Vaquero-Martín J (2016) Is the Commercial Antibiotic-Loaded Bone Cement Useful in Prophylactic and Cost Saving After Knee and Hip Joint Arthroplasty? The Transatlantic Paradox. http://dx.doi.org/10.1016/j.arth.2016.11.012

Schmolders J, Hischebeth GTR, Friedrich MJ, Randau TM, Wimmer MD, Kohlhof H, Molitor E, Gravius S (2014) Evidence of MRSE on a gentamicin and vancomycin impregnated polymethyl-methacrylate (PMMA) bone cement spacer after two-stage exchange arthroplasty due to periprosthetic joint infection of the knee. BMC Infect Dis DOI:10.1186/1471-2334-14-144

Smith DC (2005) The genesis and evolution of acrylic bone cement. Orthop Clin Am 36(1):1–10

Sprowson AP, Jensen CD, Gupta S, Parsons N, Murty AN, Jones SMG, Inman D, Reed MR (2013) The effect of high dose antibiotic impregnated cement on rate of surgical site infection after hip hemiarthroplasty for fractured neck of femur: a protocol for a double-blind quasi randomised controlled trial. BMC Muscoskelet Disord DOI:10.1186/1471-2474-14-356

Sterling GJ, Potter JM, Koerbin G, Crawford S, Crawford R (2003) The pharmacokinetics of Simplex P Tobramycin Bone Cement. A study investigating the elution characteristics of Simplex P Tobramycin Bone Cement in total hip replacement. J Bone Joint Surg Br 85(5):646–649

Styker Bone Cement http://www.stryker.com/en-us/products/Orthopaedics/BoneCementSubstitutes/index.htm

Valour F, Trouillet-Assant S, Riffard N, Tasse J, Flammier S, Rasigade JP, Chidiac C, Vandenesch F, Ferry T, Laurent F (2015) Antimicrobial activity against intraosteoblastic Staphylococcus aureus. Antimicrob Agents Chemother 59(4):2029–2036

Watanakunakorn C, Tisone JC (1982b) Effects of a vancomycin-rifampin combination on enterococci. Antimicrob Agents Chemother 22(5):915–916

Watanakunakorn C, Tisone JC (1982a) Synergism between vancomycin and gentamicin or tobramycin for methicillin-susceptible and methicillin-resistant Staphylococcus aureus strains. Antimicrob Agents Chemother 22(5):903–905

Watanakunakorn C (1982) Treatment of infections due to methicillin-resistant Staphylococcus aureus. Ann Intern Med 97(3):376–378

Weckbach S, Möricke A, Braunwarth H (2012) Octenidine in combination with polymethylmethacrylate: a new option for preventing infection? Archives of Orthopaedic and Trauma Surgery 132(1):15–20

Zahar A, Hannah P (2016) Antibiotikazumischung zum Knochenzement beim septischen Prothesenwechsel. Oper Orthop Traumatol DOI:10.1007/s00064-015-0424-6

Zimmerli W, Trampuz A, Ochsner PE (2004) Prosthetic-joint infections. N Engl J Med 351(16):1645–1654

Spacers

K.-D. Kühn (Ed.), *Management of Periprosthetic Joint Infection*
DOI 10.1007/978-3-662-54469-3_8

8.1 Spacer Management

Manuel Villanueva-Martinez, Pablo Sanz-Ruiz and Christof Berberich

8.1.1 Introduction

Infection is one of the most devastating complications of total knee arthroplasty (TKA). It is also the leading cause of early revision after knee arthroplasty ahead of instability and aseptic loosening.

The surgical treatment of choice is two-stage exchange, which, nevertheless, is an aggressive, costly and lengthy procedure. The use of an antibiotic-loaded spacer in the interim phase between explantation of the infected prosthesis and implantation of the new revision prosthesis has become generally accepted practice. The purpose of such spacers is to maintain a certain amount of joint stability and mobility and to provide high intra-articular concentrations of local antibiotics needed to eradicate the infection. In order to achieve this goal, it is of high importance to select the correct antibiotic combinations for the spacer according to the antibiogram of the causative pathogen(s).

The challenge for surgeons lies in the choice of different spacer philosophies (static vs articulating spacer), different shapes and manufacturing options (e. g. intraoperatively made spacers according to the joint anatomy left after debridement, spacers manufactured with mould systems or prefabricated spacers). Each option has its pros and cons. Some examples of customized hand-made spacers are presented in the case reports in this chapter.

8.1.2 Frequency of Orthopaedic Infections and Prosthetic Joint Infections

Fortunately, the frequency of prosthetic joint infection (PJI) is not increasing in our hospital (H. Beata María and H. Gregorio Marañón). Routine use of antibiotic-loaded cement for all our primary TKAs, revision knee arthroplasties, and cemented hips has led to a significant reduction in the frequency of infection (Parvizi et al. 2008; Hansen et al. 2014; Sanz-Ruíz et al. 2016).

We also encourage strict observance of prophylactic measures and control of the operating room environment: closed doors, proper attire for personnel directly involved in the procedure, change of gloves and disposable instruments, and adherence to the recommendations of the International Consensus Meeting on Periprosthetic Joint Infection (Parvizi et al. 2013). We wash the surgical field with antiseptic solution (iodine povidone) and saline solution every 15–20 min.

These measures have enabled us to reduce the frequency of infection from 3.3% to around 1% in primary arthroplasties at our first institution (a public general hospital with the capacity to handle emergencies and patients with multiple trauma) and to less than 0.5% at our second institution, a private hospital performing only elective surgery.

Although the frequency of PJI is increasing in most developed countries, some hospitals report lower rates than others (Kurtz et al. 2007; Villanueva-Martinez et al. 2012).

The worldwide increase in the frequency of PJI has a number of explanations, namely, more frequent indication of surgery in patients with comorbid conditions and patients who have already undergone several procedures, increased prevalence of resistant micro-organisms, and poor adherence to prophylactic measures. In addition, we now have more diagnostic tools at our disposal, and many micro-organisms considered as contaminant or defective are now considered infectious, e. g. *Propionibacterium acnes* (Parvizi et al. 2009).

Comorbid conditions and more resistant bacteria in patients who have undergone several procedures necessitate expensive, frustrating and aggressive surgical solutions, thus illustrating that arthroplasty has entered a new era. Greenhouse operating rooms may become more important, since hospitals with this type of operating room have lower rates of infection. Consequently, prevention will be the cornerstone of our approach to difficult-to-treat or untreatable infections.

8.1.3 Treatment Algorithms for PJI

We follow the *diagnostic algorithms* of the American Academy of Orthopaedic Surgeons (AAOS) and the

International Consensus Meeting (Parvizi et al. 2013) for the treatment of PJIs.

During surgery, our standard protocol is to take six to eight samples, including samples from the prosthesis, and send them to the laboratory immediately. If we cannot process samples immediately, we store them in a fridge.

We routinely perform culture and polymerase chain reaction (PCR) assay of samples. If the result is positive for a micro-organism with special requirements for growth, these may be observed in culture (Marin et al. 2012).

Sonication of implants is also a common practice in our setting, although this is not generally the case in Spain. Delayed cultures (2 weeks) also form part of our current protocol (Trampuz et al. 2007; Schafer et al. 2008).

According to the Tsukayama classification, *surgical treatment protocols* vary with the type of infection. In addition, it is important to take into consideration the infecting micro-organism and the patient's local and general condition (Tsukayama et al. 1996).

Two-stage exchange remains the treatment of choice in late infection, with good or excellent results in 80–100% of cases; nevertheless, it is aggressive, costly, and long (Jiranek et al. 2015). It is also considered the treatment of choice in fungal infection, viral infection, inflammatory diseases, immunosuppression, and re-infection after re-implantation.

The trend in Spain is towards one-stage revision in selected cases. This is also our practice. However, our preference is for two-stage revision. Strict selection criteria are key to a high success rate with one-stage revision and include reliable identification of the infecting micro-organism, a favourable oral antibiotic profile, no soft tissue damage or fistulae, and no need for bone grafting.

Surgeons with little experience in one-stage revision should begin with cases involving exchange of primary implants rather than revision implants. We consider that the patient's general status (e. g. rheumatoid arthritis, old age, comorbidities) should not be a limitation for one-stage re-implantation, but should be yet another reason for preventing limitation of function between stages (Masters et al. 2013; Jiranek et al. 2015).

Our *antibiotic protocols* are based on the guidelines of the Infectious Diseases Society of America, with specific modifications.

- As a rule, we administer parenteral antibiotics for no more than 1 week.
- In two-stage revisions, we administer antibiotics for 6 weeks (1 week parenteral and 5 weeks oral).
- In acute or late haematogenous infections treated with debridement, antibiotics, and implant retention (DAIR), we are now shortening the antibiotic protocols to 8 weeks, rather than maintaining classic protocols (3–6 months).
- The procedure for one-stage revision is the same as for acute infections.

In doubtful cases (potential Tsukayama type IV) or cases in which we suspect the causative agent but do not have a reliable diagnosis, we continue with the antibiotic regimen until we have the results of protocolized cultures (Zimmerli 2015).

8.1.4 Most Frequently Detected Pathogens

The most commonly isolated micro-organisms are Gram-positive cocci, with coagulase-negative staphylococci (CNS), *S. aureus* and enterococci accounting for 65% of cases. Gram-negative bacilli, including *Escherichia coli*, *Proteus mirabilis*, and *Pseudomonas aeruginosa*, are far less frequent causes of infection (6%). Anaerobes, including *Propionibacterium acnes*, account for 4% of infections.

Approximately 7% of cultures are negative. Polymicrobial infections account for 20% of cases (Cobo and Del Pozo 2011). In a recent study in Spanish hospitals, Gram-negative bacilli were more common than in our institution. Out of a total of 2,015 PJIs recorded over the 8-year study period, infections in 242 patients (12%) were originally caused by Gram-negative bacteria (Rodríguez-Pardo et al. 2014).

8.1.5 Use of Spacers

Whenever possible, we use antibiotic-loaded spacers (monoblock in the case of hips and articulating

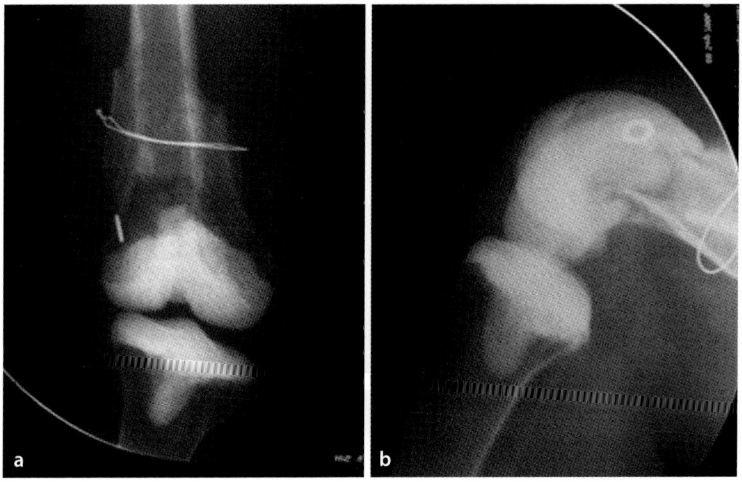

Fig. 8.1 a, b Articulating spacer in a segmental defect. Good range of motion, although some instability can be observed.

in the case of knees; see Fig. 8.1). We tailor the antibiotic protocol to the previous antibiogram, when available.

We do not use preformed spacers, although some of our colleagues use silicone moulds and tailor the type and load of antibiotic to the infecting micro-organism. Our current protocol is based on custom hand-made spacers for both the knee and the hip. We routinely use nails or intramedullary rods to build hip spacers and occasionally use them in knees affected by severe bone loss. In cases where soft tissue healing is problematic, we use a monoblock spacer or an articulating spacer and immobilize the knee in extension with an orthosis.

The choice of spacer depends on many factors, including degree of bone loss, state of soft tissue, choice of antibiotics, and financial and technical restraints. A benefit common to both articulating and non-articulating antibiotic-loaded spacers is that greater intra-articular levels of antibiotic can be delivered than with parenteral antibiotics (Alt et al. 2004).

Although this approach remains open to debate, some authors agree that using articulating spacers for the treatment of infected TKA provides better functional results and enables more efficacious eradication of infection than do non-articulating spacers. This concept is not as widely accepted as the idea of soft tissue preservation (Chiang et al. 2011; Romano et al. 2012; Park et al. 2010).

The shape and features of articulating spacers vary considerably, from fully manual spacers made in preformed moulds to modular spacers, which include plastic and metal surfaces.

Spacers differ in price, complexity, and degree of constraint. The advantages of articulating spacers are as follows: retraction of soft tissue and extensor mechanisms is prevented, high doses of antibiotics can be added between operations, bone mass is preserved better than with non-articulating spacers, the need for expanded approaches at re-implantation is reduced, and the success rate is higher (Chiang et al. 2011).

These approaches also enable more controlled mobility of the joint and application of a partial support brace, thus facilitating acceptable function between procedures.

Articulating spacers take a number of forms. The main forms are as follows:

1. Manual construction with cement in the operating room, which makes it possible to recreate the normal anatomy of the knee or build more congruent systems (ball and socket; Fig. 8.2; MacAvoy and Ries 2005; Villanueva-Martinez et al. 2008).
2. Construction of customized spacers in the operating room using prefabricated silicone or aluminium moulds or trial components to shape the spacer (Goldstein et al. 2001; Hsu et al. 2007).

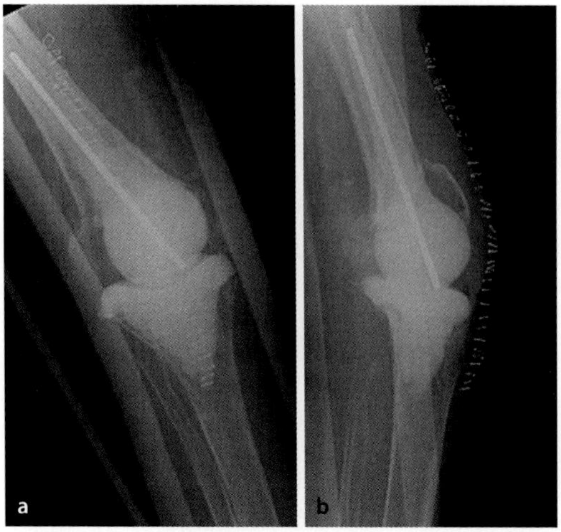

■ **Fig. 8.2 a, b** Ball and socket spacer

Cement moulds can be made during surgery using trial components, and the definitive spacer can be made using cement moulds (Ha 2006).

3. Prefabricated spacers made of cement only (Pitto et al. 2005).
4. Preformed articulating systems (PROSTALAC®). Cement components in combination with modular components made of plastic and metal (Gooding et al. 2011).
5. Spacer prosthesis. Re-sterilization of the prosthesis and insertion of a femoral component and a polyethylene insert with cement or a new prosthesis with high antibiotic loads as a spacer (Anderson et al. 2009).
6. Combinations of these approaches for moderate or massive defects (Incavo et al. 2009).

These concepts, with personal or individual variations, also apply to hip spacers. The approaches used comprise hand-made spacers, preformed spacers, silicone or aluminium moulds, PROSTALAC®, and spacer prostheses.

8.1.6 Duration of Spacer Placement in Two-Stage Procedures

We base re-implantation time on the progress of analytical parameters such as C-reactive protein (CRP) and erythrocyte sedimentation rate (ESR), which should be normal or almost normal. When in doubt, we discontinue the antibiotics and aspirate the joint.

We administer a short parenteral course of antibiotics (7 days) followed by oral therapy for a further 5 weeks. In one-stage revision, the course of antibiotics lasts 6–8 weeks; in infections treated with DAIR, the course lasts 8–12 weeks. In doubtful cases, we also consider the aggressiveness of the infecting micro-organism when deciding whether to prolong the antibiotic regimen. At re-implantation, we take standard samples for culture and freeze samples for histopathology.

8.1.7 Choice of Cement for Spacers

Antibiotic-loaded cement spacers release high concentrations of drug and enable higher intra-articular concentrations to be reached than parenteral antibiotics alone, with little effect on serum or urine concentrations and, therefore, with minimal risk of systemic damage (Springer et al. 2004).

It is essential to achieve local bactericidal concentrations that eradicate infection or prevent colonization of the new implant during the re-implantation phase (the »race for the surface«; Hanssen and Spangehl 2004).

We prefer cements that elute the highest dose of antibiotics. The only commercial presentations with a synergistic effect are Copal® G+C and Copal® G+V (gentamicin combined with clindamycin or vancomycin). Copal® enables increased release of antibiotic and better inhibits the formation of biofilm than gentamicin alone (Ensing et al. 2008).

During the past few years, we have been using Copal® G+C combined with 2–2.5 g of vancomycin powder per pack of cement. The second antibiotic enables a synergistic effect and broader spectrum. The third antibiotic covers methicillin-resistant *Staphylococcus* species, which are also resistant to clindamycin and gentamicin. Occasionally, we add cephalosporins instead of vancomycin as the third antibiotic. Extra aminoglycosides in powder can be recommended, although the combination is difficult to obtain in some countries.

Other reasons for using commercially available cements with a synergistic effect include the following (Frommelt and Kühn 2005):

- When antibiotics are added manually to the cement, the synergistic effect makes release differ significantly between bone cements. With commercial formulations, release is optimized and more predictable.
- Synergy enables the release of greater amounts of antibiotic, thus making inhibition of bacterial growth more effective and increasing the chances of winning the »race for the surface«.
- Elution rates are higher than with other commercial brands or combinations.
- With high elution rates, even organisms classified as resistant in routine antibiograms can be eradicated when the dose is increased sufficiently.
- At least part of the responsibility for the mixture is with the commercial brand, not the surgeon.

If these cements are not available, our recommendation is to use Palacos® R+G and add vancomycin powder or cephalosporins or an extra dose of aminoglycosides, depending on the infecting micro-organism and the availability of the antibiotics in powder form.

8.1.8 Choice of Antibiotic for Local Use in Spacers

Synergy between aminoglycosides + vancomycin, aminoglycosides + clindamycin, and, occasionally, a cephalosporin (ceftazidime, ceftriaxone, cefepime, and cefotaxime are available in powder forms in our setting) enables coverage of a broad spectrum of micro-organisms (Frommelt and Kühn 2005).

In cases of fungal PJI, we use fluconazole (500 mg per 40 g of polymer) combined with amphotericin B (200 mg per 40 g polymer), although elution of the combination from bone cement seems limited (Goss et al. 2007).

Effective elution from cement has also been observed with quinolones, daptomycin, and linezolid, although these agents are difficult to obtain in powder form or are too expensive. Anguita-Alonso et al. compared quinolones, cefazolin, and linezolid and found linezolid to be the most stable antibiotic after polymerization of polymethyl methacrylate (PMMA).

Daptomycin is also eluted in local bactericidal concentrations for *S. aureus* and CNS, with a release profile similar to that of vancomycin (Anguita-Alonso et al. 2006).

Therefore, antibiotics that should be taken into consideration in the coming years include linezolid, teicoplanin, and daptomycin for vancomycin-resistant *Staphylococcus* and meropenem (which also has a synergistic effect with vancomycin), amikacin, and fosfomycin for multidrug-resistant Gram-negative bacteria. These antibiotics are usually available in powder form (see ◘ Fig. 8.3 and ◘ Fig. 8.4). However, antibiotic-loaded cements containing these drugs are not commercially available (Frommelt and Kühn 2005).

Currently, our cements of choice are Copal® C+G and Copal® G+V. Copal® seems ideal for articulating spacers, which are withdrawn after a few weeks, but may not be as appropriate as Palacos® R+G for definitive re-implantation once the infection has been cured.

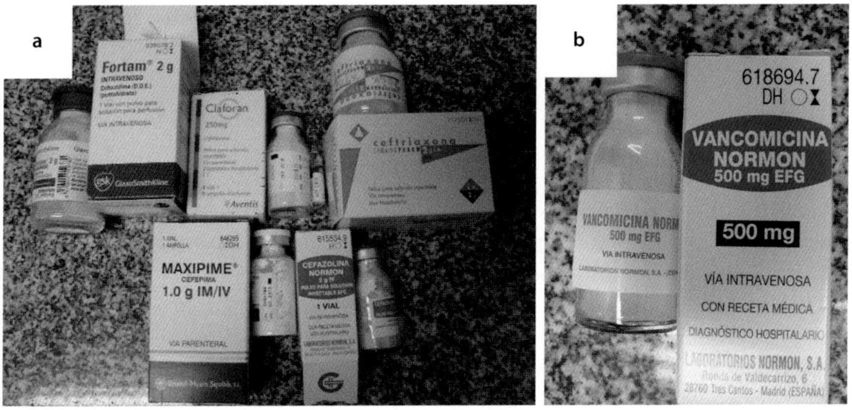

◘ **Fig. 8.3 a, b** Most cephalosporins and vancomycin are available in powder form in most countries

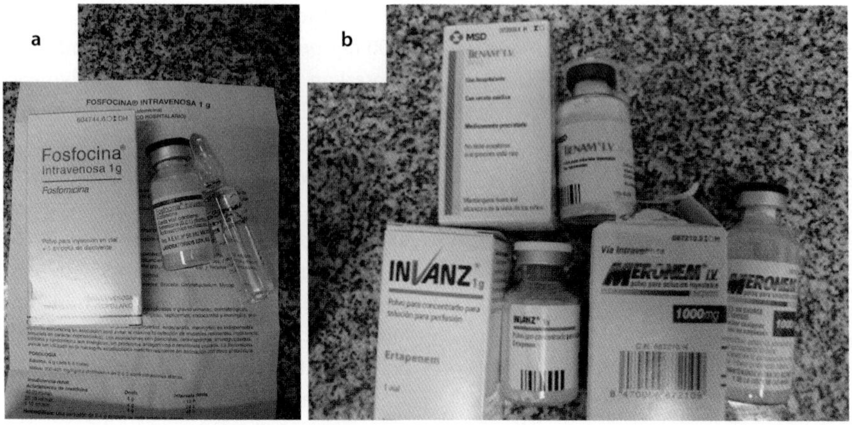

Fig. 8.4 a, b Fosfomycin and meropenem in powder form

Tab. 8.1 Authors' preferred cement and antibiotics

Infecting micro-organism	Cement	Supplements	Alternatives
MSSA, MSSE	Copal® G+C	Cefuroxime	Copal® G+V
MRSA, MRSE	Copal® G+V	Vancomycin added to Palacos® R+G or Copal® G+C if Copal® G+V not available	Teicoplanin, Daptomycin, Linezolid
Anaerobe	Copal® G+C		
Gram-negative	Copal® G+V, Copal® G+C	Ceftazidime Cefuroxime Cefotaxime Colistin	For Pseudomonas Cefoperazone Amikacin Cefepime Ceftazidime Meropenem
Multi-resistant Gram-negative	Copal® G+V	Amikacin Meropenem Fosfomycin	
Fungal	Palacos® R+G vs Copal® C+C	Fluconazole ± Amphotericin B	
TBC	Palacos® R+G vs Copal® G®C+C	Isoniazid	

Therefore, we prefer commercially available antibiotic-loaded cement, to which we often add antimicrobial drugs manually (for our choices, see Tab. 8.1). Thus, with minimum modifications, we can cover a broad spectrum of bacteria (see Fig. 8.5) and release higher doses of antibiotics at the site of infection than we would when using prefabricated spacers.

8.1.9 Adding Antibiotic to PMMA During Spacer Manufacture

We follow the method of Frommelt and Kühn, namely, fractional addition of antibiotic, which involves the gradual addition of cement and antibiotic powder (equal amounts) and mixing the two until the expected antibiotic load is reached (From-

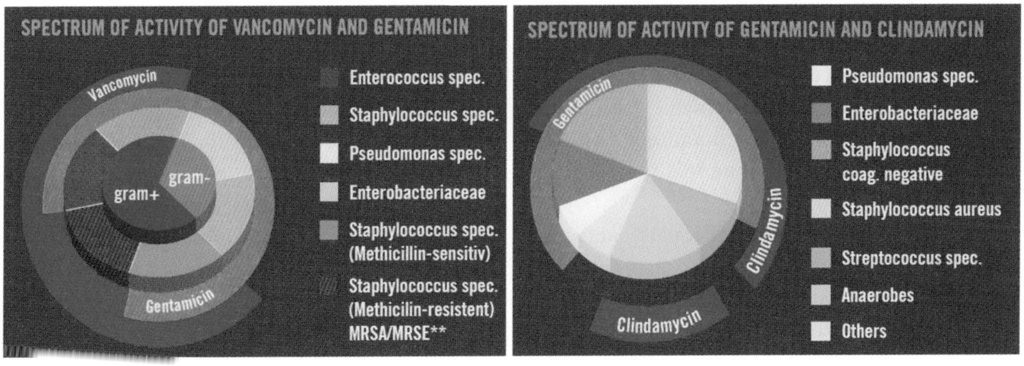

Fig. 8.5 Spectrum of activity of commercial cements (Kühn 2014; Kühn et al. 2016). *MRSA* methicillin-resistant *Staphylococcus aureus*, *MRSE* methicillin-resistant *Staphylococcus epidermidis*

melt and Kühn 2005). The mixture should be homogeneous. Then we add the liquid monomer according to the manufacturer's specifications. The cement can be mixed manually (our standard protocol) or vacuum-mixed, depending on the type of cement and the availability of vacuum systems. Once mixed, the cement is applied in the doughy phase or late phase of polymerization to prevent excessive interdigitation, thus facilitating extraction during surgery and providing the surgeon with a certain degree of freedom to shape the articulating surface of the spacer.

Applying antibiotics such as vancomycin in the doughy phase may lead to better elution of antibiotic from the cement. However, this approach is not our current practice and may limit the working time necessary for a customized spacer (Laine et al. 2011).

Whenever possible, we use premixed bone cements to ensure uniform and predictable elution and safety.

8.1.10 Techniques for Fixation of Revision Implant: Cemented vs Cementless

In the case of knee revision, cemented fixation is our first choice for primary and revision arthroplasty. We use different packs of cement for the tibia and for the femur. First, we press the cement with the fingers in order to ensure better interdigitation, mainly in the anterior and posterior femoral cuts, where interdigitation is minimal if the cement is placed only at the prosthesis, and in the metaphysis. We then place cement in the prosthesis (Pérez Mañanes et al. 2011).

We prefer to cement the surface and the metaphysis (Sanz-Ruiz et al. 2015). This is also our standard protocol in revision surgery when using constrained condylar implants or metal augments. However, in the case of rotating hinge implants, we use a plug and distal retrograde pressurization with a cement gun. Our preference in revision hip arthroplasty is not to use cement, unless the patient is very old or impaction grafting is necessary.

The conclusions of the International Consensus Meeting state that antibiotic-loaded cement reduces the incidence of PJI following TJA and should be used in patients at high risk for PJI following elective arthroplasty. Therefore, antibiotic should be added to cement in all patients undergoing cemented or hybrid fixation as part of revision arthroplasty.

The conclusions of the International Consensus Meeting make a clear difference between the various types of cement with regard to antibiotic elution. Cobalt® GHV, Palacos® R+G, Refobacin®, and SmartSet® GHV have higher cumulative delivery than other cements (Squire et al. 2008; Neut et al. 2010; Meyer et al. 2011). However, the experts do not agree on whether these differences necessarily imply variations in the incidence of PJI. We believe that PJI is a multifactorial problem in which we cannot measure the specific contribution of each single factor. Therefore, we should choose cement with higher elution rates and use all available measures to reduce the incidence of infection (adequate prophylaxis, using the cement with the highest elution rates, changing gloves and disposable instruments, washing the surgical field with antiseptic solution – iodine povidone – and saline solution every 15–20 min).

No single response is adequate, and outcome depends on several factors (e. g. prophylaxis, type of cement, surgical environment). Nevertheless, PJI is increasingly frequent, and outcome worsens as many incorrect treatments are applied without adhering to recommended protocols. In addition, outcome is poor when managing difficult-to-treat infections (Schwarzkopf et al. 2013). Therefore, all possible preventive measures should be taken.

8.1.11 Case Study 1: A Chain of Mistakes, Not Complications

A 35-year-old man sustained a complex injury of the left knee – including the anterior cruciate ligament (ACL), posterior cruciate ligament (PCL), medial collateral ligament (MCL), and tibial plateau fracture – after a traffic accident. All injuries but the PCL were reconstructed.

At the age of 45, removal of previous hardware and a TKA were indicated for knee osteoarthritis (OA). The selected implant was a NexGen® CR prosthesis (even though his PCL was torn; first mistake), which was fixed without cement despite the risk associated with the presence of previous hardware (second and third mistakes: cementless fixation, therefore no antibiotic in the cement; two screws directed towards the cancellous bone, instead of four screws directed towards the tibial cortical layer; February 2000). The femoral component was positioned in flexion, and some posterior osteophytes were not removed (fourth mistake). The range of motion (ROM) achieved was 0–80°.

In October 2000, the patient developed a fistula that was treated with DAIR 8 months after the index arthroplasty (fifth mistake). Culture revealed CNS, and the patient was treated with ciprofloxacin (sixth mistake, not combined treatment; however, this is a debatable issue, since a high bacterial load may also lead to rifampicin resistance).

The patient remained free of pain, with limited ROM. In 2003 and 2008, he developed two new fistulae, which were treated with DAIR (seventh mistake). In both episodes, cultures were negative (eighth and ninth mistakes: correct sampling? correct processing? correct treatment in the laboratory?). Although free from pain, the patient was stiff and progressively unstable.

He presented to our department for the first time in 2010. The knee was painful, unstable, with light swelling, although not warm. The ROM was 0–60°, and two scars were visible (closed at the time). The patient was a smoker and had stents. The X-rays revealed a loosened TKA (see ▪ Fig. 8.3 and ▪ Fig. 8.4).

Blood analysis disclosed the following values: WBC, normal; ESR, 18 mm/h (reference range, 2–14 mm/h); CRP, 0.6 mg/l (reference range, 0.0–0.5 mg/l). Culture of the aspirate was negative. The bone scan (WBC-Tc99m HMPAO + Tc99m) was positive. Allergy studies were negative for Cr, Ni, Co, Ti, Cu, PMMA, and ZrO.

Despite previous negative cultures, we treated the patient as infected. A two-stage protocol was necessary, as the infecting micro-organism had not been identified and we expected to gain more ROM with the spacer. Unless proven otherwise, a fistula should be considered indicative of infection (some exceptions are possible with metal-on-metal prostheses or allergies). The first stage included removal of the prosthesis and placement of a spacer made of Copal® G+C by adding 2 g of vancomycin per pack of cement (see ▪ Fig. 8.3 and ▪ Fig. 8.4). The patient reached 95° of flexion with the spacer, more than with the index TKA (see ▪ Fig. 8.3 and ▪ Fig. 8.4).

We took protocolized cultures, including sonication of the removed prosthesis. Synovial fluid and periprosthetic tissue cultures were negative at the first reading and positive at the second reading (14 days). Sonication of the implant (≥50 CFU/ml) and PCR enabled early detection of the infecting micro-organism and pointed to the need for prolonged cultures. Although this is our standard protocol and should be the rule in all laboratories treating PJI, prolonged culture is not always the rule in many laboratories in Spain. *Staphylococcus lugdunensis* was isolated. Many laboratories do not have specific procedures for identification of CNS.

The final diagnosis was sub-acute, low-grade infection after primary TKA. In addition, the diagnosis was considerably delayed.

After a short intravenous regimen and a 2-month oral antibiotic protocol, we performed re-implantation. Histopathology of periprosthetic tissue ruled out acute inflammation. Cultures were negative. We chose an Oxinium® component (Legion-Smith and Nephew) for re-implantation. Some metaphyseal grafting of the tibia was necessary. The components were cemented with Palacos® R+G. At re-implantation, we placed the tibial component in excessive internal rotation (tenth mistake). Patellofemoral tracking was not congruent.

Therefore, even though we had avoided extensile exposures with the two-stage protocol and the articulating spacer, we finally had to perform an extended tibial tubercle osteotomy and rotate and re-cement the tibial component appropriately (see ◘ Fig. 8.3 and ◘ Fig. 8.4). The consequences were as expected, namely, compromise of soft tissue resulting from the two scars and the wires. Wound dehiscence over the cerclage wires of the tibial osteotomy required surgical closure 15 days after re-implantation. New samples were taken for culture during the procedure. All results were negative, and the wound healed uneventfully.

The final ROM was 0–120° after 10 years of stiffness and an occult infection. The patient remains free from pain, and the Knee Society Score was rated as excellent. Laboratory markers remain normal 5 years later (see ◘ Fig. 8.3 and ◘ Fig. 8.4).

Learning Points

- A fistula should be considered indicative of infection unless proven otherwise.
- The best available diagnostic tools should be used, namely, sonication, PCR, and delayed cultures. PCR could point to the need for prolonged conventional cultures or specific requirements to culture the suspected infecting micro-organism.
- This case illustrates a chain of mistakes, not complications. First, a posterostabilized design should be used if the PCL is not functional. Second, an infection diagnosed late is not an indication for DAIR. Third, combined antibiotic therapy was not prescribed. Fourth, many laboratories do not have the technology to diagnose a wide variety of strains of CNS.
- Articulating spacers with antibiotic-loaded acrylic cement make it possible to preserve ROM and prevent soft tissue retraction. They also prevent bone loss and, most importantly, are associated with a high rate of eradication of the infection. In this case study, extensile exposure was related to intraoperative mistakes, not to retraction of soft tissue, which was avoided with the articulating spacer.

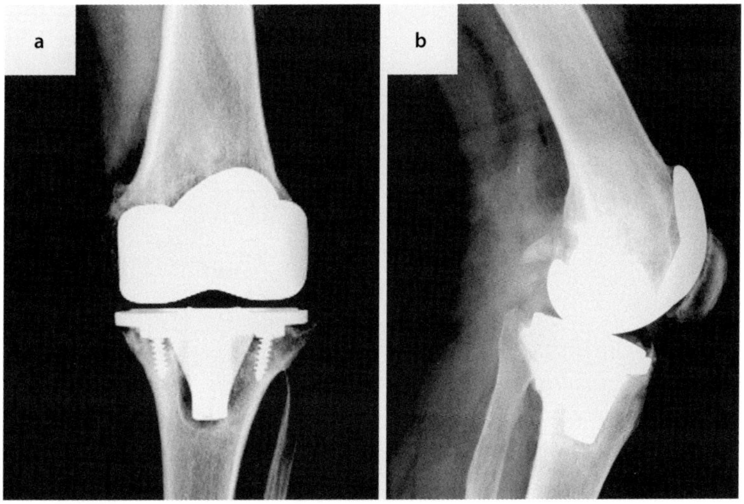

◘ **Fig. 8.6** **a, b** Case study 1: poor surgical technique and inadequate implant selection

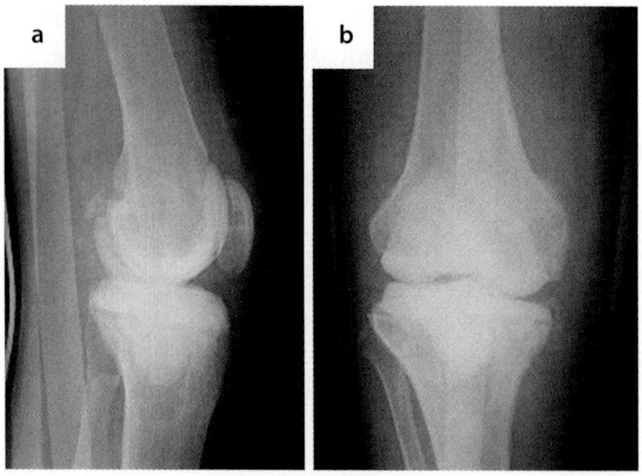

■ **Fig. 8.7 a, b** Case study 1: customized articulating spacer with Copal® G+C and added vancomycin

8.1.12 Case Study 2: Low-Grade Infection of a THA – Complications and Mistakes

A 72-year-old man underwent THR with a modular femoral component for OA. During the post-operative period, he experienced a THA dislocation that required open reduction and replacement of the modular components (neck and head). He then underwent prolonged surgical wound drainage.

The patient came to our clinic 3 years later. The physical examination revealed a 3-cm shortening and forced external rotation. He had pain, stiffness, and limited ROM, with a severe limp and function-

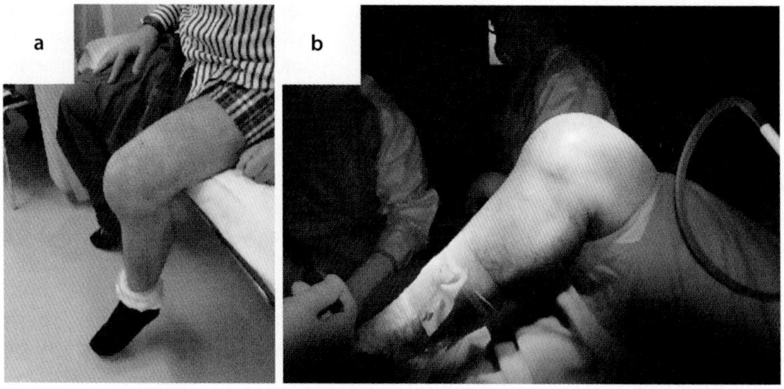

■ **Fig. 8.8 a, b** Case study 1: range of motion with the spacer

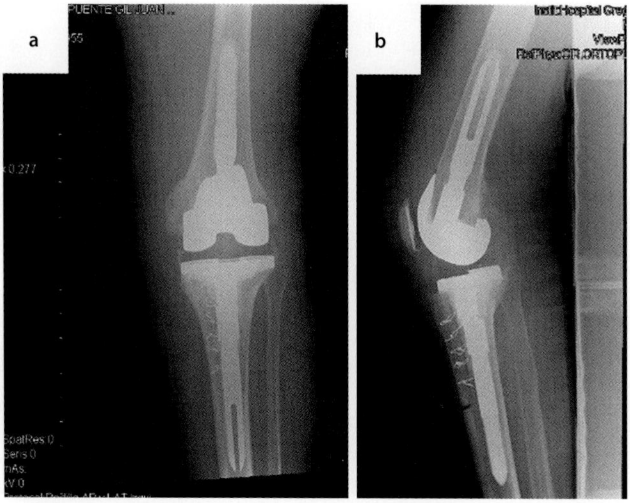

■ **Fig. 8.9 a, b** Case study 1: final X-rays

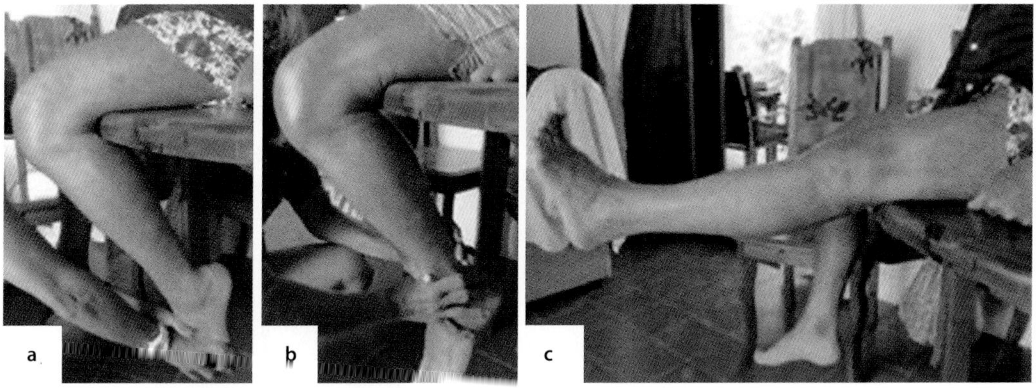

■ **Fig. 8.10** **a–c** Case study 1: final range of motion

al impairment for daily activities. The X-rays revealed a varus deformity with shortening and remodelling of the medial femoral cortex (■ Fig. 8.11).

The patient probably sustained a periprosthetic fracture that caused implant subsidence and posterior dislocation, leading to varus femoral remodelling around the implant and retroversion, until late stabilization finally occurred. The patient was unaware of this complication. The ESR and CRP levels were elevated (ESR, 22 mm/h [2–14 mm/h]; CRP, 0.8 mg/l [0–0.5 mg/l]), and culture of the fluid obtained from ultrasound-guided joint aspiration revealed methicillin-resistant CNS.

We performed a two-stage revision procedure. The first stage involved an extended trochanter osteotomy and placement of a hand-made spacer built with an Ender nail (■ Fig. 8.12). The cement used was Copal® G+C to which 2.5 g of extra vancomycin per pack was added (Copal® G+V was not available at that time; ■ Fig. 8.13. The initial intravenous protocol included meropenem and teicoplanin for 10 days, followed by a long oral course of cotrimoxazole + rifampicin for 8 weeks. Standard cultures were again positive for methicillin-resistant CNS.

Three months later, 1 week before the scheduled re-implantation, the patient experienced a double fracture after a fall (at the site of the spacer neck and at the femoral diaphysis, at the apex of the varus deformity; ■ Fig. 8.14). Therefore, we had no doubt about whether to perform a femoral osteotomy or merely align the new implant without performing an osteotomy and cerclage the trochanter over the new implant, while accepting some diastasis between the implant and the greater trochanter osteotomy.

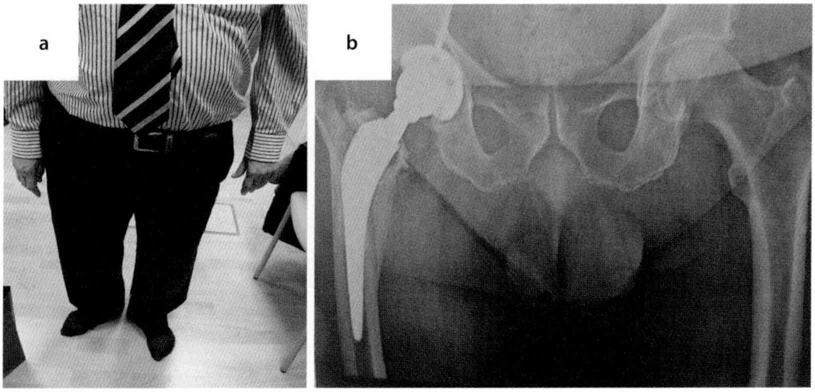

■ **Fig. 8.11** **a, b** Case study 2: photograph of the patient and preoperative X-rays

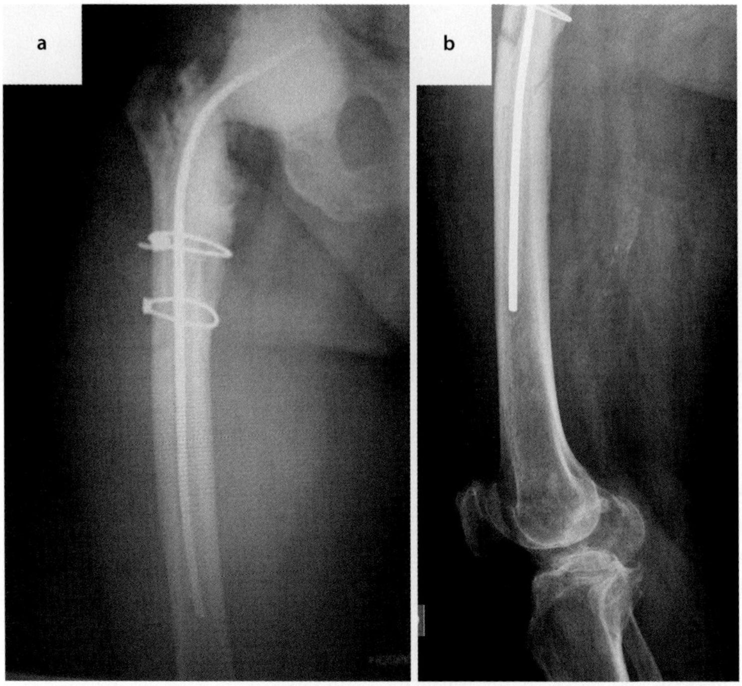

Fig. 8.12 a, b Case study 2: a long custom hand-made hip spacer bridging the femoral osteotomy

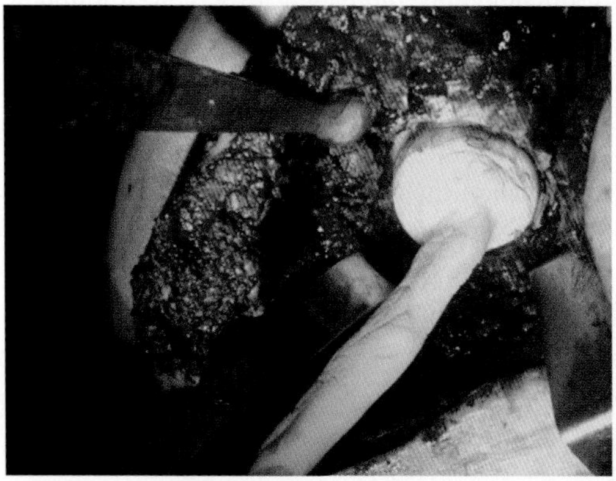

Fig. 8.13 Case study 2: the cement used was Copal® G+C with vancomycin

This complication illustrates one of the main problems of customized spacers in hip surgery. Dislocation and the steep learning curve for surgeons are additional problems.

The procedure was performed 2 days after the fall.

During re-implantation, frozen samples were sent for histopathology and standard samples for culture. Histology and cultures were all negative for acute inflammation and infection, respectively.

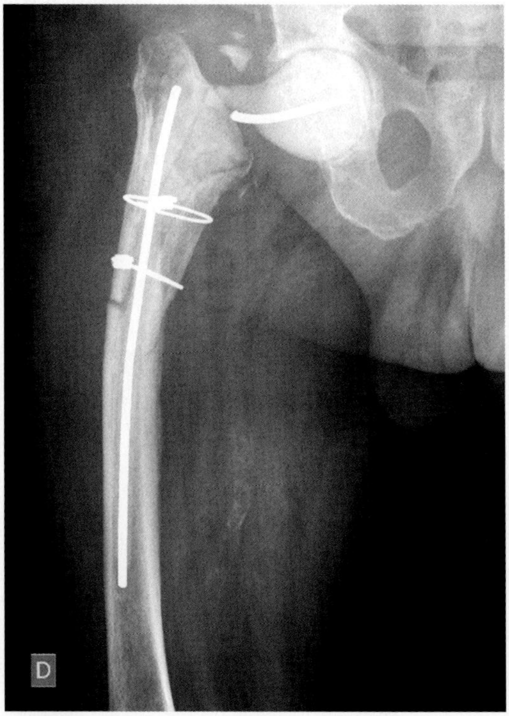

Fig. 8.14 Case study 2: double fracture at the medial femoral cortex and at the neck of the spacer

A cementless modular stem (MP-Link) was selected for the femur, and a constrained titanium tripolar cup (Stryker) was selected for the acetabulum. We tried to reduce the potential risk of dislocation in an overweight patient with poor proprioception who had undergone an extended trochanteric osteotomy and had a previous history of dislocation.

Three years after re-implantation, the patient remains free from pain, and the ROM is almost normal. The length of the limb has been restored, the varus deformity has been aligned, and the position of the leg is normal (◘ Fig. 8.15).

Critical Points for a Successful Outcome

- Lack of criteria to identify and manage an unstable periprosthetic fracture
- History and poor management of prolonged wound drainage
- Management of a varus deformity and extensile approach with a long customized spacer
- Potential complications associated with customized spacers

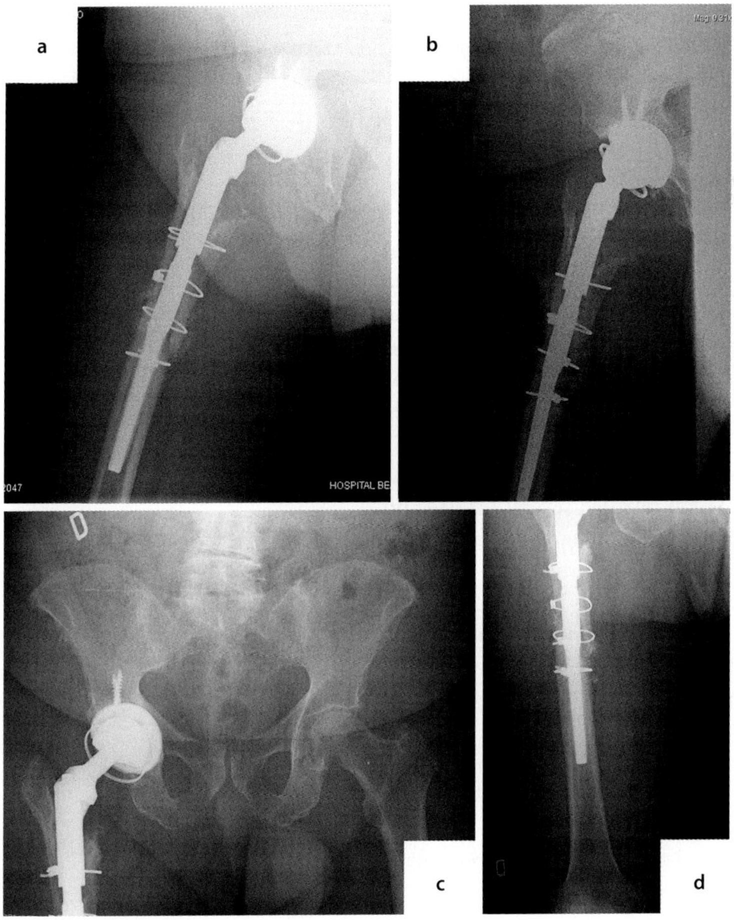

◘ **Fig. 8.15 a–d** Case study 2: final reconstruction

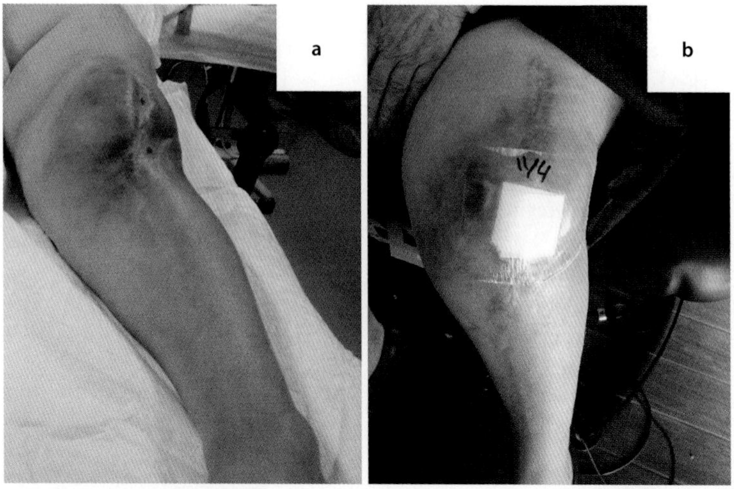

Fig. 8.16 **a, b** Case study 3: preoperative situation with multiple scars, a narrow skin bridge and two fistulae

8.1.13 Case Study 3: Three-Stage Revision – A More Realistic Approach

A 75-year-old woman underwent several surgical procedures on her left knee (open meniscectomy, tibial osteotomy, TKA, revision TKA, re-revision TKA). Diagnosis was confirmed as infection after isolation of *Enterococcus faecium*. The patient was treated with multiple DAIR procedures and erratic courses of antibiotics (linezolid, daptomycin).

The ESR and CRP levels were elevated. The physical examination revealed several fistulae and criss-crossing scars with a narrow skin bridge (Fig. 8.16). The patient was almost non-ambulant when she came to our hospital. The WBC was normal, while ESR and CRP levels were elevated (ESR, 30 mm/h [10–20 mm/h]; CRP, 13 mg/l [0–10 mg/l]). The re-revision TKA was a cemented hinge prosthesis (Fig. 8.16).

During the first stage, all previous hardware and cement were removed. Osteotomy of the femur and tibia was necessary to remove the well-fixed implant. A customized articulating spacer was made using Kirschner wires, and the osteotomy was closed with cerclage (Fig. 8.18, Fig. 8.19). The selected cement was Copal® G+C, to which 2.5 g of vancomycin per pack was added.

In this situation, the spacer was unstable, and the patient required an external orthosis to walk between procedures. The orthosis was removed several times a day and assisted flexion–extension movements were encouraged.

Three weeks after the first stage, wound healing was unsatisfactory at the critical crossing area of the previous procedures (an area of 2–3 mm had not healed). Consequently, an aggressive approach was necessary to prevent secondary contamination. Second debridement was performed, the spacer was changed for a monoblock spacer (same cement and same antibiotics), and standard samples were taken

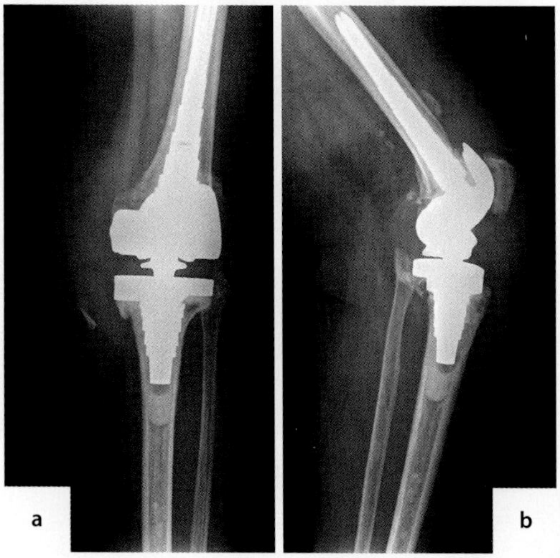

Fig. 8.17 **a, b** Case study 3: cemented hinge revision TKA

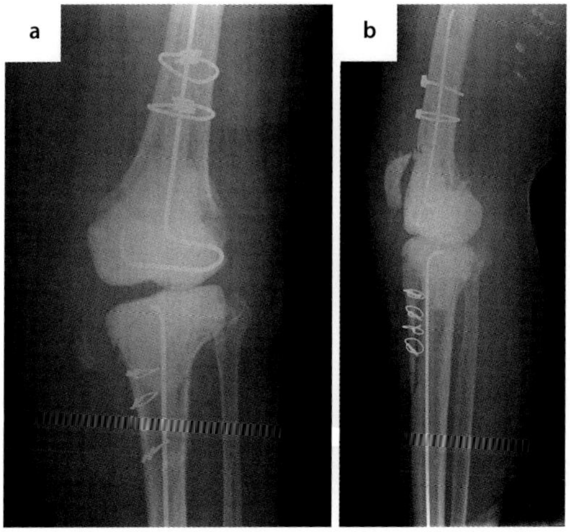

■ **Fig. 8.18 a, b** Case study 3: X-rays showing custom hand-made articulating spacer

(■ Fig. 8.20). Interestingly, all cultures were negative, indicating that either the first debridement or the combination of surgery, antibiotic-loaded acrylic cement, and systemic antibiotics was successful. The rest of the skin and soft tissue bridge was resected at this stage, and the assisted ROM interrupted. The wound healed uneventfully.

Two months later, the patient underwent a third procedure. WBC, ESR, and CRP levels were normal or almost normal. Re-implantation was performed using a modular rotating hinge, Endo-Model® prosthesis, and distal retrograde cementation with Palacos® R+G (■ Fig. 8.21). New standard samples and histology were negative for infection and acute inflammation. The patient recovered and is ambulant, with occasional mild pain. The wound has healed, and the ROM is 0–110°.

Points of Interest

Fistulae or soft tissue compromise may be a limitation for one-stage revision, despite appropriate radical debridement.

Additional limitations for one-stage re-implantation include the aggressiveness or unconfirmed identification of the infecting micro-organism and the need for bone grafting.

Although a new meta-analysis has revealed comparable results with one- and two-stage re-implantation, case selection may be subject to bias. In our current practice, we only attempt one-stage procedures in favourable cases (Masters et al. 2013).

In difficult cases, two-stage revision may become a three- or four-stage revision, as we illustrate in the present case. It is interesting that these extra procedures are not considered failures of a two-stage protocol. This finding should be emphasized in the literature when comparing rates of re-infection after a one-stage protocol (0–11%) and after a two-stage protocol (0–41%; Masters et al. 2013).

Despite the wealth of publications and guidelines, many surgeons still follow erroneous protocols (antibiotics in monotherapy at incorrect doses and times, repeated DAIR procedures in chronic infection), thus compromising outcome (Betsch et al. 2008; Schwarzkopf et al. 2013).

Surgeons should consider referring patients to units with multidisciplinary teams to ensure that treatment is administered appropriately.

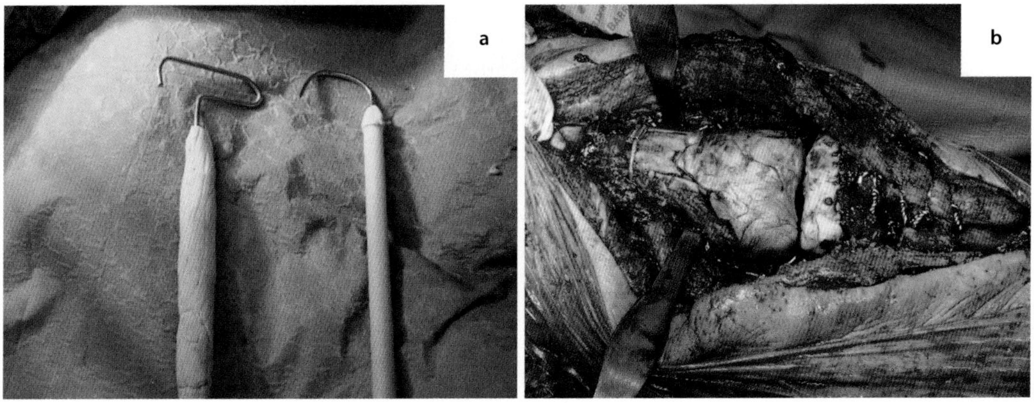

■ **Fig. 8.19 a, b** Case study 3: intraoperative pictures of custom hand-made articulating spacer

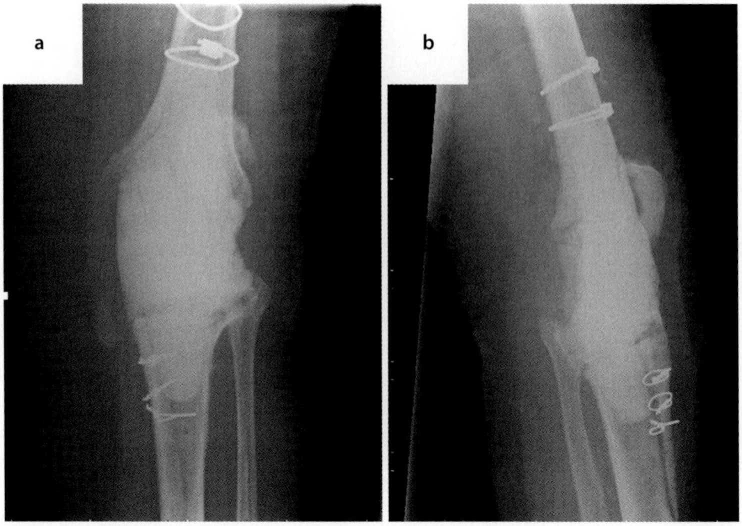

Fig. 8.20 a, b Monoblock spacer

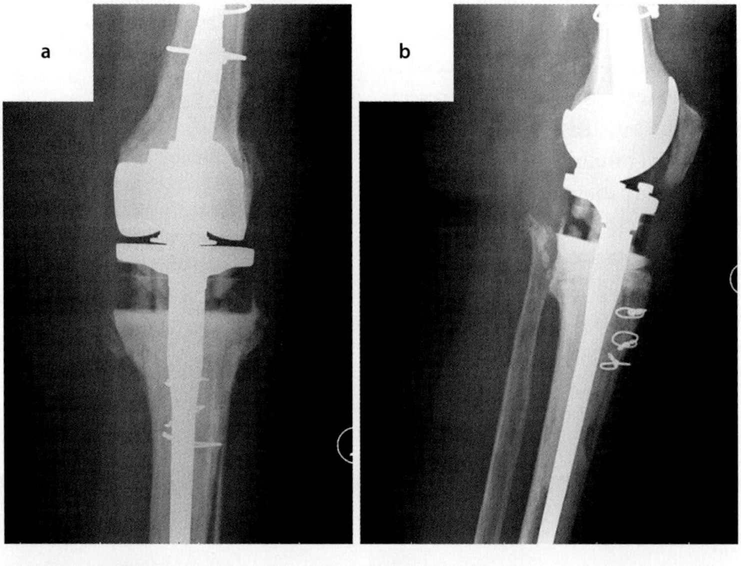

Fig. 8.21 a, b Cemented hinge revision TKA

The lack of specialization is also evident in details such as the scars in the present case. Instead of using the distal part of the lateral scar of the osteotomy, the surgeon left a narrow, more medial bridge, thus creating an area of poor vascularization that was the main reason for poor wound healing.

8.1.14 Case Study 4: Limitations for One-Stage Re-implantation

A 55-year-old woman had undergone ten operations for dysplasia of the hip. The most recent procedures were prosthesis exchange, vacuum-assisted secondary closure, and failed DAIR procedures.

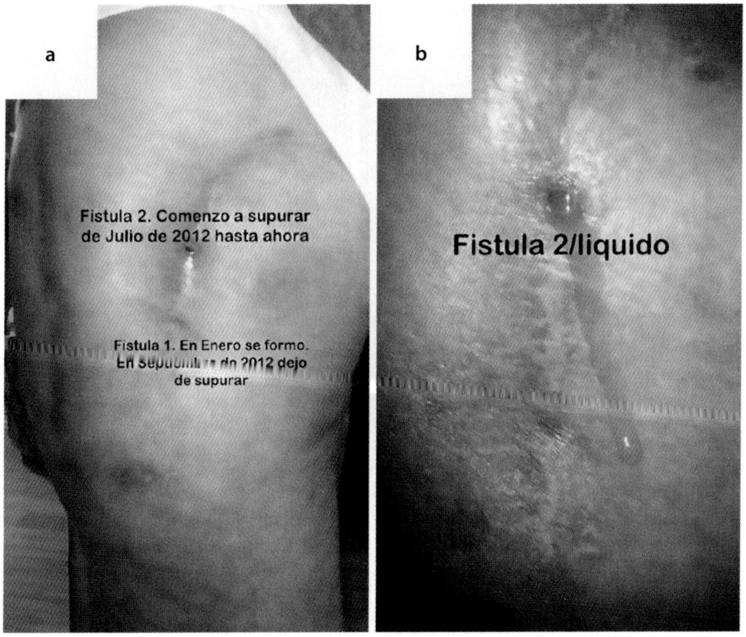

Fig. 8.22 a, b Case study 4: preoperative fistulae. (**a** Fistula 2, suppurating since July 2012. Fistula 1, developed in January, stopped suppurating in September 2012. **b** Fistula 2/discharge)

The patient came to our hospital with a productive fistula (active for the last 2 years), severe bone loss on the femoral side, and mild loss in the acetabulum (Fig. 8.22). The cemented prosthesis was loose. In addition, the cementation technique and design did not seem to be adequate. The patient was experiencing severe pain and walked with crutches and a marked limp. Previous culture had revealed *Stenotrophomonas maltophilia*. Protocolized cultures revealed *Finegoldia magna*, which was considered a defective *Peptostreptococcus* species for many years.

The fistula and the need for bone grafting made two-stage revision the protocol of choice.

During the first stage, all hardware and cement were removed and exhaustive debridement was performed. A long hand-made hip spacer was inserted, bridging the thinned lateral cortex at the apex of the previous mobilized implant (Fig. 8.23). We used Copal® G+C for the spacer and added 3 g of vancomycin per pack of cement.

Standard samples, including sonication of samples from the implant, revealed *Finegoldia magna*.

No hip orthosis was required. Partial weight-bearing was encouraged, with the help of crutches. After 10 days of intravenous antibiotic therapy, oral antibiotic therapy was started for 8 weeks (amoxicillin 1 g/8 h plus metronidazole 500 mg/8 h).

The prosthesis was re-implanted 10 weeks later (impaction bone grafting with Palacos® R+G cement; Fig. 8.24).

Three years after the operation the patient (an actress) returned to work and remains free from pain. The outcome is excellent.

Points of Interest

Incorrect treatment can compromise outcome.
Bone grafting is a limitation for one-stage re-implantation.
Manual hip spacers can be adapted to difficult situations.
The need for orthosis depends on the patient and bone status (e. g. young patient, damage to the greater trochanter, good performance with crutches).
Sonication and PCR were necessary to identify a previously defective bacterium as the causative micro-organism.

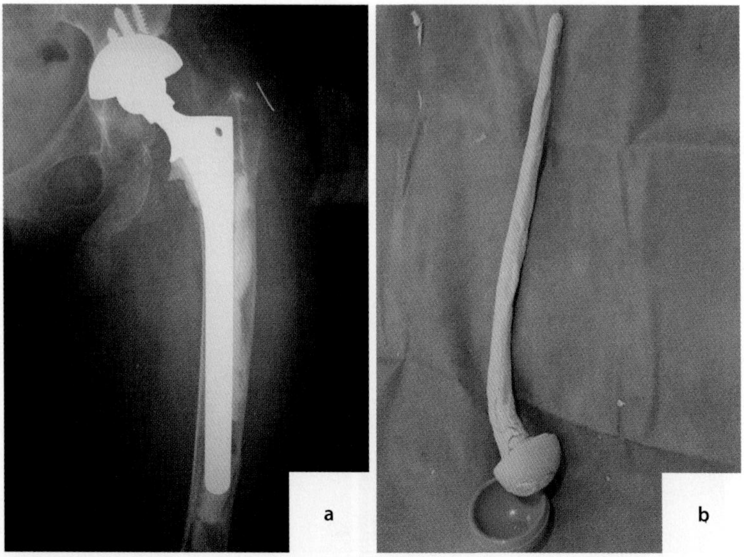

■ **Fig. 8.23** a, b Case study 4: preoperative x-rays and hand-made spacer of the hip

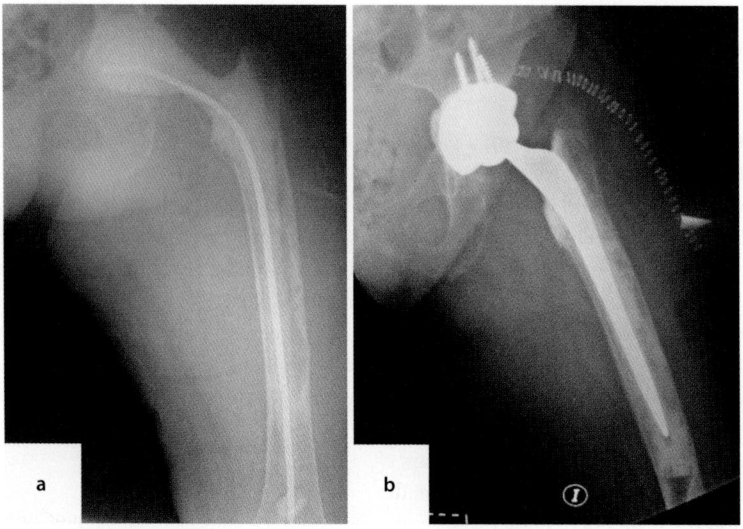

■ **Fig. 8.24** a, b Case study 4: X-rays with the spacer and after final re-implantation

8.1.15 Case Study 5: Optimizing Diagnosis

A 52-year-old man had been operated on 3 years previously for OA. The selected implant was a Corail® Stem with a Pinnacle® Cup (De Puy). The patient had occasional soreness, stiffness, and mild pain. The WBC, CRP, and ESR levels were normal.

The pain became worse after an injury to the operated hip. An ultrasound image revealed a mass over the greater trochanter measuring 15×9×5 cm (■ Fig. 8.25). The mass was aspirated using ultrasound guidance. Culture was negative but the pain persisted.

The patient was diagnosed with bursitis of the greater trochanter. Culture and PCR of the resected soft-tissue were positive for *Abiotrophia defectiva.*

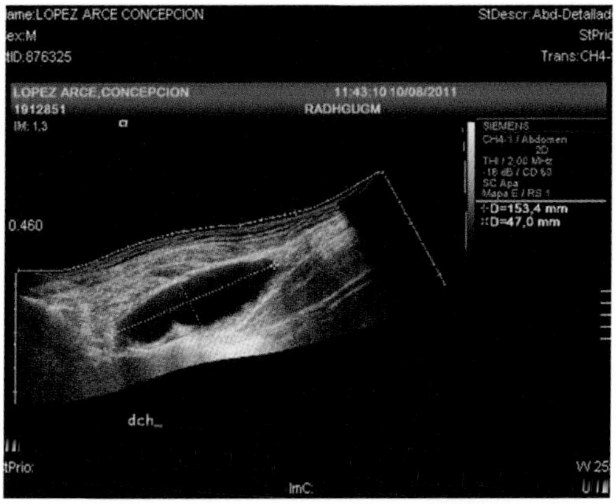

■ **Fig. 8.25** Case study 5: ultrasound mass over the greater trochanter

The pain persisted and the patient was considered infected. A two-stage revision was scheduled. Laboratory values before the first stage were as follows: WBC, normal; CRP, 0.58 mg/l (0.00–0.50 mg/l); ESR, 8 mm/h (2–14 mm/h).

The implant was well fixed. An extended trochanter osteotomy was performed and bridged with a customized spacer made of Copal® G+C combined with an extra 2.5 g of vancomycin per pack of cement (■ Fig. 8.26). Two months later, before re-implantation, the laboratory values were as follows: WBC, normal; ESR, 5 mm/h (2–14 mm/h); CRP, 0.78 mg/l (0–0.8 mg/l). Four years after re-implantation, the patient remains free of pain, with no signs of recurrence (■ Fig. 8.27).

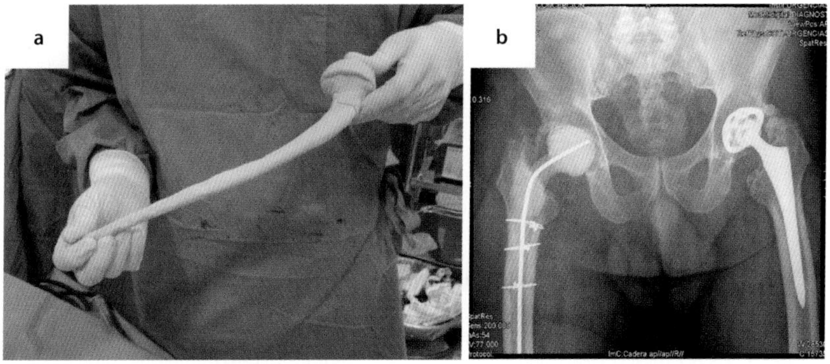

■ **Fig. 8.26 a, b** Case study 5: custom hand-made spacer of the hip and post-operative X-rays

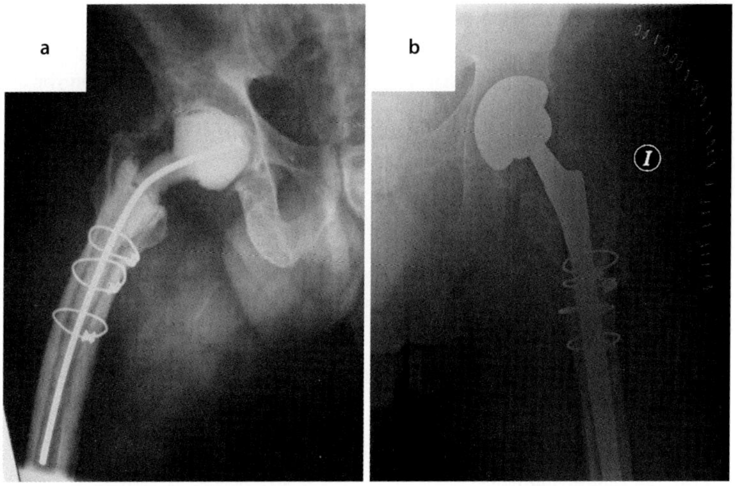

■ **Fig. 8.27 a, b** Case study 5: post-operative X-rays with the spacer and after reconstruction

Before molecular biology techniques were widely available, *Abiotrophia defectiva* was included with *Streptococcus defectivus*. This entity only grows in special media, forms satellite colonies around *S. aureus* and other bacteria, and can be confused with Gram-positive bacteria.

Learning Point

With rates of negative cultures in the literature ranging from 7% to 30% in cases treated as infection, greater efforts should be made to reduce these rates. Standard samples, fast processing, prolonged cultures, sonication, and molecular biology techniques should form part of the armamentarium of specialized multidisciplinary centres (Trampuz et al. 2007; Schafer et al. 2008; Marin et al. 2012).

Take-Home Message

- Whenever possible, we use antibiotic-loaded spacers (monoblock in the case of hips and articulating in the case of knees) and tailor the antibiotic protocol to the previous antibiogram (when available).
- We do not use preformed spacers. Many doctors in Spain use silicone moulds and tailor the type and load of antibiotic to the infecting micro-organism. Our current protocol is based on customized spacers for both the knee and the hip. We routinely use nails or intramedullary rods to build our hip spacers and occasionally use them in knees with severe bone loss.
- In cases where soft tissue healing is problematic, we use a monoblock spacer or an articulating spacer and immobilize the knee in extension with an orthosis.
- The choice of spacer depends on many factors, including degree of bone loss, state of soft tissue, choice of antibiotics, and financial and technical restraints. A benefit common to both articulating and non-articulating antibiotic-loaded spacers is that significant higher intra-articular levels of antibiotic can be delivered than with parenteral antibiotics.
- Although the better type of spacer (monoblock or articulating) remains open to debate, most authors believe that articulating spacers for the treatment of infected TKA provide better soft tissue and bone mass preservation and better functional results. Another potential advantage is a higher eradication rate when using articulating spacers.
- Antibiotic-loaded cement spacers release high concentrations of drug and enable higher intra-articular concentrations to be reached than parenteral antibiotics alone, with little effect on serum or urine concentrations and, therefore, with minimal risk of systemic damage.
- We prefer cements that elute the highest dose of antibiotics. The only commercial presentations with a synergistic effect are Copal® G+C and Copal® G+V (gentamicin combined with clindamycin or vancomycin). Copal enables increased release of antibiotic and greater ability to inhibit the formation of biofilm than gentamicin alone.
- Commercially available cements with a synergistic effect are used for other reasons:
  - When antibiotics are added manually to the cement, the synergistic effect makes antibiotic release differ significantly between bone cements. With commercial formulations, release is optimized and more predictable.
  - Synergy can enable the release of greater amounts of antibiotic, thus making inhibition of bacterial growth more effective and increasing the chances of winning the »race for the surface«.
  - Elution rates are higher than with other commercial brands or combinations.
  - By achieving high rates of antibiotic elution, even micro-organisms classed as resistant in routine antibiograms can be eradicated when the dose is increased sufficiently.
  - Elution is more predictable.
- We often manually add additional antimicrobial drugs to the commercial combination to cover a broad spectrum of bacteria and release higher doses of antibiotics at the site of infection than we would using prefabricated spacers.
- We follow the method of Frommelt and Kühn, namely, fractional addition of antibiotic.
- Synergy between aminoglycosides + vancomycin, aminoglycosides + clindamycin and, occasionally, a cephalosporin (ceftazidime, ceftriaxone, cefepime, and cefotaxime, which are available in powder form in our setting) can enable coverage of a broad spectrum of micro-organisms.
- Other antibiotics that should be taken into consideration in the coming years include linezolid, teicoplanin, and daptomycin for vancomycin-resistant *Staphylococcus* species, and meropenem (which also has a synergistic effect with vancomycin), amikacin, and fosfomycin for multidrug-resistant Gram-negative bacteria. These antibiotics are usually available in powder form. However, antibiotic-loaded cements containing these drugs are not commercially available.

References

Alt V, Bechert T, Steinrucke P, Wagener M, Seidel P, Dingeldein E, Domann E, Schnettler R (2004) In vitro testing of antimicrobial activity of bone cement. Antimicrob Agents Chemother 48(11):4084-4088

Anderson JA, Sculco PK, Heitkemper S, Mayman DJ, Bostrom MP, Sculco TP (2009) An articulating spacer to treat and mobilize patients with infected total knee arthroplasty. J Arthroplasty 24(4):631-635

Anguita-Alonso PM, Rouse S, Piper KE, Jacofsky DJ, Osmon DR, Patel R (2006) Comparative study of antimicrobial release kinetics from polymethylmethacrylate. Clin Orthop Relat Res [illegible]

Betsch BY, Eggli S, Siebenrock KA, Tauber MG, Muhlemann K (2008) Treatment of joint prosthesis infection in accordance with current recommendations improves outcome. Clin Infect Dis 46(8):1221-1226

Chiang ER, Su YP, Chen TH, Chiu FY, Chen WM (2011) Comparison of articulating and static spacers regarding infection with resistant organisms in total knee arthroplasty. Acta Orthop 82(4):460-464

Cobo J, Del Pozo JL (2011) Prosthetic joint infection:diagnosis and management. Expert Rev Anti Infect Ther 9(9):787-802

Ensing GT, van Horn JR, van der Mei HC, Busscher HJ, Neut D (2008) Copal bone cement is more effective in preventing biofilm formation than Palacos R-G. Clin Orthop Relat Res 466(6):1492-1498

Frommelt L, Kühn K.-D. (2005) Properties of bone cement: antibiotic-loaded cement. In S. Breusch and H. Malchau (eds) The well-ceemnted total hip arthroplasty. Springer, Berlin Heidelberg, pp. 86-92

Goldstei, WM, Kopplin M, Wall R, Berland K (2001) Temporary articulating methylmethacrylate antibiotic spacer (TAMMAS). A new method of intraoperative manufacturing of a custom articulating spacer. J Bone Joint Surg Am 83-A [Suppl 2]Pt 2:92-97

Gooding CR, Masri BA, Duncan CP, Greidanus NV, Garbuz DS (2011) Durable infection control and function with the PROSTALAC spacer in two-stage revision for infected knee arthroplasty. Clin Orthop Relat Res 469(4):985-993

Goss B, Lutton C, Weinrauch P, Jabur M, Gillett G, Crawford R (2007) Elution and mechanical properties of antifungal bone cement. J Arthroplasty 22(6):902-908

Ha C W (2006) A technique for intraoperative construction of antibiotic spacers. Clin Orthop Relat Res 445:204-209

Hansen EN, Adeli B, Kenyon R, Parvizi J (2014) Routine use of antibiotic laden bone cement for primary total knee arthroplasty:impact on infecting microbial patterns and resistance profiles. J Arthroplasty 29(6):1123-1127

Hanssen AD, Spangehl MJ (2004) Practical applications of antibiotic-loaded bone cement for treatment of infected joint replacements. Clin Orthop Relat Res(427):79-85

Hsu YC, Cheng HC, Ng TP, Chiu KY (2007) Antibiotic-loaded cement articulating spacer for 2-stage reimplantation in infected total knee arthroplasty:a simple and economic method. J Arthroplasty 22(7):1060-1066

Incavo SJ, Russell RD, Mathis KB, Adams H (2009) Initial results of managing severe bone loss in infected total joint arthroplasty using customized articulating spacers. J Arthroplasty 24(4):607-613

Jamsen E, Huhtala H, Puolakka T, Moilanen T (2009) Risk factors for infection after knee arthroplasty. A register-based analysis of 43,149 cases. J Bone Joint Surg Am 91(1):38-47

Jiranek WA, Waligora AC, Hess SR, Golladay GL (2015) Surgical treatment of prosthetic joint infections of the hip and knee:changing paradigms? J Arthroplasty 30(6):912-918

Kühn K-D (2014) PMMA cements. ISBN-13 978-3-642-41535-7, doi:10.1007/978-3-642-41536-4

Kühn K-D, Lieb E, Berberich C (2016). PMMA bone cement: What is the role of local antibiotics? Maitrise Orthopaedique Commission Paritaire [illegible] ISSN:11482362 (Special Issue June 2016)

Kurtz S, Ong K, Lau E, Mowat F, Halpern M (2007) Projections of primary and revision hip and knee arthroplasty in the United States from 2005 to 2030. J Bone Joint Surg Am 89(4):780-785

Laine JC, Nguyen TQ, Buckley JM, Kim HT (2011) Effects of mixing techniques on vancomycin-impregnated polymethylmethacrylate. J Arthroplasty 26(8):1562-1566

MacAvoy MC, Ries MD (2005) The ball and socket articulating spacer for infected total knee arthroplasty. J Arthroplasty 20(6):757-762

Marin M, Garcia-Lechuz JM, Alonso P, Villanueva M, Alcala L, Gimeno M, E. Cercenado, M. Sanchez-Somolinos, C. Radice and E. Bouza (2012) Role of universal 16S rRNA gene PCR and sequencing in diagnosis of prosthetic joint infection. J Clin Microbiol 50(3):583-589

Masters JP, Smith NA, Foguet P, Reed M, Parsons H, Sprowson AP (2013) A systematic review of the evidence for single stage and two stage revision of infected knee replacement. BMC Musculoskelet Disord 14:222

Meyer J, Piller G, Spiegel CA, Hetzel S, Squire M (2011). Vacuum-mixing significantly changes antibiotic elution characteristics of commercially available antibiotic-impregnated bone cements. J Bone Joint Surg Am. 93(22):2049-2056

Neut D, Kluin OS, Thompson J, van der Mei HC, Busscher HJ (2010) Gentamicin release from commercially-available gentamicin-loaded PMMA bone cements in a prosthesis-related interfacial gap model and their antibacterial efficacy. BMC Musculoskelet Disord 11:258

Park SJ, Song EK, Seon JK, Yoon TR, Park Y H (2010). Comparison of static and mobile antibiotic-impregnated cement spacers for the treatment of infected total knee arthroplasty. International Orthopaedics (SICOT) 34:1181-1186

Parvizi J, Azzam K, Ghanem E, Austin MS, Rothman RH (2009) Periprosthetic infection due to resistant staphylococci: serious problems on the horizon. Clin Orthop Relat Res 467(7):1732-1739

Parvizi J, Gehrke T, Chen AF (2013) Proceedings of the International Consensus on Periprosthetic Joint Infection. Bone Joint J 95-B(11):1450-1452

Parvizi J, Saleh KJ, Ragland PS, Pour AE, Mont MA (2008) Efficacy of antibiotic-impregnated cement in total hip replacement. Acta Orthop 79(3):335-341

Pérez Mañanes R, Vaquero Martín J, Villanueva Martínez M (2011) Influencia de la técnica de cementación sobre la calidad del manto de cemento en la artroplastia de rodilla. Estudio experimental sobre un modelo sintético. Rev Esp Cir Ortop Traumatol 55(1):39-49

Pitto RP, Castelli CC, Ferrari R, Munro J (2005) Pre-formed articulating knee spacer in two-stage revision for the infected total knee arthroplasty. Int Orthop 29(5):305-308

Rodriguez-Pardo D, Pigrau C, Lora-Tamayo J, Soriano A, del Toro MD, Cobo J, Palomino J, Euba G, Riera M, Sanchez-Somolinos M, Benito N, Fernandez-Sampedro M, Sorli L, Guio L, Iribarren JA, Baraia-Etxaburu JM, Ramos A, Bahamonde A, Flores-Sanchez X, Corona PS, Ariza J, R. G. f. t. S. o. P. Infection (2014) Gram-negative prosthetic joint infection:outcome of a debridement, antibiotics and implant retention approach. A large multicentre study. Clin Microbiol Infect 20(11):911-919

Romano CL, Gala L, Logoluso N, Romano D, Drago L (2012) Two-stage revision of septic knee prosthesis with articulating knee spacers yields better infection eradication rate than one-stage or two-stage revision with static spacers. Knee Surg Sports Traumatol Arthrosc 20(12): 2445-2453

Sanz-Ruiz P, Villanueva-Martinez M, Matas-Diez JA, Vaquero-Martin J (2015) Revision TKA with a condylar constrained prosthesis using metaphyseal and surface cementation:a minimum 6-year follow-up analysis. BMC Musculoskelet Disord 16:39

Sanz-Ruiz P, Matas-Diez JA, Sánchez-Somolinos M, Villanueva-Martínez M, Vaquero-Martin J (2016). Is the commercial antibiotic-loaded bone cement useful in prophylactic and cost saving after knee and hip joint arthroplasty? The Transatlantic Paradox. doi:http://dx.doi.org/10.1016/j.arth.2016.11.012

Schafer P, Fink B, Sandow D, Margull A, Berger I, Frommelt L (2008) Prolonged bacterial culture to identify late periprosthetic joint infection:a promising strategy. Clin Infect Dis 47(11):1403-1409

Schwarzkopf R, Oh D, Wright E, Estok DM, Katz JN (2013) Treatment failure among infected periprosthetic patients at a highly specialized revision TKA referral practice. Open Orthop J 7:264-271

Springer BD, Lee GC, Osmon D, Haidukewych GJ, Hanssen AD, Jacofsky DJ (2004) Systemic safety of high-dose antibiotic-loaded cement spacers after resection of an infected total knee arthroplasty. Clin Orthop Relat Res(427):47-51

Squire MW, Ludwig BJ, Thompson JR, Jagodzinski J, Hall D, Andes D (2008) Premixed antibiotic bone cement:an in vitro comparison of antimicrobial efficacy. J Arthroplasty 23[6 Suppl 1]:110-114

Trampuz A, Piper KE, Jacobson MJ, Hanssen AD, Unni KK, Osmon DR, Mandrekar JN, Cockerill FR, Steckelberg JM, Greenleaf JF, Patel R (2007) Sonication of removed hip and knee prostheses for diagnosis of infection. N Engl J Med 357(7):654-663

Tsukayama DT, Estrada R, Gustilo RB (1996) Infection after total hip arthroplasty. A study of the treatment of one hundred and six infections. J Bone Joint Surg Am 78(4):512-523

Villanueva-Martinez M, Hernandez-Barrera V, Chana-Rodriguez F, Rojo-Manaute J, Rios-Luna A, San Roman Montero J, Gil-de-Miguel A, Jimenez-Garcia R (2012) Trends in incidence and outcomes of revision total hip arthroplasty in Spain:a population based study. BMC Musculoskelet Disord 13:37

Villanueva-Martinez M, Rios-Luna A, Pereiro J, Fahandez-Saddi H, Villamor A (2008) Hand-made articulating spacers in two-stage revision for infected total knee arthroplasty:-good outcome in 30 patients. Acta Orthop 79(5):674-682

Zimmerli W (2015) [Orthopaedic implant-associated infections:Update of antimicrobial therapy]. Orthopade 44(12): 961-966

8

8.2 Articulating Cement Spacers for the Treatment of Hip and Knee Arthroplasty Associated Infections

David Campbell

8.2.1 Introduction

Revisions for infected hip and knee arthroplasties highlight many of the hazards and morbidities associated with complex revision procedures (Jung et al. 2009; Berend et al. 2013). Patients present with more complex skeletal and medical problems that require multidisciplinary inputs to manage their orthopaedic and medical co-morbidities. Acute or chronic sepsis, malnutrition, and the predispositions that are associated with an increased risk of infection coexist. The necessity to remove infected implants results in skeletal defects and soft tissue management issues, and necessitates enormous cost.

The use of an articulating spacer is a ubiquitous tool for revision surgeons managing these problems as it facilitates delivery of antibiotics to the source of infection, permits stabilization of the skeleton, manage soft tissues and vastly improves the morbidity of patients during the interval period between removal of the infected components and re-implantation of the definitive implant (Masri et al. 1998; Haddad et al. 2000; Meek et al. 2003, 2004; Giulieri et al. 2004; Voleti et al. 2013). With an increasing use of outpatient antibiotic administration, the ability to speed the patient's discharge from hospital is an appealing cost-saving measure. It is not uncommon for extrinsic factors to delay the definitive second-stage intervention, and the ability to retain a functional temporary implant reduces the morbidities to the patient whilst they await medical optimization and a semi-elective second surgical procedure (Lee et al. 2016). Gomez et al. (2015) reported the outcome of 504 cases of periprosthetic infections treated with resection and insertion of a spacer and reported that 14% did not proceed with a second-stage procedure and had permanent spacer retention.

There is an increasing interest in single-stage revisions for arthroplasty-associated infections. In well-selected patient groups, where a single-stage revision is appropriate, the infection control is similar but mechanical complications are decreased (Langlais 2003). It is suggested that a single-stage revision be considered where there is an identified organism sensitive to antibiotics, in a healthy host, and where a single-stage cemented revision can be achieved in the absence of excessive fibrosis, sinuses or bone loss requiring allograft (Haddad et al. 2015; Nagra et al. 2015; Ilchmann et al. 2016; Zahar and Gehrke 2016). For the majority of patients, the conditions for single-stage revisions are not met and a two-stage revision is the most common treatment pathway, and largely considered the standard of care for most patients since it was first described in 1983 by Insall et al.

8.2.2 Articulating Spacers for Hip Arthroplasty

Resection arthroplasty as a definitive or staged option for treatment of bacterial infections associated with hip arthroplasties is largely a historical option owing to its considerable morbidity. Successful removal of a femoral component without osteotomy, or limited fixation of a short femoral osteotomy, can be facilitated without extensive skeletal reconstruction and these cases could permit the use of a Girdlestone procedure as an alternative to a spacer. Removal of a well-fixed ingrown or cemented femoral component often necessitates extensive osteotomies for complete removal of the component and cement. Larger osteotomies and longer femoral components will require more extensive skeletal reconstruction with a requirement for intramedullary fixation (◘ Fig. 8.28). Non-articulating intramedullary rods made from antibiotic-loaded acrylic cement (ALAC) as popularized by the Mayo group are proven options (Hanssen and Spangehl 2004) but most surgeons will favour the addition of an articular surface to obtain the functional benefits of an articulating spacer.

Citak et al. (2014) reported the conclusions of the prosthetic joint infection work group evaluating articulating spacers. The clinician group had an 89% consensus agreement that a well-performed articulating hip spacer provided improved function for patients between stages, and were especially preferred for patients that are likely to have a spacer in place for more than 3 months. They reviewed 26 original articles analysing the functional outcome; at 2 years there was a non-significant trend towards functional improvement when an articulating spacer had been used. A few studies evaluated function between stages with a superior outcome for those receiving an articulating spacer compared with a non-articulating spacer. In all, 81% of respondents agreed that re-implantation surgery was easier at the second stage compared with a non-articulating spacer.

Infection control was reported in 65 papers including 2,063 infected total hip arthroplasty cases treated with an articulating spacer and 354 cases treated with a non-articulating spacer with a similar infection control rate of 92.5% and 90.7%, respectively. The confounding variables include the heterogeneity of organisms, comorbidities and other factors that prevent a definitive conclusion.

8.2.3 Articulating Hip Spacers Options

Several forms of articulating hip spacers are in current use and vary with their method of manufacture, femoral fixation and articulation. When a comparison of infection control and functional outcome is considered between manufactured spacers and surgeon-made dynamic spacers, there is a paucity of

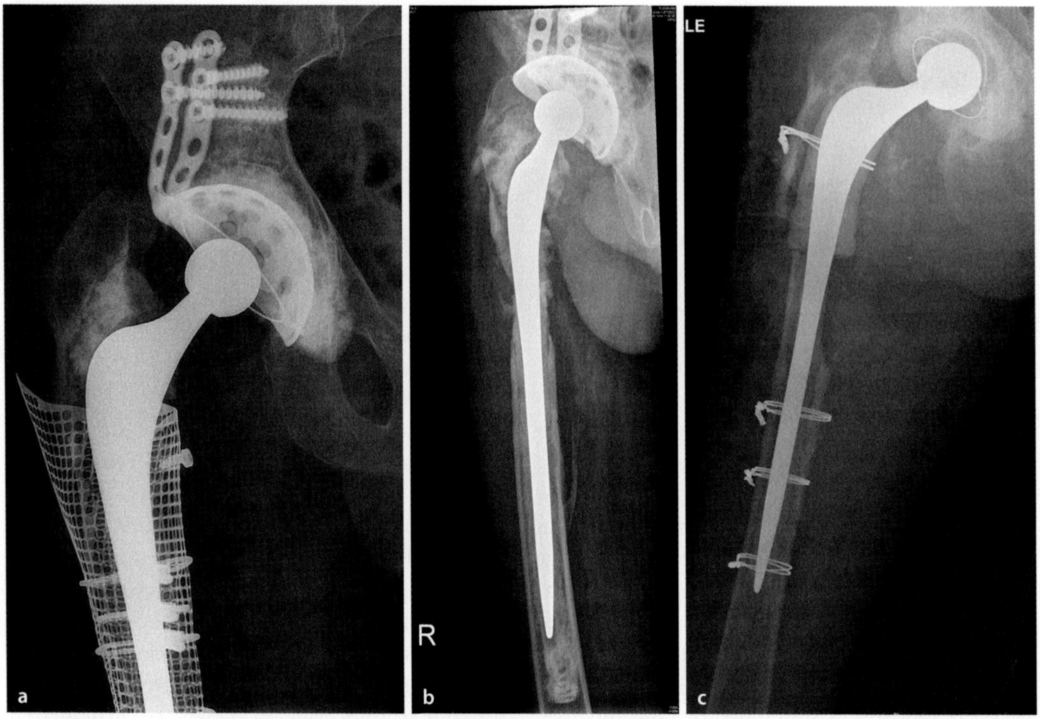

Fig. 8.28 a–c Example of infection-associated impaction-grafted revision with proximal bone deficiency. Multiply operated 58-year-old male patient with *S. aureus* infection before and after removal of mesh. Surgeon-manufactured articulating spacer incorporating proximal segment and capture cup. Definitive reconstruction was a proximal femoral replacement

direct comparative information. In 55 original articles including 1,011 hip arthroplasty cases treated with handmade spacers and 914 cases treated with manufactured spacers, similar functional outcomes were achieved (Citak et al. 2014). The prosthetic joint infection work group evaluating articulating spacers felt there was no function or infection control difference between the two groups; however, it noted that issues of cost, ease of use, and antibiotic delivery should be considered.

A favoured articulating spacer is the PROSTALAC® hip system (Depuy, Warsaw, Ind.) that is commercially available in North America and on request through the CE marking system elsewhere. It consists of an all-polyethylene constrained acetabular component that is loosely cemented combined with a press-fit femoral component that is manufactured from a metal endoskeleton surrounded by ALAC that is cured in a mould system. The surgical technique is described elsewhere (Duncan and Beauchamp 1993; Kendall et al. 1994) and briefly consists of removal of the previous components, often with an extended trochanteric osteotomy, and comprehensive soft tissue wound toilet. The acetabular component is loosely cemented late in the stage of cement polymerization and allowed to cure. Simultaneously, cement is added to a femoral mould of the selected length and size and allowed to cure. The manufactured femoral component is essentially a smooth press-fit device that is inserted into the femur either before or after closure of the osteotomies. Routine wound closure ensues, usually without drains. In the original description of the technique the patients were encouraged to continue partial weight-bearing to allow for the healing of osteotomies and prevent subsidence of the loosely press-fit femoral component (Duncan and Beauchamp 1993; Younger et al. 1997).

A definitive second-stage reconstruction was performed in a semi-elective manner when the infection was felt to be controlled at a mean interval of 4 months. Younger et al. (1997) reported infection control in 94% of 48 patients from the original series. Harris hip scores improved from 34 points preoperatively to 56 points during the interval period and 76 points following the definitive reconstruction. Notably, patients were instructed to retain partial weight-bearing, which negatively impacts upon the Harris Hips scores during the interval period. Non-design surgeons have reported similar success with this implant system (Scharfenberger et al. 2007).

Etienne et al. (2003) describe a method similar to the PROSTALAC® system utilizing standard hip arthroplasty components to minimize cost. They used a spacer consisting of a polyethylene acetabular liner and an inexpensive modular femoral component or a recycled autoclaved femoral component. The low-friction articulating surface permits function similar to a conventional hip prosthesis. In their original publication they report an infection control rate of 91% in 32 cases. The author describes a similar method that has been used for over two decades.

There are several commercially available monoblock femoral components that consist of a pre-moulded prosthesis manufactured with a standardized dose of antibiotics (Spacer G and InterSpace, Tecres, Verona, Italy) or alternatively a monoblock stem manufactured by the surgical team using a mould system (Zimmer Biomet StageOne® Select, Warsaw, Ind.). These implants are typically short-stemmed femoral components that resemble Austin–Moore-style press-fit hemiarthroplasty components. They are designed for press-fit fixation into the femur and articulate directly with the acetabulum. With minimalist femoral fixation, and a higher friction articulation within a damaged acetabulum, they are intended for expedient surgery and short-term use. It is usually recommended they be removed within 180 days. These implants are less structurally stable and prone to erode through the acetabulum into unsupported osteopoenic bone with prolonged retention or full weight-bearing. Several case series report a common practice of monoblock spacers crafted by the surgical team using readily available items such as bulb irrigators used as a mould combined with Rush pins or stout K-wires as an endoskeleton combined with ALAC (Yamamoto et al. 2003; Durbhakula et al. 2004).

The Exeter group described an articulating hip spacer referred to as the »Kiwi technique«, which utilizes a loosely cemented femoral component articulating against a polyethylene acetabular cup (Lamberton et al. 2005). The original technique involved loosely cementing the femoral and acetabular component within the patient's bone as a mould, removing it to cure and then press-fitting it in an attempt to avoid definitive fixation into the bone. The technique has evolved to include definitive fixation of the components into the patient's femur and acetabulum without the use of pressurization late in the state of cement polymerization to allow stable fixation that can be removed without bone loss. Essentially this technique is similar to a one-stage revision and the patients are encouraged to mobilize as tolerated with the intention of removing the loosely cemented components at a definitive second stage. It is not uncommon for patients to decline this second stage and retain the definitive component akin to a one-stage procedure. Tsung et al. (2014) report their experience of a similar technique using a loosely cemented Exeter monoblock stem and cemented cup with definitive retention of the implant in 34 of 76 hips.

A major advantage of the use of an articulating spacer is the management of medically challenged patients. It is common to have medical and social delays prior to the second stage, which are greatly facilitated if a patient can weight bear, in the outpatient setting, during the interval period. Some patients refuse the second stage on the basis of a successfully performed first-stage implant, and this is the genesis of the Kiwi approach. Lee et al. (2016) describe the use of a PROSTALAC® component as a definitive implant with similar infection resolution but impaired pain scores compared with patients completing the second stage. When more than 4.5 g of antibiotic is added to a 40-g mix (more than 10% by weight), the mechanical characteristics of the cement are significantly compromised and it is anticipated that the construct will be of decreased durability and longevity. To date there have been isolated reports of fixation failures of retained first-stage arthroplasties (Choi et al. 2014) and the author has experience of two patients with mechanical loosening of retained acetabular components after 5 years.

8.2.4 Complications and Developments

Complications following infection for revision are extremely frequent and are anticipated in 50–60% of this complex medical group (Jung et al. 2009). Mechanical complications will occur in approximately 16% of patients (Langlais 2003) as a consequence of initial implant removal and subsequent temporary device failure. Subsidence and implant fracture is a common mode of failure where a short-stem press-fit device is used. Femoral component fracture is associated with surgeon-made components and preformed articulating spacers (Durbhakula et al. 2004; Citak et al. 2015; ◘ Fig. 8.29). Devices with a larger diameter endoskeleton such as the PROSTALAC® (Depuy) or a revision system with an internal diameter greater than 6 mm are used to minimize the risk of component fracture and have not been associated with implant breakage. A long-stemmed femoral component usually provides adequate diaphyseal fixation that is sufficient to allow osteotomies to unite. Mid-length and long-stemmed PROSTALAC® stems are press-fit and may have rotational and axial instability. A further development is the addition of a small volume of proximal cement, which aids femoral fixation to prevent rotary instability or subsidence of a temporary femoral component and usually allows for full weight-bearing.

On the acetabular side, dislocation is a prevalent issue, partly as a consequence of press-fit femoral components that have rotatory instability (Pattyn et al. 2011; Bori et al. 2014). Large-diameter femoral head implants such as monoblock Austin–Moore-style implants impart some joint stability, but significant erosion and bone loss can occur with the use of a monoblock device articulating on osteopoenic bone (Faschingbauer et al. 2015). Drexler et al. (2016) describe the use of a supra-acetabular cement augment successfully used to prevent dislocation of monoblock components in 50 hips. The addition of a loosely cemented polyethylene acetabular component greatly facilities weight-bearing and protection of osteopoenic bone. It is common for segmental defects and anterior/posterior wall fractures to heal during the interval period in an environment of hyperaemic bone when it is loaded. However, the use of an acetabular component requires a smaller femoral head and the PROSTALAC® system utilizes a constrained acetabular implant to mitigate the increased dislocation risk.

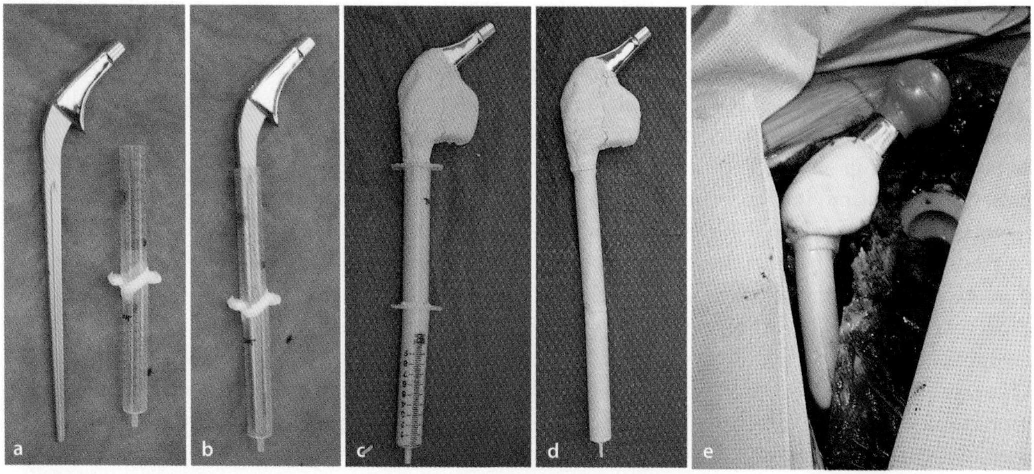

◘ **Fig. 8.29 a–e** Spacer complications. A 78-year-old female patient with infected discontinuity and intra-pelvic cement and small 8-mm femoral diaphysis. Intra-pelvic cement extraction, posterior column plate and cemented polyethylene cup. Narrow femur precluded the use of a 6–8-mm endoskeleton, manufactured with cement gun cartridge mould and Rush pin endoskeleton. At 8 weeks the weak femoral component deformed, necessitating an earlier-than-planned second-stage revision

Additionally, using a cement-stabilized femoral component allows for the use of a non-constrained polyethylene acetabular component.

8.2.5 Author's Preferred Treatment

Considering the parameters of cost, flexibility of antibiotic choice, skeletal stabilization and the ability to maximize weight-bearing, the author uses a surgeon-made spacer with an endoskeleton made of a (less expensive) mid- to long-stemmed cemented implant and an all-polyethylene acetabular component (Spectron®, Smith & Nephew, Tenn.; ◘ Fig. 8.30). When the sensitivity profiles of the infecting organism(s) are known, antibiotics are optimized for the organism(s). In the absence of a defined organism, an empirical combination of vancomycin and an aminoglycoside is preferred. Palacos cement with proprietary antibiotics is used as the base cement, which minimizes the cost of additional antibiotics. An ideal combination is 3.6 g tobramycin/gentamicin combined with 1–2 g of vancomycin with a target of 4–5 g antibiotics per 40 g cement mix.

Osteotomies are planned where necessary and the femoral component length is determined by preoperative templating. Most primary cementless stems can be removed with an intact medulla and are amenable to a short or mid-length spacer. Most cemented femoral components are managed with an extended trochanteric osteotomy to facilitate complete cement removal and will require a longer spacer to bypass the osteotomy. All components are removed and the soft tissues addressed by a comprehensive removal of infected devitalized tissue and lavage with normal saline. Multiple pathological samples are obtained from synovium and implant membranes.

Healthy acetabular bone is exposed and irrigated but no attempts at cement pressurization are made. An acetabular trial is performed to select an all-polyethylene cup of 36 mm, where size permits, and a relatively small cup to facilitate a large cement mantel increasing the volume of ALAC. Usually high-viscosity cement (e. g. Palacos® R+G, Copal®) is introduced late in the polymerization stage at approximately 6 min and is minimally pressurized.

The femoral component is prepared by removing all residual cement or membrane. The diaphysis is gently prepared with reamers of increasing diameters minimizing bone loss. The templated component length is optimized by the operative findings and a diameter 1–2 mm less than the intramedullary diameter is selected. Where possible, the osteotomy is closed prior to the implantation of the femoral component with smooth, doubled circlage wires, which minimize foreign body surface area compared with cables.

Whilst the acetabular component is being implanted, the definitive femoral component is manufactured on the back table. A cylinder of the chosen diameter is manufactured with the use of one to three sterile syringes firmly secured with hyperfix dressing tape and lubricating with paraffin oil. ALAC is inserted into the tube and a thin long-stemmed femoral component placed in the medulla of the cement-filled tube and allowed to cure. Where necessary, a collar can be moulded onto the stem. The cement is permitted to cure before removal of the plastic syringes, which results in a smooth cylindrical cementless implant. Usually a total of one to two mixes of cement are used for both the acetabulum fixation and femoral component manufacture. Approximately 20 g of the cement and monomer is held in reserve for secondary femoral fixation.

The femoral component is press-fit into the femur. To permit full weight-bearing, the remaining cement that was held in reserve is mixed and the proximal femur is cemented to aid rotational and vertical stability of the femoral component. Any minor adjustments of length and offset are made with modular femoral head components. Routine hip closure is performed without the use of a drain.

An assessment of bone defect(s) is recorded with a preliminary plan of the requirements for the second-stage reconstruction.

Post-operatively the patients are permitted weight-bearing within the constraints of the osteotomy fixation and full weight-bearing is preferred. Supplementary parenteral antibiotics are administered with guidance from an infectious disease specialist. Patients are followed up with serial inflammatory marker assessments and a definitive second-stage reconstruction is planned when there is a likely infection resolution determined by falling

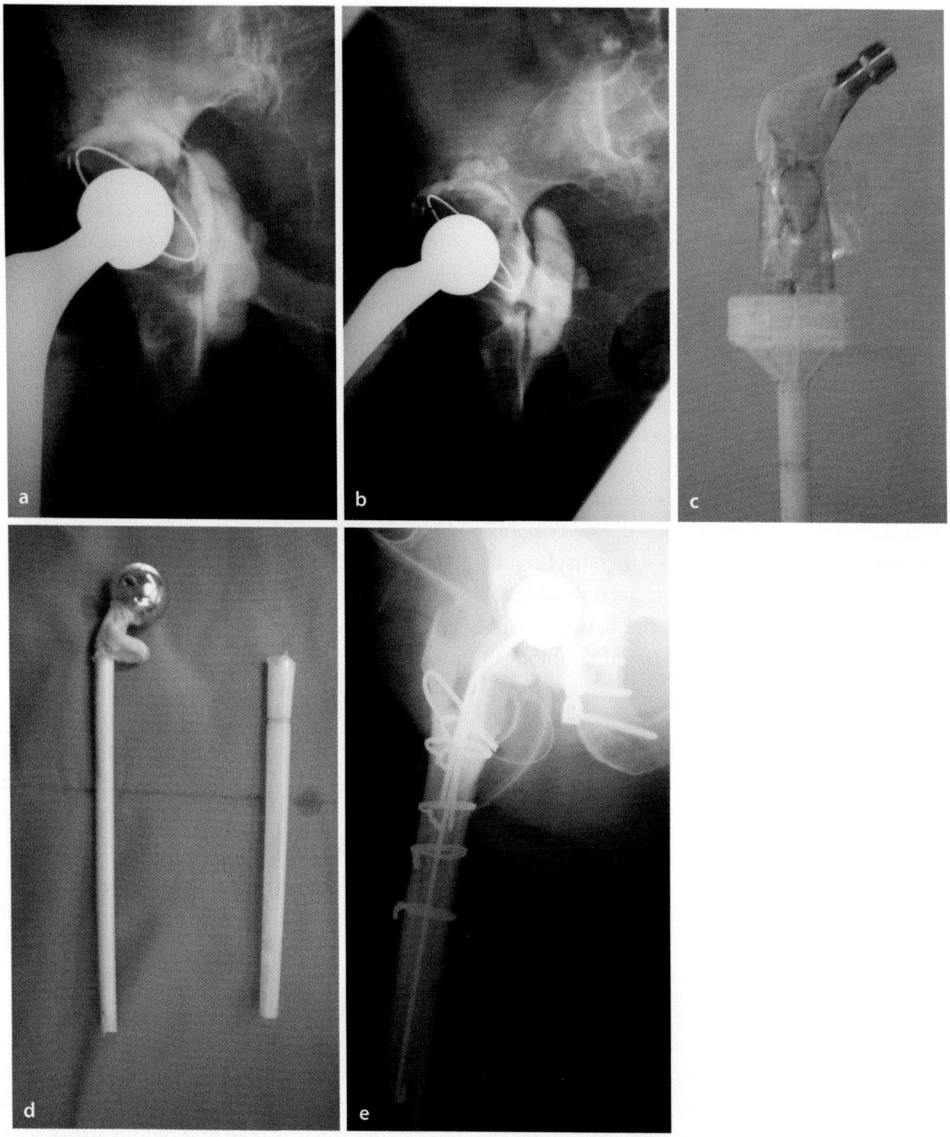

Fig. 8.30 a–e Surgeon-manufactured articulating hip spacer. A cylinder made of two hypodermic syringes is filled with ALAC and a thin-diameter long-stemmed revision component used as an endoskeleton. The proximal calcar region is adapted for defect management and allowed to polymerize. The press-fit implant is liberated from the plastic mould and press-fit into the femur. Osteotomies are closed and a small volume of retained cement inserted into the proximal femur for supplementary fixation

inflammatory markers (Ghanem et al. 2009). At the second procedure, the loosely cemented acetabular component is removed. The femoral component is easily extracted after removal of the proximal femoral cement; the smooth cylindrical diaphyseal portion of the femoral implant should afford little resistance to removal. Most osteotomies have healed by 3–4 months permitting a definitive reconstruction with a short to mid-length stem for the majority.

8.2.6 Articulating Spacers for Infected Total Knee Arthroplasty

Two-stage revision arthroplasty for infection without the use of a spacer is largely a historical procedure, especially for knee arthroplasty where soft tissue contractures, fibrosis and joint instability compromise the second-stage procedure (Booth and Lotke 1989). The addition of ALAC facilitates a local depot of antibiotics, manages dead space and enables skeletal stabilization. The further adaptation to use articulating spacers has been described in the knee since 1995 (Scott et al. 1993; Hofmann et al. 1995; McPherson et al. 1995).

The original description of two-stage revisions for infected knee arthroplasties by Insall et al. (1983) involved the use of ALAC blocks loosely inserted into the knee without fixation and supported by an external splint. With this technique a period of non-weight-bearing was required resulting in osteopoenia and considerable patient morbidity. Soft tissue contractures and stiffness were the norm, making the definitive reconstruction a complex and difficult procedure, often requiring extended approaches and a stiff knee was a common outcome (Faschingbauer et al. 2016). Carlton et al. (1997) reported 40% of patients sustained additional tibial bone loss and 44% of patients sustained further femoral bone loss as a consequence of erosion from the cement spacers.

The prosthetic joint infection work group evaluating articulating spacers reported on the evidence relating to the use of functional spacers for the management of infected total knee arthroplasties (Citak et al. 2014). There are no reported studies specifically examining the surgical ease of use of a non-articulating spacer but there was 80% agreement amongst the reviewers that re-implantation surgery was easier when a patient received an articulating spacer. There is invariably an increased range of motion before the second stage that facilitates the exposure, usually with maintenance of more normal soft tissue tension, ligament preservation, lack of osteopoenic bone and restoration of the anatomy. When the patient is permitted weight-bearing, the osteopoenia observed with an infected knee arthroplasty often resolves. It is not uncommon for segmental defects or fractures to heal converting a segmental defect to a more simply managed cavitatory defect. The prosthetic joint infection work group examined 46 original articles examining the mid-term functional outcome of patients with re-implanted articulating spacers compared with non-articulating spacers, and most report a superior outcome for patients receiving articulating spacers. At 2 years there was a non-significant trend for an improved range in motion when an articulating spacer had been used.

Direct comparisons of treatment protocols and implants are confounded by difference in organism, patient and treatment variables. The use of spacers has not been identified as a significant variable related to infection eradication. The working group reviewed 59 articles that included 1,557 cases treated with articulating spacers and 601 cases treated with non-articulating spacers, reporting eradication rates of 91.5% and 87.0%, respectively. There are no level 1 studies comparing infection control between difference types of articulating spacers, but the literature does include a report of 304 cases treated by the PROSTALAC® method, 410 with the Hoffman method, 716 with cemented moulds and 52 with Spacer K custom pre-made spacers. The eradication rate was comparable in all cases at 91.1%, 93.7%, 91.6% and 94.2%, respectively.

8.2.7 Articulating Knee Spacers Options

A number of different types of articulating spacers have been used to mitigate patient morbidity including stiffness and instability. Broadly there are three groups of articulating knee spacers in frequent usage including cement-on-cement components that are prefabricated or made intraoperatively with moulds, a low-friction implant utilizing a new or sterilized explanted femoral component, and specific low-friction stabilized PROSTALAC® devices.

The articulating surface of temporary knee spacers varies considerably. A common implant is a high-friction arthroplasty utilizing femoral and tibial components made of ALAC that are loosely cemented and allowed to articulate one on the other. Implants include pre-manufactured components such as Spacer K (Tecres) or manufactured by the surgical team free-hand (McPherson et al. 1995; MacAvoy and Ries 2005; Villanueva-Martinez et al. 2008) or using a mould system (StageOne™, Zimmer Biomet) or Copal® knee moulds (Heraeus Medical). These devices permit active and passive flexion of the knee and have a variable articular constraint usually with a non-constrained round-on-flat articulation. The articulation surface is a high-friction interface that erodes the cement surfaces and has been associated with persisting cement-induced synovitis (Fink et al. 2011); consequently, a defined period of implantation, such as 8 weeks, is usually recommended for cement-on-cement devices.

The introduction of the Hofmann technique (Hofmann et al. 1995), or the subsequent modification of using a new femoral component, allows for the use of a more robust metal femoral component that prevents femoral component fracture and enable a more conforming low-friction articulation. Briefly, the technique involves sterilizing the explanted femoral component. The sterilized explanted femoral component and a thin polyethylene liner are loosely cemented with ALAC. This technique has been successfully reported for over two decades by the innovator (Hofmann et al. 2005) and independent series (Emerson et al. 2002; Jamsen et al. 2006; Anderson et al. 2009) with infection resolution and clinical outcomes equal to any described technique. Sadly this technique has been prohibited by many institutional directives that have barred the re-use of explanted components and necessitates the use of more expensive alternatives (Kalore et al. 2012). This directive is the genesis of a technique of cementing a new femoral component of the same, or approximate, size. There are understandable concerns of impaired infection control due to the larger volume of metal and polyethylene that does not elute antibiotics, but to date these concerns have not been founded (Jamsen et al. 2006; Kalore et al. 2012). The bone–cement interface remains protected from infection by the ALAC that secures the temporary device in situ and it is typical to use one or two mixes of ALAC for fixation, which does permit the inclusion of a large depot of antibiotic.

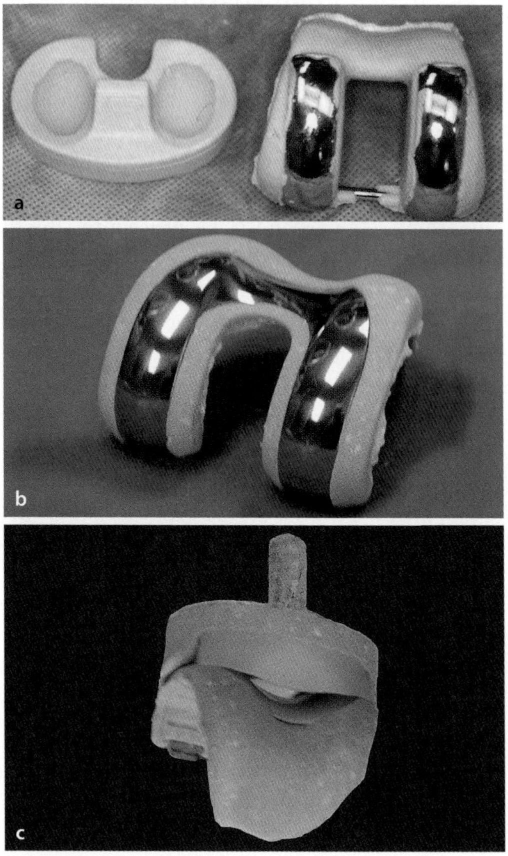

Fig. 8.31 a–c Low-friction stabilized knee spacers. **a** PROSTALAC® implants incorporate a posterior cruciate cam and post mechanism. **b, c** Signature implants incorporate a deep-dished articulation with an elevated anterior lip for PCL substitution. Both implants have a femoral endoskeleton that stabilizes the two femoral condyles and articulate against small polyethylene inserts

The PROSTALAC® system (Depuy; Fig. 8.31) is a further refinement of an infection-specific implant incorporating the elements of a low-friction arthroplasty with posterior implant constraint that is manufactured mostly from ALAC (Haddad et al. 2000). This system is available in a variety of sizes and thickness of implants and is commercially available in North America. ALAC is customized for the sensitivities of the organism(s) in question and inserted into a size specific metal mould. The articular surface of the tibial component includes two small polyethylene components. The femoral component includes two thin metal femoral articular surfaces that are linked posteriorly and strengthen the ALAC femoral component. The posterior bar of the femoral component facilitates posterior ligament stabilization similar to a posterior cruciate ligament (PCL)-replacing a primary knee implant.

A similar device from Signature Orthopaedics (Sydney, Australia; ◘ Fig. 8.31) utilizes silicone moulds to manufacture a tibial component of chosen thickness including a dished polyethylene tibial component with an anterior lip. The femoral component has a metal bicondylar articular insert that stabilizes the condyles preventing fracture and articulates against the deep dish of the tibial component resulting in coronal stabilization, similar to a PCL-replacing primary knee implant.

8.2.8 Complications and Developments

The articular surface of the temporary device is an important determent of the ability to weight bear and the range of motion of the knee. Cement-on-cement articulations are associated with persisting synovitis as a consequence of cement-on-cement wear of the articular surface (Fink et al. 2011). The incorporation of a metal-on-polyethylene implant from a primary or custom implant greatly facilitates knee range of motion in the absence of friction.

Early designs of round-on-flat implants would occasionally dislocate posteriorly, and this is especially prevalent when associated with a deficiency with the extensor mechanism. Knee dislocation and instability are more common with less constrained devices and a supplementary splint is often used (Struelens et al. 2013). More constrained devices such as the PROSTALAC® or Signature custom (◘ Fig. 8.31) can mitigate this risk and it is rare to require supplementary bracing. In the presence of a grossly incompetent soft tissue envelope, additional support with a hinged brace may be required, particularly for collateral ligament instability or extensor deficiency. It is anticipated these problems will necessitate increased constraint at the time of the second-stage revision (Lau et al. 2016).

Fracture of an unsupported femoral component made of ALAC is an occasional sequel and may occur at the time of surgical impaction or with subsequent weight-bearing. To prevent fracture or dislocation (some) manufactures recommend partial weight-bearing during the spacer interval. If detected at the time of surgery, the cement used for fixation is usually sufficient to allow for continued use of the device without clinical compromise (◘ Fig. 8.32). The use of a metal femoral component (Hofmann technique) or a custom device that includes a metal endoskeleton, such as the PROSTALAC® or Signature devices, mitigate this risk and permit unrestricted weight-bearing.

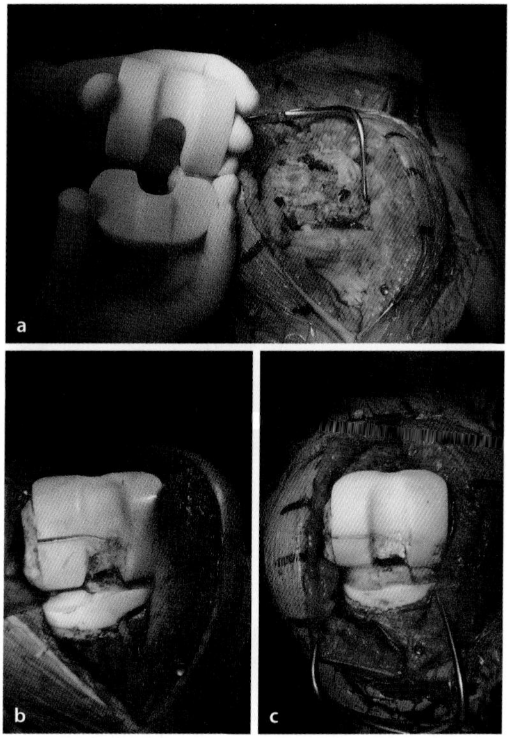

◘ **Fig. 8.32 a–c** Cement-on-cement knee spacer. Spacer K implant is loosely cemented in situ with fracture of the unsupported femoral component during impaction. Defect repaired and filled with cement. Components recommended to be explanted before 8 weeks to minimize cement synovitis and cement fractures

Failure of fixation will occasionally occur, especially on the tibial side where a loosely cemented component has minimal micro or macro fixation. A degree of component loosening, tilt or subluxation can be tolerated leading up to the second-stage intervention with a reduction of weight-bearing or increased splintage (Struelens et al. 2013). Coronal subluxation is associated with a need for increased constraint of the definitive reconstruction and sag-

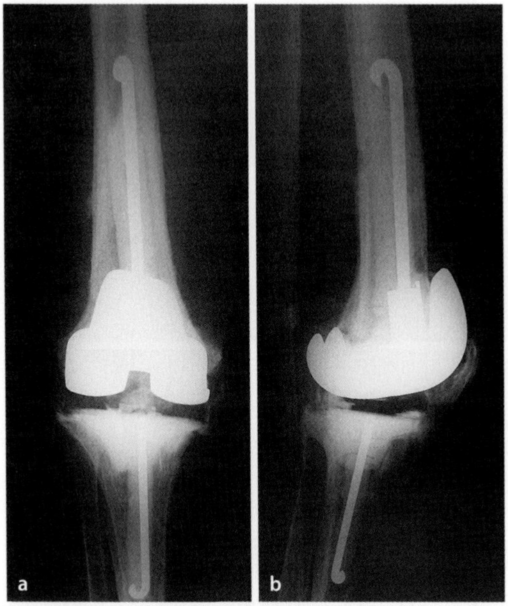

Fig. 8.33 a,b Stemmed re-sterilized revision components. Example of surgeon-manufactured intramedullary stems used to stabilize an infected revision component. Hofmann technique of re-sterilizing the existing femoral component, cementing a new polyethylene insert, and replacing the original diaphyseal stems with press-fit ALAC stems. Stems are manufactured with moulds made from hypodermic syringes and supported with Rush pins to facilitate fixation to the metaphyseal components

ittal subluxation is associated with greater tibial bone defects (Lau et al. 2016).To mitigate loss of fixation of the device, the addition of an intramedullary rod may be a useful adjunct (Fig. 8.33).

8.2.9 Author's Preferred Treatment

Preoperative planning involves isolation of the organism(s) and selection of a heat-stable antibiotic combination for manufacture of the ALAC. It is preferred to use an antibiotic cement combination that exceeds the MIC of the known organisms and usually 10–15% of antibiotic by weight is selected. Palacos cement is the preferred cement because of its documented cement elution characteristics, and the green chlorophyll colouration facilitates identification at the time of secondary surgical removal of implants.

Patient evaluation including skin, ligament stability, and neurovascular examination is required and particular attention is paid to the presence of sinuses, anticipated ligament stability, and bone defects once the implants have been removed. An articulating spacer is considered where reasonable implant fixation can be achieved and there is adequate ligament stability with a preserved extensor mechanism. Where there are gross bone deficiencies or ligament instability, an alternative technique such as a temporary arthrodesis may be more appropriate.

Previous incisions are utilized where possible. It is usually possible to extract the existing implants after a medial and lateral gutter clearance without the need for additional extensor mobilization. The ability to remove tibial inserts assists the exposure when a tight extensor mechanism is encountered. The existing components are removed with minimization of additional bone loss. A total synovectomy is performed and all necrotic bone is removed. Cultures are taken from multiple sites.

It is the author's previous preference to use the Hoffman technique, re-sterilizing the existing femoral component, which facilitates the sizing of implants and minimizing cost. The re-sterilized femoral component and the thinnest sized polyethylene tibial insert are used with an estimation of tibial cement thickness to approximate gap balance and stability. This technique can be utilized for a failed revision implant in the context of significant bone defects, and the substitution of a stemmed implant with a custom-made intramedullary stem made of ALAC is a helpful addition (Fig. 8.31).

More recently, institutional directives have prevented the (off-label) use of re-sterilized explanted components and a custom implant is a cost-competitive alternative (Signature Orthopaedic, Sydney Australia; Fig. 8.29). When a custom-made implant is utilized, the implants are trailed for size and manufactured in a dedicated silicon mould system. The polyethylene tibial articular surface and the femoral articular component are placed in the moulds with two mixes of ALAC. Pressurization is applied as the cement cures and excessive cement is removed following polymerization.

The knee is comprehensively irrigated but attempts to achieve dry cement for pressurization are avoided with the intention of loosely cementing the components. An additional mix of ALAC is added and the tibial component is loosely cemented in situ followed by the femoral component. In cases where the extensor mechanism is profoundly stiff, it is possible to cement the femoral component and then manipulate a thin tibial component in position followed by tibial cement whilst holding the knee in an approximate position of alignment.

Once the cement has cured, the knee is placed through a range of motion and an assessment of ligament stability and balance is made. It is not imperative to have perfect stabilization of the knee but the goal is to achieve sufficient stability to allow full weight-bearing without support. Where there is gross ligament instability, a hinged knee brace can be applied in the post-operative period. The knee is closed without the aid of a wound drain where possible and the patient is allowed weight- bearing as tolerated and encouraged to continue flexion and extension exercises to maintain flexion and muscle tone. During the first-stage procedure, bone defects and ligament stability are assessed and a provisional plan of the definitive second stage can be predicted and recorded in the operative note.

8.2.10 Preparation of an Intramedullary Rod

Where there is deficient metaphyseal fixation, intramedullary rods in varying diameter and length can be manufactured with the use of a Rush pin as an endoskeleton. The length and diameter required are assessed with the use of cylindrical reamers and a rod of 1–2 mm less diameter is selected. Frequently a 10-ml or 20-ml hypodermic syringe is used which approximates the diameter of the tibial and femoral diaphysis, respectively. Hyperfix or similar stout adhesive dressing is used to secure one or more syringes to manufacture a smooth-walled cylindrical mould. Liquid paraffin oil is used to lubricate the inner surface of the mould, which is filled with ALAC. A Rush pin is inserted into the centre of the tube with the hooked end distally, which ensures removal of the cement column at the second stage. About 1–2 cm of Rush pin is left protruding to allow fixation to the articular components, or in the case of a knee arthrodesis, to a contralateral femoral or tibial pin. When the cement has polymerized, the sleeve is removed revealing a smooth press-fit device. The rod is press-fit into the medulla of the tibia or femur and additional cement is used to secure the intramedullary rod against the femoral or tibial component. At the time of removal of the definitive device, an osteotome is used to dislodge the bond between the rod and the metaphyseal implant. Stout instruments are used to grasp the protruding Rush pin and extract the rod, which should have minimal boding on the adjacent bone.

8.2.11 Conclusion

The use of articulating spacers has been widely adopted and considered by many to be the standard of care during the interval period of a two-stage revision for periprosthetic infections. Surgeons overwhelmingly believe the use of a temporary implant facilitates the subsequent definitive reconstruction but study designs to examine this hypothesis are problematic, and supportive literature is limited. There is sufficient literature to conclude the use of an articulating spacer for hip or knee infections is at least as efficacious as other methods when considering infection resolution.

During the interval period there is significant patient morbidity, and the use of an articulating spacer improves the patient's mobility and independence. The ability to manage patients in an outpatient setting is a cost advantage, which overshadows the surgical and implants costs. There are several implants available with competing costs and functional advantage and none has been proven to have superiority in all domains of fixation, bone preservation, joint stability and cost. Choosing an implant within the surgeon's skill set that most effectively prepares the joint for the definitive second-stage procedure and normalizes the patient's function during the interval period is a logical and probably cost-effective decision.

Take-Home Message

- Revision for infection: patients present with more complex skeletal and medical problems.
- Articulating spacers are a ubiquitous tool for revision surgeons because they facilitate the delivery of antibiotics.
- In absence of a definition of the pathogens (PJI), ALBC spacers loaded with vancomycin are preferred.
- The ability to manage patients in an outpatient setting is a cost advantage.
- Articulating spacers improve the patient's mobility and independence.

References

Anderson JA, Sculco PK, Heitkemper S, Mayman DJ, Bostrom MP, Sculco TP (2009) An articulating spacer to treat and mobilize patients with infected total knee arthroplasty. J Arthroplasty 24(4):631-635

Berend KR, Lombardi AV, Jr., Morris MJ, Bergeson AG, Adams JB, Sneller MA (2013) Two-stage treatment of hip periprosthetic joint infection is associated with a high rate of infection control but high mortality. Clin Orthop Relat Res 471(2):510-518

Booth RE, Jr, Lotke PA (1989) The results of spacer block technique in revision of infected total knee arthroplasty. Clin Orthop Relat Res 248:57-60

Bori G, Garcia-Oltra E, Soriano A, Rios J, Gallart X, Garcia S (2014) Dislocation of preformed antibiotic-loaded cement spacers (Spacer-G): etiological factors and clinical prognosis. J Arthroplasty 29(5):883-888

Calton TF, Fehring TK, Griffin WL (1997) Bone loss associated with the use of spacer blocks in infected total knee arthroplasty. Clinical Orthop Relat Res 345:148-154

Choi HR, Freiberg AA, Malchau H, Rubash HE, Kwon YM (2014) The fate of unplanned retention of prosthetic articulating spacers for infected total hip and total knee arthroplasty. J Arthroplasty 29(4):690-693

Citak M, Argenson JN, Masri B, Kendoff D, Springer B, Alt V, et al (2014) Spacers. J Arthroplasty 29[2 Suppl]:93-99

Citak M, Citak M, Kendoff D (2015) [Dynamic versus static cement spacer in periprosthetic knee infection: A meta-analysis]. Der Orthopade 44(8):599-606

Drexler M, Kuzyk PR, Koo K, Gross AE, Kosashvili Y, Reischl N, et al (2016) The use of a supra-acetabular antibiotic-loaded cement shelf to improve hip stability in first-stage infected total hip arthroplasty. J Arthroplasty 31(11): 2574-2578

Duncan CP, Beauchamp C (1993) A temporary antibiotic-loaded joint replacement system for management of complex infections involving the hip. Orthop Clinics North Am 24(4):751-759

Durbhakula SM, Czajka J, Fuchs MD, Uhl RL (2004) Spacer endoprosthesis for the treatment of infected total hip arthroplasty. J Arthroplasty 19(6):760-767

Emerson RH, Jr, Muncie M, Tarbox TR, Higgins LL (2002) Comparison of a static with a mobile spacer in total knee infection. Clin Orthop Relat Res. 404:132-138

Etienne G, Waldman B, Rajadhyaksha AD, Ragland PS, Mont MA (2003) Use of a functional temporary prosthesis in a two-stage approach to infection at the site of a total hip arthroplasty. J Bone Joint Surg Am 85A[Suppl 4]: 94-96

Faschingbauer M, Reichel H, Bieger R, Kappe T (2015) Mechanical complications with one hundred and thirty eight (antibiotic-laden) cement spacers in the treatment of periprosthetic infection after total hip arthroplasty. Int Orthop 39(5):989-994

Faschingbauer M, Bieger R, Reichel H, Weiner C, Kappe T (2016) Complications associated with 133 static, antibiotic-laden spacers after TKA. Knee Surg Sports Traumatol Arthrosc 24(10):3096-3099

Fink B, Rechtenbach A, Buchner H, Vogt S, Hahn M (2011) Articulating spacers used in two-stage revision of infected hip and knee prostheses abrade with time. Clin Orthop Relat Res 469(4):1095-1102

Ghanem E, Azzam K, Seeley M, Joshi A, Parvizi J (2009) Staged revision for knee arthroplasty infection: what is the role of serologic tests before reimplantation? Clin Orthop Relat Res 467(7):1699-1705

Giulieri SG, Graber P, Ochsner PE, Zimmerli W (2004) Management of infection associated with total hip arthroplasty according to a treatment algorithm. Infection 32(4): 222-228

Gomez MM, Tan TL, Manrique J, Deirmengian GK, Parvizi J (2015) The fate of spacers in the treatment of periprosthetic joint infection. J Bone Joint Surg Am 97(18):1495-1502

Haddad FS, Masri BA, Campbell D, McGraw RW, Beauchamp CP, Duncan CP (2000) The PROSTALAC functional spacer in two-stage revision for infected knee replacements. Prosthesis of antibiotic-loaded acrylic cement. J Bone Joint Surg Br 82(6):807-812

Haddad FS, Sukeik M, Alazzawi S (2015) Is single-stage revision according to a strict protocol effective in treatment of chronic knee arthroplasty infections? Clin Orthop Relat Research 473(1):8-14

Hanssen AD, Spangehl MJ (2004) Practical applications of antibiotic-loaded bone cement for treatment of infected joint replacements. Clin Orthop Relat Res 427: 79-85

Hofmann AA, Kane KR, Tkach TK, Plaster RL, Camargo MP (1995) Treatment of infected total knee arthroplasty using an articulating spacer. Clin Orthop Relat Res. 321:45-54

Hofmann AA, Goldberg T, Tanner AM, Kurtin SM (2005) Treatment of infected total knee arthroplasty using an articulating spacer: 2- to 12-year experience. Clin Orthop Relat Res 430:125-131

Ilchmann T, Zimmerli W, Ochsner PE, Kessler B, Zwicky L, Graber P, et al (2016) One-stage revision of infected hip arthroplasty: outcome of 39 consecutive hips. Int Orthop 40(5):913-918

Insall JN, Thompson FM, Brause BD (1983) Two-stage reimplantation for the salvage of infected total knee arthroplasty. J Bone Joint Surg Am 65(8):1087-1098

Jamsen E, Sheng P, Halonen P, Lehto MU, Moilanen T, Pajamaki J, et al (2006) Spacer prostheses in two-stage revision of infected knee arthroplasty. Int Orthop 30(4):257-261

Jung J, Schmid NV, Kelm J, Schmitt E, Anagnostakos K (2009) Complications after spacer implantation in the treatment of hip joint infections. Int J Med Sci 6(5):265-273

Kalore NV, Maheshwari A, Sharma A, Cheng E, Gioe TJ (2012) Is there a preferred articulating spacer technique for infected knee arthroplasty? A preliminary study. Clin Orthop Relat Res 470(1):228-235

Kendall RW, Masri BA, Duncan CP, Beauchamp CP, McGraw RW, Bora B (1994) Temporary antibiotic loaded acrylic hip replacement: a novel method for management of the infected THA. Sem Arthroplasty 5(4):171-177

Lamberton TD, Hubble MJ, Kenny PJ, Timperley AJ, Gie GA (2005) Management of infection of THJR with the Kiwi prostalac technique. J Bone Joint Surg Br 87B [Suppl I]:32

Langlais F (2003) Can we improve the results of revision arthroplasty for infected total hip replacement? J Bone Joint Surg Br 85(5):637-640

Lau AC, Howard JL, Macdonald SJ, Teeter MG, Lanting BA (2016) The effect of subluxation of articulating antibiotic spacers on bone defects and degree of constraint in revision knee arthroplasty. J Arthroplasty 31(1):199-203

Lee WY, Hwang DS, Kang C, Shin BK, Zheng L (2016) Usefulness of prosthesis made of antibiotic-loaded acrylic cement as an alternative implant in older patients with medical problems and periprosthetic hip infections: a 2- to 10-year follow-up study. J Arthroplasty 32:228-233

MacAvoy MC, Ries MD (2005) The ball and socket articulating spacer for infected total knee arthroplasty. J Arthroplasty 20(6):757-762

Masri BA, Duncan CP, Beauchamp CP (1998) Long-term elution of antibiotics from bone-cement: an in vivo study using the prosthesis of antibiotic-loaded acrylic cement (PROSTALAC) system. J Arthroplasty 13(3):331-338

McPherson EJ, Lewonowski K, Dorr LD (1995) Techniques in arthroplasty. Use of an articulated PMMA spacer in the infected total knee arthroplasty. J Arthroplasty 10(1):87-89

Meek RM, Dunlop D, Garbuz DS, McGraw R, Greidanus NV, Masri BA (2004) Patient satisfaction and functional status after aseptic versus septic revision total knee arthroplasty using the PROSTALAC articulating spacer. J Arthroplasty 19(7):874-879

Meek RM, Masri BA, Dunlop D, Garbuz DS, Greidanus NV, McGraw R, et al (2003) Patient satisfaction and functional status after treatment of infection at the site of a total knee arthroplasty with use of the PROSTALAC articulating spacer. J Bone Joint Surg Am 85a(10):1888-1892

Nagra NS, Hamilton TW, Ganatra S, Murray DW, Pandit H (2015) One-stage versus two-stage exchange arthroplasty for infected total knee arthroplasty: a systematic review. Knee Surg Sports Ttraumatol Arthrosc 24: 3106-3114

Pattyn C, De Geest T, Ackerman P, Audenaert E (2011) Preformed gentamicin spacers in two-stage revision hip arthroplasty: functional results and complications. Int Orthop 35(10):1471-1476

Scharfenberger A, Clark M, Lavoie G, O'Connor G, Masson E, Beaupre LA (2007) Treatment of an infected total hip replacement with the PROSTALAC system. Part 2: Health-related quality of life and function with the PROSTALAC implant in situ. Canadian J Surg 50(1):29-33

Scott IR, Stockley I, Getty CJ (1993) Exchange arthroplasty for infected knee replacements. A new two-stage method. J Bone Joint Surg Br 75(1):28-31

Struelens B, Claes S, Bellemans J (2013) Spacer-related problems in two-stage revision knee arthroplasty. Acta Orthop Belgica 79(4):422-426

Tsung JD, Rohrsheim JA, Whitehouse SL, Wilson MJ, Howell JR (2014) Management of periprosthetic joint infection after total hip arthroplasty using a custom made articulating spacer (CUMARS); the Exeter experience. J Arthroplasty 29(9):1813-1818

Villanueva-Martinez M, Rios-Luna A, Pereiro J, Fahandez-Saddi H, Villamor A (2008) Hand-made articulating spacers in two-stage revision for infected total knee arthroplasty: good outcome in 30 patients. Acta Orthop 79(5): 674-682

Voleti PB, Baldwin KD, Lee GC (2013) Use of static or articulating spacers for infection following total knee arthroplasty: a systematic literature review. J Bone Joint Surg Am 95(17):1594-1599

Yamamoto K, Miyagawa N, Masaoka T, Katori Y, Shishido T, Imakiire A (2003) Clinical effectiveness of antibiotic-impregnated cement spacers for the treatment of infected implants of the hip joint. J Orthop Sci 8(6):823-828

Younger AS, Duncan CP, Masri BA, McGraw RW (1997) The outcome of two-stage arthroplasty using a custom-made interval spacer to treat the infected hip. J Arthroplasty 12(6):615-623

Zahar A, Gehrke TA (2016) One-stage revision for infected total hip arthroplasty. Orthop Clinics North Am 47(1): 11-8

8.3 Spacer Management in the Treatment of Late Periprosthetic Infections of the Hip

Bernd Fink

Periprosthetic infections occur with an incidence of less than 1% but, nevertheless, are a serious complication of hip arthroplasties (Garvin and Hanssen 1995; Fitzgerald 1995). When early infections occur, within 4 weeks of implantation, the implant can be left in place with a high probability of cure, whereas late infections require prosthesis revision to eradicate the infection (Cui et al. 2007; Hanssen and Osmon 2002). In such cases, one can differentiate between one-stage and two-stage revisions. Two-stage revision involves an initial operation to remove all foreign materials followed by an interim phase of mostly 6–12 weeks, either left as a Girdlestone situation or with the implantation of a cement spacer.

Two-stage septic revision surgery is the most common method for treating infected endoprostheses. A general advantage of the two-stage concept is that the surgical debridement is carried out twice whereby the second operation allows for the eradication of residual organisms following the initial debridement. The cement of the spacer is not intended as a means of fixing the prosthesis, and therefore the mechanical characteristics of the cement are not of primary importance at this stage. Thus, large amounts of antibiotics can be mixed into the cement before the spacer is formed. It has been possible to achieve a survival rate using two-stage revision concepts for infected hip arthroplasties of between 90% and 100% (Garvin et al. 1994; Garvin and Hanssen 1995; Burnett et al. 2007; Lieberman et al. 1994; Fink et al. 2009).

In most two-stage revisions, an antibiotic-containing spacer is usually placed in position for a certain period of time before the final prosthesis is implanted (Evans 2004; Burnett et al. 2007; Hofmann et al. 2005; Goldman et al. 1996; Fink et al. 2009). The function of the spacer is on the one hand to release the antibiotic into the infected bed of the prosthesis and on the other to minimize soft-tissue contractures, retain soft-tissue tension and thereby maintain reasonable functionality until a prosthesis can be re-implanted (Burnett et al. 2007).

There are many questions pertaining to both one-stage and two-stage revisions that still have to be answered, and existing procedures are based more on empirical findings than on data from prospective studies with a high level of evidence. It is for this reason that the following aspects of two-stage revision have been treated very differently by different groups: the type of spacer, the type of antibiotic used in the spacer, the duration of the spacer period, the duration of systemic antibiotic treatment, aspiration before re-implantation, and the type of re-implantation (cemented or cementless).

8.3.1 Type of Spacer

There are several different types of spacer: static and mobile spacers, monoblock and two-part mobile spacers, as well as commercially available and customized mobile spacers made in the operating theatre.

Antibiotic-loaded beads form a kind of spacer that does not have a specific articulating surface and thereby is a more or less static spacer that only fills the gap of the removed artificial joint. The disadvantage of this procedure is that manufactured beads are usually employed and these only contain gentamicin or vancomycin (Fehring et al. 1999; Haddad et al. 2000). Leg shortening and instability still occur and cause problems with mobilization. Re-implantation of a prosthesis is also often made more difficult because of scarring, tissue shrinkage and osteoporosis caused by inactivity (Leunig et al. 1998; Mitchell et al. 2003; Hsieh et al. 2004a, 2004b). In addition, abrasion of zirconium dioxide particles is to be expected during mobilization and this could lead to third-body wear following re-implantation of the prosthesis. Disch et al. (2007) decided therefore not to use local antibiotic carriers following removal of the prosthesis during two-stage revisions and found a reinfection rate of 6.3% in 32 hips 41.3 months after re-implantation although there was a considerable reduction in the quality of life during the Girdlestone phase, which lasted 13 months on average.

Mobile spacers can be differentiated into monoblock and two-part spacers. The potential disadvantages of the monoblock spacers are spacer fracture and bone resorption (Hsieh et al. 2005; Leunig et al. 1998). The monoblock spacer induces bone resorption at the acetabulum because the hard cement has to articulate against the osteoporotic bone caused by the infection. This is avoided in the two-part spacer by the spacer having its own articulation surface. However, this cement-based articulation surface in the two-part spacer can lead to the release of abraded cement particles (Disch et al. 2007; Fink et al. 2011a).

The femoral component of the monoblock and two-part spacers is associated with the risk of spacer fracture. This risk is particularly high when the femoral component is composed of cement alone. It is therefore recommended that the spacer consist of a metal core encased in cement, as is the case in commercially available spacers. A further risk is the potential for dislocation of the spacer out of the bone (either with or without fracture). In order to avoid this complication, it is recommended that, instead of simply inserting the spacer into the femur, the prepared spacer is fixed in position by applying cement at the metaphysis.

We use a two-part spacer where the cup-shaped acetabulum spacer is formed out of antibiotic-loaded cement (with a specific mixture of antibiotics recommended by the microbiologist). The spacer stem component consists of old prosthesis stem models, monoblock devices in most cases and no longer used for primary implantations, which are encased in antibiotic-supplemented cement and, just before implantation, coated in the patient's own blood in order to facilitate easier removal. The two components of the spacer are connected by a metal headpiece (◘ Fig. 8.34, ◘ Fig. 8.35; Fink et al. 2009). However, a recent analysis of synovial membranes obtained during the operation to remove the spacer and to implant the new prosthesis revealed the presence of abraded cement debris, in particular, zirconium dioxide particles (Fink et al. 2011a). Thus it must be concluded that all types of spacer will produce abraded cement particles and this only goes to emphasize the necessity for a radical debridement of the joint area at the time of prosthesis implantation during the second stage of the revision (Fink et al. 2011a). The use of zirconium-free spacer cement (Heraeus Medical GmbH, Wehrheim, Germany) is aimed at circumventing this problem associated with abraded particle.

A further important factor in deciding the type of spacer to be used is the amount of damage to the bone caused by the explantation of the infected prosthesis. The removal of a well-fixed cemented or cementless infected femoral implant is a challenge for the surgeon. The infected prosthetic bed has to be radically debrided while sparing as much as possible the functionally important areas of bone such as the trochanter major as the attachment area for the gluteal musculature. It is for that reason that we favour the transfemoral approach for removal of well-fixed infected femoral components. This approach enables an effective debridement of the infected femoral component bed and of the osteolytic areas that are often present, while limiting any injury to the trochanter major, the vasto-gluteal muscle loop and the isthmus femoris, which represents the area of fixation for the cementless revision stem implanted during the second stage. The endofemoral approach for removing the femoral component does not always enable a reproducible debridement of the osteolytic areas and has a higher risk of femoral fracture. The transfemoral approach avoids this risk. However, it is important that the femoral spacer is long enough to extend beyond the boundaries of the resulting bony flap and that the whole is sufficiently stable.

In this procedure, using the transfemoral approach, we favour the closure of the bony flap with cerclage wires in order to avoid migration of the flap, or its dislocation, as described by Morshed et al. (2005; ◘ Fig. 8.34, ◘ Fig. 8.35). We re-open the flap during the second stage by removing the cerclage wires so that we can carry out a second radical debridement of the prosthetic bed and ensure that the distally fixed, cementless, modular revision stem is correctly positioned in the isthmus of the femur with the fixation zone distal to the osteotomy (◘ Fig. 8.34, ◘ Fig. 8.35). To analyse the results of the transfemoral approach for revision of infected hip prostheses, 76 septic two-stage revisions involving fixation of the bony flap in the first stage with cerclage wires and reopening of the flap at the time of re-implantation were followed prospectively, with clinical and radiological assessment, for a mean period of 51.2±23.2 months (24–118 months;

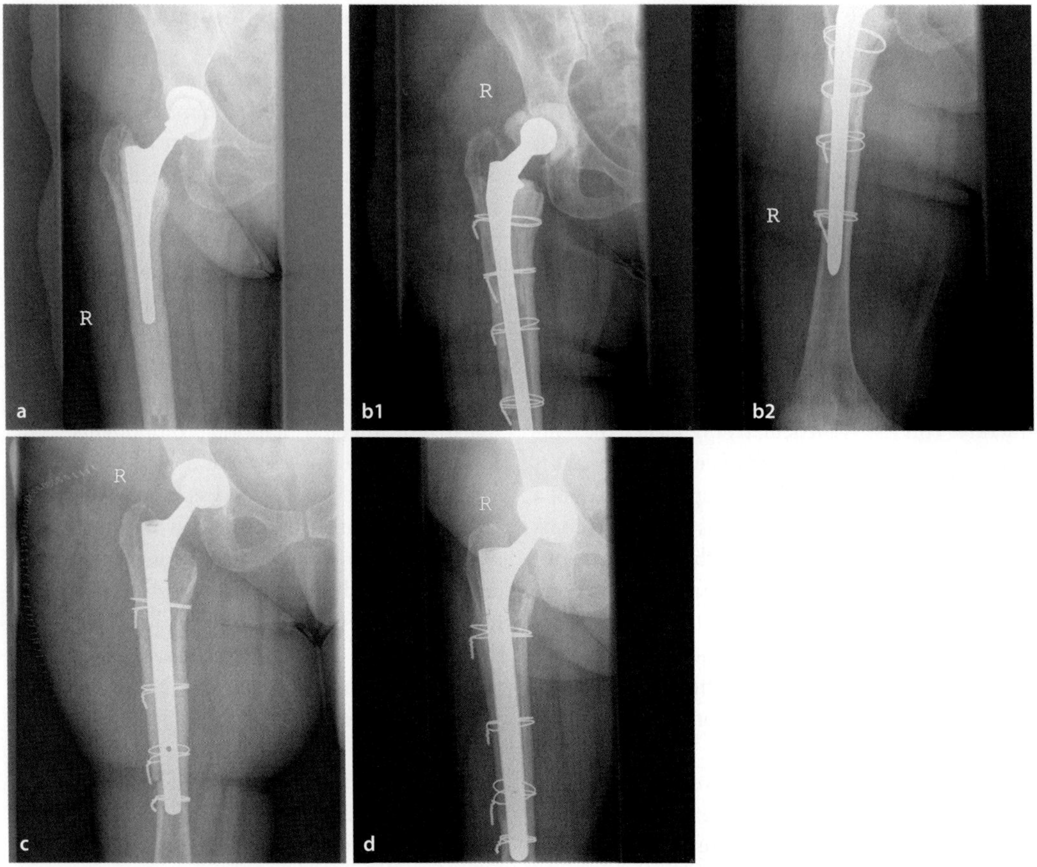

■ **Fig. 8.34 a–d** Two-stage revision via a transfemoral approach of an infected total hip prosthesis with a well-fixed cemented stem. **a** Infected hip arthroplasty with a well-fixed cemented stem with long cement mantle. **b1, b2** Interims prosthesis with a cement cup and cemented monoblock femoral stem after transfemoral revision of the infected hip arthroplasty. **c** Re-implantation of a cementless revision stem and cementless cup in the second stage. **d** Follow-up after 2 years

Fink and Oremek 2016). The rate of complete union of the bony flap after re-implantation was 98.7% and a successful outcome with no recurrence of reinfection was recorded in 93.4% of all cases. Subsidence of the stem occurred at a rate of 6.6 %, dislocation at a rate of 6.6 %, and there was no aseptic loosening of the implants. The Harris Hip Score was 62.2±12.6 points with the spacer and 86.6±15.5 points 2 years after re-implantation of the new implant. Nine fractures (11.8%) of the flap occurred during the operation due to osteolytic or osteoporotic weakness of the flap itself but these all healed without further intervention (Fink and Oremek 2016). Our data demonstrate that the transfemoral approach is a safe method for septic revision of well-fixed cemented or cementless hip prostheses and that the use of cerclage wires for closing the osteotomy flap in the first stage does not lead to higher reinfection rates.

Acetabular bone defects are another problem associated with spacer implantation. These can lead to situations where a stable fixation of the cement cup is not possible. In such cases, and when the infecting organism can be identified, we carry out a one-stage revision whereby the acetabular defect is stabilized by use of the Ganz reinforcement ring or the Burch–Schneider cage into which the cup is then cemented (■ Fig. 8.36). However, it is sometimes necessary to carry out a two-stage revision of the femoral component using the transfemoral ap-

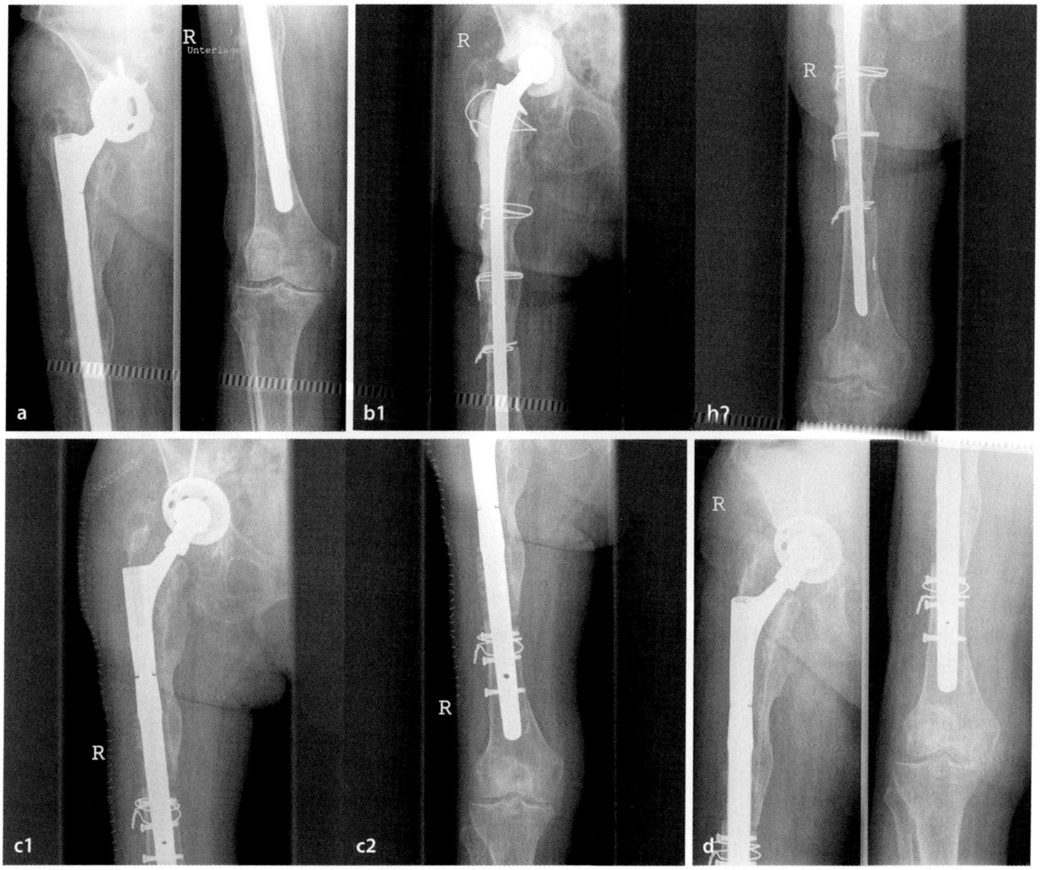

Fig. 8.35 a–d Two-stage revision via a transfemoral approach of an infected total hip prosthesis with a well-fixed long cementless revision stem. **a** Infected hip arthroplasty with a well-fixed cementless revision stem. **b1, b2** Interims prosthesis with a cement cup and cemented femoral stem after transfemoral revision of the infected hip arthroplasty. **c1, c2** Re-implantation of a cementless revision stem with distal interlocking screws and cementless cup in the second stage. **d** Follow-up after 2 years

proach for explantation of a septic prosthesis. In such cases, we carry out a so-called hybrid septic revision that involves a one-stage revision of the acetabular component and a two-stage revision of the femoral component (Fig. 8.37).

8.3.2 Local Antibiotics in the Spacer

It is important for the antibiotic effect of the spacer that the local antibiotic concentration is greater than the minimal inhibitory concentration for the pathogens that cause the periprosthetic infection and that it remains so for the whole spacer period. Otherwise there would be a danger of a recurrence of the infection and of the emergence of resistant micro-organisms. There have been very few publications concerning the elution of antibiotics from spacer cement in vivo over a period of several weeks. Masri et al. (1998) followed up 49 patients for an average period of 118 days after spacer explantation and found sufficiently high concentrations of the antibiotics vancomycin and tobramycin. Similarly, Hsieh et al. (2006) studied 46 patients for an average period of 107 days and found sufficient levels of vancomycin and aztreonam. Bertazzoni Minelli et al. (2004) investigated 20 patients and demonstrated a substantial elution of the antibiotics gentamicin

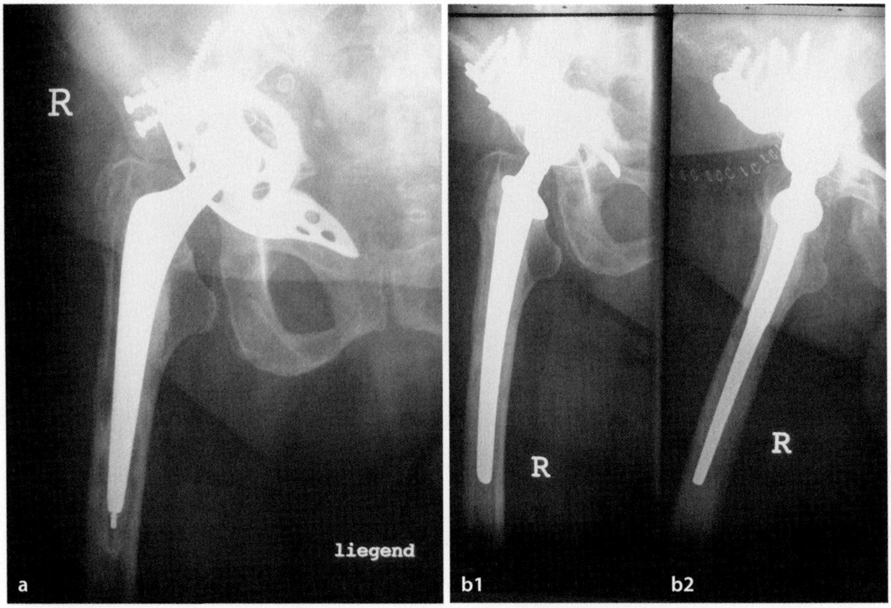

Fig. 8.36 One-stage revision of an infected total hip arthroplasty with acetabular bone defect, Paprosky IIIA. **a** Infected total hip arthroplasty with a cemented stem and a Burch–Schneider cage. **b1, b2** One-stage revision with implantation of a cemented stem and a new Burch–Schneider cage

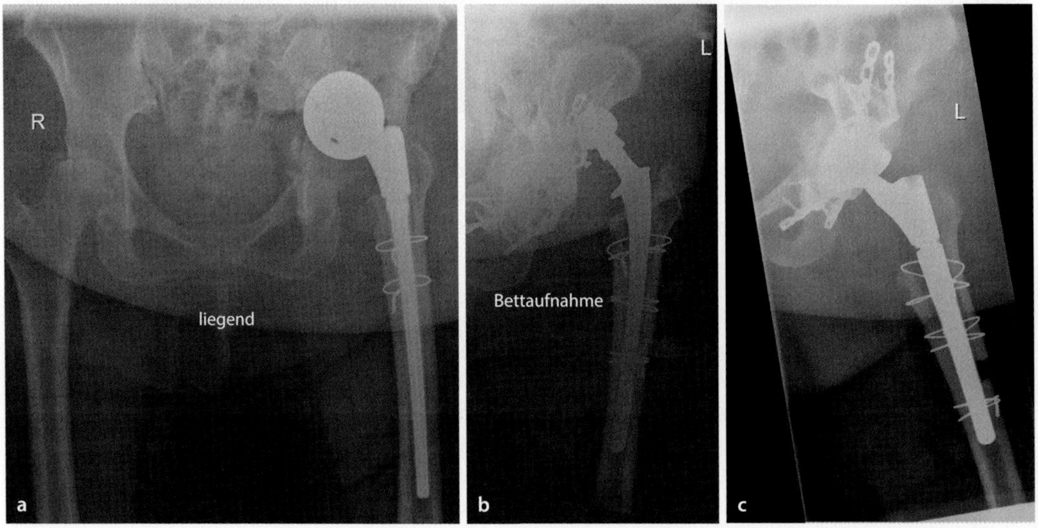

Fig. 8.37 **a–c** Hybrid revision with one-stage revision of the acetabulum and two-stage revision via a transfemoral approach of the femoral stem. a Infected hip arthroplasty with **a** well-fixed cementless revision stem and a loose cup on the acetabular side with pelvic discontinuity. **b** Reconstruction of the acetabular side with reconstructions plates, a Ganz ring and a cemented cup, and on the femoral side with a cemented interims prosthesis. Dislocation of the hip 6 weeks after the first operation. **c** Second-stage revision with implantation of a cementless revision stem via the transfemoral approach and a dual-mobility cup by leaving the reconstruction plates and the Ganz ring on the acetabulum

and vancomycin directly after spacer implantation, followed by a constant level of release over periods ranging from 3 to 6 months.

Our own in vivo study revealed antibiotic levels in the tissues surrounding the spacer 6 weeks after implantation that were higher than the minimal inhibitory concentration for the bacteria that had caused the periprosthetic infection. This was demonstrated in 14 two-stage revision septic arthroplasties using spacers containing gentamicin and clindamycin in the cement and also in cases where vancomycin was included (Fink et al. 2011b). Ours was the first study to measure antibiotic concentrations in the tissues surrounding the spacer and thus to assess the amount of antibiotic at the site of the later implantation of the new prosthesis.

Not all antibiotics can be used for mixing into the cement because they must be available in powder form, be water-soluble, and be thermostable. The most commonly used are gentamicin, clindamycin, vancomycin, tobramycin, aztreonam, ampicillin, and ofloxacin (Anagnostakos et al. 2005; Hofmann et al. 2005). Most published studies always include the same antibiotics in the cement. Some authors use vancomycin and tobramycin as local antibiotics on a regular basis because they have a broad spectrum of activity (Fehring et al.1999; Kraay et al. 2005). However, not all bacteria can be successfully treated with these agents (e. g. some Gram-negative organisms). This is also the disadvantage of commercially manufactured spacers that, like the beads, only contain gentamicin or vancomycin as a single antibiotic. Therefore this is an argument for investigating the antibiotic resistance pattern of the isolated bacteria and selecting a specific antibiotic for the treatment. Masri et al. (2007) reported a success rate of 89.7% in their retrospective study involving bacteria-specific antibiotic mixed into the cement of a PROSTALAC® spacer (DePuy Orthopaedics, Inc., Warsaw, Ind.) and we saw no re-infection of 36 cases with a minimum follow-up of 2 years using this concept for handmade spacers (Fink et al. 2009).

Different antibiotics are released at different rates from the spacers and affect each other when in combination with other antibiotics (Cui et al. 2007). The use of two antibiotics results in a synergistic effect and the elution of the individual components is better than that of the single antibiotics on its own (Simpson et al. 2005; Baleani et al. 2008; Anagnostakos et al. 2005; Ensing et al. 2003; Penner et al. 1996). Many surgeons now use cement with gentamicin and clindamycin in combination (Copal®, Heraeus Medical GmbH, Wehrheim, Germany) rather than gentamicin alone because of the better antibiotic elution kinetics exhibited by the former; a third antibiotic (usually vancomycin) is often added according to organism specificity defined by an antibiogram (Fink et al. 2009; Ensing et al. 2003). This concept enabled us and others to achieve an eradication rate of between 93.5% and 100%, which implies that an adequate level of antibiotic was available in the tissues surrounding the spacer (Fink et al. 2009; Hsieh et al. 2005; Fink and Oremek 2016). However, in our in vivo study, the addition of vancomycin did not result in an increase in the release of the antibiotics present in Copal® G+C, namely gentamicin and clindamycin (Fink et al. 2011b). Moreover, hand-mixed cement results in a better elution of antibiotics than cement mixed under vacuum. This is because there are air bubbles in the hand-mixed cement that increase the total area of the antibiotic-eluting surface. However, the mechanical properties (e. g. resistance to breakage) of the hand-mixed cement are poorer than that of the vacuum-mixed cement. The mechanical properties of the spacer cement do not necessarily have to be equivalent to those of the cement used to fix primary endoprosthetic implants, however. Thus, we recommend the addition of several organism-specific antibiotics to the spacer cement and, applying this concept, we were able to show that the local antibiotic concentrations 6 weeks after implantation were still above the relevant minimal inhibitory concentrations (Fink et al. 2011b). In addition, we observed a very low rate of recurrence – at or around 0% – in the clinical setting (Fink et al. 2009). Thus, the antibiotic-containing spacer not only fulfils a mechanical function, it also plays an important role in the treatment of periprosthetic infections.

8.3.3 Duration of the Spacer Period and Systemic Antibiotic Therapy

The period of time between the two operations of a two-stage revision and the time of systemic antibiotic therapy are highly variable between the studies, ranging from a few days to several years for the spacer period and from 2 weeks to several months for the systemic antibiotic therapy after re-implantation (◘ Tab. 8.2 and ◘ Tab. 8.3). Many authors determine the time of re-implantation of a prosthesis according to clinical parameters and clinical chemistry data and carry out an aspiration of the area before surgery is performed (Lieberman et al. 1994; McDonald et al. 1989; Hsieh et al. 2005; Masri et al. 2007). Other authors have a more or less rigid procedural plan (Haddad et al. 2000; Garvin et al. 1994; Evans 2004). These differences in procedure, not only between studies but also within studies, mean that it cannot be decided which time period between the two steps and spacer phase is the most suitable. This also appears to underscore the importance of the surgical debridement for therapeutic success of the two-stage revision. However, most surgeons choose a spacer period of 6–12 weeks and a systemic therapy of 6–12 weeks after re-implantation (◘ Tab. 8.2 and ◘ Tab. 8.3).

8.3.4 Aspiration Before Re-implantation

There are no comparative studies that consider this aspect of the therapeutic concept either. In order to reproducibly assess the validity of aspiration of the joint when deciding whether or not to carry out a re-implantation, the antibiotic treatment has to be discontinued for a period of at least 2 weeks, if not 4 weeks (Mont et al. 2000). Since the recommended bacterial cultivation period is 2 weeks, aspiration of the joint before implantation leads to a delay in re-implantation of between 4 and 6 weeks (Schäfer et al. 2008). In our study of the local concentrations of antibiotics in the tissue around the prosthesis bed, we were able to show that local antibiotic levels were higher than the minimal inhibitory concentrations 6 weeks after spacer implantation, but whether this would also be true after a further 4–6 weeks is debatable. However, the fact that there is an effective level of antibiotic in the tissues at the time of the aspiration means that, in our opinion, the prognostic value of the whole aspiration procedure is overrated. For this reason, we do without this procedure and rely entirely on clinical observation and monitoring of C-reactive protein (CRP) levels. Previous experience has shown that CRP decreases to a level between 10 and 30 mg/l within 2 or 3 weeks of surgery. A normal level of less than 5 mg/l cannot be expected when a spacer has been implanted. If the CRP level does not decrease to the afore-mentioned level within the 3-week period, or there is persistent wound secretion, or there are other signs and symptoms that suggest the presence of a deep infection, we do not carry out a re-implantation but rather renew the spacer with accompanying debridement of the prosthesis bed.

8.3.5 Type of Prosthesis Used for Re-implantation

Although the use of a cemented prosthesis for re-implantation has the advantage that antibiotics can be added to the cement, there are no obvious differences in re-infection rate between cemented and cementless prostheses (◘ Tab. 8.2 and ◘ Tab. 8.3). Thus the procedures adopted during the first stage of the operation, involving radical debridement and local and systemic antibiotic treatment to maintain freedom from infection, appear to be more meaningful for the treatment of periprosthetic infections than the type of implant used for the re-implantation. Since the optimal interdigitation of the cement requires a spongiform structure to the bone, and this is not found after debridement, especially in the femoral component, it is likely that the quality of the long-term fixation of the cemented prosthesis will be diminished by the presence of smooth bone surfaces. Although there are no reports concerning aseptic loosening of cemented re-implants following two-stage septic revision arthroplasty, we know that the rate of loosening of cemented revision stems is much higher than that of cementless stems (Wirtz et al. 1997; Fink et al. 2005). We therefore use cementless revision stems for re-implantation, and it is the disadvantages of cemented re-implantations that have persuaded us to choose a two-stage procedure over the one-stage procedure for hip joint revision, although not for knee revisions.

Using the concept we have described, we have been able to achieve study outcomes of 100% and

Tab. 8.2 Results of two-stage cemented revision of periprosthetic infection of the hip

Author	N	Follow-up	Spacer/ beads	Local antibiotics	Duration of intravenous antibiotics	Interval until re-implantation	Antibiotics after implantation	Eradication rate	Aseptic loosening
McDonald et al. 1989	82	5.5 years	Resection arthroplasty	No	26.1 (4–59 days)	1.5 years (6 days–6.2 years)	No antibiotics in cement	87%	
Colyer and Capello 1994	37	2.7 years	Resection arthroplasty	No	6 weeks parenteral	6 weeks (4–214 weeks)	2 weeks parenteral, 3 months oral	84%	
Garvin et al. 1994	32	≥ 2 years, 4.1 years	Beads	Gentamicin	6 weeks parenteral	6 weeks		91%	0%
Lieberman et al. 1994	32	40 (24–80) months	Beads Spacer	Gentamicin Tobramycin Vancomycin	6 weeks (20–49 days)	8 weeks (3 weeks–32 months)		91%	
Younger et al. 1997	48	43 (24–63) months	Spacer	Gentamicin	3 weeks parenteral, 3 weeks oral	13 weeks (5–42 weeks)	3 weeks parenteral, 3 weeks oral	94%	0%
Leunig et al. 1998	12	2.2 years	Spacer	Gentamicin		4 (2–7) months		100%	
Evans 2004	23		Spacer	Gentamicin	6 weeks	12 weeks	No	95.7%	
Hsieh et al. 2005	24	4.2 years	Spacer	Specific: Vancomycin Piperacillin Aztreonam Teicoplanin	2 weeks parenteral, 4 weeks oral	11–17 weeks, when CRP normal	1 week parenteral	100%	0%

Tab. 8.3 Results of two-stage cementless revision of periprosthetic infection of the hip

Author	N	Follow-up	Spacer/ Beads	Local antibiotics	Duration of intravenous antibiotics	Interval until re-implantation	Antibiotics after implantation	Eradication rate	Aseptic loosening
Wilson and Lorr 1989	13/ 22[a]	≥3 years, 48 months	Resection arthroplasty	No	3 weeks parenteral	6–12 weeks	3 days parenteral	91% / 100% cementless	7.6% stem loosening
Nestor et al. 1994	34	47 (24–72) months	Resection arthroplasty	No	≥ 4 weeks parenteral	8 (3–19) months	Different	82%	18% stem loosening
Fehring et al. 1999	25	41 (24–98) months	Beads	Tobramycin in 16 cases	6 weeks parenteral	4.8 months		92%	0 %
Haddad et al. 2000	50	5.8 (2–8.7) years	Beads + cement ball	Gentamicin	5 days parenteral and then oral	3 weeks	≥3 months	92%	8% stem subsidence
Koo et al. 2001	22	41 (24–78) months	Spacer Beads	Vancomycin Gentamicin Cefotaxime	6 weeks	6–12 weeks		95%	5% cup loosening 30% stem subsidence
Hofmann et al. 2005	27	76 (28–148) months	Old stem and new polyethylene cup	Tobramycin	6 weeks parenteral, in 17 cases additional oral administration for 6 weeks			94%	0%
Kraay et al. 2005	33	≥2 years	Spacer in 16 cases	Tobramycin in 16 cases	≥6 weeks parenteral	7.4 (3–37) months		92%	9% cup 0% stem
Masri et al. 2007	29	≥2 years	Prostalac spacer	Tobramycin Vancomycin Cefuroxime Penicillin[b]	6 weeks parenteral or in combination with oral	12 weeks	5 days intravenous	90%	0%
Yamamoto et al. 2009	17	38 months	Spacer	Gentamicin Vancomycin	>3 weeks		1 week parenteral, oral until CRP normal	100%	
Fink et al. 2009	36	≥2 years	Spacer	Specific: Gentamicin Clindamycin Vancomycin Ampicillin Ofloxacin	2 weeks parenteral, 4 weeks oral	6 weeks	2 weeks parenteral, 4 weeks oral	100%	6% stem subsidence 0% loosening

[a] Thirteen of 22 re-implantations without cement
[b] Combination of another local antibiotic with tobramycin

93.5% freedom from infection (Fink et al. 2009, Fink and Oremek 2016). These results suggest that our concept for septic revision surgery will continue to produce reproducible good clinical outcomes.

Take-Home Messages

- Two-stage septic revision surgery is the most common method for treating infected endoprostheses.
- It is important for the antibiotic effect of the spacer that the local antibiotic concentration is greater than the minimal inhibitory concentration for the pathogens that cause the periprosthetic infection and remains so for the whole spacer period.
- Antibiotic-containing spacers not only fulfil a mechanical function they also play an important role in the treatment of periprosthetic infections.
- The procedures adopted during the first stage of the operation, involving radical debridement and local and systemic antibiotic treatment to maintain freedom from infection, appear to be more meaningful for the treatment of periprosthetic infections than the type of implant used for the reimplantation.

References

Anagnostakos K, Kelm J, Regitz T, Schmitt E, Jung W (2005) In vitro elution of antibiotic release from and bacteria growth inhibition by antibiotic-loaded acrylic bone cement spacers. J Biomed Mater Res 72–B:373-378

Baleani M, Persson C, Zolezzi C, Andollina A, Borelli AM, Tigani D (2008) Biological and biomechanical effects of Vancomycin and Meropenem in acrylic bone cement. J Arthroplasty 23:1232-1238

Bertazzoni Minelli E, Benini A, Magnan B, Bartolozzi P (2004) Release of gentamicin and vancomycin from temporary human hip spacers in two-stage revision of infected arthroplasty. J Antimicrob Chemother 53:329-334

Burnett RSJ, Kelly MA, Hanssen AD, Barrack RL (2007) Technique and timing of two-stage exchange for infection in TKA. Clin Orthop Relat Res 464:164-178

Colyer RA, Capello WN (1994) Surgical treatment of the infected hip implant. Two-stage reimplantation with a one-month interval. Clin Orthop Relat Res 298:75-79

Cui Q, Mihalko WM, Shields JS, Ries M, Saleh HJ (2007) Antibiotic-impregnated cement spacers for the treatment of infection associated with total hip or knee arthroplasty. J Bone Joints Surg Am 89–A:871-882

Disch AC, Matziolis G, Perka C (2007) Two-stage operative strategy without local antibiotic treatment for infected hip arthroplasty: clinical and radiological outcome. Arch Orthop Trauma Surg 127:691-697

Ensing GT, van Horn JR, van der Mei HC, Busscher HJ, Neut D (2003) Copal bone cement is more effective in preventing biofilm formation than Palacos R-G. Clin Orthop Relat Res 466:1492-1498

Evans RP (2004) Successful treatment of total hip and knee infection with articulating antibiotic components: a modified treatment method. Clin Orthop Relat Res 427:37-46

Fehring TK, Calton TF, Griffin WL (1999) Cementless fixation in 2-stage reimplantation for periprosthetic sepsis. J Arthroplasty 14:175-181

Fink B, Oreme D (2016) The transfemoral approach for removal of well-fixed femoral stems in two-stage septic hip revision. J Arthroplasty 31:1065-1071

Fink B, Hahn M, Fuerst M, Thybaut L, Delling G (2005) Principle of fixation of the cementless modular revision stem Revitan. Unfallchirurg 108:1029-1037

Fink B, Grossmann A, Fuerst M, Schäfer P, Frommelt L (2009) Two-stage cementless revision of infected hip endoprostheses. Clin Orthop Relat Res 467:1848-1858

Fink B, Rechtenbach A, Büchner H, Vogt S, Hahn M (2011) Articulating spacers used in two-stage revision of infected hip and knee prostheses abrade with time. Clin Orthop Relat Res 469:1095-1102

Fink B, Vogt S, Reinsch M, Büchner H (2011) Sufficient release of antibiotic by a spacer 6 weeks after implantation in two-stage revision of infected hip prostheses. Clin Orthop Relat Res 469:3141-3147

Fitzgerald RH Jr (1995) Infected total hip arthroplasty: Diagnosis and treatment. J Am Acad Orthop Surg 3: 249-262

Garvin KL, Evans BG, Salvati EA, Brause BD (1994) Palacos gentamicin for the treatment of deep periprosthetic hip infections. Clin Orthop Relat Res 298:97-105

Garvin KL, Hanssen AD (1995) Current concepts review: Infection after total hip arthroplasty. J Bone Joint Surg Am 77–A:1576-1588

Goldman RT, Scuderi GR, Insall JN (1996) 2-stage reimplantation for infected total knee replacement. Clin Orthop Relat Res 331:118-124

Haddad FS, Muirhead-Allwood SK, Manktelow AR, Bacarese-Hamilton I (2000) Two-stage uncemented revision hip arthroplasty for infection. J Bone Joint Surg Br 82:689-694

Hanssen AD, Osmon DR (2002) Evaluation of a staging system for infected hip arthroplasty. Clin Orthop Rel Res 403 16-22

Hofmann AA, Goldberg TD, Tanner AM, Cook TM (2005) Ten-year experience using an articulating antibiotic cement hip spacer for the treatment of chronically infected total hip. J Arthroplasty 20:874-879

Hsieh PH, Shih CH, Chang YH, Lee MD, Shih HN, Yang WE (2004a) Two-stage revision hip arthroplasty for infection: comparison between the interim use of antibiotic-loaded cement beads and a spacer prosthesis. J Bone Joint Surg Am 86:1989–1997

Hsieh PH, Chen LH, Chen CH, Lee MS, Yand WE, Shih CH (2004b) Two-stage revision hip arthroplasty for infection

with a custom-made, antibiotic-loaded, cement prosthesis as an interim spacer. J Trauma 56:1247-1252
Hsieh PH, Shih CH, Chang YH, Lee MS, Yang WE, Shih HN (2005) Treatment of deep infection of the hip associated with massive bone loss. Two-stage revision with an antibiotic-loaded interim cement prosthesis followed by reconstruction with allograft. J Bone Joint Surg Br 87-B:770-775
Hsieh PH, Chang YH, Chen SH, Ueng SW, Shih CH (2006) High concentration and bioactivity of vancomycin and aztreonam eluted from Simplex cement spacers in two-stage revision of infected hip implants: a study of 46 patients at an average follow-up of 107 days. J Orthop Res 24:1615-1621
Koo KH, Yang JW, Cho SH, Song HR, Park HB, Ha YC, Chang JD, Kim SY, Kim YH (2001) Impregnation of vancomycin, gentamicin, and cefotaxime in the cement spacer for two-stage cementless reconstruction in infected total hip arthroplasty. J Arthroplasty 16:882-892
Kraay MJ, Goldberg VM, Fitzgerald SJ, Salata MJ (2005) Cementless two-staged total hip arthroplasty for deep periprosthetic infection. Clin Orthop Relat Res 441:243-249
Leunig M, Chosa E, Speck M, Ganz R (1998) A cement spacer for two-stage revision of infected implants of the hip joint. Int Orthop 22:209-214
Lieberman JR, Callaway GH, Salvati EA, Pellici PM, Brause BD (1994) Treatment of the infected total hip arthroplasty with a two staged reimplantation protocol. Clin Orthop Relat Res 301:205-212
Masri BA, Duncan CP, Beauchamp CP (1998) Long-term elution of antibiotics form bone-cement. An in vivo study using the prosthesis of antibiotic-loaded acrylic cement (PROSTALAC) system. J Arthroplasty 13:331-338
Masri BA, Panagiotopoulos KP, Greidanus NV, Garbuz DS, Duncan CP (2007) Cementless two-stage exchange arthroplasty for infection after total hip arthroplasty. J Arthroplasty 22:72-78
McDonald DJ, Fitzgerald RA, Ilstrup DM (1989) Two-stage revision of the total hip arthroplasty because of infection. J Bone Joint Surg 71–A:828-832
Mitchell PA, Masri BA, Garbuz DS, Greidanus NV, Duncan CP (2003) Cementless revision for infection following total hip arthroplasty. Instr Course Lect 52:323-330
Mont MA, Waldman BJ, Hungerford DS (2000) Evaluation of preoperative cultures before second-stage reimplantation of a total knee prosthesis complicated by infection: a comparison-group study. J Bone Joint Surg Am 82:1552-1557
Morshed S, Huffman R, Ries M (2005) Extended trochanteric osteotomy for 2-stage revision of infected total hip arthroplasty. J Arthroplasty 20:294-301
Nestor BJ, Hanssen AD, Ferrer-Bonzalez R, Fitzgerald RH (1994) The use of porous prostheses in delayed reconstruction of total hip replacements that have failed because of infection. J Bone Joint Surg Am 76:349-359
Neut D, van Horn JR, van Kooten TG, van der Mei HC, Busscher HJ (2003) Detection of biomaterial-associated infections in orthopaedic joint implants. Clin Orthop Rel Res 413:261-268
Penner MJ, Masri BA, Duncan CP (1996) Elution characteristics of Vancomycin and Tobramycin combined in acrylic bone-cement. J Arhtroplasty 11:939-944
Schäfer P, Fink B, Sandow D, Margull A, Berger I, Frommelt L (2008) Prolonged bacterial culture to identify late periprosthetic joint infection: A promising strategy. Clin Inf Dis 47:1403-1409
Simpson PMS, Dall GF, Breusch SJ, Heisel C (2005) In vitro elution and mechanical properties of antibiotic-loaded SmartSet HV and Palocor R acrylic bone cements. Orthopäde 34:1255-1262
Wilson MG, Dorr LD (1989) Reimplantation of infected total hip arthroplasties in the absence of antibiotic cement. J Arthroplasty 4:263-269
Wirtz DC, Niethard FU (1997) Etiology, diagnosis and therapy of aseptic hip prosthesis loosening - a status assessment. Z Orthop Ihre Grenzgeb 135:270-280
Yamamoto K, Miyagawa N, Masaoka T, Katori Y, Shishido T, Imakiire A (2009) Cement spacer loaded with antibiotics for infected implants of the hip joint. J Arthroplasty 24:83-89
Younger ASE, Duncan CP, Masri BA, McGraw RW (1997) The outcome of two-stage arthroplasty using a custom-made interval spacer to treat the infected hip. J Arthroplasty 12:615-623

8

8.4 Spacer Management

Kiran Singisetti and Ian Stockley

8.4.1 Evaluation of a Suspected Case of PJI

Simple blood tests in the form of C-reactive protein (CRP), erythrocyte sedimentation rate (ESR) and white blood cell count (WBC) are routinely taken. They are usually elevated in cases of periprosthetic joint infection (PJI) but not necessarily so.

We have a low threshold for aspirating a prosthetic joint if there is any suspicion of infection, as we believe it is imperative to obtain accurate bacteriology results at this stage (◘ Fig. 8.38; Ali et al. 2006). Improved accuracy of this technique is possible if the patient is not taking antibiotics; hence, we strongly recommend patients stop them at least 2 weeks prior to the procedure. Furthermore, incubating the cultures for 14 days increases the sensitivity and specificity of the result (Schäfer et al. 2008). A negative aspiration result does not exclude

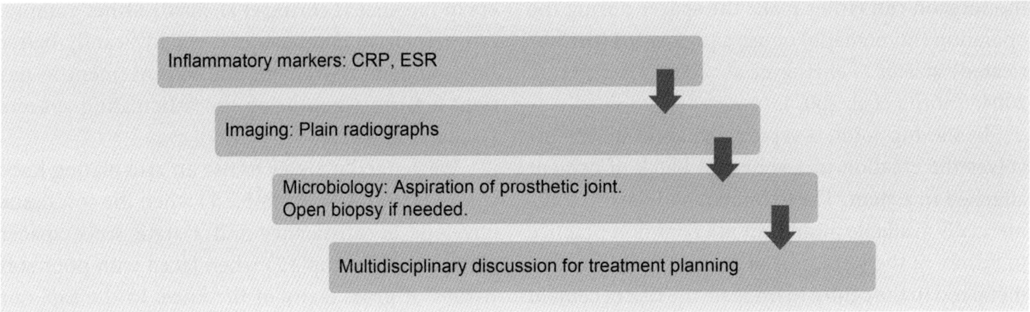

Fig. 8.38 Algorithm for evaluation of suspected PJI

infection and if still suspicious, repeat aspiration is undertaken.

8.4.2 Commonly Encountered Pathogens

The common pathogens in our practice tend to be the Gram-positive organisms; coagulase-negative staphylococcus, *Staphylococcus aureus* and Streptococcus. Over the last 5 years, however, we have being seeing an increasing number of Gram-negative organisms. Fungal infections, although relatively uncommon, present regularly and are usually associated with patients who have had multiple revision procedures and those with medical co-morbidities such as rheumatoid arthritis.

8.4.3 One-Stage Versus Two-Stage Procedure

Whilst there are many different management options available for the patient with a chronically infected prosthesis, the best option in terms of improving overall function post-operatively is that of exchange surgery, whether it be a one- or two-stage procedure.

Whilst there continues to be debate about the relative merits of one- versus two-stage procedures, we believe that better functional outcome is achieved following a single stage but accept that, theoretically at least, control of infection may be better with a two-stage procedure. There is currently a lack of good-quality evidence, e. g. randomized controlled studies, to demonstrate a significant difference in outcome between the two procedures. Baker et al have reported on there being no significant difference in the patient-reported outcome measures (PROMS) in comparing the single-stage versus two-stage revisions when using the National Joint Registry data (Baker et al. 2013). Currently, our default position is to perform a single-stage but will resort to a two-stage procedure if we do not know the identity of the infecting organism or if the patient is systemically unwell with sepsis. The quality of the soft tissues does not necessarily determine what we do, as we have found that during the debridement, the overall quality of the tissues improves. In particular the presence of a sinus, which historically meant a two-stage procedure, we regard as irrelevant and will often proceed to a single-stage procedure in these cases. The sinus by its presence »decompresses«' the soft tissues.

8.4.4 Spacer Types

Antibiotic-loaded bone cement (ALBC) spacers have been used for a long time in an attempt to create and maintain a temporary joint space in the interval between stages of a two-staged procedure. In addition, they help in the management of PJI by acting as a depot of antibiotic. Antibiotic elutes from the surface in high concentration (Booth and Lotke 1989; Senthi et al. 2011).

The terminology around the different types of spacers used today can be confusing. Generally speaking, spacers can be described as being static or dynamic (articulating or functional). In addition, the surgeon can either make the spacer during the operation (homemade) or use a preformed (prefabricated) spacer (Fehring et al. 2000; Hsieh et al. 2004; Cabrita et al. 2007).

In the hip joint, a typical dynamic spacer involves the creation of a spherical block of cement attached to a stem. These can be made using commercially available moulds. It is a common practice to reinforce the stem part of cement mould with a metal rod in the centre to mitigate the risk of cement fracture. Potential complications of articulating spacers include dislocation, breakage and adverse local tissue reactions secondary to the cement debris (Barreira et al. 2015). Poorer clinical outcomes have been noted where spacers have dislocated out the hip joint (Bori et al. 2014; Barreira et al. 2015). There are now proprietary formulations of low-abrasive cement specifically developed for making cement spacers (Copal® spacem). Issues with preformed spacers are the associated cost that is not insignificant, possible limitations with size and more importantly the quantity of antibiotic added to the cement as one has no intraoperative flexibility of changing this.

We tend to use antibiotic-loaded cement beads as a depot source of antibiotic. These are made by moulding by hand the cement to form small biconcave-shaped discs, which are then placed on 8-gauge braided wire to form chains prior to polymerization of the cement. These can then be inserted down the femoral canal or rolled up and placed into the acetabulum. This method of producing a depot of local antibiotic has been shown to give much higher local concentrations of antibiotic than that which can be achieved by intravenous administration of antibiotics (Wahlig et al. 1978; Stockley et al. 2008).

In 2014, the international consensus statement on PJI gave the opinion that there was no difference in the efficacy of infection eradication, irrespective of the type of spacer used, whether it be an articulating or non-articulating spacer in the hip or knee joint(Parvizi et al. 2011).

There is also the question of range of movement after the second-stage procedure: Does an articulating spacer lead to a better range as compared with a static spacer? Fehring et al. have suggested there is no significant difference in the final range of movement when comparing static versus dynamic spacers in the knee (Fehring et al. 2000). Other authors, however, have demonstrated a significantly better final range of movement and improvement in patient activity when using the articulating spacers (Jaekel et al. 2012).

We generally prefer to use an articulating knee spacer (■ Fig. 8.39; Example 1) when the soft tissue envelope is satisfactory and a static knee spacer (■ Fig. 8.40; Example 2) when faced with poor soft tissues or gross laxity of the knee. In the hip, our practice is to use a non-articulating spacer like the homemade beads when the bone stock is satisfactory (■ Fig. 8.41; Example 3) and to use a block spacer (■ Fig. 8.42; Example 4) when there is femoral bone loss; which in addition helps maintain leg length and a good soft tissue bed in preparation for subsequent second-stage implantation of a definitive prosthesis.

8.4.5 Antibiotics to Be Added to Bone Cement

As long as the sterile antibiotic powder is heat stable, any antibiotic in theory can be added to the cement powder prior to mixing with the monomer. Gentamicin is the most commonly preloaded antibiotic added to bone cement (e. g. Palacos® R+G). Various other factory-added antibiotic bone cement formulations are available with gentamicin and clindamycin (e. g. Copal® G+C), gentamicin with vancomycin (e. g. Copal® G+V) and tobramycin (e. g. Simplex® P with tobramycin) being the more commonly used combinations today.

Our practice is to add the additional antibiotics in theatre. The choice is determined by the antibiogram of the infecting organism identified at the preoperative aspiration or the first-stage cultures. This allows us flexibility to tailor specific local antibiotic delivery in high dose following advice from a musculoskeletal microbiologist. Fungal periprosthetic infections are becoming an increasing problem and we have experience of adding antifungal agents like voriconazole or fluconazole to the bone cement with good success (Fehring et al. 2000; Bruce et al. 2001).

Hand mixing of the bone cement with additional antibiotics may lead to even higher local elution of antibiotic, but this can lead to inferior mechanical

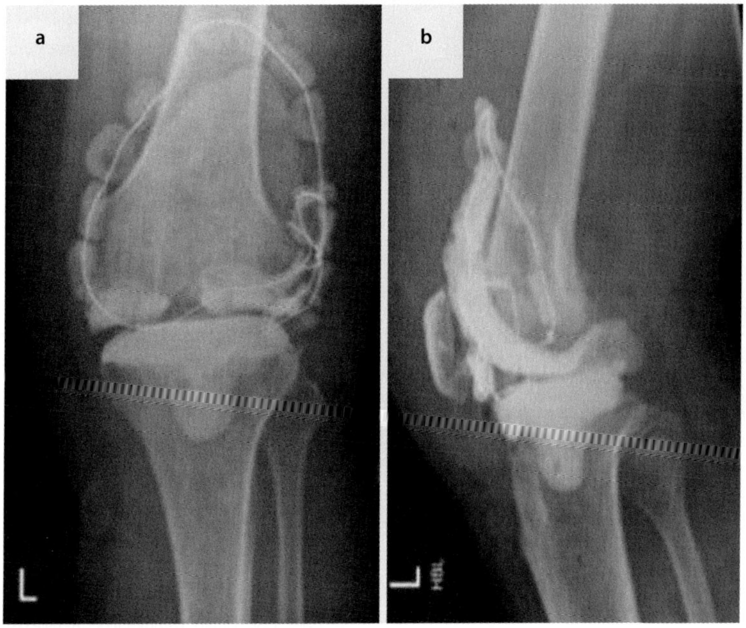

Fig. 8.39 a, b Case example 1: Articulating spacer in the knee joint. Antibiotic-loaded cement was moulded to the shape of the distal femur and proximal tibia. In addition, a string of cement beads was placed in the supra-patellar pouch and para-patellar gutters to allow for further elution of antibiotic and also to maintain distention of the soft tissues

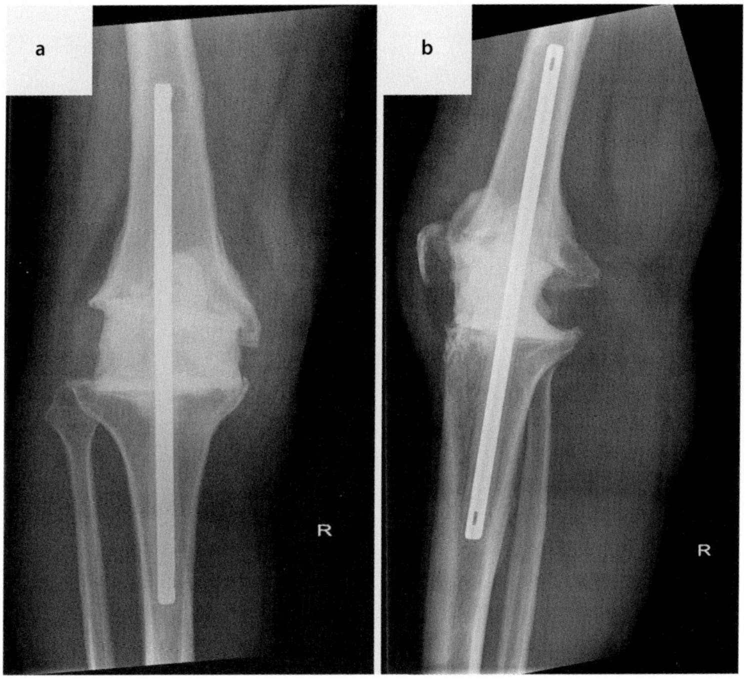

Fig. 8.40 a, b Case example 2: Static spacer in the knee joint. A contoured block of antibiotic-loaded cement, reinforced with an intramedullary rod, was used to reduce the risk of fracture and dislocation in this case where there was significant bone loss and soft tissue instability

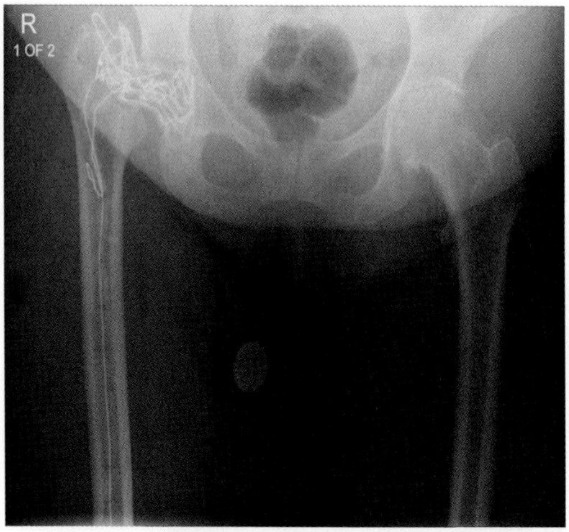

■ **Fig. 8.41** Case example 3: Static spacer in the hip joint. In this case antibiotic-loaded cement beads were used in hip joint where there was relatively good bone stock

properties of the cement compared with a commercially manufactured mix. However, as long as 10% of the weight of the powder is not exceeded by the weight of the antibiotic powder no significant effects are seen (Lautenschlager et al. 1976). In vitro studies have shown that cyclical loading of articulating knee spacers can increase the elution of antibiotic (Rogers et al. 2011).

8.4.6 Prostheses Used for Revision

The type of prosthesis fixation, whether it be cemented or uncemented, has not been shown to affect the incidence of PJI following primary surgery. There is some agreement that the use of antibiotic-impregnated cement compared with plain bone cement in primary as well as revision surgery decreases the risk for PJI (Bourne 2004; Jämsen et al. 2010).

We use both cemented and uncemented prostheses at the time of revision surgery depending upon the reasons for failure of the primary reconstruction. If sepsis is the cause and we know the antibiotic sensitivities of the infecting organism,

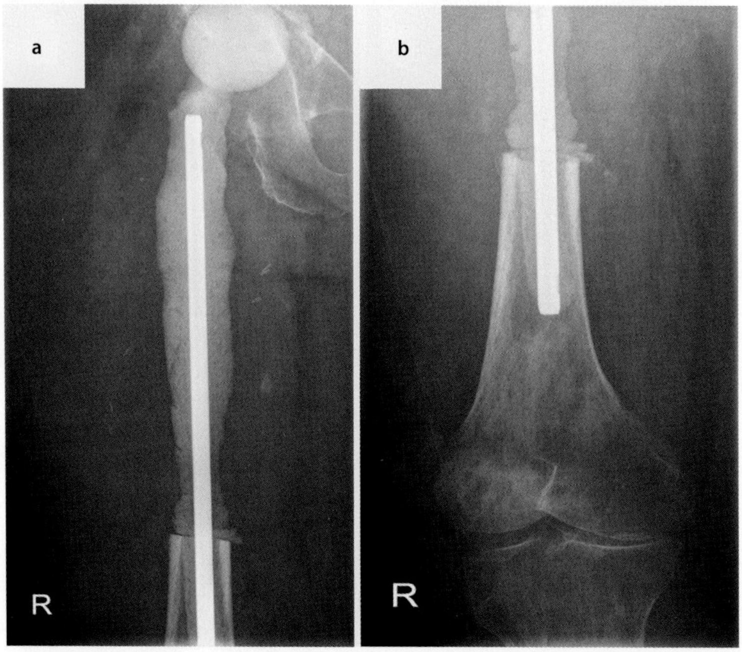

■ **Fig. 8.42 a, b** Case example 4: Articulating/block spacer for the hip joint. A block spacer, contoured for the femoral head proximally, reinforced with central metal rod for improved mechanical stability, was used to maintain soft tissue tension as a consequence of extensive bone loss

then in most cases we will offer a single-stage exchange using antibiotic-loaded bone cement. Otherwise, it will be a two-stage procedure with either cemented or uncemented prostheses being used at the second stage depending upon the individual circumstances; for example, quantity and quality of the remaining bone stock and the patient's age and general well-being. If it is primarily an aseptic revision, uncemented or cemented components may be used just like in the second stage of a staged exchange procedure.

Take-Home Message

- Common pathogens tend to be the Gram-positive organisms, coagulase-negative staphylococcus, *Staphylococcus aureus* and Streptococcus.
- Over the past 5 years an increasing number of Gram-negative organisms have been seen.
- The best option in terms of improving overall function post-operatively is that of exchange surgery.
- We use both cemented and uncemented prostheses at the time of revision surgery depending upon the reasons for failure of the primary reconstruction.
- We opt for single-stage exchange using antibiotic-loaded bone cement in cases of sepsis and known antibiotic sensitivities of the infecting organism.
- We opt for the two-stage procedure if we do not know the identity of the infecting organism or if the patient is systemically unwell with sepsis

References

Ali F, Wilkinson JM, Cooper JR, Kerry RM, Hamer AJ, Norman P, Stockley I (2006) Accuracy of joint aspiration for the preoperative diagnosis of infection in total hip arthroplasty. J Arthroplasty 21(2):221-226

Baker P, Petheram TG, Kurtz S, Konttinen YT, Gregg P, Deehan D (2013) Patient reported outcome measures after revision of the infected TKR: comparison of single versus two-stage revision. Knee Surg Sports Traumatol Arthrosc 21(12):2713-20

Barreira P, Leite P, Neves P, Soares D, Sousa R (2015) Preventing mechanical complications of hip spacer implantation: technical tips and pearls. Acta Orthop Belg 81(2):344-348

Booth RE Jr, Lotke PA (1989) The results of spacer block technique in revision of infected total knee arthroplasty. Clin Orthop Relat Res 248:57-60

Bori G, García-Oltra E, Soriano A, Rios J, Gallart X, Garcia S (2014) Dislocation of preformed antibiotic-loaded cement spacers (Spacer-G): etiological factors and clinical prognosis. J Arthroplasty 29(5):883-888

Bourne RB (2004) Prophylactic use of antibiotic bone cement: an emerging standard – in the affirmative. J Arthroplasty 19[4 Suppl 1]:69-72

Bruce AS, Kerry RM, Norman P, Stockley I (2001) Fluconazole-impregnated beads in the management of fungal infection of prosthetic joints. J Bone Joint Surg Br 83(2):183-184

Cabrita HB, Croci AT, Camargo OP, Lima AL (2007) Prospective study of the treatment of infected hip arthroplasties with or without the use of an antibiotic-loaded cement spacer. Clinics (Sao Paulo) 62(2):99-108

Fehring TK, Odum S, Calton TF, Mason JB (2000) Articulating versus static spacers in revision total knee arthroplasty for sepsis. The Ranawat Award. Clin Orthop Relat Res 380:9-16

Hsieh PH, Shih CH, Chang YH, Lee MS, Shih HN, Yang WE (2004) Two-stage revision hip arthroplasty for infection: comparison between the interim use of antibiotic-loaded cement beads and a spacer prosthesis. J Bone Joint Surg Am 86A(9):1989-1897

Jaekel DJ, Day JS, Klein GR, Levine H, Parvizi J, Kurtz SM (2012) Do dynamic cement-on-cement knee spacers provide better function and activity during two-stage exchange? Clin Orthop Relat Res. 2012 Sep ;470(9):2599-604

Jämsen E, Furnes O, Engesaeter LB, Konttinen YT, Odgaard A, Stefánsdóttir A, Lidgren L (2010) Prevention of deep infection in joint replacement surgery. Acta Orthop 81(6):660-666

Lautenschlager EP, Jacobs JJ, Marshall GW, Meyer PR Jr (1976) Mechanical properties of bone cements containing large doses of antibiotic powders. J Biomed Mater Res 10(6):929-938

Parvizi J, Gehrke T (2013) Proceedings of the International Consensus Meeting on Periprosthetic Joint Infection. Data Trace Publishing Company

Rogers BA, Middleton FR, Shearwood-Porter N, Kinch S, Roques A, Bradley NW, Browne M (2011) Does cyclical loading affect the elution of antibiotics from articulating cement knee spacers? J Bone Joint Surg Br 93(7):914-920

Schäfer P, Fink B, Sandow D, Margull A, Berger I, Frommelt L (2008) Prolonged bacterial culture to identify late periprosthetic joint infection: a promising strategy. Clin Infect Dis 47:1403-1409

Senthi S, Munro JT, Pitto RP (2011) Infection in total hip replacement: meta-analysis. Int Orthop 35(2):253-260

Stockley I, Mockford BJ, Hoad-Reddick A, Norman P (2008) The use of two-stage exchange arthroplasty with depot antibiotics in the absence of long-term antibiotic therapy in infected total hip replacement. J Bone Joint Surg Br 90(2):145-148

Wahlig H, Dingeldein E, Bergmann R, Reuss K (1978) The release of gentamicin from polymethacrylate beads: an experimental and pharmacokinetic study. J Bone Joint Surg Br 60B:270-275

Coating

K.-D. Kühn (Ed.), *Management of Periprosthetic Joint Infection*
DOI 10.1007/978-3-662-54469-3_9

9.1 Antibacterial Coating of Implants in Orthopaedics and Trauma

Finding the Right Pathway to a More Effective Surgical Site Infection Prevention

Carlo Luca Romanò, Enrico Gallazzi, Sara Scarponi, Ilaria Morelli and Lorenzo Drago

9.1.1 Introduction

The importance of asepsis and antisepsis in surgery was first recognized by Ingac Semmelweiss in 1847. Since then, several effective infection prevention methods have been introduced, but surgical site infection (SSI) still remains one of the most important reasons for failure in orthopaedics and trauma; up to 2.5% of primary hip and knee replacements and up to 20% of joint revision procedures may in fact be complicated by periprosthetic joint infection (PJI; Lentino 2003; Dale et al. 2009; Aggarwal 2014a). Moreover multi-drug resistant pathogens are more and more involved in PJI, thus reducing treatment options. Indeed, most PJIs require implant removal, with increased morbidity and even mortality (Zmistowski et al. 2013) and high associated social and economic costs (Kurtz et al. 2012).

PJI occurs as a result of the interaction of different factors. Bacterial load or contamination at the surgical site plays an initial role; even with the most cautious antisepsis procedures, elective surgery may in fact not be performed in a completely bacterial-free environment (An and Friedman 1996; Humphreys 2012). Another factor to take in consideration are the host's immune defences; while the bacterial load at the surgical site is usually low and easily overcome by the immune system and antibiotic prophylaxis (Jamsen et al. 2010), if the host immune defences are impaired, such as in diabetes or chronic renal failure, the risk of infection increases greatly (Illingworth et al. 2013; Pruzansky et al. 2014; Aggarwal et al. 2014b). The complexity of the surgical procedures also influences the risk of infection (Namba et al. 2012). In this context, implanted device characteristics such as size, shape, material, surface finishing and intended use also play an important role (Moriarty et al. 2010).

On the bright side, recent evidence pointed out how local prophylaxis using antibiotic-loaded bone cement or bone grafts may reduce the incidence of implant-related infections (Jamsen et al. 2010; van de Belt et al. 2001a). In line with this, in a recent international consensus meeting on PJI, a strong recommendation was delivered concerning the need for developing effective antibacterial coatings in order to prevent bacterial adhesion and colonization of implants and proliferation into the surrounding tissues (Cats-Baril 2013).

In this chapter we provide an overview and a classification of the various technologies under study or currently on the market. Classifying different technologies may be useful in order to better compare different solutions, to improve the design of validation tests and, hopefully, to improve and speed up the regulatory process in this promising and rapidly evolving field.

9.1.2 Antibacterial Coatings: Rationale and Pathophysiology of Implant-Related Infections

The concept of a »race for the surface« in implant-related infection was proposed by Anthony Gristina more than three decades ago. According to this model, host and bacterial cells compete in determining the ultimate fate of the implant, with a very low probability of attachment of bacterial cells to the implant when the host cells colonize the implant surface first, and vice versa (Gristina et al. 1988). While this is probably a rather simplistic model, it has stimulated technological progress and fuelled the idea of modifying the surface of implants in order to favour host cells and prevent bacterial adhesion.

The process of bacterial adhesion can be divided into two basic phases: reversible and irreversible. Bacterial cells express a wide range of adhesins, which are able to interact with many of the biomaterial surface receptor sites, thus making them able to adhere and survive on virtually all natural and artificial surfaces (Costerton et al. 2003; Busscher and van der Mei 2012). Environmental and surface characteristics of a biomaterial such as surface roughness, hydrophobicity and electrostatic charge play only conditional roles (Chen et al. 2011). Moreover, implanted biomaterials are immediately covered by a protein film, composed of complement, albumin and several other host proteins and lipids (Jenney and Anderson 2000; Thevenot et al. 2008; Costerton et al. 1999). This conditional cover acts as a reservoir of several receptors for bacterial adhesive ligands, mediating adhesion of free-floating bacteria to the surface of the biomaterials (Wagner et al. 2011; Wang et al. 2012; Ribeiro et al. 2012). This first, reversible phase of bacterial adhesion is mechanically and biologically unstable and relies on nonspecific interactions between implant surface and bacterial adhesins. The second phase is mediated by molecular and cellular interactions closely associated with the expression of biofilm-specific gene clusters in reversibly attached bacteria (Costerton et al. 1999; Stoodley et al. 2011; Laverty et al. 2013; Foster et al. 2014).

From the host's perspective, the details of implant osteointegration and tissue integration are also only partially elucidated (Anderson et al. 2008; Gardner et al. 2013). The attachment of the host cell on the implant surface leads to periprosthetic bone regeneration and remodelling, and this may be protective against bacterial colonization (Busscher et al. 2012). However, bacterial micro-colonies survive even in osteointegrated implants, and peri-implant fibrous barriers can prevent contact between host immunity sentinel cells and bacterial molecules, thus limiting the host's immune response (Zimmerli et al. 1984; Higgins et al. 2009; Zimmerli and Sendi 2011).

As a result, there is a strong need for intrinsic implant surface antibacterial functionality to overcome the implant-induced defects in the local immune response and to prevent the striking ability of bacteria to quickly adhere on a substrate and immediately produce a protective biofilm barrier, providing a competitive advantage to the host's cells over the contaminating micro-organisms. At the same time any coating technology should prove to be safe, should not interfere with osteointegration or induce bacterial resistance in the long run. The basic requirements that an »ideal« coating technology should fulfil to meet the needs for widespread clinical use are summarized in ◘ Tab. 9.1.

Moreover, the entire bacterial colonization process, from microbial adhesion on an implant surface to the production of an established mature biofilm layer, may only take a few hours (◘ Fig. 9.1; Holá et al. 2006), so any implant antibacterial functionality should act at the exact time of surgery, that is, from the moment the implant is extracted from the sterile package to at least until the very next few hours after it is inserted into the body and the skin closed, or, in other words, just before bacteria can adhere on the implant and start producing biofilms.

A mature biofilm layer is completely built in less than 24 h, and therefore correct timing of systemic antibiotic prophylaxis and the possible application of a local antibacterial protection play a key role in overcoming the ability of bacteria to adhere on the implant and quickly protect them-

◘ **Tab. 9.1** List of requirements for »ideal« antibacterial implant coating strategy

Requirements	Fulfilments			
Safety	No systemic toxicity	No local toxicity	No detrimental effects on bone healing	No unwanted long-term side effects
In vitro activity	No cytotoxicity or genotoxicity	Proven bactericidal and antibiofilm activity on different surfaces	Large spectrum	No induction of resistance
Efficacy	Proven in vivo	Case series	Multicentre trials	Randomized trials
Ease-of-use	Easy handling	Versatility	Resistance to press-fit insertion	Storage
Market	Acceptable cost	Wide availability	Easy to manufacture	Overcomes regulatory issues

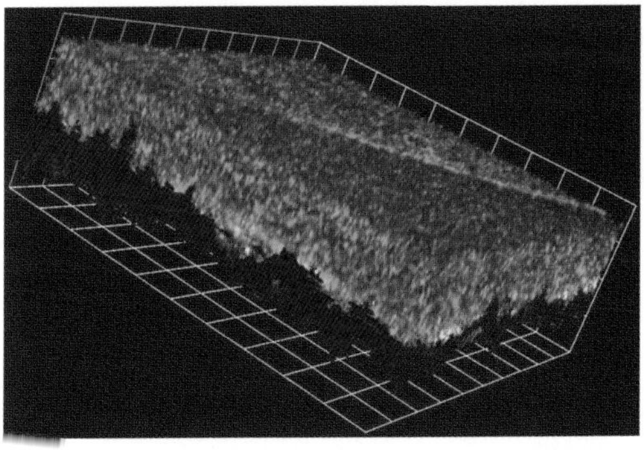

Fig. 9.1 Confocal laser microscopy three-dimensional reconstruction of *Staphylococcus aureus* biofilm grown for 72 h (in *green*, stained with Syto9®) on a sanded titanium alloy surface (in *blue*)

selves with biofilms from the host's immune system and antibiotics.

9.1.3 Coating Classification and Mechanism of Action

Many different approaches have been followed in order to obtain antibacterial implant protection. Based on their mechanism of action, antibacterial coatings can be classified as follows (cf. Tab. 9.2):

1. *Passive surface finishing/modification.* This strategy is aimed at preventing or reducing bacterial adhesion on implants through surface chemistry and/or structure modifications, without the use of any pharmacologically active substance. Examples of this approach include modified titanium dioxide surface or polymer coatings.
2. *Active surface finishing/modification.* In this strategy, pharmacologically active pre-incorporated bactericidal agents such as antibiotics, antiseptics, metal ions or other organic and inorganic substances are actively released from the implant, in order to reduce bacteria adhesion. Examples of this approach are »contact killing« active surface with silver- or iodine-coated joint implants.
3. *Perioperative antibacterial local carriers or coatings.* This strategy employs local antibacterial carriers, or coatings, that are not built in the device, but rather are applied during surgery, immediately prior of the implant; they may have direct or synergistic antibacterials activity, or deliver high local concentrations of loaded antibiotics or antibacterials.

While necessarily schematic, this classification may be helpful both from the clinical point of view, helping the clinician in the choice of correct coating, and from the regulatory point of view, which may differ substantially for different coating classes.

Passive Surface Finishing/Modification

Several lines of evidence showed how the surface characteristics of the implant, i.e. roughness, hydrophilicity, surface energy, potential and conductivity, play an important role in initial bacterial adhesion to implant and subsequently biofilm formation (Moriarty et al. 2010; Chen et al. 2011). Thus, by modifying surface characteristics of the implant, a reduction in bacterial adhesion can be achieved.

For example, ultraviolet light irradiation can lead to an increase in »»spontaneous« wettability on titanium dioxide, which can inhibit bacterial adhesion without compromising osteogenesis on titanium alloy implants (Gallardo-Moreno et al. 2009; Yu et al. 2003). A bacterial anti-adhesive surface can also be achieved by modifying the crystalline structure of the surface oxide layer (Del Curto et al. 2005).

Other than by a direct modification of the titanium dioxide surface, passive antibacterial finishing can be obtained by applying certain polymer coatings, such as hydrophilic polymethacrylic acid, polyethylene oxide or protein-resistant polyethylene glycol (Zhang et al. 2008; Harris et al. 2004; Kaper et al. 2003). The downside of the passive finishing technique is that some of these coatings reduce osteoblast function on the implant surface. This issue has been overcome by using additional bioactive molecules, such as sericin and RGD motifs, with the immobilization technique, thus achieving a normal or even improved osteoblast function (Harris et al. 2004). Moreover, recent studies showed how hydrophobic and superhydrophobic surface finishing greatly reduces bacterial adhesion on implant surfaces (Zhu et al. 2014; Braem et al. 2013).

As discussed earlier, surfaces and/or protein–bacteria interactions play a crucial role in the early phases of implant placement. Thus, treating these interactions could be a successful strategy to reduce bacterial adhesion (Campoccia et al. 2013). The host's first substances that interact with the implant are various plasma proteins, such as albumin, fibro-

Tab. 9.2 Classification of antibacterial implant protection strategies

Strategy	Features	Examples	Development stage	Limits
Passive surface finishing/ modifications (PSM)	Prevention of bacterial adhesion	Hydrophilic surface	Preclinical	Limited antibacterial and antibiofilm activity Possible interference with osteointegration Unknown long-term effects Regulatory issues
		Super-hydrophobic surface		
		Anti-adhesive polymers		
		Nano-patterned surface		
		Albumin		
		Hydrogels		
		Biosurfactants		
Active surface finishing/ modifications (ASM)	Inorganic	Silver ions and nanoparticles	Market	Incomplete implant coating Questionable long-term toxicity Limited versatility and applicability Limited large-scale applications Possible bacterial resistance induction Costs
		Other metals (copper, zinc, titanium dioxide etc.)	Preclinical	Questionable long-term toxicity Regulatory issues.
		Non-metals: iodine	Clinical	Incomplete implant coating Questionable long-term toxicity Challenging large-scale application Regulatory issues
		Other non-metal ions (selenium, grapheme, etc.)	Preclinical	Poorly studied compounds. Coating resistance to press-fit insertion. Questionable long-term toxicity Challenging large scale application. Regulatory issues.
	Organic	Coated/linked antibiotics	Market	Unique application to nail coating Long-term effects on osteointegration Single antibiotic (gentamicin)
		Covalently linked antibiotics	Preclinical	Incomplete implant coating Questionable long-term toxicity Challenging large-scale application Regulatory issues
		Antimicrobial peptides		No data on in vivo or clinical effects Coating resistance to press-fit insertion Questionable long-term toxicity Challenging large-scale application Regulatory issues
		Cytokines		
		Enzymes and biofilm disrupting agents		
		Chitosan derivatives		
	Synthetic	Non-antibiotic antimicrobial compounds		
		»Smart« coatings		
	Combined	Multilayer coating		

Tab. 9.2 (Continued)

Strategy	Features	Examples	Development stage	Limits
Perioperative antibacterial local carriers or coatings (LCC)	Non-biodegradable	Antibiotic-loaded polymethyl methacrylate	Market	Resistance and small-colony variants induction No antibiofilm effect Incomplete implant coating May not be used for cementless implants
	Biodegradable	Antibiotic-loaded bone grafts and substitutes	Market	Limited availability Not proven efficacy as implant coating Cost
		Fast-resorbable hydrogel	Market	Medium term results available from two multicenter clinical trials.

nectin, fibrinogen, laminin, collagen and some lipids. The reduction of conditional protein lipid layer deposition and the formation of a protective protein layer could be achieved either by changing the surface physico-chemical characteristics (Yeo et al. 2012) or by modifying the surface micro-morphology (Bacakova et al. 2011; Lu et al. 2012).

The former strategy was employed by Friedman et al. using a rabbit model. They demonstrated a reduced bacterial adherence on pure titanium samples and decreased infection rates of implants coated with cross-linked albumin (An et al. 1997).

The latter strategy was investigated by several authors, and consists in obtaining the anti-adhesion effect by changing the surface at a nanometrical scale, i.e. by increasing the roughness of the surface. It has been shown that this nanometric increase in roughness facilitates the formation of a thick protein layer on the surface, which greatly reduces bacterial adhesion (Bacakova et al. 2011; Lu et al. 2012; Singh et al. 2011).

More recently, novel strategies include production of self-assembled mono- or multilayers, surface grafting or hydrogels, or the use of biosurfactants and microbial amphiphilic compounds with excellent anti-adhesive properties (Rivardo et al. 2009; Rodrigues et al. 2006).

Recently a different approach to passive finishing was investigated. This approach is based on the assumption that a three-dimensional nanostructure finishing, other than reducing bacterial adhesion by increasing the surface's roughness, can be used as a reservoir for perioperative loaded antibiotic. This novel approach is of particular interest because it combines the advantages of the perioperative loading strategy with the antibacterial passive finishing. In a recent study a silk fibroin/hyaluronic acid coating engineered to increase surface roughness was tested in vitro (Arpacay et al. 2015). In another in vitro study titanium implants were finished with a three-dimensional nanostructuring designed to be loaded with tannic acid/gentamicin, showing a significant decrease in *Staphylococcus aureus* adhesion and growth (Hizal et al. 2015).

In summary, to date a number of passive anti-adhesive tactics have been proposed for different purposes. However, passive surface modification has several limitations that reduce its effectiveness in clinical practice. First of all, currently a universal surface treatment that can be applied to all surfaces, all bacterial species, and all implants does not exist. Moreover, passive coating methods should be preferred as long as their antibacterial ability is strong enough to prevent biofilm formation. However, the effectiveness of passive coatings for decreasing bacterial adhesion is limited and varies greatly depending on the bacterial species (Hetrick et al. 2006). Furthermore, in some situations the use of a strong anti-adhesive layer is not feasible, such as in total hip arthroplasty, because it could prevent host bone osseointegration and lead to early mechanical failure (Lu et al. 2012; Singh et al. 2011). Finally, the long-term effects of these new technologies both on the host's cells and on bacterial resistance are poorly understood and need to be further investigated before widespread clinical applications would be possible.

Active Surface Finishing/Modification

Active surface finishing/modification may include pharmacologically active pre-incorporated antibacterial agents or compounds, like antibiotics, antiseptics, metal ions and organic molecules. Such pharmacologically activated coatings may change the implant from a passive, inert biomaterial, to an active material capable of defending itself from bacterial colonization. The disadvantages of this approach are the difficult to predict long-term effects and challenging regulatory issues, as will be discussed, which have prevented clinical application of many otherwise promising technologies.

Two main strategies have been proposed for effective antibacterial surface treatment: either »contact killing« or drug eluting. In the former, the surface is finished with substances that can kill bacteria when they try to colonize the implant; in killing bacteria they rely on diverse mechanisms of action, which may interfere with cell respiration or division, cell wall formation or bacterial signalling network (e.g. quorum sensing) as well as inhibition of the transition of the planktonic phenotype of bacteria into a sessile type (Stoodley et al. 2013). In the latter strategy the finishing allows for the slow release of antibiotics from the implant, in order to reach an antibiotic concentration around the implant higher than the minimum inhibitory concentration (MIC) for the most common pathogens. Those tactics are aimed at protecting the implant long enough to allow both prophylactic antibiotic activity and the host immune response to kill bacteria.

In terms of durability, we can distinguish between degradable and non-degradable coatings. Antibacterial surface technologies can employ metals (silver, zinc, copper, etc.), non-metal elements (e.g. iodine, selenium), organic substances (antibiotics, anti-infective peptides, chitosan, other substances), and their combinations.

The antibacterial activity of the majority of metal coatings is closely linked to the ionic or nano form rather than to the bulk material (Lemire et al. 2013). The most prevalent metals used as antibacterial coatings are silver, copper and zinc. Silver is currently the most diffuse. Silver antibacterial activity is well known, and mostly depends on the ability of dissolved cations to interfere with bacterial cell membrane permeability and cellular metabolism. Moreover, when released in an aqueous medium, silver cations also contribute to formation of reactive oxygen species and other mechanisms that potentially influence prokaryotic cells (Chernousov and Epple 2013). Despite the demonstrated clinical efficacy and safety in recent comparative studies (Wafa et al. 2015; Hardes et al. 2010), routine using of silver-coated implants remains rather limited. The main concerns have been about the toxicity of silver ions: The same activity that interferes with prokaryotic cells could also interfere with eukaryotic cells, exerting cytotoxicity on bone cells, and the silver ions released could accumulate and cause harm in distant locations (Mijnendonckx et al. 2013). Research efforts have focused on the development of silver coating technologies that reduce or even eliminate toxicity while maintaining constructive antibacterial effects (Noda et al. 2009; Panacek et al. 2009). A recent study showed how a combination of silver and hydroxyapatite coating could even promote osteoblast activity (Eto et al. 2015). Copper and zinc also have potent antibacterial effects on a wide spectrum of bacterial species (Grass et al. 2011; Petrini et al. 2006); however, the potential toxic side effects of these metals remain a strong concern (Hodgkinson and Petris 2012). Proposed solutions include copper- and zinc-based nanomaterials or, alternatively, controlled release (Pelgrift and Friedman 2013).

The main limiting factors to the widespread clinical use of such finishing were the risk of bacterial resistance to metallic coatings (Moseke et al. 2011), the mechanical properties of implant nanocoatings since damage may occur during surgical implantation especially in cementless implants inserted via press-fit methods (Shtansky et al. 2006), and, eventually, cost issues and the inability to apply the technology to a variety of prosthetic implants and devices.

A different approach in active finishing is to modify commonly used alloys, like titanium, by rendering it capable of exerting an antibacterial activity. The anti-infective potential of titanium dioxide layers has been widely investigated and proven effective in vitro both alone (Arenas et al. 2013) or in combination with other substances (Hu et al. 2012).

Selenium bound covalently onto the surface of titanium or titanium alloy implant discs has been shown to prevent *S. aureus* and *S. epidermidis* attachment without affecting osteoblast viability (Holinka et al. 2013). Selenium catalyzes the formation of superoxide radicals and subsequently inhibits bacterial adhesion and viability. In addition, selenium nanoparticles can inhibit bacterial growth and biofilm formation (Tran and Webster 2011).

Ongoing research is also directed to determine the clinical applicability of carbon substances like graphene or carbon nanotubes, which can be synthesized in multifunctional layers (Martynkova and Valaskova 2014). One of the most interesting technologies under study today, related to non-metal elements, is iodine coating of titanium alloys, which has recently demonstrated clinical efficacy in a continuous series of 222 patients with excellent results (Tsuchiya et al. 2012).

Active finishing with antibiotics can basically be approached in two different ways: by covalently binding antibiotics to the surface of implants, thus conferring antibacterial properties to the implant surface; or by covering the implant's surface with an antibiotic-eluting system, such as specific antibiotic formulations capable of adhering to surfaces even when sterilized, and to release antibiotics only when implanted. Regarding the first approach, a large number of studies have investigated the efficacy of surfaces coated with covalently linked antibiotics (Antoci et al. 2007b; Alt et al. 2006; Schmidmaier et al. 2006; Fei et al. 2011; Neut et al. 2012). The limitations of this technique are mainly the limited clinical effectiveness of such implants for infections caused by bacteria that are resistant to the coupled antibiotic. In addition, strong forces such as covalent binding are insufficiently sensitive to react to weak external stimuli, thus limiting the killing activity potential of bacteria which might not be directly adjacent to the implant (Shchukin and Mohwald 2013).

To overcome these issues, combinations of antibiotics with other compounds have been proposed either alone or in association with a particular mechanism of controlled release (Vogt et al. 2005). Antibiotics such as gentamicin are natively water-soluble salts. However, with a simple ion exchange reaction they can be converted to lipophilic substances, such as gentamicin palmitate (GP; Vogt et al. 2005). The new obtained antibiotic formulation has a waxy appearance, and can be used directly on the surfaces of various types of implants, such as cementless endoprosthesis or titanium intramedullary nails. The GP coating can undergo sterilization processes and maintain its drug-eluting proprieties (Kühn 2010); moreover, some studies showed how this particular formulation can be used in bank bone tissue and can maintain antibiotic-eluting proprieties even after freezing for bone storage (Coraca-Huber et al. 2014). The in vitro antibiotic elution profile of GP coatings is similar to the one of antibiotic-loaded PMMA, with a peak in the first 24 h and a sustained release of antibiotics for around 30 days (Fölsch et al. 2015). This elution profile is designed to allow for surface protection in the critical first few hours after the implant (see above). Moreover, it has been suggested that the hydrophobic quality of palmitate could hinder bacterial adhesion on the surface by itself, thus providing an additional anti-biofilm effect (Kittinger et al. 2011). The GP coating has proven to be effective in preventing infection in a rat model (Fölsch et al. 2015); however, further studies are needed to demonstrate the clinical efficacy of this new, yet promising approach.

Biodegradable polymers and sol-gel coatings are also utilized to form controlled release antibiotic-laden coatings on titanium implants (Guillaume et al. 2012; Tang et al. 2012). Clinical applications of antibiotic-loaded D-poly-lactate acid/gentamicin intramedullary coated nails have been recently reported with early positive results (Fuchs et al. 2011).

Some antiseptic agents such as chlorhexidine, chloroxylenol or poly-hexamethylene biguanide have demonstrated efficacy and might be an alternative in avoiding the risk of drug resistance. Chlorhexidine can be adsorbed to the TiO_2 layer on titanium surfaces and is released gradually over several days (Campbell et al. 2000). Its release pattern is similar to that of antibiotic-laden coatings with an initial rapid release rate followed by slower but sustained release (Kozlovsky et al. 2006).

Another promising approach involves coating implants with antimicrobial peptides, cytokines or other molecules critical for host response to bacterial invasion. This heterogeneous group of substances has proven experimentally their efficacy against a wide range of pathogens (Yount et al. 2012). Antimicrobial peptides, like antibiotics, function via damage of the cell wall and inhibition of key bacterial protein synthesis. In addition, they exert an influence on inflammation, tissue healing, and apoptotic events (Haney et al. 2013); resistance to antimicrobial peptides has been reported less frequently than to antibiotics (Dobson et al. 2013). Initial experiments demonstrated that a thin layer of antimicrobial peptides affixed onto the surfaces of metal alloys exhibits excellent antibacterial effects against typical pathogens related to PJI (Holmberg et al. 2013).

Chitosan (CS) is a polycationic polymer derived from chitin that exhibits antibacterial and antifungal activity. The exact mechanism of action remains poorly understood. There is some evidence that CS derivatives can be firmly anchored to titanium alloys and that they have a protective effect against some bacterial species either alone or in combination with other antimicrobial substances such as antibiotics or antimicrobial peptides (Costa et al. 2014; Pérez-Anes et al. 2015). CS derivatives secured to external fixator pins have been studied as a method of preventing pin tract infections (Jennison et al. 2014). However, we are not aware of a study to date reporting data from a clinical setting.

Most of the research in this field, as discussed earlier, has focused on metal surface coatings. However, in total knee replacement and total hip replacement wearable surfaces such as polyethylene (PE) cover a large part of the prosthesis exposed to body tissues, while being unprotected against infections. In this context, some researchers focused on developing an antibacterial coating for PE by incorporating silver nanoparticles. The silver-coated PE showed in vitro antibacterial activity while maintaining intact its mechanical proprieties. While preliminary, these results support further research in this promising field (Harrasser et al. 2015).

The long-term impact of permanently coated implants with antibiotics and other organic compounds, never used before either for local or general administration, does raise concerns regarding the possible induction of bacterial resistance, local and general toxicity and possible detrimental effects on implant osteointegration, which have ultimately prevented clinical applications to date.

Other fascinating but complex and futuristic research pathways involve the development of multifunctional surface layers, like functional polymer brush coating, which combine anti-adhesive and antimicrobial substances and other compounds able to enhance tissue integration (Muszanska et al. 2014), and »smart coatings«, sensitive and responsive to a variety of stimuli, including the presence of bacteria (Yu et al. 2013). This research poses a number of open issues, such as feasible coating manufacturing process, non-adverse reactions in vivo, mechanical resistance and preservation of intended functionalities throughout the life of the device, etc.

Perioperative Antibacterial Carriers or Coatings

Passive and active surface modifications of implants have been traditionally studied in order to provide long-term or permanent antibacterial protection of coated devices. However, the pathogenesis of biofilm-related infections points out how the destiny of an implant, regarding bacterial colonization, is decided within the very first hours after insertion into the human body, as discussed earlier. This also explains the equal efficacy of short- and long-term systemic prophylaxis to prevent PJIs (Heydemann and Nelson 1986).

In this context, a new and different approach to implant protection from bacterial colonization is to provide a traditional implant with an antibacterial carrier or coating at the time of surgery, instead of pre-manufacturing implants with surface modifications. This approach could allow for the applicability of a universal antibacterial coating to many different already existing implants and biomaterials.

Protecting implants with antibiotics at the time of surgery has always attracted much attention in orthopaedics. Buchholz et al. first popularized the incorporation of antibiotics into polymethyl methacrylate (PMMA) bone cement for local antibiotic prophylaxis in cemented total joint arthroplasty (Buchholz and Engelbrecht 1970). Antibiotic-loaded bone cement can decrease deep infection rates of cemented total hip arthroplasties and revision rates due to supposed »aseptic« loosening when combined with systemic antibiotic administration (Engesaeter et al. 2003), and this solution has been found both effective and economically sound, especially in high-risk patients (Gutowski et al. 2014; Dunbar 2009). The main issue with using PMMA as a coating is that it was not designed as a local delivery carrier of antibiotics: the elution profile of PMMA, even when loaded with antibiotics, is not designed to prevent biofilm formation and thus can favour the development of antibiotic-resistant »small-colony variants« (van den Belt et al. 2001b; Neut et al. 2005).

Other porous materials for local antibiotic delivery like collagen sponges (De Grood 1951), cancellous bone (Buttaro et al. 2005) and calcium phosphate cements (Gautier et al. 2000; Yamamura et al. 1992) were also not specifically designed to protect implanted biomaterials, and have several limitations when used with this goal: First, there is a lack of in vitro, in vivo and clinical evidence of efficacy in this specific application; second, they cannot be applied as a coating to all implant surfaces; third, they have relatively high costs; and fourth, they could possibly interfere with primary implant fixation and long-term osteointegration.

Based on these considerations, a challenging option is to design specific, effective and easy-to-use antibacterial coatings that can be applied at the time of surgery directly on the implant by the surgeon, either pre-loaded or loaded intraoperatively with antibacterials. In recent years biocompatible hydrogels emerged as a possible attractive solution: They have shown capabilities to deliver local pharmacological agents and may be designed to meet the desired elution pattern (Overstreet et al. 2015). Recently, a fast-resorbable hydrogel coating, composed of covalently linked hyaluronan and poly-D,L-lactide, Defensive Antibacterial Coating (DAC®, Novagenit Srl, Mezzolombardo, Italy; ◘ Fig. 9.2), was introduced in the European market and may open a novel perspective in the field of antibacterial coatings.

This coating undergoes complete hydrolytic degradation in vivo and is able to completely release a variety of different antibacterials at concentrations ranging from 2% to 10%, including glycopeptides, aminoglycosides, fluoroquinolones, etc., within 48–72 h (Pitarresi et al. 2013).

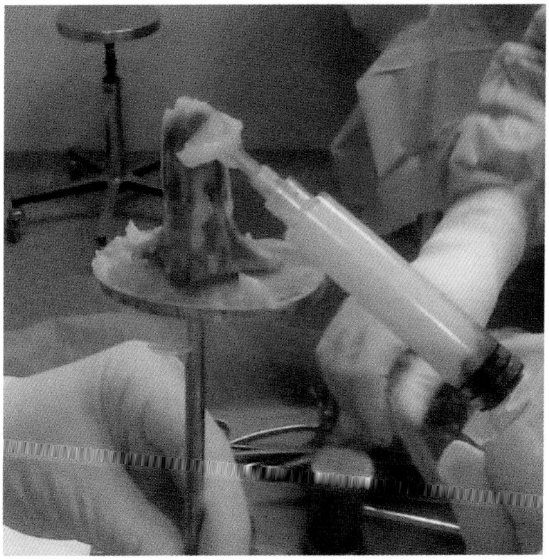

◘ **Fig. 9.2** Defensive Antibacterial Coating (DAC®; Novagenit Srl, Mezzolombardo, Italy) is a fast-resorbable hydrogel, which can be loaded intraoperatively with antibiotics and/or antibiofilm agents, is applied during surgery on a cementless knee joint prosthesis

It was engineered as a short-term local delivery system, with efficacy in early bacterial colonization, providing complete protection of the implant for the time needed to win the »race to the surface,« i.e. in the first hours after surgery. In principle, the ideal antibiotic delivery coating should release antibiotics at optimal bactericidal levels for a sufficiently long period of time to prevent potential infection, i.e. a few hours after surgery as far as post-surgical infections are concerned and then subsequently antibiotic release should cease quickly to eliminate the risk of developing antibiotic resistance. In addition, any untoward effects of antibiotics on tissue integration of the implant should be minimized (Antoci et al. 2007a). The hydrogel showed a synergistic antibacterial activity with various antibiotics and an antibiofilm effect could be demonstrated in vitro on different substrates and against different common pathogens involved in orthopaedic implant-related infections. This adds an extremely high versatility, through intraoperative mixing with a choice of different antibacterial agents and possible application to virtually all currently used implants and biomaterials.

Moreover, once applied on titanium standard joint prosthesis, the hydrogel coating showed resistance to press-fit insertion both in the animal model and in human femurs. Also, histocompatibility studies showed the absence of inflammatory or degenerative signs and physiological bone growth in animal models (Drago et al. 2014). Finally, in vivo studies have recently demonstrated, for the first time, the efficacy of the short-term local prophylaxis offered by vancomycin-loaded DAC® hydrogel in an animal model of highly contaminated implants both with (Giavaresi et al. 2014) and without systemic prophylaxis (Boot et al. 2015). Currently, the clinical results of two multicentre European trials, partially funded by the European Commission under the Seventh Framework Programme on Research Technological Development and Demonstration, allow to confirm the safety and the efficacy of the DAC® hydrogel coating device, that has received the CE mark (Romanò et al. 2016; Malizos et al. 2017).

9.1.4 Coating Technologies: Validation and Regulatory Issues

It is a common knowledge that the pathway to regulatory approval and commercialization of medical products may often be expensive and time-consuming. However, when antimicrobial technologies and devices are concerned, reaching the market can become a real challenge. Non-standardized in vitro assays and preclinical animal models, the lack of feasible and affordable clinical validation procedures, the questionable definition of medical devices with »ancillary« drugs all limit access to the market and hence to the clinical application of a number of potentially highly effective technologies, thus also preventing many patients from taking advantage of the most recent discoveries.

To bridge the gap between the clinical need for technologies aimed at reducing/preventing bacterial adhesion and biofilm formation and the ability of the regulatory requirements to set realistic standards, a stepwise pathway can be proposed, in which preclinical strategies, predictive of ultimate clinical efficacy, should serve as a control point for effective translation of new technologies to clinical applications.

1. In the proposed pathway, given the intrinsic technical limitations of animal models or clinical tests to evaluate bacterial adhesion and/or biofilm formation, standardized in vitro testing should be accepted as a demonstration of the efficacy of antibacterial coatings of implantable medical devices, even if including drugs with only local effects and a known safety profile for systemic administration.
2. In vitro microbiological testing of safety, antibacterial activity, anti-adhesive properties and anti-biofilm effects may be currently performed in a controlled experimental setting. In particular, to test the ability of a coating to reduce/prevent biofilm formation there is a wide range of tests, from the easiest and cheapest to the most accurate and sophisticated. The oldest and one of the most widely used techniques for biofilm quantification is spectrometry on crystal violet staining (Christensen et al. 1985). Even if burdened by several limitations, including being a semi-quantitative assay with a limited specificity and the inability to give information on the three-dimensional structure of hydrated biofilms (Gomes et al. 2013), crystal violet staining is still widely used, mainly for its ease of use and low cost and it can be a useful first screening test for many technologies. More recently, the introduction of confocal laser scanning microscopy (CLSM; Bridier et al. 1993; Khajotia et al. 2013) has significantly increased the accuracy of biofilm assessment. Advantages of CLSM are the possibility to focus lasers with high precision on the sample and to select the light beam for each excitation frequency required, in order to increase resolution and depth of the field. Furthermore, the images can be elaborated with different colours for each frequency, allowing one to appreciate the three-dimensionality of the sample. Advances in software technology and the introduction of fluorescence staining currently allow for the quantification of various biofilm components, such as living and dead cells and the exopolysaccharide matrix (Heydorn et al. 2000), while further technical improvements allow for the simultaneous visualization of biofilms and of the substrate used as support for biofilm formation (e.g. titanium; Drago et al. 2016) (◻ Fig. 9.1).
3. In vivo assessment of the amount of bacterial colonization of coated implants and signs of infection, both of which are the final by-product of bacterial adhesion and biofilm formation, should represent, together with in vivo safety evaluation, a further validation step before receiving a pre-approval to perform clinical trials.

4. Clinical trials should then be focused on further assessing the safety of the coating technology, while efficacy should be the object of a well-defined and mandatory post-marketing surveillance procedure, managed by a credited independent private or public institution.

9.1.5 Conclusion

Examination of antibacterial coating technologies suggests a striking discrepancy between the proposed strategies of antibacterial surface treatment and the ultimate completion of in vitro and in vivo experimentation. In fact, it appears that little progress is being made in the translation of the aforementioned modalities into clinically useful technologies. Barriers to translational medicine in this field are most likely related to economic, medico-legal, regulatory and biotechnological issues.

Most of the studied coatings in fact are not suitable for surface treatment of orthopaedic implants owing to problems with cytotoxicity, immunoreactivity and genotoxicity (Daghighi et al. 2013), while clinical application of those successfully tested in vitro and in vivo may be limited by a number of various concerns. Improving collaborative efforts amongst governments, regulatory agencies, industry leaders and health-care payers will probably allow more patients to benefit from these technologies (Romanò et al. 2015; Moriarty et al. 2014).

Take-Home Message

- Implant-related and surgical-site infections represent one of the most difficult medical-outcome problems in orthopaedics and trauma.
- Virtually all implant-related infections are »biofilm-related« and, given the striking ability of bacteria to immediately produce the biofilm matrix once attached to a surface, a rational modern approach should be directed at preventing bacterial adhesion and biofilm formation at the very time of surgery.
- Antibacterial coatings or surface modifications of orthopedic implants are a promising solution
- Their primary goal should be to prevent bacterial adhesion to the implant surface and to favour host cells responsible for bone in-growth and vascularization.
- Various combinations of materials and substances acting as a physical barrier to biofilm formation, chemically or pharmacologically, have been tested in vitro and in vivo.
- Clinical trials to exclude adverse side effects such as pharmatoxicity, impaired osseointegration and formation of resistance of pathogens to active ingredients have recently shown the safety and efficacy of some technology, while many others are in the pipeline.
- To foster the timely introduction of safe and efficient solutions to the market, scientists and medical doctors offer their cooperation to the regulatory authorities to establish validated in vitro and in vivo models.
- Once effective antibacterial coatings become available on the market for large-scale use, unprotected implants will probably be regarded as a thing of the past.

References

Aggarwal VK, Bakhshi H, Ecker NU, Parvizi J, Gehrke T, Kendoff D (2014a) Organism profile in periprosthetic joint infection: Pathogens differ at two arthroplasty infection referral centers in Europe and in the United States. J Knee Surg 10. doi:10.1055/s-0033-1364102

Aggarwal VK, Tischler EH, Lautenbach C, Williams GR Jr, Abboud JA, Altena M, Bradbury TL, Calhoun JH, Dennis DA, del Gaizo DJ, et al (2014b) Mitigation and education. J Arthroplasty 29:19–25

Alt V, Bitschnau A, Osterling J, Sewing A, Meyer C, Kraus R, Meissner SA, Wenisch S, Domann E, Schnettler R (2006) The effects of combined gentamicin-hydroxyapatite coating for cementless joint prostheses on the reduction of infection rates in a rabbit infection prophylaxis model. Biomaterials 27:4627–4634

An YH, Friedman RJ (1996) Prevention of sepsis in total joint arthroplasty. J Hosp Infect 33:93–108

An YH, Bradley J, Powers DL, Friedman RJ (1997) The prevention of prosthetic infection using a cross-linked albumin coating in a rabbit model. J Bone Joint Surg Br 79: 816–819

Anderson JM, Rodriguez A, Chang DT (2008) Foreign body reaction to biomaterials. Semin Immunol 20:86–100

Antoci V Jr, Adams CS, Hickok NJ, Shapiro IM, Parvizi J (2007a) Antibiotics for local delivery systems cause skeletal cell toxicity in vitro. Clin Orthop Relat Res 462:200-206

Antoci V Jr, King SB, Jose B, Parvizi J, Zeiger AR, Wickstrom E, Freeman TA, Composto RJ, Ducheyne P, Shapiro IM et al (2007b) Vancomycin covalently bonded to titanium alloy prevents bacterial colonization. J Orthop Res 25:858–866

Arenas MA, Perez-Jorge C, Conde A, Matykina E, Hernandez-Lopez JM, Perez-Tanoira R, de Damborenea JJ, Gómez-Barrena E, Esteba J (2013) Doped TiO2 anodic layers of enhanced antibacterial properties. Colloids Surf. B Biointerfaces 105:106–112

Arpacay P, Turkan U (2015) Development of antibiotic-loaded silk fibroin/hyaluronic acid polyelectrolyte film coated CoCrMo alloy. Biomedizinische Technik Biomedical Engineering

Bacakova L, Filova E, Parizek M, Ruml T, Svorcik V (2011) Modulation of cell adhesion, proliferation and differentiation on materials designed for body implants. Biotechnol Adv 29:739–767

Boot W, Vogely HCh, Nikkels PGJ, Pouran B, van Rijen M, Dhert WJA, Gawlitta D (2015) Local prophylaxis of implant-related infections using a hydrogel as carrier. Proceeding of eCM XVI Congress on Bone and Implant Infection

Braem A, van Mellaert L, Mattheys T, Hofmans D, de Waelheyns E, Geris L, Anné J, Schrooten J, Vleugels J (2013) Staphylococcal biofilm growth on smooth and porous titanium coatings for biomedical applications. J Biomed Mater Res. A. doi:10.1002/jbm.a.34688

Bridier A, Meylheuc T, Briandet R (1993) Realistic representation of Bacillus subtilis biofilms architecture using combined microscopy (CLSM, ESEM and FESEM). Micron (England) 48:65–69

Buchholz HW, Engelbrecht H (1970) Depot effects of various antibiotics mixed with Palacos resins. Der Chirurg 41: 511e5

Busscher HJ, van der Me, HC, Subbiahdoss G, Jutte PC, van den Dungen JJ, Zaat SA, Schultz MJ, Grainger DW (2012) Biomaterial-associated infection: Locating the finish line in the race for the surface. Sci Transl Med 4:153rv10

Busscher HJ, van der Mei HC (2012) How do bacteria know they are on a surface and regulate their response to an adhering state? PLoS Pathog 8:e1002440

Buttaro MA, Pusso R, Piccaluga F (2005) Vancomycin-supplemented impacted bone allografts in infected hip arthroplasty. Two-stage revision results. J Bone Joint Surg Br 87:314e9

Campbell AA, Song L, Li XS, Nelson BJ, Bottoni C, Brooks DE, et al (2000) Development, characterization, and anti-microbial efficacy of hydroxyapatitechlorhexidine coatings produced by surface-induced mineralization. J Biomed Mater Res 53:400e7

Campoccia D, Montanaro L, Arciola CR (2013) A review of the biomaterials technologies for infection-resistant surfaces. Biomaterials 34:8533–8554

Cats-Baril W, Gehrke T, Huff K, Kendoff D, Maltenfort M, Parvizi J (2013) International consensus on periprosthetic joint infection: Description of the consensus process. Clin Orthop Relat Res 471:4065–4075

Chen Y, Busscher HJ, van der Mei HC, Norde W (2011) Statistical analysis of long- and short-range forces involved in bacterial adhesion to substratum surfaces as measured using atomic force microscopy. Appl Environ Microbiol 77:5065–5070

Chernousova S, Epple M (2013) Silver as antibacterial agent: Ion, nanoparticle, and metal. Angew Chem Int Ed Engl 52:1636–1653

Christensen GD, Simpson WA, Younger JJ et al (1985) Adherence of coagulase-negative staphylococci to plastic tissue culture plates: a quantitative model for the adherence of staphylococci to medical devices. J Clin Microbiol 22:996–1006

Coraca-Huber DC, Wurm A, Fille M, Hausdorfer J, Nogler M, Kühn KD (2014) Effect of freezing on the release rate of gentamicin palmitate and gentamicin sulfate from bone tissue. J Orthop Res 32:842–847

Costa F, Maia S, Gomes P, Martins MC (2014) Characterization of hLF1-11 immobilization onto chitosan ultrathin films, and its effects on antimicrobial activity. Acta Biomater doi:10.1016/Jactbio.2014.02.028

Costerton JW, Stewart PS, Greenberg EP (1999) Bacterial biofilms: A common cause of persistent infections. Science 284:1318–1322

Costerton W, Veeh R, Shirtliff M, Pasmore M, Post C, Ehrlich G (2003) The application of biofilm science to the study and control of chronic bacterial infections. J Clin Investig 112:1466–1477

Daghighi S, Sjollema J, van der Mei HC, Busscher HJ, Rochford ET (2013) Infection resistance of degradable versus non-degradable biomaterials: An assessment of the potential mechanisms. Biomaterials 34:8013–8017

Dale H, Hallan G, Hallan G, Espehaug B, Havelin LI, Engesaeter LB (2009) Increasing risk of revision due to deep infection after hip arthroplasty. Acta Orthop 80:639–645

De Grood MP (1951) Pathology, diagnosis and treatment of subdural empyema. Arch Chir Neerl 3:128e38

Del Curto B, Brunella MF, Giordano C, Pedeferri MP, Valtulina V, Visai L et al (2005) Decreased bacterial adhesion to surface-treated titanium. Int J Artif Organs 28:718e30

Dobson AJ, Purves J, Kamysz W, Rolff J (2013) Comparing selection on S. aureus between antimicrobial peptides and common antibiotics. PLoS One 8:e76521

Drago L, Boot W, Dimas K, Malizos K, Hänsch GM, Stuyck J, Gawlitta D, Romanò CL (2014) Does implant coating with antibacterial-loaded hydrogel reduce bacterial colonization and biofilm formation in vitro ? Clin Orthop Relat Res 472(11):3311–3323

Drago L, Agrappi S, Bortolin M, Toscano M, Romano CL, De Vecchi E (2016) How to study biofilms after microbial colonization of materials used in orthopaedic implants. Int J Molec Sci 17

Dunbar MJ (2009) Antibiotic bone cements: their use in routine primary total joint arthroplasty is justified. Orthopedics 32(9)

Engesaeter LB, Lie SA, Espehaug B, Furnes O, Vollset SE, Havelin LI (2003) Antibiotic prophylaxis in total hip arthroplasty: effects of antibiotic prophylaxis systemically and in bone cement on the revision rate of 22,170 primary hip replacements followed 0-14 years in the Norwegian Arthroplasty Register. Acta Orthop Scand 74: 644e51

Eto S, Miyamoto H, Shobuike T, Noda I, Akiyama T, Tsukamoto M, Ueno M, Someya S, Kawano S, Sonohata M, Mawatari M (2015) Silver oxide-containing hydroxyapatite coating supports osteoblast function and enhances implant anchorage strength in rat femur. J Orthop Res 33(9): 1391–1397

Fei J, Liu GD, Pan CJ, Chen JY, Zhou YG, Xiao SH, Wang Y, Yu HJ (2011) Preparation, release profiles and antibacterial properties of vancomycin-loaded Ca-P coating titanium alloy plate. J Mater Sci Mater Med 22:989–995

Fölsch C, Federmann M, Kühn KD et al (2015) Coating with a novel gentamicinpalmitate formulation prevents implant-associated osteomyelitis induced by methicillin-susceptible Staphylococcus aureus in a rat model. Int Orthop 39:981–988

Foster TJ, Geoghegan JA, Ganesh VK, Hook M (2014) Adhesion, invasion and evasion: The many functions of the surface proteins of Staphylococcus aureus. Nat Rev Microbiol 12:49–62

Fuchs T, Stange R, Shmidmaier S, Raschke MJ (2011) The use of gentamicin-coated nails in the tibia: preliminary results of a prospective study Arch Orthop Trauma Surg 131(10):1419–1425

Gallardo-Moreno AM, Pacha-Olivenza MA, Saldana L, Perez-Giraldo C, Bruque JM, Vilaboa N, et al (2009). In vitro biocompatibility and bacterial adhesion of physico-chemically modified Ti6Al4V surface by means of UV irradiation. Acta Biomater 5:181e92

Gardner AB, Lee SK, Woods EC, Acharya AP (2013) Biomaterials-based modulation of the immune system. Biomed Res Int. doi:10.1155/2013/732182

Gautier H, Merle C, Auget JL, Daculsi G (2000) Isostatic compression, a new process for incorporating vancomycin into biphasic calcium phosphate: comparison with a classical method. Biomaterials 21:243e9

Giavaresi G, Meani E, Sartori M, Ferrari A, Bellini D, Sacchetta AC, Meraner J, Sambri A, Vocale C, Sambri V, Fini M, Romanò CL (2014) Efficacy of antibacterial-loaded coating in an in vivo model of acutely highly contaminated implant. Int Orthop 38(7):1505–1512

Gomes LC, Moreira JM, Miranda JM, Simoes M, Melo LF, Mergulhao FJ (2013) Macroscale versus microscale methods for physiological analysis of biofilms formed in 96-well microtiter plates. J Microbiol Methods 95:342–349

Grass G, Rensing C, Solioz M (2011) Metallic copper as an antimicrobial surface. Appl Environ Microbiol 77:1541–1547

Gristina AG, Naylor, P, Myrvik, Q (1988) Infections from biomaterials and implants: A race for the surface. Med Prog Technol 14:205–224

Guillaume O, Garric X, Lavigne JP, Van Den Berghe H, Coudane J (2012) Multilayer, degradable coating as a carrier for the sustained release of antibiotics: preparation and antimicrobial efficacy in vitro. J Control Release 162:492–501

Gutowski CJ, Zmistowski BM, Clyde CT, Parvizi J (2014) The economics of using prophylactic antibiotic-loaded bone cement in total knee replacement. Bone Joint J 96B(1): 65–69

Haney EF, Hancock RE (2013) Peptide design for antimicrobial and immunomodulatory applications. Biopolymers 100:572–583

Hardes J, von Eiff C, Streitbuerger A, Balke M, Budny T, Henrichs MP, Hauschild G, Ahrens H (2010) Reduction of periprosthetic infection with silver-coated megaprostheses in patients with bone sarcoma. J Surg Oncol 101(5):389–395

Harrasser N, Jussen S, Banke IJ, Kmeth R, von Eisenhart-Rothe R, Stritzker B, Gollwitzer H, Burgkart R (2015) Antibacterial efficacy of ultrahigh molecular weight polyethylene with silver containing diamond-like surface layers. AMB Express 64

Harris LG, Tosatti S, Wieland M, Textor M, Richards RG (2004) Staphylococcus aureus adhesion to titanium oxide surfaces coated with non-functionalized and peptide-functionalized poly(L-lysine)-grafted poly(ethylene glycol) copolymers. Biomaterials 25:4135–4148

Hetrick EM, Schoenfisch MH (2006) Reducing implant-related infections: active release strategies. Chem Soc Rev 35:780–789

Heydemann JS, Nelson CL (1986) Short-term preventive antibiotics. Clin Orthop Relat Res 205:184–187

Heydorn A, Nielsen AT, Hentzer M et al (2000) Quantification of biofilm structures by the novel computer program COMSTAT. Microbiology (England) 146(Pt10):2395–2407

Higgins DM, Basaraba RJ, Hohnbaum AC, Lee EJ, Grainger DW, Gonzalez-Juarrero M (2009) Localized immunosuppressive environment in the foreign body response to implanted biomaterials. Am J Pathol 175:161–170

Hizal F, Zhuk I, Sukhishvili S, Busscher HJ, van der Mei HC, Choi CH (2015) Impact of 3D Hierarchical nanostructures on the antibacterial efficacy of a bacteria-triggered self-defensive antibiotic coating. ACS Appl Mater Interfaces 7:20304–20313

Hodgkinson V, Petris MJ (2012) Copper homeostasis at the host-pathogen interface. J Biol Chem 287:13549–13555

Holá V, Růžička F, Votava M (2006) The dynamics of staphylococcus epidermis biofilm formation in relation to nutrition, temperature, and time. Scripta Medica 79:169–174

Holinka J, Pilz M, Kubista B, Presterl E, Windhager R (2013) Effects of selenium coating of orthopaedic implant surfaces on bacterial adherence and osteoblastic cell growth. Bone Joint J 95:678–682

Holmberg KV, Abdolhosseini M, Li Y, Chen X, Gorr SU, Aparicio C (2013) Bio-inspired stable antimicrobial peptide coatings for dental applications. Acta Biomater 9:8224–8231

Hu H, Zhang W, Qiao Y, Jiang X, Liu X, Ding C (2012) Antibacterial activity and increased bone marrow stem cell functions of Zn-incorporated TiO2 coatings on titanium. Acta Biomater 8:904–915

Humphreys H (2012) Surgical site infection, ultraclean ventilated operating theatres and prosthetic joint surgery: Where now? J Hosp Infect 81:71–72

Illingworth KD, Mihalko WM, Parvizi J, Sculco T, McArthur B, el Bitar Y, Saleh KJ (2013) How to minimize infection and thereby maximize patient outcomes in total joint arthro-

plasty: a multicenter approach: AAOS exhibit selection. J Bone Joint Surg Am 95:e50
Jamsen E, Furnes O, Engesaeter LB, Konttinen YT, Odgaard A, Stefansdottir A, et al (2010a) Prevention of deep infection in joint replacement surgery. Acta Orthop 81:660e6
Jenney CR, Anderson JM (2000) Adsorbed serum proteins responsible for surface dependent human macrophage behavior. J Biomed Mater Res 49:435–447
Jennison T, McNally M, Pandit H (2014) Prevention of infection in external fixator pin sites. Acta Biomater 10:595–603
Kaper HJ, Busscher HJ, Norde W (2003) Characterization of poly(ethylene oxide) brushes on glass surfaces and adhesion of Staphylococcus epidermidis. J Biomat Sci Polym Ed 14:313–324
Khajotia SS, Smart KH, Pilula M, Thompson DM (2013) Concurrent quantification of cellular and extracellular components of biofilms. JoVE e50639
Kittinger C, Marth E, Windhager R et al (2011) Antimicrobial activity of gentamicin palmitate against high concentrations of Staphylococcus aureus. J Mater Science Mater Med 22:1447–1453
Kozlovsky A, Artzi Z, Moses O, Kamin-Belsky N, Greenstein RB (2006) Interaction of chlorhexidine with smooth and rough types of titanium surfaces. J Periodontol 77:1194e200
Kühn KD (2010) Part I: In-vitro release of gentamicinpalmitate coating in uncemented titanium implants. Int J Nano Biomaterials 3:94–105
Kurtz SM, Lau E, Watson H, Schmier JK, Parvizi J (2012) Economic burden of periprosthetic joint infection in the United States. J Arthroplasty 27:61–6 Lemire JA, Harrison JJ, Turner RJ (2013) Antimicrobial activity of metals: Mechanisms, molecular targets and applications. Nat Rev Microbiol 11:371–384
Laverty G, Gorman SP, Gilmore BF (2013) Biomolecular mechanisms of staphylococcal biofilm formation. Future Microbiol 8:509–524
Lemire JA, Harrison JJ, Turner RJ (2013) Antimicrobial activity of metals: Mechanisms, molecular targets and applications. Nat Rev Microbiol 11:371–384
Lentino JR (2003) Prosthetic joint infections: Bane of orthopedists, challenge for infectious disease specialists. Clin Infect Dis 36:1157–1161
Lu T, Qiao Y, Liu X (2012) Surface modification of biomaterials using plasma immersion ion implantation and deposition. Interface Focus 2:325–336
Malizos K, Blauth M, Danita A, Capuano N, Mezzoprete R, Logoluso N, Drago L, Romanò CL (2017) Fast-resorbable antibiotic-loaded hydrogel coating to reduce post-surgical infection after internal osteosynthesis: a multicenticenter randomized controlled trial. J Orthop Traum. doi:10.1007/s10195-017-0442-2
Martynkova GS, Valaskova M (2014) Antimicrobial nanocomposites based on natural modified materials: A review of carbons and clays. J Nanosci Nanotechnol 14:673–693
Mijnendonckx K, Leys N, Mahillon J, Silver S, van Houdt R (2013) Antimicrobial silver: Uses, toxicity and potential for resistance. Biometals 26:609–621
Moriarty TF, Schlegel U, Perren S, Richards RG (2010) Infection in fracture fixation: can we influence infection rates through implant design? J Mater Sci Mater Med 21:1031e5
Moriarty TF, Grainger DW, Richards RG (2014) Challenges in linking preclinical anti-microbial research strategies with clinical outcomes for device-associated infections. Eur Cell Mater 28:112–128
Moseke C, Gbureck U, Elter P, Drechsler P, Zoll A, Thull R, Ewald A (2011) Hard implant coatings with antimicrobial properties. J Mater Sci Mater Med 22:2711–2720
Muszanska AK, Rochford ET, Gruszka A, Bastian AA, Busscher HJ, Norde W, van der Mei HC, Herrmann A (2014) Anti-adhesive polymer brush coating functionalized with antimicrobial and rgd peptides to reduce biofilm formation and enhance tissue integration. Biomacromolecules 15:2019–2026
Namba RS, Inacio MC, Paxton EW (2012) Risk factors associated with surgical site infection in 30,491 primary total hip replacements. J Bone Joint Surg Br 94:1330e8
Neut D, Hendriks JG, van Horn JR, van der Mei HC, Busscher HJ (2005) Pseudomonas aeruginosa biofilm formation and slime excretion on antibiotic-loaded bone cement. Acta Orthop 76(1):109–114
Neut D, Dijkstra RJ, Thompson JI, van der Mei HC, Busscher HJ (2012) A gentamicin-releasing coating for cementless hip prostheses-Longitudinal evaluation of efficacy using in vitro bio-optical imaging and its wide-spectrum antibacterial efficacy. J Biomed Mater Res A 100:3220–3226
Noda I, Miyaji F, Ando Y, Miyamoto H, Shimazaki T, Yonekura Y, Miyazaki M, Mawatari M, Hotokebuchi T (2009) Development of novel thermal sprayed antibacterial coating and evaluation of release properties of silver ions. J Biomed Mater Res B Appl Biomater 89:456–465
Overstreet D, McLaren A, Calara F, Vernon B, McLemore R (2015) Local gentamicin delivery from resorbable viscous hydrogels is therapeutically effective. Clin Orthop Relat Res 473(1):337–347
Panacek A, Kolar M, Vecerova R, Prucek R, Soukupova J, Krystof V, Hamal P, Zboril R, Kvítek L (2009) Antifungal activity of silver nanoparticles against Candida spp. Biomaterials 30:6333–6340
Pelgrift RY, Friedman AJ (2013) Nanotechnology as a therapeutic tool to combat microbial resistance. Adv Drug Deliv Rev 65:1803–1815
Pérez-Anes A, Gargouri M, Laure W, Van Den Berghe H, Courcot E, Sobocinski J, Tabary N, Chai F, Blach JF, Addad A, Woisel P, Douroumis D,Martel B, Blanchemain N, Lyskawa J (2015) Bioinspired titanium drug eluting platforms based on a poly-β-cyclodextrin-chitosan layer-by-layer self-assembly targeting infections. ACS Appl Mater Interfaces 7(23):12882–128893
Petrini P, Arciola CR, Pezzali I, Bozzini S, Montanaro L, Tanzi MC, Speziale P, Visai L (2006) Antibacterial activity of zinc modified titanium oxide surface. Int J Artif Organs 29:434–442
Pitarresi G, Palumbo FS, Calascibetta F, Fiorica C, Di Stefano M, Giammona G (2013) Medicated hydrogels of hyaluronic

9

acid derivatives for use in orthopedic field. Int J Pharm 449(1-2):84–94
Pruzansky JS, Bronson MJ, Grelsamer RP, Strauss E, Moucha CS (2014) Prevalence of modifiable surgical site infection risk factors in hip and knee joint arthroplasty patients at an urban academic hospital. J Arthroplasty 29:272–276
Ribeiro M, Monteiro FJ, Ferraz MP (2012) Infection of orthopedic implants with emphasis on bacterial adhesion process and techniques used in studying bacterial-material interactions. Biomatter 2:176–194
Rivardo F, Turner RJ, Allegrone G, Ceri H, Martinotti MG (2009) Anti-adhesion activity of two biosurfactants produced by Bacillus spp. prevents biofilm formation of human bacterial pathogens. Appl Microbiol Biotechnol 83:541–553
Roach P, Eglin D, Rohde K, Perry CC (2007) Modern biomaterials: A review—Bulk properties and implications of surface modifications. J Mater Sci Mater Med 18:1263–1277
Rodrigues L, Banat IM, Teixeira J, Oliveira R (2006) Biosurfactants: potential applications in medicine. J Antimicrob Chemother 57:609–618
Romanò CL, Scarponi S, Gallazzi E, Romanò D, Drago L (2015) Antibacterial coating of implants in orthopaedics and trauma: a classification proposal in an evolving panorama. J Orthop Surg Res 10:157. doi:10.1186/s13018-015-0294-5
Romanò CL, Malizos K, Capuano N, Mezzoprete R, D'Arienzo M, Van Der Straeten C, Scarponi S, Drago L (2016) Does an antibiotic-loaded hydrogel coating reduce early post-surgical infection after joint arthroplasty ? J Bone Joint Infect 1:34–41
Schmidmaier G, Lucke M, Wildemann B, Haas NP, Raschke M (2006) Prophylaxis and treatment of implant-related infections by antibiotic-coated implants: A review. Injury 37:S105–S112
Shchukin D, Mohwald H (2013) Materials science. A coat of many functions. Science 341:1458–1459
Shi, X, Wu, H, Li, Y, Wei, X, Du, Y. Electrical signals guided entrapment and controlled release of antibiotics on titanium surface. J Biomed. Mater. Res. A 2013, 101, 1373–1378
Shtansky DV, Gloushankova NA, Bashkova IA, Kharitonova MA, Moizhess TG, Sheveiko AN, Kiryukhantsev-Korneev FV, Petrzhik MI, Levashov EA (2006) Multifunctional Ti-(Ca,Zr)-(C,N,O,P) films for load-bearing implants. Biomaterials 27:3519–3531
Singh AV, Vyas V, Patil R, Sharma V, Scopelliti PE, Bongiorno G, Podestà A, Lenardi C, Gade WN, Milani P (2011) Quantitative characterization of the influence of the nanoscale morphology of nanostructured surfaces on bacterial adhesion and biofilm formation. PLoS One 6:e25029
Stoodley P, Ehrlich GD, Sedghizadeh PP, Hall-Stoodley L, Baratz ME, Altman DT, Sotereanos NG (2011) Orthopaedic biofilm infections. Curr Orthop Pract 22:558–563
Stoodley P, Hall-Stoodley L, Costerton B, DeMeo P, Shirtliff M, Gawalt E, Kathju S (2013) Biofilms, biomaterials, and device-related infections. In Ratner BD, Hoffman AS, Schoen FJ, Lemons JE (eds) Biomaterials science: an introduction to materials in medicine. Academic Press (Elsevier), Waltham, pp. 565–583
Tang Y, Zhao Y, Wang H, Gao Y, Liu X, Wang X, et al (2012) Layer-by-layer assembly of antibacterial coating on interbonded 3D fibrous scaffolds and its cytocompatibility assessment. J Biomed Mater Res A 100:2071–2078
Thevenot P, Hu W, Tang L (2008) Surface chemistry influences implant biocompatibility. Curr Top Med Chem 8:270–280
Tran PA, Webster TJ (2011) Selenium nanoparticles inhibit Staphylococcus aureus growth. Int J Nanomed 6: 1553–1558
Tsuchiya H, Shirai T, Nishida H, Murakami H, Kabata T, Yamamoto N, Watanabe K, Nakase J (2012) Innovative antimicrobial coating of titanium implants with iodine. J Orthop Sci 17(5):595–604
van de Belt H, Neut D, Schenk W, van Horn JR, van der Mei HC, Busscher HJ (2001a) Infection of orthopedic implants and the use of antibiotic-loaded bone cements. A review. Acta Orthop Scand 72:557e71
van de Belt H, Neut D, Schenk W, van Horn JR, van Der Mei HC, Busscher HJ (2001b) Staphylococcus aureus biofilm formation on different gentamicin-loaded polymethylmethacrylate bone cements. Biomaterials 22(12):1607–1611
Vogt S, Kühn KD, Gopp U, Schnabelrauch M (2005) Resorbable antibiotic coatings for bone substitutes and implantable devices. Materialwissenschaft und Werkstofftechnik 36:814–819
Wafa H, Grimer RJ, Reddy K, Jeys L, Abudu A, Carter SR, Tillman RM (2015) Retrospective evaluation of the incidence of early periprosthetic infection with silver-treated endoprostheses in high-risk patients: case-control study. 97B(2):252–257
Wagner C, Aytac S, Hansch GM (2011) Biofilm growth on implants: Bacteria prefer plasma coats. Int J Artif Organs 34:811–817
Wang Y, Subbiahdoss G, de Vries J, Libera M, van der Mei HC, Busscher HJ (2012) Effect of adsorbed fibronectin on the differential adhesion of osteoblast-like cells and Staphylococcus aureus with and without fibronectin-binding proteins. Biofouling 28:1011–1021
Yamamura K, Iwata H, Yotsuyanagi T (1992) Synthesis of antibiotic-loaded hydroxyapatite beads and in vitro drug release testing. J Biomed Mater Res 26:1053e64
Yeo IS, Kim HY, Lim KS, Han JS (2012) Implant surface factors and bacterial adhesion: A review of the literature. Int J Artif Organs 35:762–772
Yount NY, Yeaman MR (2012) Emerging themes and therapeutic prospects for anti-infective peptides. Annu Rev Pharmacol Toxicol 52:337–360
Yu JC, Ho W, Lin J, Yip H, Wong PK (2003) Photocatalytic activity, antibacterial effect, and photoinduced hydrophilicity of TiO2 films coated on a stainless steel substrate. Environ Sci Technol 37:2296e301
Yu Q, Cho J, Shivapooja P, Ista LK, Lopez GP (2013) Nanopatterned smart polymer surfaces for controlled attachment, killing, and release of bacteria. ACS Appl Mater Interfaces 5:9295–9304

Zhang F, Zhang Z, Zhu X, Kang ET, Neoh KG (2008) Silk-functionalized titanium surfaces for enhancing osteoblast functions and reducing bacterial adhesion. Biomaterials 29:4751–4759
Zhu H, Guo Z, Liu W (2014) Adhesion behaviors on superhydrophobic surfaces. Chem Commun (Camb) 18: 3900–3913
Zimmerli W, Lew PD, Waldvogel FA (1984) Pathogenesis of foreign body infection. Evidence for a local granulocyte defect. J Clin Investig 73:1191–1200
Zimmerli W, Sendi P (2011) Pathogenesis of implant-associated infection: The role of the host. Semin Immunopathol 33:295–306
Zmistowski B, Karam JA, Durinka JB, Casper DS, Parvizi J (2013) Periprosthetic joint infection increases the risk of one-year mortality. J Bone Joint Surg Am 95:2177–2184

9.2 Anti-infective Coating to Prevent Prosthetic Joint Infection

Hiroyuki Tsuchiya and Tamon Kabata

9.2.1 Overview of General Strategies for the Anti-infective Coating of Endoprostheses

Improvements in medical technology now enable us to perform major joint implant surgery for patients with poor general status, elderly patients who formerly would not have been considered for surgery, and for other high-risk patients. With the development of tumour chemotherapies and biological therapies that utilize monoclonal antibodies, the number of immunosuppressive patients has been increasing. These patients are highly susceptible to prosthesis infections, and therefore new appropriate technologies and creative solutions are urgently needed. Anti-infective biomaterials have attracted attention as an adjunctive measure to reduce the rate of medical device-related infections in all cases, but especially in those for which the risks of contamination are high (Campoccia et al. 2013).

Standard antibiotic therapies that are effective against other bacterial infections such as pneumonia generally fail to cure periprosthetic infections (Hendriks et al. 2004). One reason for this is that bacteria adhere to the surface of the implant, forming an infectious biofilm which is highly resistant to antibiotics (Mah and O'Toole 2001). The presence of biofilms, combined with the poor vascularization of the bone/implant interface, makes the infections extremely difficult to treat (Kazemzadeh-Narbat et al. 2010). Since the first critical step in the pathogenesis of medical device-associated infections is the adhesion and adsorption of contaminant bacteria on biomaterial surfaces, inhibiting this microbial adhesion and colonization is one of the most straightforward strategies for preventing implant infections. Thus, anti-infective coating for implant surfaces is a promising area for research. Over the past few years, several new strategies have been proposed to control and prevent the microbial contamination of implants.

Current orthopaedic implants with anti-infective properties can be obtained using a number of different strategies, for example, developing biomaterials that have self-sterilizing coatings or are able to deliver antimicrobial substances (Gallo et al. 2014; Romanò et al. 2015). As Romano et al. have noted, anti-infective coatings can be classified into at least three groups:

1. Passive surface finishing/modification
2. Active surface finishing/modification
3. Perioperative antibacterial local carriers or coatings (Romanò et al. 2015)

The first strategy employs an anti-adhesive approach. The material characteristics of implants, such as surface roughness, chemistry, hydrophilicity, surface energy or potential, and conductivity, play crucial roles in bacterial adhesion and subsequent biofilm formation (Romanò et al. 2015). Passive surface finishing/modification is aimed at preventing or reducing bacterial adhesion, without releasing bactericidal agents to the surrounding tissue. Examples for passive surface finishing/modification are:

- Albumin (An et al. 1996)
- Anti-adhesive polymers (Neoh and Kang 2011; Follmann et al. 2012; Muszanska et al. 2014)
- Nano-patterned surfaces (Truong et al. 2010; Singh et al. 2011; Shida et al. 2013)

- Super-hydrophobic surfaces (Stallard et al. 2012; Zhu et al. 2014)
- Hydrogels (Pandit et al. 2013; Drago et al. 2014)

However, a strong anti-adhesive layer is unsuitable for sites in which bone in-growth is anticipated, since it could also interfere with implant osteointegration (Bacakova et al. 2011).

The second strategy is to apply an antibacterial material to the implant surface to kill the adherent bacteria or to elute an antibiotic drug in order to sterilize the surface and inhibit bacterial adhesion and proliferation. Such active surface finishing/modifications can employ

- Metals (silver, zinc, copper, etc.)
- Non-metal elements (e.g. selenium, iodine)
- Organic substances (antibiotics, anti-infective peptides, chitosan, other substances)
- Combinations of all three (Massè et al. 2000; Coester et al. 2006; Fu et al. 2006; Antoci et al. 2007; Parvizi et al. 2007; Huang et al. 2008; Shirai et al. 2009; Aydin Sevinç and Hanley 2010; Hardes et al. 2010; Fuchs et al. 2011; Haenle et al. 2011; Kim et al. 2011; Li and McKeague 2011; Norowski et al. 2011; Shirai et al. 2011; Glinel et al. 2012; Tsuchiya et al. 2012; Akiyama et al. 2013; Glehr et al. 2013; Hans et al. 2013; Holinka et al. 2013; Holzapfel et al. 2013; Huang et al. 2013; Koseki et al. 2013; Rodríguez-Valencia et al. 2013; Thallinger et al. 2013; Cheng et al. 2014; Elizabeth et al. 2014; Gao et al. 2014; Magetsari et al. 2014; Shirai et al. 2014a, 2014b; Sörensen et al. 2014; Zhou et al. 2014; Demura et al. 2015; Kabata et al. 2015; Metsemakers et al. 2015a, 2015b; Neut et al. 2015; Wafa et al. 2015; Eto et al. 2016; Shirai et al. 2016; Wilding et al. 2016).

Metals have been used as antimicrobial agents since antiquity. Silver compounds have been used for thousands of years as disinfectant agents in a range of medical applications (Clement and Jarrett 1994). We know that silver kills many different strains of bacteria, but the exact fatal mechanism remains unknown. While silver is currently the most prevalent metal used in biomedical applications and the most intensively studied (Massè et al. 2000; Coester et al. 2006; Hardes et al. 2010; Akiyama et al. 2013; Glehr et al. 2013; Gao et al. 2014; Cheng et al. 2014; Wafa et al. 2015; Eto et al. 2016; Wilding et al. 2016), other metals such as zinc, copper, and so on, are also being considered for their potential anti-biofilm efficacy (Huang et al. 2008; Shirai et al. 2009; Haenle et al. 2011; Aydin Sevinç and Hanley 2010; Hans et al. 2013; Kim et al. 2011; Koseki et al. 2013; Elizabeth et al. 2014). Zinc oxide is thought to disrupt the cell walls of both Gram-positive and Gram-negative bacteria, eventually leading to elevated membrane permeability and cell damage (Huang et al. 2008). However, most work to date has investigated the use of zinc oxide against planktonic bacteria; against dental pathogens, zinc oxide showed less ability to inhibit biofilms than silver did (Aydin Sevinç and Hanley 2010). Copper has shown some promise as an anti-biofilm agent for hospital and public surfaces; however, potential toxicity issues involving copper nanoparticles may limit its use for internal devices (Kim et al. 2011).

The main obstacles to using anti-infective metals are cytotoxicity and resultant decreased biocompatibility. Therefore, most coating technology research efforts have focused on reducing or even eliminating toxicity while maintaining antibacterial effects.

Local delivery of antibiotics following trauma or orthopaedic surgery or for the treatment of chronic osteomyelitis is used to produce high antibiotic concentrations in the bone (Klemm 1979). Antibiotic-loaded polymethylmethacrylate (PMMA) is currently being used in cemented total joint arthroplasty (TJA; Buchholz and Engelbrecht 1970) and has significantly reduced post-operative infection rates (Engesaeter 2003). However, this method has not yet been implemented for cementless TJA. One possible approach is a controlled antibiotic delivery coating based on mesoporous materials (Antoci et al. 2007; Sörensen et al. 2014; Neut et al. 2015). Directly tethering antibiotics to metal implants could kill bacteria when they first come into contact with the prosthesis, thus halting the formation of biofilm. There have been several reported antibiotics which can be used as coatings (Antoci et al. 2007; Sörensen et al. 2014; Metsemakers et al. 2015a; Metsemakers et al. 2015b; Neut et al. 2015). While the reservoir of deliverable antibiotics is limited, using an antibiotic tethering approach to protect the implant surface against colonizing bacteria immediately following implantation might be enough to significantly reduce the risk of infection. However, such an effect is likely to be limited to the immediate vicinity of the implant surface, and to the bacteria within the range of the antibacterial spectrum. It may be said that this method is the most realistic and safe, and has the highest expectations for validity.

Some non-metal elements like selenium, iodine, and so on, also have anti-infective properties. Covalently binding selenium onto the surface of titanium or titanium alloy implants has been shown to prevent the attachment of *Staphylococcus aureus* and *Staphylococcus epidermidis* without affecting osteoblast viability (Holinka et al. 2013; Rodríguez-Valencia et al. 2013). Iodine is a component of thyroid hormones and is the heaviest essential element needed by all living organisms. It has a broad antibacterial spectrum and does not cause drug resistance, as might be induced by the administration of antibiotics. Anodized povidone–iodine-containing surfaces that can be directly supported on existing implants have excellent antibacterial activity, biocompatibility, and no cytotoxicity (Shirai et al. 2011). In Japan, iodine-coated orthopaedic implants have already been used in clinical trials, and the results were excellent (Tsuchiya et al. 2012; Shirai et al. 2014a, 2014b; Demura et al. 2015; Kabata et al. 2015; Shirai et al. 2016).

The third strategy is to apply antibacterial coatings perioperatively (Romanò et al. 2015). Clinically, antibiotic-loaded PMMA and impaction bone grafting with antibiotic-loaded allografts or bone substitutes can be seen as perioperative antibacterial coating in the wide sense (Klemm 1979; Buchholz and Engelbrecht 1970; Buttaro et al. 2005). Recently, a fast-resorbable hydrogel that can be loaded intraoperatively with various antibacterials and coated just before implant insertion has been introduced in the European market (Drago et al. 2014). This method has several advantages: It is simple, inexpensive, can be modified intraoperatively, does not modify the properties of the implant, enables free antibiotics selection, and so on. However, its effects are likely to be limited to the immediate vicinity of the implant surface, and distribution of the coated hydrogel may become uneven at the biomaterial–bony tissues interface.

In ◘ Tab. 9.3 a summary is given of the technologies and features of the major anti-infective coatings previously reported, according to the three strategy-based classifications described earlier. All of the coating technologies mentioned must be proven to be safe in the short and long term, should not interfere with osteointegration or induce bacterial resistance in the long run, and should be easy to implement in clinical practice and at an affordable cost. Issues related to the mechanical properties of these technologies, the longevity of the coatings, and the potential for detrimental side effects such as toxicity and interference with osseointegration all require further investigation.

9.2.2 Clinical Trials with Coated Implants

There have been many ideas for making antibacterial implants and a significant number of fundamental experiments have been reported. However, only a few clinical trial reports have been published about the actual application of this fundamental research.

The antibacterial effects of silver have been known for a long time; Ambroise Paré, surgeon to the French royal family, performed plastic surgery of the face using a silver clip in the 1500s (Wikipedia). In Europe, silver coating has been used for external fixator pins and tumour prostheses (Massè et al. 2000; Hardes et al. 2010; Glehr et al. 2013; Wafa et al. 2015). Several reports of clinical trials using silver-coated orthopaedic devices have appeared since the early 2000s (Massè et al. 2000; Coester et al. 2006; Hardes et al. 2010; Glehr et al. 2013; Wafa et al. 2015; Eto et al. 2016; Wilding et al. 2016). Massè et al. reported a prospective randomized study carried out to compare silver-coated external fixator pins and normal uncoated pins (Massè et al. 2000). The clinical behaviour and the rate of pin tract infection of the coated pins did not differ from that of the uncoated pins. Furthermore, the implant of silver-coated pins resulted in a significant increase in silver serum levels. A similar randomized controlled trial in the United States produced similar results (Coester et al. 2006). Long-term antibacterial effects are necessary to prevent pin tract infec-

Tab. 9.3 Classification and features of anti-infective implant coatings (modified from Gallo et al. 2014, Romanò et al. 2015)

Strategy	Features	Examples	Development stage	References
Passive surface finishing/modifications	Prevention of bacterial adhesion	Albumin	Preclinical	An et al. 1996
		Anti-adhesive polymers	Preclinical	Neoh and Kang 2011; Follmann et al. 2012; Muszanska et al. 2014
		Nano-patterned surface	Preclinical	Truong et al. 2010; Singh et al. 2011; Shida et al. 2013
		Super-hydrophobic surface	Preclinical	Stallard et al. 2012; Zhu et al. 2014
		Hydrogels	Preclinical	Pandit et al. 2013; Drago et al. 2014
Active surface finishing/modification	Inorganic	Silver ions Silver nanoparticles	Market	Massè et al. 2000; Coester et al. 2006; Hardes et al. 2010; Akiyama et al. 2013; Glehr et al. 2013; Gao et al. 2014; Cheng et al. 2014; Wafa et al. 2015; Eto et al. 2016; Wilding et al. 2016
		Titanium dioxide	Preclinical	Haenle et al. 2011; Koseki et al. 2013
		Zinc ion	Preclinical	Huang et al. 2008; Aydin Sevinç et al. 2010; Elizabeth et al. 2014
		Cooper ion	Preclinical	Shirai et al. 2009; Kim et al. 2011; Hans et al. 2013
		Selenium ion	Preclinical	Holinka et al. 2013; Rodríguez-Valencia et al. 2013
		Iodine	Clinical	Shirai et al. 2011; Tsuchiya et al. 2012; Shirai et al. 2014a, 2014b; Demura et al. 2015; Kabata et al. 2015; Shirai et al. 2016
	Organic	Coated antibiotics	Market	Fuchs et al. 2011; Metsemakers et al. 2015a; Metsemakers et al. 2015b
		Covalently linked antibiotics	Preclinical	Antoci et al. 2007; Sörensen et al. 2014; Metsemakers et al. 2015a; Metsemakers et al. 2015b; Neut et al. 2015
		Chitosan derivatives	Preclinical	Norowski et al. 2011; Magetsari et al. 2015
		Cytokines	Preclinical	Li and McKeague 2011
		Enzymes	Preclinical	Thallinger et al. 2013
	Synthetic	Non-antibiotic antimicrobial compounds	Preclinical	Glinel et al. 2012
	Combined	Multilayer coating	Preclinical	Fu et al. 2006; Huang et al. 2013; Zhou et al. 2014
		Smart coating	Preclinical	Holzapfel et al. 2013; Parvizi et al. 2007

Tab. 9.3 (Continued)

Strategy	Features	Examples	Development stage	References
Perioperative antibacterial local carriers or coatings	Non-biodegradable	Antibiotic-loaded polymethylmethacrylate	Market	Buchholz and Engelbrecht 1970; Klemm 1979
	Biodegradable	Antibiotic loaded bone grafts and substitutes	Market	Buttaro et al. 2005
		Resorbable hydrogel	Market	Drago et al. 2014

tions of the external fixator because external fixation periods are usually quite long. Silver, which has a relatively short-term antibacterial effect, might be unsuitable for such long-term prevention.

Wafa et al. applied a silver coating to tumour prostheses and conducted a case-control study to examine its merits (Wafa et al. 2015). The overall post-operative infection rate of the silver-coated group was significantly lower than that of the normal control group. Hardes et al. reported similar results (Hardes et al. 2010). However, the development of local argyria became a major problem as a post-operative adverse reaction. Glehr et al. reported that seven (23 %) of 32 patients developed local argyria after a median of 25.7 months following implantation of the megaprostheses with silver coatings (Glehr et al. 2013).

Recently, the results of clinical trials on a silver coating arthrodesis nail for unsalvageable infected total knee arthroplasty and a silver oxide-containing hydroxyapatite (Ag-HA) coated cementless hip implant were reported (Eto et al. 2015; Wilding et al. 2016). Arthrodesis of the knee using a -coating intramedullary nail was successful in eradicating infection and allowing limb conservation, which can be an alternative to amputation for patients with severely infected total knee arthroplasty (Wilding et al. 2016). The second study used 3% Ag-HA-coated cementless hip implants, which have both antibacterial activity from the silver ions and osteoconductivity from the HA. No adverse reaction to the silver was noted, and argyria was not observed in any of the cases. No patients developed infections after surgery (Eto et al. 2016). However, the Ag-HA coating was applied only to cylindrical fully coated stems. Therefore, remarkable stress shielding after several years is a concern.

As for antibiotic coatings, the first clinical trial was performed using a gentamicin-coated intramedullary nail for tibial open fractures (Fuchs et al. 2011). Two clinical trials using gentamicin-coated tibial nails have been reported to date (Fuchs et al. 2011; Metsemakers et al. 2015a; Metsemakers et al. 2015b). No deep infections were noted in either clinical trial.

Clinical trials in Japan have been performed using several kinds of iodine-coated implants for external fixator pins, spinal instrumentations, tumour megaprostheses, internal fixation devices (plates, nails and screws), and hip replacement implants (Tsuchiya et al. 2012; Demura et al. 2015; Kabata et al. 2015; Shirai et al 2014a, 2014b, 2016). Iodine coating is applicable for almost all titanium orthopaedic implants; it has a broad antibacterial spectrum without resistant bacteria, a long-lasting effect, and is non-cytotoxic (Tsuchiya et al. 2012). Short-term clinical results have shown it to be effective in the prevention or treatment of periprosthetic infections with no subsequent abnormalities of thyroid gland function (Tsuchiya et al. 2012; Kabata et al. 2015; Demura et al. 2015).

9.2.3 Advantages and Disadvantages of Different Coating Strategies

Affinity of Orthopaedic Materials and Anti-Infective Coatings

All coating technology is not applicable to all orthopaedic implant materials. From the viewpoint of coating properties and engineering, some materials are applicable for coating, but some are not. Certain coating technologies are applicable for all kind of materials, but others are applicable for only limited materials. For example, iodine coating cannot currently be applied to anything other than titanium implants because of technological limitations (Tsuchiya et al. 2012).

Anti-infective Duration

The duration of the anti-infective effect varies according to the differences in coating technology and coated materials. A relatively long effective period is reported for the iodine coating (more than 1 year) whereas the effective period is short (usually a few days to at most a few weeks) for silver or antibiotics coatings (Tsuchiya et al. 2012; Cheng et al. 2014; Gallo et al. 2014; Sörensen et al. 2014; Metsemakers et al. 2015a; Metsemakers et al. 2015b; Romanò et al. 2015). The typical release profile of antibiotics from conventional polymer coating systems is a high initial release of drugs followed by a very short period (a few days) of reduced release (Gallo et al. 2014; Romanò et al. 2015). By improving the coating matrix, some coating technologies have achieved much longer effective periods (Cheng et al. 2014). The clinical purpose should inform the selection of coating properties. For example, to prevent an acute infection in primary TJA, a coating with a short effective period, such as silver or antibiotics, is sufficient. To treat cases with a severely compromised host or those at high risk of recurrence infection, such as revision surgery of periprosthetic joint infection, it is considered more desirable to choose a coating with long-term effects, such as iodine. A coating with long-term effects is also theoretically feasible for the prevention of pin tract infection after the application of external fixation.

Adverse Reactions

The anti-infective properties of biomedical materials are often achieved by loading or coating them with powerful bactericides. However, these bioactive molecules can damage the host cells at the biomaterial–tissues interface and, sometimes, even produce systemic toxic effects (Gallo et al. 2014; Romanò et al. 2015). High concentrations of silver ions have been reported to be cytotoxic, and silver-coated implants may develop localized cutaneous argyria (Glehr et al. 2013). To address these issues, basic research inspections have been carried out for almost all of the coating materials with regard to both their antibacterial and cytotoxic effects. These have demonstrated in vitro and in vivo the effectiveness of several potentially promising technologies. However, we do not know whether or not an adverse reaction will actually occur when they are clinically used. Any coating material is capable of inducing allergic reactions. Thus, inspection by clinical trial is necessary.

Size Variation of the Implants

Mass-produced implants are available in an abundance of sizes for size adjustment during surgery. However, the special anti-infective implants are not always available in enough sizes. When special coating is needed, the size of the implant to be coated must be selected before surgery, which requires perfect preoperative planning. In clinical trials of iodine-coated prostheses for total hip arthroplasty, a 3D templating system was routinely used in the preoperative planning to select an appropriate implant design and size (Kabata et al. 2015).

Costs

Special coating procedures are usually costly and time-consuming. An important consideration in designing implants with antibacterial coatings relates to the characterization of reasonable and justifiable cost.

Change in Implant Performance with the Coating

A change in the surface chemistry and/or structure of the implants can be achieved by chemically or physically altering the surface layer in the existing biomaterial (e.g. oxidation or mechanical modifications like roughening/polishing/texturing). Another method involves over-coating the existing surface with a new thin layer of material having a different composition (e.g. hydroxyapatite coating on titanium alloys, antibiotics bound covalently to the substrate, fixation of other antimicrobial compounds; Gallo et al. 2014). These kinds of changes in surface character may result in a change of implant strength and bone affinity. For example, a special coating could be used to change a polished surface, upon which it is difficult to grow bone, into a rough surface that makes bone ongrowth possible, which in turn may change design concepts for implant fixation in hip and knee implants (Kabata et al. 2015).

9.2.4 Conclusion

In the near future, there is no doubt that using excellent anti-infective-coated implants to establish a new preventive strategy for PJI can greatly contribute to a lower incidence of PJIs. Further improvement will be obtained in areas such as the mechanical properties of these devices, cytotoxicity, the duration of the anti-infective effect, and the antibacterial spectrum. It will be necessary to execute clinical trials on a more ample scale to test these anti-infective technologies. Concerns about the long-term durability of such new anti-infective implants as compared with traditional implants also can only be addressed through clinical trials.

Take-Home Message

- Anti-infective biomaterials residing on implants for the purpose of arthroplasty, trauma, and tumour therapy can reduce the rate of device-related infections.
- The prevention or reduction of biofilm formation follows anti-adhesive or antibacterial strategies, while preventing cytotoxicity and bacterial resistance, or impairment in osteointegration.
- Preclinical and a few clinical trials show promising – yet inconclusive results – for the safety and efficacy of active ingredients in coatings made of metal elements or non-metal elements such as silver or iodine, respectively.
- Perioperatively applied coatings such as hydrogel may have the advantage that surgeons can tailor the admixture of active ingredients to the individual medical need.
- Clinical studies for iodine-coated implants in Japan aim at collecting convincing evidence for broad applicability whenever prostheses, plates, nails and screws are concerned.

References

Akiyama T, Miyamoto H, Yonekura Y, Tsukamoto M, Ando Y, Noda I, Sonohata M, Mawatari M (2013) Silver oxide-containing hydroxyapatite coating has in vivo antibacterial activity in the rat tibia. J Orthop Res 31(8):1195–1200

Ambroise Paré (2016) Wikipedia, The Free Encyclopedia. https://en.wikipedia.org/wiki/Ambroise_Par%C3%A9

An YH, Stuart GW, McDowell SJ, McDaniel SE, Kang Q, Friedman RJ (1996) Prevention of bacterial adherence to implant surfaces with a crosslinked albumin coating in vitro. J Orthop Res 14(5):846–849

Antoci V Jr, Adams CS, Parvizi J, Ducheyne P, Shapiro IM, Hickok NJ (2007) Covalently attached vancomycin provides a nanoscale antibacterial surface. Clin Orthop Relat Res 461:81–87

Aydin Sevinç B, Hanley L (2010) Antibacterial activity of dental composites containing zinc oxide nanoparticles. J Biomed Mater Res B Appl Biomater 94(1):22–31

Bacakova L, Filova E, Parizek M, Ruml T, Svorcik V (2011) Modulation of cell adhesion, proliferation and differentiation on materials designed for body implants. Biotechnol Adv 29(6):739–767

Buchholz HW, Engelbrecht H (1970) [Depot effects of various antibiotics mixed with Palacos resins]. Chirurg 41(11):511–515

Buttaro MA, Pusso R, Piccaluga F (2005) Vancomycin-supplemented impacted bone allografts in infected hip arthroplasty. Two-stage revision results. J Bone Joint Surg Br 87(3):314–319

Campoccia D, Montanaro L, Arciola CR (2013) A review of the clinical implications of anti-infective biomaterials and infection-resistant surfaces. Biomaterials 34(33):8018–8029

Cheng H, Li Y, Huo K, Gao B, Xiong W (2014) Long-lasting in vivo and in vitro antibacterial ability of nanostructured titania coating incorporated with silver nanoparticles. J Biomed Mater Res A 102(10):3488–3499

Clement JL, Jarrett PS (1994) Antibacterial silver. Met Based Drugs 1(5–6):467–482

Coester LM, Nepola JV, Allen J, Marsh JL (2006) The effects of silver coated external fixation pins. Iowa Orthop J 26: 48–53

Demura S, Murakami H, Shirai T, Kato S, Yoshioka K, Ota T, Ishii T, Igarashi T, Tsuchiya H (2015) Surgical treatment for pyogenic vertebral osteomyelitis using iodine-supported spinal instruments: initial case series of 14 patients. Eur J Clin Microbiol Infect Dis 34(2):261–266

Drago L, Boot W, Dimas K, Malizos K, Hänsch GM, Stuyck J, Gawlitta D, Romanò CL (2014) Does implant coating with antibacterial-loaded hydrogel reduce bacterial colonization and biofilm formation in vitro? Clin Orthop Relat Res 472(11):3311–3323

Elizabeth E, Baranwal G, Krishnan AG, Menon D, Nair M (2014) ZnO nanoparticle incorporated nanostructured metallic titanium for increased mesenchymal stem cell response and antibacterial activity. Nanotechnology doi:10.1088/0957-4484/25/11/115101

Engesaeter LB, Lie SA, Espehaug B, Furnes O, Vollset SE, Havelin LI (2003) Antibiotic prophylaxis in total hip arthroplasty: effects of antibiotic prophylaxis systemically and in bone cement on the revision rate of 22,170 primary hip replacements followed 0-14 years in the Norwegian Arthroplasty Register. Acta Orthop Scand 74(6):644–651

Eto S, Kawano S, Someya S, Miyamoto H, Sonohata M, Mawatari M (2016) First Clinical Experience With Thermal-Sprayed Silver Oxide-Containing Hydroxyapatite Coating Implant. J Arthroplasty 31(7):1498–1503

Follmann HD, Martins AF, Gerola AP, Burgo TA, Nakamura CV, Rubira AF, Muniz EC (2012) Antiadhesive and antibacterial multilayer films via layer-by-layer assembly of TMC/heparin complexes. Biomacromolecules 13(11): 3711–3722

Fu J, Ji J, Fan D, Shen J (2006) Construction of antibacterial multilayer films containing nanosilver via layer-by-layer assembly of heparin and chitosan-silver ions complex. J Biomed Mater Res A 79(3):665–674

Fuchs T, Stange R, Schmidmaier G, Raschke MJ (2011) The use of gentamicin-coated nails in the tibia: preliminary results of a prospective study. Arch Orthop Trauma Surg 131(10):1419–1425

Gallo J, Holinka M, Moucha CS (2014) Antibacterial surface treatment for orthopaedic implants. Int J Mol Sci 15(8):13849–13880

Gao A, Hang R, Huang X, Zhao L, Zhang X, Wang L, Tang B, Ma S, Chu PK (2014) The effects of titania nanotubes with embedded silver oxide nanoparticles on bacteria and osteoblasts. Biomaterials 35(13):4223–4235

Glehr M, Leithner A, Friesenbichler J, Goessler W, Avian A, Andreou D, Maurer-Ertl W, Windhager R, Tunn PU (2013) Argyria following the use of silver-coated megaprostheses: no association between the development of local argyria and elevated silver levels. Bone Joint J 95–B(7):988–992

Glinel K, Thebault P, Humblot V, Pradier CM, Jouenne T (2012) Antibacterial surfaces developed from bio-inspired approaches. Acta Biomater 8(5):1670–1684

Haenle M, Fritsche A, Zietz C, Bader R, Heidenau F, Mittelmeier W, Gollwitzer H (2011) An extended spectrum bactericidal titanium dioxide (TiO2) coating for metallic implants: in vitro effectiveness against MRSA and mechanical properties. J Mater Sci Mater Med 22(2):381–387

Hans M, Erbe A, Mathews S, Chen Y, Solioz M, Mücklich F (2013) Role of copper oxides in contact killing of bacteria. Langmuir 29(52):16160–16166

Hardes J, von Eiff C, Streitbuerger A, Balke M, Budny T, Henrichs MP, Hauschild G, Ahrens H (2010) Reduction of periprosthetic infection with silver-coated megaprostheses in patients with bone sarcoma. J Surg Oncol 101(5):389–395

Hendriks JG, van Horn JR, van der Mei HC, Busscher HJ (2004) Backgrounds of antibiotic-loaded bone cement and prosthesis-related infection. Biomaterials 25(3):545–556

Holinka J, Pilz M, Kubista B, Presterl E, Windhager R (2013) Effects of selenium coating of orthopaedic implant surfaces on bacterial adherence and osteoblastic cell growth. Bone Joint J 95–B(5):678–682

Holzapfel BM, Reichert JC, Schantz JT, Gbureck U, Rackwitz L, Nöth U, Jakob F, Rudert M, Groll J, Hutmacher DW (2013) How smart do biomaterials need to be? A translational science and clinical point of view. Adv Drug Deliv Rev 65(4):581–603

Huang W, Li X, Xue Y, Huang R, Deng H, Ma Z (2013) Antibacterial multilayer films fabricated by LBL immobilizing lysozyme and HTCC on nanofibrous mats. Int J Biol Macromol 53:26–31

Huang Z, Zheng X, Yan D, Yin G, Liao X, Kang Y, Yao Y, Huang D, Hao B (2008) Toxicological effect of ZnO nanoparticles based on bacteria. Langmuir 24(8):4140–4144

Kabata T, Maeda T, Kajino Y, Hasegawa K, Inoue D, Yamamoto T, Takagi T, Ohmori T, Tsuchiya H (2015) Iodine-Supported Hip implants: Short Term Clinical Results. Biomed Res Int doi:10.1155/2015/368124

Kazemzadeh-Narbat M, Kindrachuk J, Duan K, Jenssen H, Hancock RE, Wang R (2010) Antimicrobial peptides on calcium phosphate-coated titanium for the prevention of implant-associated infections. Biomaterials 31(36): 9519–9526

Kim JS, Adamcakova-Dodd A, O'Shaughnessy PT, Grassian VH, Thorne PS (2011) Effects of copper nanoparticle exposure on host defense in a murine pulmonary infection model. Part Fibre Toxicol doi:10.1186/1743-8977-8-29

Klemm K (1979) [Gentamicin-PMMA-beads in treating bone and soft tissue infections (author's transl)]. Zentralbl Chir 104(14):934–942

Koseki H, Asahara T, Shida T, Yoda I, Horiuchi H, Baba K, Osaki M (2013) Clinical and histomorphometrical study on titanium dioxide-coated external fixation pins. Int J Nanomedicine 8:593–599

Li B, McKeague AL (2011) Emerging ideas: Interleukin-12 nanocoatings prevent open fracture-associated infections. Clin Orthop Relat Res 469(11):3262–3265

Magetsari R, Dewo P, Saputro BK, Lanodiyu Z (2014) Cinnamon Oil and Chitosan Coating on Orthopaedic Implant Surface for Prevention of Staphylococcus Epidermidis Biofilm Formation. Malays Orthop J 8(3):11–14

Mah TF, O'Toole GA (2001) Mechanisms of biofilm resistance to antimicrobial agents. Trends Microbiol 9(1):34–39

Massè A, Bruno A, Bosetti M, Biasibetti A, Cannas M, Gallinaro P (2000) Prevention of pin track infection in external fixation with silver coated pins: clinical and microbiological results. J Biomed Mater Res 53(5):600–604

Metsemakers WJ, Reul M, Nijs S (2015a) The use of gentamicin-coated nails in complex open tibia fracture and revision cases: A retrospective analysis of a single centre case series and review of the literature. Injury 46(12):2433–2437

Metsemakers WJ, Emanuel N, Cohen O, Reichart M, Potapova I, Schmid T, Segal D, Riool M, Kwakman PH, de Boer L, de Breij A, Nibbering PH, Richards RG, Zaat SA, Moriarty TF (2015b) A doxycycline-loaded polymer-lipid encapsulation matrix coating for the prevention of implant-related

osteomyelitis due to doxycycline-resistant methicillin-resistant Staphylococcus aureus. J Control Release 209:47–56
Muszanska AK, Rochford ET, Gruszka A, Bastian AA, Busscher HJ, Norde W, van der Mei HC, Herrmann A (2014) Antiadhesive polymer brush coating functionalized with antimicrobial and RGD peptides to reduce biofilm formation and enhance tissue integration. Biomacromolecules 15(6):2019–2026
Neoh KG, Kang ET (2011) Combating bacterial colonization on metals via polymer coatings: relevance to marine and medical applications. ACS Appl Mater Interfaces 3(8): 2808–2819
Neut D, Dijkstra RJ, Thompson JI, Kavanagh C, van der Mei HC, Busscher HJ (2015) A biodegradable gentamicin-hydroxyapatite-coating for infection prophylaxis in cementless hip prostheses. Eur Cell Mater 29:42–55
Norowski PA, Courtney HS, Babu J, Haggard WO, Bumgardner JD (2011) Chitosan coatings deliver antimicrobials from titanium implants: a preliminary study. Implant Dent 20(1):56–67
Pandit V, Zuidema JM, Venuto KN, Macione J, Dai G, Gilbert RJ, Kotha SP (2013) Evaluation of multifunctional polysaccharide hydrogels with varying stiffness for bone tissue engineering. Tissue Eng Part A 19(21–22):2452–2463
Parvizi J, Antoci V Jr, Hickok NJ, Shapiro IM (2007) Selfprotective smart orthopedic implants. Expert Rev Med Devices 4(1):55–64
Rodríguez-Valencia C, López-Álvarez M, Cochón-Cores B, Pereiro I, Serra J, González P (2013) Novel selenium-doped hydroxyapatite coatings for biomedical applications. J Biomed Mater Res A 101(3):853–861
Romanò CL, Scarponi S, Gallazzi E, Romanò D, Drago L (2015) Antibacterial coating of implants in orthopaedics and trauma: a classification proposal in an evolving panorama. J Orthop Surg Res doi:10.1186/s13018-015-0294-5
Shida T, Koseki H, Yoda I, Horiuchi H, Sakoda H, Osaki M (2013) Adherence ability of Staphylococcus epidermidis on prosthetic biomaterials: an in vitro study. Int J Nanomedicine 8:3955–3961
Shirai T, Tsuchiya H, Shimizu T, Ohtani K, Zen Y, Tomita K (2009) Prevention of pin tract infection with titanium-copper alloys. J Biomed Mater Res B Appl Biomater 91(1): 373–380
Shirai T, Shimizu T, Ohtani K, Zen Y, Takaya M, Tsuchiya H (2011) Antibacterial iodine-supported titanium implants. Acta Biomater 7(4):1928–1933
Shirai T, Tsuchiya H, Nishida H, Yamamoto N, Watanabe K, Nakase J, Terauchi R, Arai Y, Fujiwara H, Kubo T (2014a) Antimicrobial megaprostheses supported with iodine. J Biomater Appl 29(4):617–623
Shirai T, Watanabe K, Matsubara H, Nomura I, Fujiwara H, Arai Y, Ikoma K, Terauchi R, Kubo T, Tsuchiya H (2014b) Prevention of pin tract infection with iodine-supported titanium pins. J Orthop Sci 19(4):598–602
Shirai T, Tsuchiya H, Terauchi R, Tsuchida S, Mizoshiri N, Igarashi K, Miwa S, Takeuchi A, Kimura H, Hayashi K, Yamamoto N, Kubo T (2016) The outcomes of reconstruction using frozen autograft combined with iodine-coated implants for malignant bone tumors: compared with non-coated implants. Jpn J Clin Oncol 46(8):735–740
Singh AV, Vyas V, Patil R, Sharma V, Scopelliti PE, Bongiorno G, Podestà A,Lenardi C, Gade WN, Milani P (2011) Quantitative characterization of the influence of the nanoscale morphology of nanostructured surfaces on bacterial adhesion and biofilm formation. PLoS One doi:10.1371/journal.pone.0025029
Sörensen JH, Lilja M, Sörensen TC, Åstrand M, Procter P, Fuchs S, Strømme M, Steckel H (2014) Biomechanical and antibacterial properties of Tobramycin loaded hydroxyapatite coated fixation pins. J Biomed Mater Res B Appl Biomater 102(7):1381–1392
Stallard CP, McDonnell KA, Onayemi OD, O'Gara JP, Dowling DP (2012) Evaluation of protein adsorption on atmospheric plasma deposited coatings exhibiting superhydrophilic to superhydrophobic properties. Biointerphases 7(1–4):31
Thallinger B, Prasetyo EN, Nyanhongo GS, Guebitz GM (2013) Antimicrobial enzymes: an emerging strategy to fight microbes and microbial biofilms. Biotechnol J 8(1): 97–109
Truong VK, Lapovok R, Estrin YS, Rundell S, Wang JY, Fluke CJ, Crawford RJ, Ivanova EP (2010) The influence of nano-scale surface roughness on bacterial adhesion to ultrafine-grained titanium. Biomaterials 31(13):3674–3683
Tsuchiya H, Shirai T, Nishida H, Murakami H, Kabata T, Yamamoto N, Watanabe K, Nakase J (2012) Innovative antimicrobial coating of titanium implants with iodine. J Orthop Sci 17(5):595–604
Wafa H, Grimer RJ, Reddy K, Jeys L, Abudu A, Carter SR, Tillman RM (2015) Retrospective evaluation of the incidence of early periprosthetic infection with silver-treated endoprostheses in high-risk patients: case-control study. Bone Joint J 97–B(2):252–257
Wilding CP, Cooper GA, Freeman AK, Parry MC, Jeys L (2016) Can a Silver-Coated Arthrodesis Implant Provide a Viable Alternative to Above Knee Amputation in the Unsalvageable, Infected Total Knee Arthroplasty? J Arthroplasty 31(11):2542–2547
Zhou B, Li Y, Deng H, Hu Y, Li B (2014) Antibacterial multilayer films fabricated by layer-by-layer immobilizing lysozyme and gold nanoparticles on nanofibers. Colloids Surf B Biointerfaces 116:432–438
Zhu H, Guo Z, Liu W (2014) Adhesion behaviors on superhydrophobic surfaces. Chem Commun 50(30):3900–3913

9.3 Aspects of Antimicrobial Implant Coating

Andreas Kolb, Susann Klimas, Thomas Kluge and Klaus-Dieter Kühn

9.3.1 Introduction

In recent decades, the quality of life of many patients has been considerably improved by the increased use of medical implants. As a consequence of the growing use of implants, a parallel trend toward more infections has been observed. In particular, older and multimorbid patients, who benefit the most from new treatment options, also face the highest risk of infection, and therefore the majority of cases of infections in critically ill patients are related to medical devices (Darouiche 2001; von Eiff et al. 2005). Such implant-associated infections still represent a serious problem and an increasing risk, especially in arthroplasty, which is devastating for the patient and costly for any health-care system (Kim 2008).

The main cost generators of periprosthetic joint infections (PJI) are additional surgical procedures, increased length of hospitalization, prolonged treatment with antibiotics, implantation of new, often expensive devices, and consideration of increased risk factors (Bozic and Ries 2005; Ferguson et al. 1996; Kirkland et al. 1999; Warren et al. 2006).

The treatment costs per case can easily exceed US $50,000. As a consequence, health authorities aim to minimize their expenses in terms of potentially avoidable infections or to stop reimbursing hospital-acquired infections. Therefore, additional reimbursement is not provided for any infection acquired during the current hospitalization. The same is true for cases where substantial documentation is missing to determine if the condition was already present at admission. Furthermore, hospitals will receive reduced payments if they do not report such an event.

One of the most efficient and practical approaches aimed at reducing the frequency of PJI is to avoid the biofilm formation on the surface of the implants because pathogens are optimally protected from the body's own immune defence in this biofilm matrix (Kühn 2014).

9.3.2 Interaction of Germs and Implants

Implants may harbour bacteria that may persevere on the surface in organized biofilms over many years. However, all foreign bodies such as medical implants are not capable of actively combating the bacteria and thus the formation of the biofilm. The human organism consists of billions of cells and exists in peaceful cohabitation with a significantly greater amount of micro-organisms (approx. by the power of 10). Many of these micro-organisms take on vital tasks for the host. Evolution has successfully moulded this cohabitation of micro-organisms and humans over millions of years and ensured the formation of a symbiotic connection of the highest precision and quality, ensuring mutual survival.

9.3.3 Biofilm Formation

The developmental stages of biofilm formation are shown in ◘ Fig. 9.3. In the proliferation stage and in the mature biofilm, the bacteria surround themselves with a matrix comprising water and biopolymers. This protects them from desiccation and toxic substances (i.e. antibiotics; Stewart and Costerton 2001). Therefore, the prevention of biofilm formation by tackling bacteria in the planktonic and sessile stages is the only reasonable vantage point.

The irreversible adhesion of bacteria to a surface occurs within seconds to minutes, while the next steps happen on a timescale of hours to days after implantation (Gristina and Costerton 1985). A resorbable coating (without antibiotic) should therefore be in place on the implant for at least 24–72 h. By constantly renewing its surface, possibly adhering bacteria are washed away from the bulk material. The coating will first of all delay the »race to the (implant) surface« between the host cells and bacteria by this time. However, this delay is thought to enable the systemically administered antibiotics and the host immune system to clear the microbial burden introduced during the operation; i.e. the endogenous cells can outnumber the bacteria once the race starts with delay and normal osseointegration can occur.

Preventing the formation of a biofilm in this time span can be a major contributing factor in

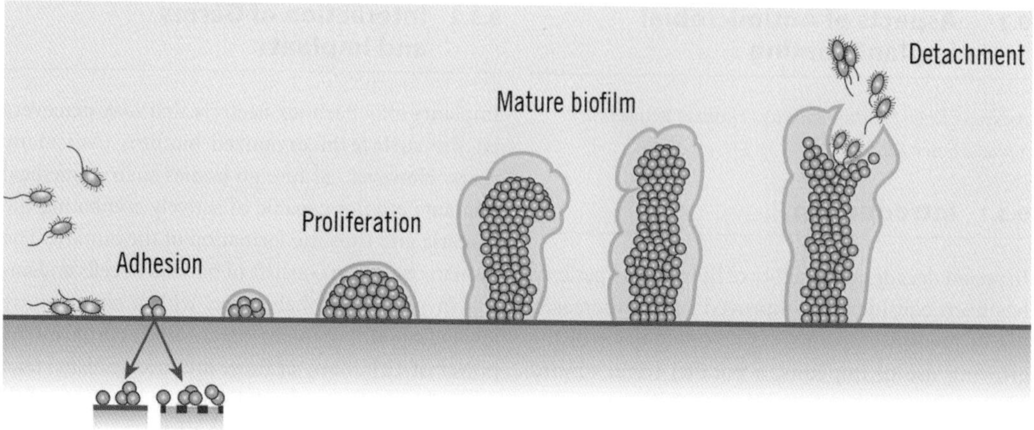

Fig. 9.3 Developmental stages of biofilm

avoiding chronic implant infection, loosening and revision surgery (Song et al. 2013). The minimum inhibitory concentration (MIC) defines the susceptibility breakpoint of planktonically grown bacteria. However, bacteria that grow within a biofilm are significantly more resistant to antibiotics. Thus, to effectively fight bacteria within a biofilm, levels of antibiotics way above the MIC are required at the surgical site.

The minimum anti-infective dose of active ingredients that are able to prevent biofilm formation is defined as the minimum biofilm inhibiting concentration (MBIC), while the minimum concentration able to destroy germs within an existing biofilm is defined as the minimum biofilm eliminating concentration (MBEC). Both values are of great importance for the assessment of the true antibiotic susceptibility of bacteria grown in biofilm, and are of particular interest for the development of implant surface coatings.

Especially in bone and joint-related infections, this cannot always be achieved by normally dosed systemic administration alone. Because higher systemic doses may lead to severe side effects, the local release of drugs should be considered as a desirable secondary mode of action that can also be provided by the implant coating (cf. Fig. 9.9).

9.3.4 Antimicrobial Protection

Medical implants consist of diverse materials which support and/or replace various bodily functions of a special type in medicine and are in direct interaction with the human biological systems. The affinity toward micro-organisms is quite different and depends on the material and its surface on one hand and the location of the implant within the body on the other (Thull 2004). Bacteria such as *Staphylococcus epidermidis* can obviously colonize polymers and, for example, hydroxylapatite a little easier than metals, which in turn are colonized more easily by *Staphylococcus aureus*. The rougher a polymer or metallic surface, the greater the likelihood of it being colonized by micro-organisms.

To date, the local antimicrobial protection of the surface of especially cementless prostheses has been somewhat disregarded. The same is true for several steel alloys, especially titanium, which represents a particularly interesting and suitable implant material for such endoprostheses owing to its relatively low E-modulus and the passivation layer on the surface.

Antimicrobial Agents

Several medical devices were successfully combined with anti-infective agents in vitro. Unfortunately, only few of these combination products are approved as medical devices. Since most combinations are not commercially available, surgeons often prepare customized combinations manually and perioperatively. The legal consequence is that they become the responsible manufacturer and thus assume liability for the product.

Antiseptics like heavy metal ions, agents containing halogens, organic ammonium salts, phenols and phenol derivatives and alcohols are possible agents.

Although *heavy metal ions*, such as of silver, copper, mercury or zinc, possess an excellent broad antimicrobial impact, they prefer to randomly attack S-H groups, not being capable of differentiating whether it belongs to a bacterial or a vital protein of the host cell. Therefore, heavy metal ions are characterized by a non-specific mode of action. This random mechanism has to be considered a disadvantage. Furthermore, the statement that there are no resistance mechanisms against heavy metal ions is not sustainable (Hasman et al. 2006). The mode of action of heavy metal ions is non-specific against germs.

In addition, *chlorine-, bromine- or iodine-containing solutions* can be utilized for antiseptic surface treatment and are used topically for smaller wounds and wound dressings. Iodine-containing antiseptics typically used for the disinfection of skin were developed based on their capability to quickly kill germs by completely encapsulating them.

Further, *halogen-containing antiseptics* like octenidine or chlorhexidine are of interest for coating processes. Octenidine is characterized by a broad-spectrum effectiveness against Gram-positive and Gram-negative germs, yeasts, fungal infections and encapsulated viruses. Furthermore, it is sufficiently active against MRSA in very low doses. Chlorhexidine is also characterized by its extremely broad active spectrum and is almost completely discharged without being metabolized. Its effect is the destruction of the bacterial cell membrane. The mode of action of octenidine and chlorhexidine is non-specific.

Phenols and phenol derivatives are also of interest for implant coatings. For example, triclosan as a derivative of phenol, since it is already on the market in a licensed medical device (suture material) as a combination product. It possesses an active spectrum that is effective against Gram-positive germs. Microbiologically, it does not have a broad spectrum and is linked to increased allergies and asthma. Triclosan is also likely to promote bacterial resistance and induce cross-resistance. It may degrade into dioxin (Rule et al. 2005), which is toxic and has to be highly pre-purified to prevent formation of chlorinated benzo-dioxins.

Isopropanol, ethanol and propanol can be utilized as antiseptics. A certain content of water is required in the case of ethanol 70–80% to be an optimal disinfectant. It is regarded as an ideal means for the disinfection of hands. Proteins are encapsulated by alcohol and unfurl, which causes their protective cover to disintegrate, denaturing the proteins in the process. The mode of action of triclosan and alcohols is non-specific against germs.

Organisms developed a broad spectrum of mechanisms to combat bacterial infection. One mechanism is the production of *antimicrobial peptides (AMPs)*, to actively combat bacterial infection. To date, about 750 different AMPs are known and can be reproduced synthetically, equipped with specific qualities. AMPs have bactericidal, fungicidal, virucidal and tumouricidal properties. They can bind to the negatively charged bacterial membranes and destroy their stability. Within the peptide, the active group of defensins is of particular interest, since it can destroy even matured biofilms. In combination with anti-infective substances, they function as a »door opener«, can penetrate deeply into a mature biofilm, and eradicate bacteria located within.

Thus, AMPs have features that can potentially be used for implant surface coatings (Costa et al. 2011). The mode of action of AMPs is non-specific against germs.

Antibiotics work selectively against bacteria and hereby attack various positions of the micro-organism: inhibition of cell wall biosynthesis (beta-lactam antibiotics, glycopeptides, fosfomycin), blocking of protein synthesis (aminoglycoside, tetracycline, chloramphenicol, macrolide, lincosamide), suppression of nucleic acid synthesis [rifampicin (ansamycin antibiotic), sulfonamide, gyrase inhibitors], interference with permeability of cytoplasmic membrane (polyene antibiotics, polypeptide antibiotics). Antibiotics can inhibit the growth and/or reproduction of bacteria (bacteriostatic) or ensure the destruction of the micro-organisms (bactericidal).

In surgery, bactericidally and bacteriostatically effective antibiotics play an important role as an adjuvant treatment to support the body's own immune system. Both operating principles reduce the bacterial count, which enables the macrophages immune response to succeed.

In contrast to chemical antimicrobial agents, especially from antiseptics, antibiotics are antibacterial substances that attack a specific target in the bacterial cell. This is unique in nature! For example, they specifically block an important metabolic process of the bacterial organism. As a consequence, the bacteria are no longer viable. Therefore, the mode of action of antibiotics is specific against bacteria.

9.3.5 Antimicrobial Resistance

Clinical reporting often depicts resistance in combination with antibiotics, which is one of the reasons why antibiotics are perceived rather critically when applied for diverse indications. Especially a prophylactic antibiotic treatment is broadly recognized as a risk. However, the development of resistance is a fundamental bacterial quality and enables them to adapt to changes in the environment for survival. Given time, bacteria can develop survival strategies that basically allow them to adapt to any sort of anti-infective agents. As a result, the application of anti-infective agents can always lead to bacteria that acquire resistance and survive. Thus, the risk of inducing resistance in bacteria is certainly not limited to antibiotics, but must be taken into account for every available anti-infective agent.

In medical practice, particularly in surgery, antibiotics are commonly administered prophylactically prior to surgery. The adjuvant treatment is applied to significantly decrease the total germ count and to support the immune response of the body. Nevertheless, if a total hip arthroplasty (THA) or total knee arthroplasty (TKA) needs to be performed, the systemic treatment alone is insufficient to reduce the local germ count, since additional germs invade the operational field perioperatively. Increased germ invasion due to a low local drug concentration amplifies the risk of biofilm formation on implant surfaces. This holds particularly true for exchange operations and for operations of multimorbid elderly patients.

The fundamental therapeutic measure is surgery, whereas the adjuvant treatment with antibiotics or anti-infectives is only meant to additionally protect the operating area and the revised implant. The agents reduce the local germ number and thus support the immune system to eradicate invasive germs.

In this complex interplay, an anti-infective coating of implants can provide an adjuvant protection of the implant surface from colonization, while supporting the immune system to reduce local germs.

9.3.6 Coating Strategies

In principle, it is possible to prevent germ colonization of the implant by manipulating its surface. These anti-adhesive coatings can be manufactured physically, chemically or biologically. If the coating consists partly or completely of anti-infective agents, germs are meant to be killed upon implant surface contact. If the anti-infective agent is eluted from the coating, the resulting eluate protects not only the implant surface, but the surrounding tissues as well. Both coating technologies can be intelligently combined, depending on the intended use.

There are innovative solutions (see ◘ Tab. 9.4) for the local antimicrobial protection of metallic implant surfaces with or without a carrier matrix, degradable or non-degradable:

1. Passive surface modifications (e.g. super-hydrophobic, anti-adhesive)
2. Carrier systems with incorporated antimicrobial agents
3. Antimicrobial agents included in porous organic or inorganic surfaces (e.g. hydroxylapatite or calcium phosphate coatings)
4. Antimicrobial heavy metals or heavy metal salts with or without an additional layer
5. Antimicrobial non-metal surfaces (iodine, selenium, peptides, enzymes)
6. Self-adhesive antimicrobiotical coatings (low-soluble antimicrobial fatty salts, AntibiotiCoat®, Heraeus Medical)

Tab. 9.4 Overview of coating strategies

Concept	Function/Claim	Carrier	Examples	References
Manipulating implant surfaces (passive surface modification)	Physical, chemical or biological adaptations that prevent/reduce bacterial adhesions	w/o Fig. 9.4a)	Albumin	An et al. 1996
			Hydrogels	Rivardo et al. 2009; Pandit et al. 2013
			Bio-surfactants	Rodrigues et al. 2006
			Super-hydrophobic surface	Stallard et al. 201[illegible]; Braem et al. 2014; Zhu et al. 2014
			Nano-patterned surface	Truong et al. 201[illegible]; Xue et al. 2010; Bacakova et al. 2011; Singh et al. 201[illegible]; Lu et al. 2012; Shida et al. 2013
		w Fig. 9.4b)	Anti-adhesive polymers	Kaper et al. 200[illegible]; Harris et al. 2004; Zhang et al. 2008; Neoh and Kang 2011; Follmann et al. 2012; Muszanska et al. 2014
			Albumin	An et al. 1996
			Hydrogels	Pandit et al. 2013; Zhao et al. 2013; Drago et al. 2014
			Bio-surfactants	Rodrigues et al. 2006
The various coating strategies depicted above can be combined in many different variations (e.g. hydrogels and antibiotics).				Rodrigues et al. 2006; Zhao et al. 2013; Drago et al. 2014
Antimicrobial agents (active surface finishing/modification)	Pharmacologically activated coatings supposed to kill microorganisms upon »contact killing«	w/o Fig. 9.5a)	Antimicrobial heavy metal or heavy metal salts anorganic, non-specific):	
			Silver (ions)	Massè et al. 2000; Coester et al. 2006; Hardes et al. 2010; Glehr et al. 2013; Wafa et al. 2015; Wilding et al. 2016
			Copper (ions)	Grass et al. 2011; Hans et al. 2013; Hoene et al. 2013
			Zinc (ions)	Petrini et al. 2006
			Titanium dioxide	Kosek et al. 2013
			Antimicrobial non-metal surfaces (anorganic, non-specific):	
			Antiseptics (chlorhexidine, octenidine)	Obermeier et al. 2015

Tab. 9.4 (Continued)

Concept	Function/Claim	Carrier	Examples	References
Antimicrobial agents (active surface finishing/ modification)	Pharmacologically activated coatings supposed to kill micro-organisms upon »contact killing«	w/o Fig. 9.5a)	Ions (iodine, selenium, grapheme)	Shirai et al. 2011; Tran and Webster 2011; Tsuchiya et al. 2012; Holinka et al. 2013; Shirai et al. 2014; Demura et al. 2015; Kabata et al. 2015; Shirai et al. 2016
			Radicals (nitric oxide)	Choi and Hu 2008
Active elution of antimicrobial agents (perioperative modification)	Pharmacologically activated coatings that elute biocides and kill micro-organisms in the local environment	w Fig. 9.5b)	Carrier systems with incorporated antimicrobial agents (organic):	
			Synthetically produced antimicrobial peptides (AMPs; e.g. defensin, protegrin, magainin, indolicin, cytokines, chitosan derivatives)	Costa et al. 2011; Li and McKeague 2011; Norowski et al. 2011; Yount and Yeaman 2012; Renoud et al. 2012; Holmberg et al. 2013 Thallinger et al. 2013; Costa et al. 2014; Magetsari et al. 2014; Pérez-Anes et al. 2015; Onaizi and Leong 2016
			Antibiotics	Gollwitzer et al. 2003; Alt et al. 2006; Schmidmaier et al. 2006; Antoci et al. 2007; Fei et al. 2011; Neut et al. 2012; Shchukin and Mohwald 2013; Sörensen et al. 2014; Metsemakers et al. 2015; Neut et al. 2015
			Antibodies (immunoglobulin G, IgG)	Lim et al. 2011
			Lytic bacteriophages	Thallinger et al. 2013
			Antimicrobial agents included in porous organic or inorganic surfaces:	
			Hydroxyapatite	Darouiche et al. 1998; Campbell et al. 2000; Kozlovsky et al. 2006; Matl et al. 2009; Akiyama et al. 2013; Obermaier et al. 2014; Zhou et al. 2014; Eto et al. 2015
			Calcium phosphate coatings	Yamamura et al. 1992; Gautier et al. 2000
			Antimicrobial heavy metal or heavy metal salts (anorganic, non-specific):	
			Silver (ions)	Cheng et al. 2014; Gao et al. 2014; Eto et al. 2016
			Copper (ions)	Shirai et al. 2009; Kim et al. 2011
			Zinc (ions)	Huang et al. 2008; Aydin Sevinç and Hanley 2010; Elizabeth et al. 2014

			Titanium dioxide	Haenle et al. 2011
			Antimicrobial non-metal surfaces (anorganic, non-specific):	
			Antiseptics (chlorhexidine, octenidine)	Obermeier et al. 2015
			Ions (iodine, selenium, grapheme)	Rodríguez-Valencia et al. 2013; Martynkova et al. 2014
			Radicals (nitric oxide)	Page et al. 2009; Xue et al. 2010
		w (Fig. 9.6a)	Self-adhesive antimicrobial coating that completely degrades (organic):	
			Fast-resorbable hydrogel coatings, »Defensive Antibacterial Coating« (DAC®)	Drago et al. 2014
			Self-adhesive antibimicrobial coating that remains in the body(organic, AntibiotiCoat®)	
			Sol-gel coatings loaded with antibiotics	Tang et al. 2012
			Non-biodegradable polymethylmethacrylate (PMMA) loaded with antibiotics	Buchholz and Engelbrecht 1970; Klemm 1979; Guillaume et al. 2012; Kühn 2013; Kühn et al. 2016
		w/o (Fig. 9.6b)	Self-adhesive antimicrobial coating that completely degrades (organic):	
			Low-soluble antimicrobial fatty salts	Vogt et al. 2005; Matl et al. 2008; Obermaier et al. 2012; Kühn 2014
			Bone chips	Coraca-Huber et al. 2014, 2015
The various coating strategies depicted above can be combined in many different variations.				Buchholz and Engelbrecht 1970; Klemm 1979; Guillaume et al. 2012; Tang et al. 2012; Kühn 2013; Costa et al. 2014; Magetsari et al. 2014; Metsemakers et al. 2015; Neut et al. 2015; Pérez-Anes et al. 2015; Eto et al. 2016; Kühn et al. 2016; Onaizi and Leong 2016

Coating concepts with (*w*) or without (*w/o*) carrier. Most of the current strategies are only scientifically proven and further clinical tests are necessary. From a legal regulatory point of view, carrier systems might be problematic, since they remain in the body even after the agents are long gone and since it is not known what side effects they might cause in the long term

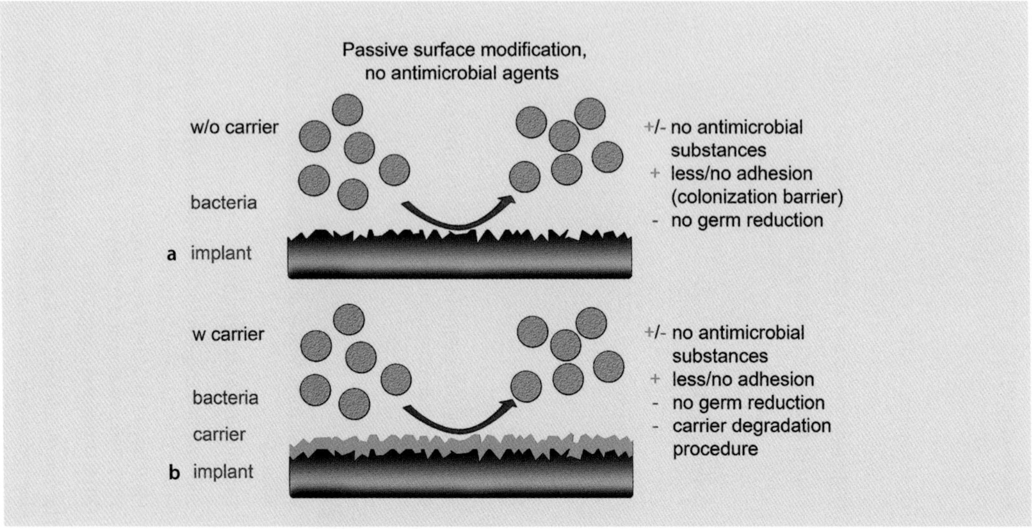

▪ **Fig. 9.4 a,b** Manipulating implant surfaces (passive surface modification). *w/o* without, *w* with

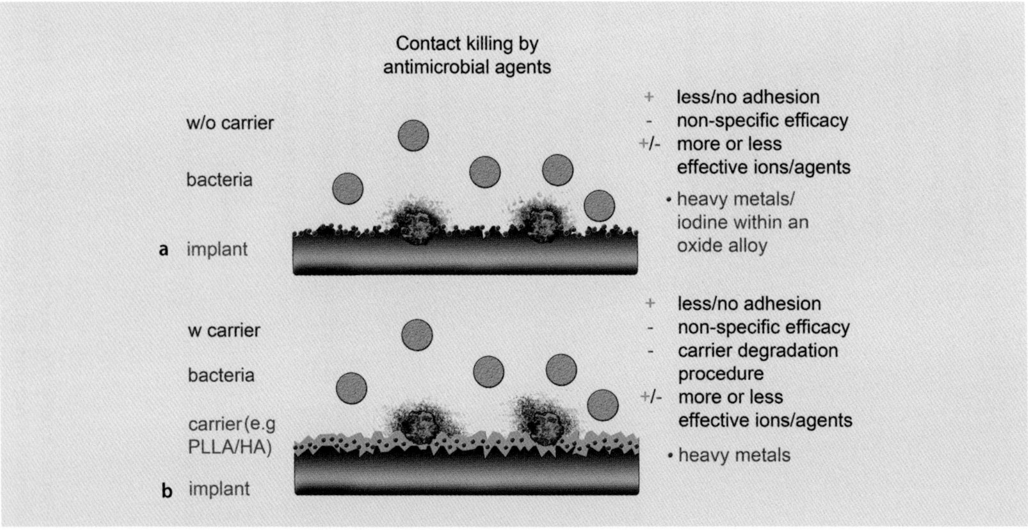

▪ **Fig. 9.5 a,b** Coatings containing antimicrobial agents (active surface finishing/modification); *PLLA* Poly-L-lactide acid *HA* hydroxyapatite

In the following section, regulatory aspects, a novel coating strategy and in vitro as well as in vivo evaluation test methods will be presented.

9.3.7 Regulatory Aspects of Antibiotic Coatings

The intraoperative management of implant-associated infections represents an important clinical problem that still awaits a solution (Adams et al. 2009; Jennings et al. 2015; Qayyum and Khan 2016). There are certainly products on the market that address this problem.

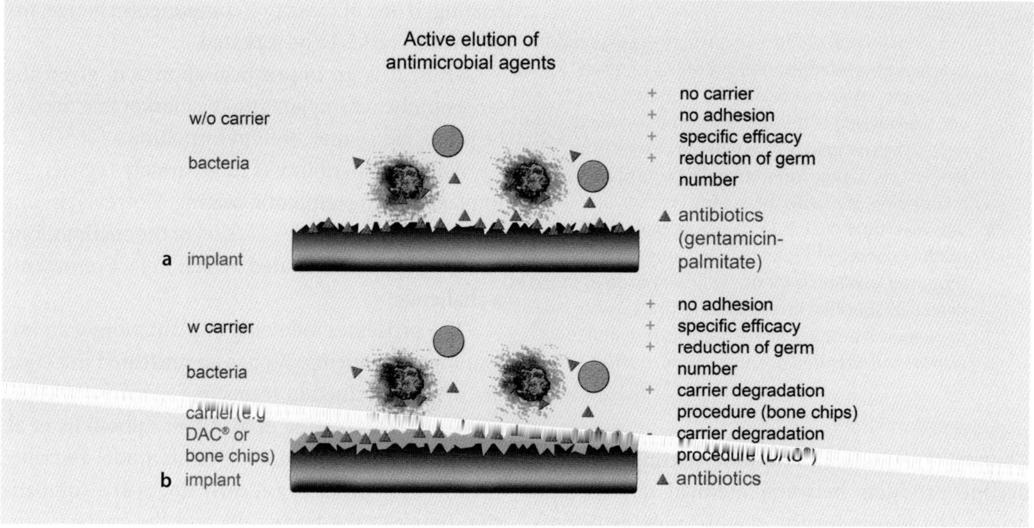

Fig. 9.6 a,b Coatings that actively elute antimicrobial agents (perioperative modification). *w/o* without, *w* with

The most widespread and evident example for a successful symbiosis of biomaterials and antimicrobials is antibiotic-loaded PMMA bone cement (ALBC), an acrylic material for the fixation of metallic implants in the body. The addition of antibiotics to PMMA cement began in 1969 (Buchholz and Engelbrecht 1970; Wahlig and Buchholz 1972). The principle of ALBCs as a colonization barrier for germs (Frommelt and Kühn 2005; Kühn et al. 2016) is an excellent basis for the medical implant coating concept. As a proof of concept for the anti-infective properties of antibiotic-loaded cement, a recent meta-analysis with a large sample size in the United States founds a significant reduction of infection risk when bone cements containing antibiotics were used in primary or revision surgery (Parvizi et al. 2008).

ALBCs elute antibiotics locally, thus preventing side effects that are normally associated with systemic administration of these drugs.

From a legal perspective, these products are classified as medical devices and are approved as combination products due to their pharmaceutical component.

9.3.8 What Is a Combination Product?

In general, combination products consist of a combination of drugs, devices, and/or biological products. Since they contain components usually regulated under different types of regulatory authorities, it remains a challenge to categorize them. However, an exact definition of combination products is needed, especially because the regulations related to the different components have an impact on further processes such as preclinical testing, marketing, and so on.

According to 21 CFR 3.2 (e), a combination product is defined by:

1. A product comprising two or more regulated components (i.e. drug/device, biologic/device, drug/biologic, or drug/device/biologic) that are physically, chemically, or otherwise combined or mixed and produced as a single entity
2. Two or more separate products packaged together in a single package or as a unit and comprising drug and device products, device and biological products, or biological and drug products
3. A drug, device, or biological product packaged separately that according to its investigational plan or proposed labelling is intended for use only with an approved individually specified drug, de-

vice, or biological product where both are required to achieve the intended use, indication, or effect and where, upon approval of the proposed product, the labelling of the approved product would need to be changed (e.g. to reflect a change in intended use, dosage form, strength, route of administration, or significant change in dose)

4. Any investigational drug, device, or biological product packaged separately that according to its proposed labelling is for use only with another individually specified investigational drug, device, or biological product where both are required to achieve the intended use, indication, or effect

Thus by their nature, antibiotic coatings are borderline products between medical devices and drugs. The reason for the classification as devices lies in their primary mode of action, namely, the mechanical fixation of the prosthesis. If this is mechanical in nature and the function of the drug is only ancillary, then the product can be registered as a medical device, which is of course favourable for the manufacturer in most cases in view of time to market and regulatory requirements. If this primary mechanical function is missing, as in the case of PMMA chains for the treatment of osteomyelitis for the sake of argument, the product has to be regarded as a drug.

9.3.9 Primary Mode of Action

If the implant is not mechanically anchored by a polymer matrix, as in the case of cemented arthroplasty, the biofilm protection cannot be combined with this mechanical fixation effect. This is the case if the implant is coated by an antibiotic or antimicrobial formulation in order to protect its surface against biofilm formation. In these situations, there are two potential pathways to get the product approved as a medical device. One rather obvious route would be to combine the coating with the implant and use the mechanical function of the implant as primary mode of action and the protection of the surface by the antimicrobial agent as ancillary pharmaceutical effect. The disadvantage of this approach is that, strictly speaking, it is only valid for the very combination of the described implant and coating. If any of these two components change, the procedure needs to be repeated.

Thus, it is an impractical approach, given the large number of implants on the market that need to be protected against biofilm formation.

Another possibility is to separately register the implant and the antibiotic coating. However, in this case the primary mode of action of the coating alone needs to be demonstrated, which in fact represents a challenge.

The processes following implantation of an implant into a patient who has an untreated infection are often described in terms of a »race for the surface« model (Gristina et al. 1988; Tsibouklis et al. 2000; Subbiahdoss et al. 2009). This model describes the infection processes at early stages as a competition between the bone cells and the bacteria surrounding the implant for adhering to the newly implanted surface. If the bone cells are faster in covering this surface, the osseointegration of the new implant proceeds normally. If the bacteria manage to adhere to the surface first, the processes of biofilm formation starts, leading to septic failure of the implantation. By coating the implant, the colonization of the surface can be prevented effectively (Ivanova et al. 2015). From a regulatory perspective, the question remains regarding which is the primary mode of action in this case.

From ◘ Fig. 9.7, one can derive the two major functions such a coating combines.

Mode of action of coating implants (combination products)

1. Barrier function of the coating (primary mode of action)
2. Pharmacological function of the antibiotic (ancillary function)

The second function is clearly a pharmacological (adjuvant) effect, while the first one is physical in nature. The challenge is now to demonstrate the relative contribution of each effect to the total biofilm prevention function of the coating. The goal is to prove that the physical barrier function is dominant and the pharmacological function of the antibiotic substance is ancillary to this effect. To address this issue, we developed an experimental function model, which is described in the next section.

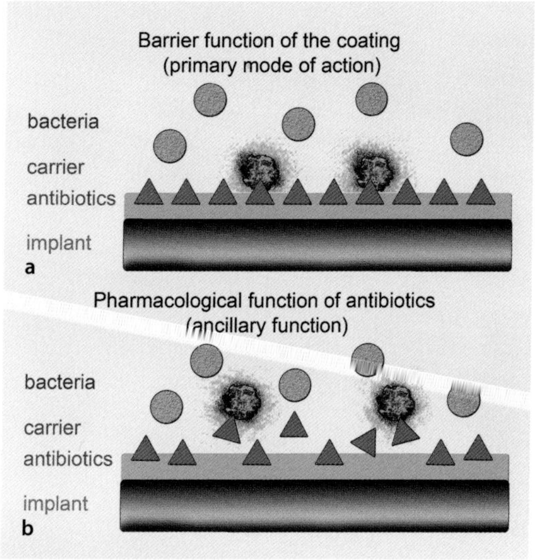

Fig. 9.7 Antibiotic coating functions: **a** barrier function of the coating (primary mode of action); **b** pharmacological function of the antibiotic (ancillary function)

9.3.10 Experimental Function Model

To prove that the primary mode of action of a coating formulation is to function as a physical barrier, an adhesion assay can be performed. In a general test set-up, the samples are firstly incubated with a germ solution. Afterwards, the loose non-adherent cells are rinsed off in a washing step. Finally, the remaining germs are labelled and detected by ELISA (Fig. 9.8).

The result thus obtained is the relative adherence of bacteria on coated implants compared with the uncoated reference (Fig. 9.9). In the depicted example, it was proven that the tested plain AB-free coating lowered the bacterial adhesion capability by 47%. The same material containing 10% gentamicin sulphate further improved this result to a 70% reduced bacterial adhesion. As a proof of concept, the primary mode of action of the tested coating formulations is a physical barrier.

Another method for examining the barrier function is applied, for example, for wound dressings and might be adapted to coatings (Fig. 9.10):

> » In this method, the test material is clamped between two flanged glass chambers, each filled with a liquid culture medium. A broth culture, containing a very small rod-shaped species of bacteria, is added to the fluid in one of the chambers and the apparatus incubated for a period of up to 7 days. During this time the culture medium is examined daily for evidence of bacterial transfer through the test material, as shown by turbidity of the liquid medium in the other chamber.« (http://www.smtl.co.uk/testing-services/46-biological/133-bacterial-and-bacteriophage-barrier-testing.html)

Such primary tests for barrier capabilities need further optimization in order to demonstrate the fate of remaining adherent bacteria or those that were able to penetrate the coating. In a functional physical barrier, the bacteria should be absent below the coating and ideally not even located within it. If bacteria were able to penetrate through the coating, the coating should provide protection against biofilm formation on the implant surface.

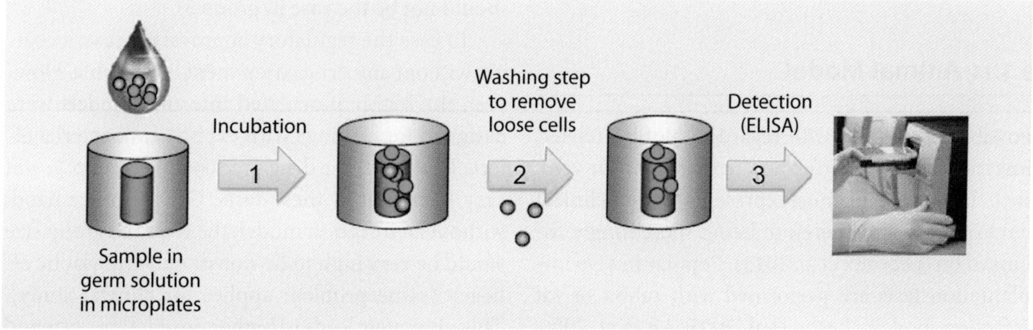

Fig. 9.8 Schematic test set-up of an adhesion assay (image courtesy of QualityLabs BT GmbH, Nuremberg, Germany)

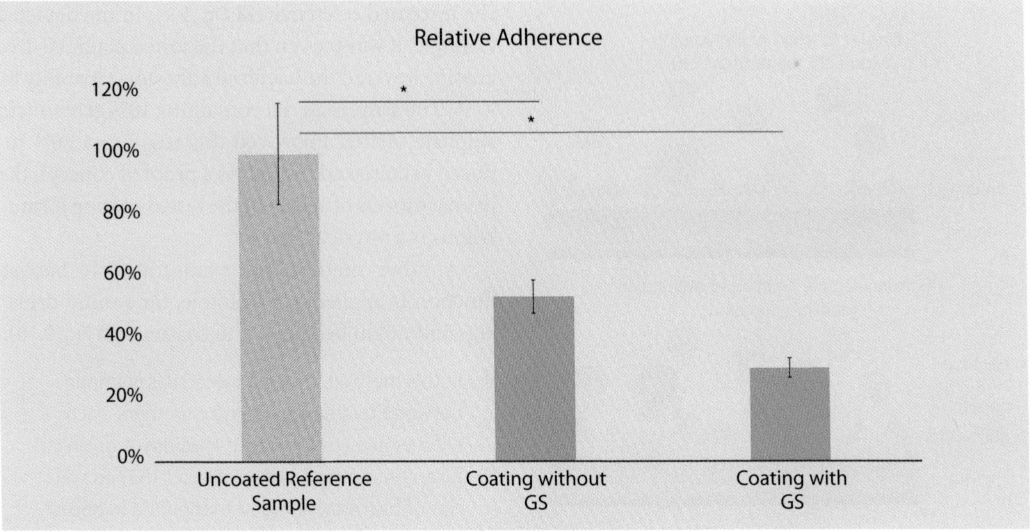

Fig. 9.9 Relative adherence of *S. aureus* to the surface of titanium screws. *Left*: uncoated reference; *centre*: coating without gentamicin sulphate (*GS*); *right*: coating with 10% gentamicin sulphate. *Error bars*: SEM; *$p<0.01$ (ANOVA, post hoc Dunnett's test); $N=7$

9

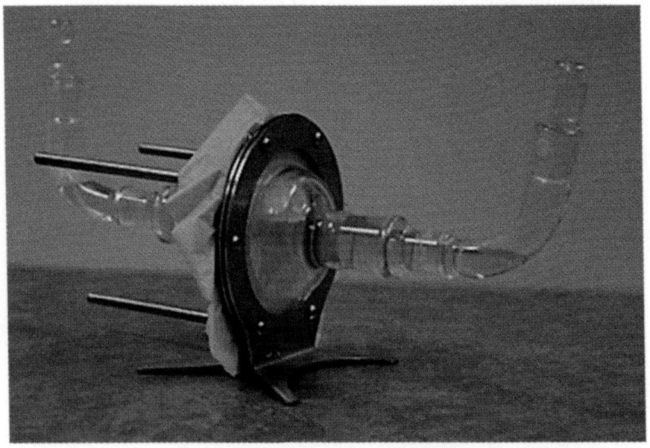

Fig. 9.10 Test set-up for evaluation of the bacterial barrier properties of wound dressings (image courtesy of the Surgical Materials Testing Laboratory, SMTL, Bridgend, UK)

9.3.11 Animal Model

Possible test set-ups with regard to biofilm-related infections can be performed in vitro and in vivo, with the latter being more representative of a clinical environment and therefore being increasingly focussed on (Lebeaux et al. 2013). Popular in vivo implantation tests are performed with rabbit or rat infection models (Lucke et al. 2005; Alt et al. 2006; Giavaresi et al. 2014; Neut et al. 2015; Fölsch et al. 2015, 2016). With respect to the regulatory requirements, we recommend to generally include three test groups.

Animal Test Groups

1. Uncoated implant
2. Implant with antibiotic-free coating
3. Implant with antibiotic-containing coating

Ideally, (control) group 1 should show the formation of a biofilm, while on group 2 implants, significantly less viable/no bacteria should be found. If any viable bacteria were detected in group 2, this should not be the case in group 3.

To ease the regulatory approval process, a coating without any drug component is desirable. However, the highly inoculated infection models were designed for coatings with explicit antibacterial effect. Therefore, the drug-free coating (group 2) will very likely fail in these tests. On the other hand, without an infection model, the required group size would be very high to demonstrate prophylactic efficacy (same problem applies for clinical study). This ultimately leads to higher production costs and may prevent the development of promising prod-

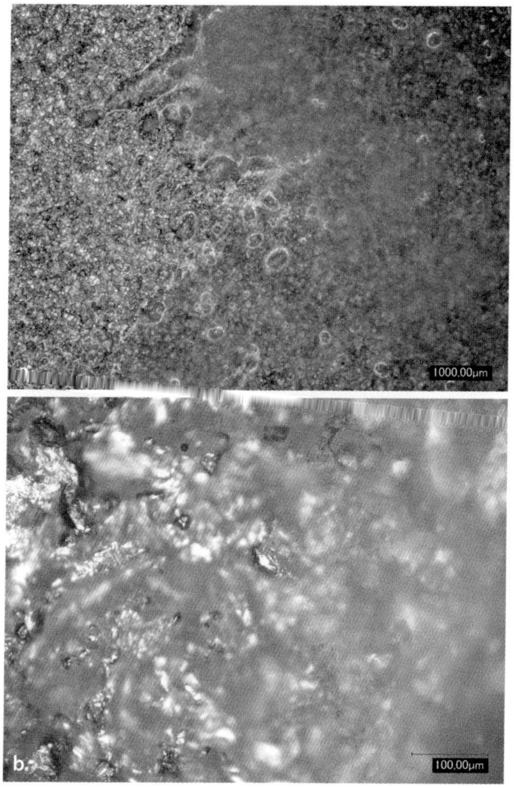

Fig. 9.11 **a**,**b** Microscopic images showing an implant with ×50 (**a**) and ×500 (**b**) magnification. The *left side* of each image shows an uncoated and the *right side* a coated region

ucts at all owing to commercial reasons. The authors denote a conflict of interest between regulatory bodies and medical device companies, to the chagrin of patients.

9.3.12 Osseointegration

A resorbable coating should not negatively influence the osseointegration of implants. In liquid or semi-liquid coatings of rough implants (Fig. 9.11), the majority of the applied material flows in the valleys, while a thinner layer remains on the pikes (Fig. 9.12). Thus, the coating will be firstly resorbed at the spikes, thereby allowing the host cells to attach and start bone ingrowth. It is of utmost importance to investigate this process in vivo. This has been addressed in the form of a pull-out test in a canine condylar defect model (Neut et al. 2015), as

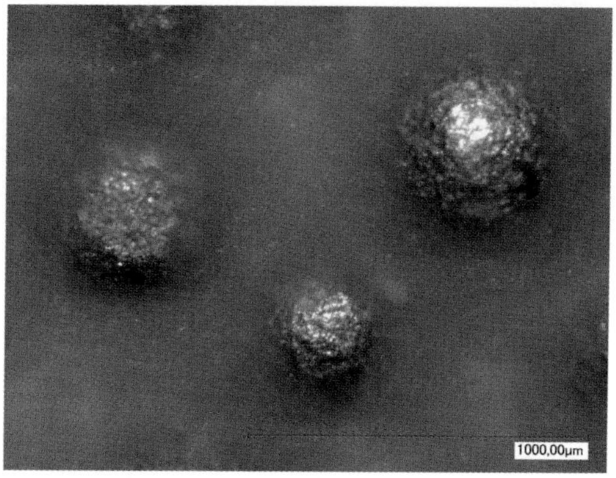

Fig. 9.12 Microscopic image of a coated implant with ×2,000 magnification

well as in a histological and histomorphometrical approach (Giavaresi et al. 2014). Recent progress has been made in monitoring osseointegration in live animals using acoustic sound analysis (Ruther et al. 2014).

We examined gentamicin palmitate (GP)-coated implants in an animal model on rabbits 4 weeks after implantation and found no osteolysis, no inflammation and no differences in osseointegration between the coated (54.5 %) and uncoated (55.5 %) test design.

Generally, more work needs to be done in this direction in order to provide the basis for a widely acceptable model of the efficacy of antibiotic coatings for implants.

9.3.13 Elution Profile

For antimicrobial examinations, the use of standardized flat discs (diameter of 15.6 mm), the amount of dissolution medium and the sample analysis points were recommended. Uncoated titanium discs as well as ALBC discs were used as references.

9.3.14 Coating Principles for Gentamicin Palmitate

The technique of transferring water-soluble gentamicin sulphate into low-soluble gentamicin fatty acid salts is a prerequisite for using it as a pure coat-

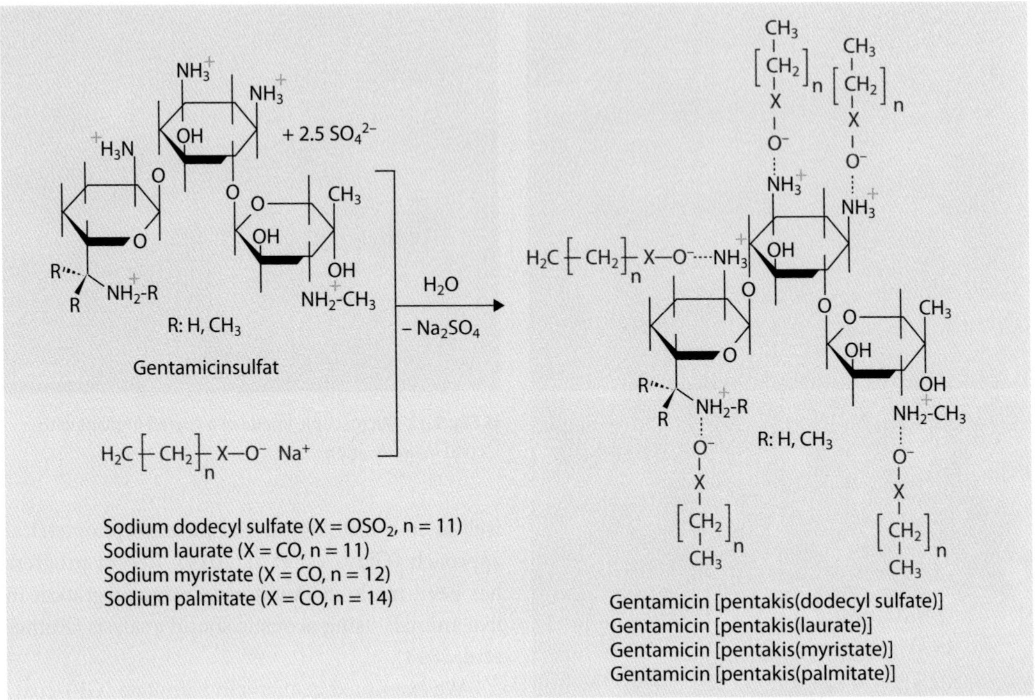

Fig. 9.13 Gentamicin fatty acids (Vogt et al. 2005)

ing material without an additional matrix. Ion exchange easily facilitates the conversion of gentamicin sulphate into gentamicin fatty acid salts. This process replaces sulphate ions with fatty acid anions (Fig. 9.13). Suitable fatty acid anions include laurate, myristate and palmitate. During the ion exchange process, the protonated gentamicin base (GB) remains unchanged. The process does not chemically alter the antimicrobial active GB (Kühn et al. 2003; Vogt et al. 2005). Furthermore, the ratio of gentamicin C1 to C1a and C2a+b is not modified. Gentamicin fatty acid salts are waxy solids exhibiting extensive adhesion properties on a multitude of surfaces in thin layers. Fatty acid anions are non-toxic and are metabolized in the human organism by beta-oxidation, thereby generating carbon dioxide and aqua (Kühn and Vogt 2007).

Solid GP is characterized as a white-to-yellow coloured fine crystalline, free-flowing powder. The GP powder is chemically based on gentamicin sulphate powder as described in the *European Pharmacopoeia*, and was dissolved in an ethanol solution. This solution was utilized in a spray or as a dipping process for the coating of implants. Evenly thin coatings can be placed by spraying, provided the endoprostheses are warmed at approx. 80–90°C before coating. The GP coating hereby proved to be a waxy solid matter, which adhered easily to the surfaces. Load content of approx. 50–250 µg of gentamicin base per cm^2 surface were easily produced on titanium endoprosthesis surfaces.

The discs – e.g. coated with GP according to Vogt et al. (2005) – were coated with different amounts of gentamicin (low and high level, e.g. 100 µg and 220 µg GB/cm^2) by using a special process described by Matl et al. (2008). The coating content of each separate sample was determined by weight.

All samples used as test samples were sterilized The flat discs were stored at 37°C in 4.33 ml dissolution medium (0.1 M phosphate buffer, pH 7.4). Aliquots were taken and dissolution medium was renewed at the following sampling points: 1 h, 6 h and after 24 h daily, until no more elution was detectable. The dissolution medium samples were stored at –20°C until analysis.

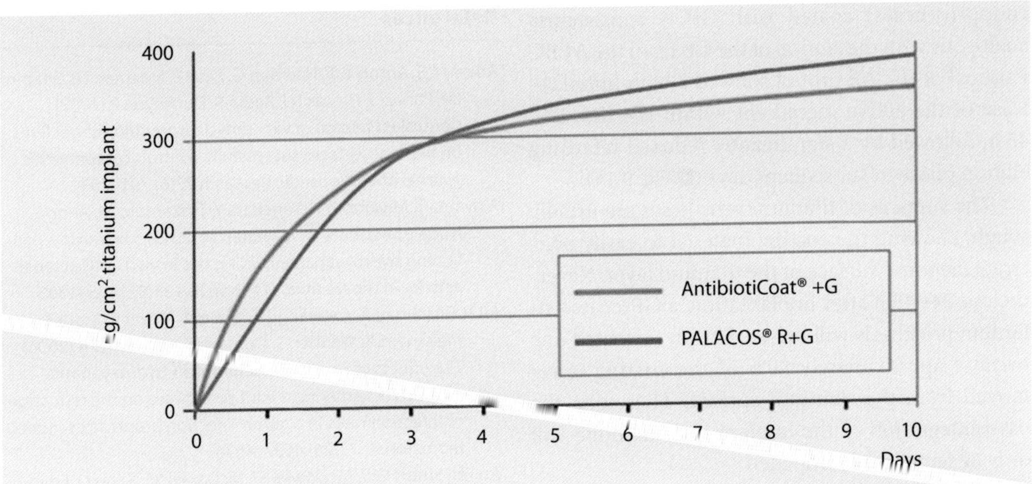

Fig. 9.14 Gentamicin release Palacos® R+G versus Gentamicin palmitate-coated (AntibiotiCoat® +G) titanium discs (Kühn 2014)

To determine the amount of the eluted active ingredient (Analytisches Zentrum Berlin) according to Heller et al. (2005), 100 µl of the eluate was analyzed via fluorescent polarization in the TDx system (Figureott TDx system, Figureott Park, Ill.). The data of the eluted gentamicin (as base) are in µg/test sample.

Ten calibration standards from 100 to 7,500 ng/ml for gentamicin including a zero (blank without internal standard) as well as a blank sample (blank with internal standard) were prepared by spiking 200 µl of working solutions (containing different gentamicin concentrations, respectively) with corresponding internal standard working solutions (18 µl for gentamicin). These solutions were used for liquid chromatography–tandem mass spectrometry (LC-MS/MS) analysis.

The study samples were diluted by a factor of 20 and prepared according to the calibration standards by adding internal standard working solution. Every sample was analysed three times.

Concerning the LC-MS/MS conditions, chromatographic separation was performed on a modular HPLC 1200 Series (Agilent Technologies, Waldbronn, Germany) using a Luna C18 (II) column, 150×2 mm, with two C18, 4×2 mm, guard columns (Phenomenex, Aschaffenburg, Germany) thermostated at 25°C. Injection volume was 2 µl. For gentamicin, the mobile phase A was 0.11 M trifluoroacetic acid/methanol (50:50) and the mobile phase B was acetonitrile. For gentamicin, an isocratic separation was achieved with an A:B ratio of 95:5 at a flow rate of 0.25 ml/min. The run time was 2.5 min and the total cycle time was less than 3 min.

Under the described conditions, the four gentamicin components C1, C2, C2a and C1a co-eluted. The HPLC method was previously used by Heller et al. (2005) to determine gentamicin in biopsy samples. The co-eluted gentamicin components were detected by using an API 4000 QTrap system (Applied Biosystems, Darmstadt, Germany). Ionization was carried out with an electrospray interface (positive polarity) using the mass selective detector in the multiple reaction monitoring mode (MRM). The extracted ion chromatograms of the following ion transitions were stored and calculated: 478.4 → 322.3 m/z (gentamicin C1), 464.4 → 322.3 m/z (gentamicin C2 and C2a), 450.3 → 322.3 m/z (gentamicin C1a.) and 468.4 → 163.1 m/z (internal standard). The three ion transitions of gentamicin components were summed using the software Analyst 1.4.2 (Applied Biosystems, Darmstadt, Germany) and calculated with Excel (Microsoft, Unterschleißheim, Germany).

Scanning electron microscopy (SEM) pictures of the coated and uncoated titanium discs were indicated.

We found that the release behaviour of GB from titanium surfaces (discs sample from cementless endoprostheses) coated with GP is consistently analogous with the elution of the GB from the ALBC Palacos® R+G. All probes showed a high initial release of the active ingredient within the first 24–48 h, followed by a significantly reduced retarding elution phase in subsequent days (▣ Fig. 9.14).

The surfaces of titanium prostheses are usually rough, allowing the coating material to easily penetrate the inner surface of the titanium layer. Nevertheless, 24–48 h after implantation, a GP-coated titanium prosthesis will behave like an uncoated one because approximately 90% of the coating is removed from the titanium surface. Therefore, the osseointegration of the implant into the bone will only be temporarily impeded.

Take-Home Message

- From a regulatory perspective, ALBC as well as coated implants are classified as medical devices and are approved as combination products due to their pharmaceutical component.
- For antimicrobial coating products sold separately, registration as medical device is very challenging.
- Comprehensive experimental models addressing the regulatory requirements are not yet available.
- Preventing biofilm formation on implants is the key of success of antimicrobial implant coatings.
- An anti-infective coating acts as a colonization barrier for germs.
- The principle of ALBCs as a colonization barrier for germs is an excellent basis for the medical implant coating concept.
- An anti-infective coating influences the »race for the surface« for a short period of time and supports the immune system with germ eradication.
- Claim of antimicrobial coating: help to reduce the risk of infection.
- The mode of action of antiseptics, heavy metals, phenols, alcohols and AMPs is non-specific against bacteria.
- Only the mode of action of antibiotics is specific against bacteria.
- The legal consequence of a customized combination product is that the surgeon becomes the responsible manufacturer and thus assumes liability for the product.
- In revision THR/TKR, the fundamental therapeutic measure is the surgery, the adjuvant treatment with antibiotics reduces the number of germs and supports the immune system.

9

References

Adams CS, Antoci V Jr, Harrison G, Patal P, Freeman TA, Shapiro IM, Parvizi J, Hickok NJ, Radin S, Ducheyne P (2009) Controlled release of vancomycin from thin sol-gel films on implant surfaces successfully controls osteomyelitis. Journal of Orthopaedic Research 27(6):701–709

Akiyama T, Miyamoto H, Yonekura Y, Tsukamoto M, Ando Y, Noda I, Sonohata M, Mawatari M (2013) Silver oxide-containing hydroxyapatite coating has in vivo antibacterial activity in the rat tibia. J Orthop Res 31(8):1195–1200

Alt V, Bitschnau A, Osterling J, Sewing A, Meyer C, Kraus R, Meissner SA, Wenisch S, Domann E, Schnettler R (2006) The effects of combined gentamicin-hydroxyapatite coating for cementless joint prostheses on the reduction of infection rates in a rabbit infection prophylaxis model. Biomaterials 27(26):4627–4634

An YH, Stuart GW, McDowell SJ, McDaniel SE, Kang Q, Friedman RJ (1996) Prevention of bacterial adherence to implant surfaces with a crosslinked albumin coating in vitro. J Orthop Res 14(5):846–849

Antoci V Jr, Adams CS, Parvizi J, Ducheyne P, Shapiro IM, Hickok NJ (2007) Covalently attached vancomycin provides a nanoscale antibacterial surface. Clin Orthop Relat Res 461:81–87

Aydin Sevinç B, Hanley L (2010) Antibacterial activity of dental composites containing zinc oxide nanoparticles. J Biomed Mater Res B Appl Biomater 94(1):22–31

Bacakova L, Filova E, Parizek M, Ruml T, Svorcik V (2011) Modulation of cell adhesion, proliferation and differentiation on materials designed for body implants. Biotechnol Adv 29:739–767

Bacterial and Viral Barrier Testing (2014) SMTL, South Wales. http://www.smtl.co.uk/testing-services/46-biological/133-bacterial-and-bacteriophage-barrier-testing.html

Bozic KJ, Ries MD (2005) The impact of infection after total hip arthroplasty on hospital and surgeon resource utilization. J Bone Joint Surg Am 87(8):1746–1751

Braem A, van Mellaert L, Mattheys T, Hofmans D, de Waelheyns E, Geris L, Anné J, Schrooten J, Vleugels J (2014) Staphylococcal biofilm growth on smooth and porous titanium coatings for biomedical applications. J Biomed Mater Res A 102(1):215–224

Buchholz HW, Engelbrecht H (1970) [Depot effects of various antibiotics mixed with Palacos resins]. Chirurg 41:511–515

Campbell AA, Song L, Li XS, Nelson BJ, Bottoni C, Brooks DE, et al (2000) Development, characterization, and anti-microbial efficacy of hydroxyapatitechlorhexidine coatings produced by surface-induced mineralization. J Biomed Mater Res 53(4):400–407

CFR - Code of Federal Regulations Title 21 (2011) FDA, Silver Spring. http://www.fda.gov/CombinationProducts/AboutCombinationProducts/ucm118332.htm

Cheng H, Li Y, Huo K, Gao B, Xiong W (2014) Long-lasting in vivo and in vitro antibacterial ability of nanostructured titania coating incorporated with silver nanoparticles. J Biomed Mater Res A 102(10):3488–3499

Choi O, Hu Z (2008) Size dependent and reactive oxygen species related nanosilver toxicity to nitrifying bacteria. Environ Sci Technol 42(12):4583–4588

Coester LM, Nepola JV, Allen J, Marsh JL (2006) The effects of silver coated external fixation pins. Iowa Orthop J 26: 48–53

Coraca-Huber DC, Ammann CG, Nogler M, Wurm A, Fille M, Frommelt L, Kühn KD, Fölsch C (2015) Lyophilized allogeneic bone tissue as an antibiotic carrier. Cell Tissue Bank doi:10.1007/s10561-016-9582-5

Coraca-Huber DC, Wurm A, Fille M, Hausdorfer J, Nogler M, Kühn KD (2014) Effect of freezing on the release rate of gentamicin palmitate and gentamicin sulfate from bone tissue. J Orthop Res 32(6):842–847

Costa F, Carvalho IF, Montelaro RC, Gomes P, Martins MC (2011) Covalent immobilization of antimicrobial peptides (AMPs) onto biomaterial surfaces. Acta Biomaterialia 7(4):1431–1440

Costa F, Maia S, Gomes P, Martins MC (2014) Characterization of hLF1-11 immobilization onto chitosan ultrathin films, and its effects on antimicrobial activity. Acta Biomater 10(8):3513–3521

Darouiche RO (2001) Device-Associated Infections: A Macroproblem that Starts with Microadherence. Clin Infect Dis 33:1567–1572

Darouiche RO, Green G, Mansouri MD (1998) Antimicrobial activity of antiseptic-coated orthopaedic device. Int J Antimicrob Agents 10(1):83–86

Demura S, Murakami H, Shirai T, Kato S, Yoshioka K, Ota T, Ishii T, Igarashi T, Tsuchiya H (2015) Surgical treatment for pyogenic vertebral osteomyelitis using iodine-supported spinal instruments: initial case series of 14 patients. Eur J Clin Microbiol Infect Dis 34(2):261–266

Drago L, Boot W, Dimas K, Malizos K, Hänsch GM, Stuyck J, Gawlitta D, Romanò CL (2014) Does implant coating with antibacterial-loaded hydrogel reduce bacterial colonization and biofilm formation in vitro? Clin Orthop Relat Res 472(11):3311–3323

Elizabeth E, Baranwal G, Krishnan AG, Menon D, Nair M (2014) ZnO nanoparticle incorporated nanostructured metallic titanium for increased mesenchymal stem cell response and antibacterial activity. Nanotechnology doi:10.1088/0957-4484/25/11/115101

Eto S, Miyamoto H, Shobuike T, Noda I, Akiyama T, Tsukamoto M, Ueno M, Someya S, Kawano S, Sonohata M, Mawatari M (2015) Silver oxide-containing hydroxyapatite coating supports osteoblast function and enhances implant anchorage strength in rat femur. J Orthop Res 33(9): 1391–1397

Eto S, Kawano S, Someya S, Miyamoto H, Sonohata M, Mawatari M (2016) First Clinical Experience With Thermal-Sprayed Silver Oxide-Containing Hydroxyapatite Coating Implant. J Arthroplasty 31(7):1498–1503

Fei J, Liu GD, Pan CJ, Chen JY, Zhou YG, Xiao SH, Wang Y, Yu HJ (2011) Preparation, release profiles and antibacterial properties of vancomycin-loaded Ca-P coating titanium alloy plate. J Mater Sci Mater Med 22:989–995

Ferguson TB Jr, Ferguson CL, Crites K, Crimmins-Reda P (1996) The additional hospital costs generated in the management of complications of pacemaker and defibrillator implantations. J Thorac Cardiovasc Surg 111(4):742–752

Follmann HD, Martins AF, Gerola AP, Burgo TA, Nakamura CV, Rubira AF, Muniz EC (2012) Antiadhesive and antibacterial multilayer films via layer-by-layer assembly of TMC/heparin complexes. Biomacromolecules 13(11): 3711–3722

Fölsch C, Federmann M, Kühn KD, Kittinger C, Kogler S, Zarfel G, Kerwat M, Braun S, Fuchs-Winkelmann S, Paletta JR, Roessler PP (2015) Coating with a novel gentamicinpalmitate formulation prevents implant-associated osteomyelitis induced by methicillin-susceptible Staphylococcus aureus in a rat model. Int Orthop 39(5): 981–988

Fölsch C, Federmann M, Lakemeier S, Kühn KD, Kittinger C, Kerwat M, Fuchs-Winkelmann S, Paletta JR, Roessler PP (2016) Systemic antibiotic therapy does not significantly improve outcome in a rat model of implant-associated osteomyelitis induced by Methicillin susceptible Staphylococcus aureus. Arch Orthop Trauma Surg 136(4): 585–592

Frommelt L, Kühn KD (2005) Properties of bone cement: antibiotic-loaded cement. In: Breusch S, Malchau H (eds) The well cemented hip arthroplasty, Springer, Heidelberg, p 86–92

Gao A, Hang R, Huang X, Zhao L, Zhang X, Wang L, Tang B, Ma S, Chu PK (2014) The effects of titania nanotubes with embedded silver oxide nanoparticles on bacteria and osteoblasts. Biomaterials 35(13):4223–4235

Gautier H, Merle C, Auget JL, Daculsi G (2000) Isostatic compression, a new process for incorporating vancomycin into biphasic calcium phosphate: comparison with a classical method. Biomaterials 21(3):243–249

Giavaresi G, Meani E, Sartori M, Ferrari A, Bellini D, Sacchetta AC, Meraner J, Sambri A, Vocale C, Sambri V, Fini M, Romanò CL (2014) Efficacy of antibacterial-loaded coating in an in vivo model of acutely highly contaminated implant. International orthopaedics 38(7):1505–1512

Glehr M, Leithner A, Friesenbichler J, Goessler W, Avian A, Andreou D, Maurer-Ertl W, Windhager R, Tunn PU (2013) Argyria following the use of silver-coated megaprostheses: no association between the development of local argyria and elevated silver levels. Bone Joint J 95–B(7): 988–992

Gollwitzer H, Ibrahim K, Meyer H, Mittelmeier W, Busch R, Stemberger A (2003) Antibacterial poly(D,L-lactic acid) coating of medical implants using a biodegradable drug delivery technology. J Antimicrob Chemother 51(3): 585–591

Grass G, Rensing C, Solioz M (2011) Metallic copper as an antimicrobial surface. Appl Environ Microbiol 77: 1541–1547

Gristina AG, Costerton JW (1985) Bacterial adherence to biomaterials and tissue. The significance of its role in clinical sepsis. J Bone Joint Surg Am 67(2):264–273

Gristina AG, Naylor P, Myrvik Q (1988) Infections from biomaterials and implants: a race for the surface. Med Prog Technol 14(3-4):205–224
Guillaume O, Garric X, Lavigne JP, Van Den Berghe H, Coudane J (2012) Multilayer, degradable coating as a carrier for the sustained release of antibiotics: preparation and antimicrobial efficacy in vitro. J Control Release 162:492–501
Haenle M, Fritsche A, Zietz C, Bader R, Heidenau F, Mittelmeier W et al (2011) An extended spectrum bactericidal titanium dioxide (TiO2) coating for metallic implants: in vitro effectiveness against MRSA and mechanical properties. J Mater Sci Mater Med 22(2):381–387
Hans M, Erbe A, Mathews S, Chen Y, Solioz M, Mücklich F (2013) Role of copper oxides in contact killing of bacteria. Langmuir 29(52):16160–16166
Hardes J, von Eiff C, Streitbuerger A, Balke M, Budny T, Henrichs MP, Hauschild G, Ahrens H (2010) Reduction of periprosthetic infection with silver-coated megaprostheses in patients with bone sarcoma. J Surg Oncol 101(5):389–395
Harris LG, Tosatti S, Wieland M, Textor M, Richards RG (2004) Staphylococcus aureus adhesion to titanium oxide surfaces coated with non-functionalized and peptide-functionalized poly(L-lysine)-grafted-poly(ethylene glycol) copolymers. Biomaterials 25:4135–4148
Hasman H, Kempf I, Chidaine B, Cariolet R, Ersbøll AK, Houe H, Bruun Hansen HC, Aarestrup FM (2006) Copper resistance in Enterococcus faecium, mediated by the tcrB gene, is selected by supplementation of pig feed with copper sulfate. Appl Environ Microbiol 72(9):5784–5789
Heller DN, Peggins JO, Nochetto CB, Smith ML, Chiesa OA, Moulton K (2005) LC/MS/MS measurement of gentamicine in bovine plasma, urine, milk, and biopsy samples taken from kidneys of standing animals. J Chromatogr B 821:22–30
Hoene A, Prinz C, Walschus U, Lucke S, Patrzyk M, Wilhelm L et al (2013) In vivo evaluation of copper release and acute local tissue reactions after implantation of copper-coated titanium implants in rats. Biomedical Mater doi:10.1088/1748-6041/8/3/035009
Holinka J, Pilz M, Kubista B, Presterl E, Windhager R (2013) Effects of selenium coating of orthopaedic implant surfaces on bacterial adherence and osteoblastic cell growth. Bone Joint J 95-B(5):678–682
Holmberg KV, Abdolhosseini M, Li Y, Chen X, Gorr SU, Aparicio C (2013) Bio-inspired stable antimicrobial peptide coatings for dental applications. Acta Biomater 9:8224–8231
Huang Z, Zheng X, Yan D, Yin G, Liao X, Kang Y, Yao Y, Huang D, Hao B (2008) Toxicological effect of ZnO nanoparticles based on bacteria. Langmuir 24(8):4140–4144
Ivanova K, Fernandes MM, Mendoza E, Tzanov T (2015) Enzyme multilayer coatings inhibit Pseudomonas aeruginosa biofilm formation on urinary catheters. Applied Microbiology and Biotechnology 99(10):4373–4385
Jennings JA, Carpenter DP, Troxel KS, Beenken KE, Smeltzer MS, Courtney HS, Haggard WO (2015) Novel Antibiotic-loaded Point-of-care Implant Coating Inhibits Biofilm. Clinical Orthopaedics and Related Research 473(7): 2270–2282
Kabata T, Maeda T, Kajino Y, Hasegawa K, Inoue D, Yamamoto T, Takagi T, Ohmori T, Tsuchiya H (2015) Iodine-Supported Hip Implants: Short Term Clinical Results. Biomed Res Int doi:10.1155/2015/368124
Kaper HJ, Busscher HJ, Norde W (2003) Characterization of poly(ethylene oxide) brushes on glass surfaces and adhesion of Staphylococcus epidermidis. J Biomat Sci Polym Ed 14:313–324
Kim JS, Kuk E, Yu KN, Kim JH, Park SJ, Lee HJ et al (2007) Antimicrobial effects of silver nanoparticles. Nanomed Nanatechnol Biol Med 3(1):95–101
Kim JS, Adamcakova-Dodd A, O'Shaughnessy PT, Grassian VH, Thorne PS (2011) Effects of copper nanoparticle exposure on host defense in a murine pulmonary infection model. Part Fibre Toxicol doi:10.1186/1743-8977-8-29
Kim S (2008) Changes in Surgical Loads and Economic Burden of Hip and Knee Replacements in the US: 1997-2004. Arthritis Rheum 59(4):481–488
Kirkland KB, Briggs JP, Trivette SL, Wilkinson WE, Sexton DJ (1999) The Impact of Surgical-Site Infections in the 1990s: Attributable Mortality, Excess Length of Hospitalization, and Extra Costs. Infect Control Hosp Epidemiol 20(11):725–730
Klemm K (1979) [Gentamicin-PMMA-beads in treating bone and soft tissue infections-(author's transl)]. Zentralbl Chir 104(14):934–942
Koseki H, Asahara T, Shida T, Yoda I, Horiuchi H, Baba K, Osaki M (2013) Clinical and histomorphometrical study on titanium dioxide-coated external fixation pins. Int J Nanomedicine 8:593–599
Kozlovsky A, Artzi Z, Moses O, Kamin-Belsky N, Greenstein RB (2006) Interaction of chlorhexidine with smooth and rough types of titanium surfaces. J Periodontol 77(7):1194–1200
Kühn KD (2013) PMMA Cements. Springer, Heidelberg. ISBN: 978-3-642-41535-7
Kühn KD (2014) Antimicrobial Implant Coating. In: Scholz M (ed) Biofunctional surface engineering, Pan Stanford Publishing, Singapore, p 121–189
Kühn KD, Vogt S (2007) Antimicrobial Implant Coating in Arthroplasty. In: Walenkamp GHIM (ed) Local Antibiotics in Arthroplasty: State of the Art from an Interdisciplinary Point of View, Thieme, Stuttgart, p 23–30
Kühn KD, Vogt S, Schnabelrauch M (2003) Porous implants with antibiotic coating, their preparation and use. EP Patent 1374923 B1, 28 May 2003
Kühn KD, Lieb E, Berberich C (2016) PMMA bone cement: what is the role of local antibiotics? Maîtrise Orthopédique 255:12–18
Lebeaux D, Chauhan A, Rendueles O, Beloin C (2013) From in vitro to in vivo models of bacterial biofilm-related infections. Pathogens 2(2):288–356
Li B, McKeague AL (2011) Emerging ideas: Interleukin-12 nanocoatings prevent open fracture-associated infections. Clin Orthop Relat Res 469(11):3262–3265

9

Lim WH, Seo WW, Choe WS, Kang CK, Park J, Cho HJ, Kyeong S, Hur J, Yang HM, Cho HJ, Lee YS, Kim HS (2011) Stent Coated With Antibody Against Vascular Endothelial-Cadherin Captures Endothelial Progenitor Cells, Accelerates Re-Endothelialization, and Reduces Neointimal Formation. Arterioscler Thromb Vasc Biol 31(12): 2798–2805

Lu T, Qiao Y, Liu X (2012) Surface modification of biomaterials using plasma immersion ion implantation and deposition. Interface Focus 2:325–336

Lucke M, Wildemann B, Sadoni S, Surke C, Schiller R, Stemberger A et al (2005) Systemic versus local application of gentamicin in prophylaxis of implant-related osteomyelitis in a rat model. Bone 36(5):770–778

Magetsari R, Dewo P, Saputro BK, [illegible] (2014) Cinnamon Oil and Chitosan Coating on Orthopaedic Implant Surface for Prevention of Staphylococcus Epidermidis Biofilm Formation. Malays Orthop J 8(3):11–14

Martynkova GS, Valaskova M (2014) Antimicrobial nanocomposites based on natural modified materials: A review of carbons and clays. J Nanosci Nanotechnol 14:673–693

Massè A, Bruno A, Bosetti M, Biasibetti A, Cannas M, Gallinaro P (2000) Prevention of pin track infection in external fixation with silver coated pins: clinical and microbiological results. J Biomed Mater Res 53(5):600–604

Matl FD, Obermeier A, Repmann S et al (2008) New anti-infective coatings of medical implants. Antimicrob Agents Chemother 52(6):1957–1963

Matl FD, Zlotnyk J, Obermeier A, Friess W, Vogt S, Büchner H, Schnabelrauch H, Stemberger A, Kühn KD (2009) New anti-infective coatings of surgical sutures based on a combination of antiseptics and fatty acids. J Biomater Sci Polym Ed 20(10):1439–1449

Metsemakers WJ, Emanuel N, Cohen O, Reichart M, Potapova I, Schmid T, Segal D, Riool M, Kwakman PH, de Boer L, de Breij A, Nibbering PH, Richards RG, Zaat SA, Moriarty TF (2015) A doxycycline-loaded polymer-lipid encapsulation matrix coating for the prevention of implant-related osteomyelitis due to doxycycline-resistant methicillin-resistant Staphylococcus aureus. J Control Release 209:47–56

Muszanska AK, Rochford ET, Gruszka A, Bastian AA, Busscher HJ, Norde W et al (2014) Antiadhesive polymer brush coating functionalized with antimicrobial and RGD peptides to reduce biofilm formation and enhance tissue integration. Biomacromolecules 15(6):2019–2026

Neoh KG, Kang ET (2011) Combating bacterial colonization on metals via polymer coatings: relevance to marine and medical applications. ACS Appl Mater Interfaces 3(8):2808–2819

Neut D, Dijkstra RJ, Thompson JI, van der Mei HC, Busscher HJ (2012) A gentamicin-releasing coating for cementless hip prostheses-Longitudinal evaluation of efficacy using in vitro bio-optical imaging and its wide-spectrum antibacterial efficacy. J Biomed Mater Res A 100:3220–3226

Neut D, Dijkstra RJ, Thompson JI, Kavanagh C, van der Mei HC, Busscher HJ (2015) A biodegradable gentamicin-hydroxyapatite-coating for infection prophylaxis in cementless hip prostheses. Eur Cell Mater 29:42–55

Norowski PA, Courtney HS, Babu J, Haggard WO, Bumgardner JD (2011) Chitosan coatings deliver antimicrobials from titanium implants: a preliminary study. Implant Dent 20(1):56–67

Obermeier A, Matl FD, Schwabe J, Zimmermann A, Kühn KD, Lakemeier SV, Eisenhart-Rothe R, Stemberger A, Burgkart R (2012) Novel fatty acid gentamicin salts as slow-release drug carrier systems for anti-infective protection of vascular biomaterials. J Mater Sci Mater Med 23(7):1675–1683

Obermeier A, Schneider J, Wehner S, Matl FD, Schieker M, von Eisenhart-Rothe R, Stemberger A, Burgkart R (2014) Novel high efficient coatings for anti-microbial surgical sutures using chlorhexidine in fatty acid slow-release carrier systems. PLoS One doi:10.1371/journal.pone.0101126

Obermeier A, Schneider J, Föhr P, Wehner S, Kühn KD, Stemberger A, Schieker M, Burgkart R (2015) In vitro evaluation of novel antimicrobial coatings for surgical sutures using octenidine. BMC Microbiology doi:10.1186/s12866-015-0523-4

Onaizi SA, Leong SSJ (2011) Tethering Antimicrobial Peptides. Biotech Advances 29(1):67–74

Overstreet D, McLaren A, Calara F, Vernon B, McLemore R (2015) Local gentamicin delivery from resorbable viscous hydrogels is therapeutically effective. Clin Orthop Relat Res 473(1):337–347

Page K, Wilson M, Parkin IP (2009) Antimicrobial surfaces and their potential in reducing the role of the inanimate environment in the incidence of hospital-acquired infections. J Mater Chem 19:3819–3831

Pandit V, Zuidema JM, Venuto KN, Macione J, Dai G, Gilbert RJ et al (2013) Evaluation of multifunctional polysaccharide hydrogels with varying stiffness for bone tissue engineering. Tissue Eng Part A 19(21–22):2452–2463

Parvizi J, Saleh KJ, Ragland PS, Pour AE, Mont MA (2008) Efficacy of antibiotic-impregnated cement in total hip replacement. Acta Orthop 79(3):335–341

Pérez-Anes A, Gargouri M, Laure W, Van Den Berghe H, Courcot E, Sobocinski J, Tabary N, Chai F, Blach JF, Addad A, Woisel P, Douroumis D,Martel B, Blanchemain N, Lyskawa J (2015) Bioinspired Titanium Drug Eluting Platforms Based on a Poly-β-cyclodextrin-Chitosan Layer-by-Layer Self-Assembly Targeting Infections ACS Appl Mater Interfaces 7(23):12882–12893

Petrini P, Arciola CR, Pezzali I, Bozzini S, Montanaro L, Tanzi MC, Speziale P, Visai L (2006) Antibacterial activity of zinc modified titanium oxide surface. Int J Artif Organs 29:434–442

Pitarresi G, Palumbo FS, Calascibetta F, Fiorica C, Di Stefano M, Giammona G (2013) Medicated hydrogels of hyaluronic acid derivatives for use in orthopedic field. Int J Pharm 449(1–2):84–94

Qayyum S, Khan AU (2016) Nanoparticles vs. biofilms: a battle against another paradigm of antibiotic resistance. MedChemComm 7(8):1479–1498

Renoud P, Toury B, Benayoun S, Attik G, Grosgogeat B (2012) Functionalization of titanium with chitosan via silanation: evaluation of biological and mechanical performances. PloS one doi:10.1371/journal.pone.0039367

Rivardo F, Turner RJ, Allegrone G, Ceri H, Martinotti MG (2009) Anti-adhesion activity of two biosurfactants produced by Bacillus spp. prevents biofilm formation of human bacterial pathogens. Appl Microbiol Biotechnol 83:541–553

Rodrigues L, Banat IM, Teixeira J, Oliveira R (2006) Biosurfactants: potential applications in medicine. J Antimicrob Chemother 57:609–618

Rodríguez-Valencia C, López-Álvarez M, Cochón-Cores B, Pereiro I, Serra J, González P (2013) Novel selenium-doped hydroxyapatite coatings for biomedical applications. J Biomed Mater 101(3):853–861

Rule KL, Ebbett VR, Vikesland PJ (2005) Formation of chloroform and chlorinated organics by free-chlorine-mediated oxidation of triclosan. Environ Sci Technol 39(9): 3176–3185

Ruther C, Gabler C, Ewald H, Ellenrieder M, Haenle M, Lindner T, Mittelmeier W, Bader R, Kluess D (2014) In vivo monitoring of implant osseointegration in a rabbit model using acoustic sound analysis. Journal of Orthopaedic Research 32(4):606–612

Schmidmaier G, Lucke M, Wildemann B, Haas NP, Raschke M (2006) Prophylaxis and treatment of implant-related infections by antibiotic-coated implants: A review. Injury 37:S105–S112

Shchukin D, Mohwald H (2013) Materials science. A coat of many functions. Science 341(6153):1458–1459

Shida T, Koseki H, Yoda I, Horiuchi H, Sakoda H, Osaki M (2013) Adherence ability of Staphylococcus epidermidis on prosthetic biomaterials: an in vitro study. Int J Nanomedicine 8:3955–3961

Shirai T, Tsuchiya H, Shimizu T, Ohtani K, Zen Y, Tomita K (2009) Prevention of pin tract infection with titanium-copper alloys. J Biomed Mater Res B Appl Biomater 91(1):373–380

Shirai T, Shimizu T, Ohtani K, Zen Y, Takaya M, Tsuchiya H (2011) Antibacterial iodine-supported titanium implants. Acta Biomater 7(4):1928–1933

Shirai T, Tsuchiya H, Nishida H, Yamamoto N, Watanabe K, Nakase J, Terauchi R, Arai Y, Fujiwara H, Kubo T (2014) Antimicrobial megaprostheses supported with iodine. J Biomater Appl 29(4):617–623

Shirai T, Tsuchiya H, Terauchi R, Tsuchida S, Mizoshiri N, Igarashi K, Miwa S, Takeuchi A, Kimura H, Hayashi K, Yamamoto N, Kubo T (2016) The outcomes of reconstruction using frozen autograft combined with iodine-coated implants for malignant bone tumors: compared with non-coated implants. Jpn J Clin Oncol 46(8):735–740

Singh AV, Vyas V, Patil R, Sharma V, Scopelliti PE, Bongiorno G et al (2011) Quantitative characterization of the influence of the nanoscale morphology of nanostructured surfaces on bacterial adhesion and biofilm formation. PloS one doi:10.1371/journal.pone.0025029

Song Z, Borgwardt L, Høiby N, Wu H, Sørensen TS, Borgwardt A (2013) Prosthesis infections after orthopedic joint replacement: the possible role of bacterial biofilms. Orthopedic reviews (Pavia) 5(2):65–71

Sörensen JH, Lilja M, Sörensen TC, Åstrand M, Procter P, Fuchs S, Strømme M, Steckel H (2014) Biomechanical and antibacterial properties of Tobramycin loaded hydroxyapatite coated fixation pins. J Biomed Mater Res B Appl Biomater. 102(7):1381–1392

Stallard CP, McDonnell KA, Onayemi OD, O'Gara JP, Dowling DP (2012) Evaluation of protein adsorption on atmospheric plasma deposited coatings exhibiting superhydrophilic to superhydrophobic properties. Biointerphases 7(1–4):31

Stewart PS, Costerton JW (2001) Antibiotic resistance of bacteria in biofilms. The lancet 358(9276):135–138

Subbiahdoss G, Kuijer R, Grijpma DW, van der Mei HC, Busscher HJ (2009) Microbial biofilm growth vs. tissue integration: »The race for the surface« experimentally studied. Acta Biomaterialia 5(5):1399–1404

Tang Y, Zhao Y, Wang H, Gao Y, Liu X, Wang X et al (2012) Layer-by-layer assembly of antibacterial coating on interbonded 3D fibrous scaffolds and its cytocompatibility assessment. J Biomed Mater Res A 100:2071–2078

Thallinger B, Prasetyo EN, Nyanhongo GS, Guebitz GM (2013) Antimicrobial enzymes: an emerging strategy to fight microbes and microbial biofilms. Biotechnology journal 8(1):97–109

Thull R (2004) Implantatoberfläche und Biofilm. In: Hendricht C, Frommelt L, Eulert J (eds) Septische Knochen- und Gelenkchirurgie, Springer Verlag, Heidelberg, p 203–210

Tran PA, Webster TJ (2011) Selenium nanoparticles inhibit Staphylococcus aureus growth. Int J Nanomed 6:1553–1558

Truong VK, Lapovok R, Estrin YS, Rundell S, Wang JY, Fluke CJ, Crawford RJ, Ivanova EP (2010) The influence of nanoscale surface roughness on bacterial adhesion to ultrafine-grained titanium. Biomaterials 31(13):3674–3683

Tsibouklis J, Stone M, Thorpe AA, Graham P, Nevell TG, Ewen RJ (2000). Inhibiting bacterial adhesion onto surfaces: the non-stick coating approach. International Journal of Adhesion and Adhesives 20(2):91–96

Tsuchiya H, Shirai T, Nishida H, Murakami H, Kabata T, Yamamoto N et al (2012) Innovative antimicrobial coating of titanium implants with iodine. J Orthop Sci 17(5):595–604

Vogt S, Kühn KD, Gopp U, Schnabelrauch M (2005) Resorbable antibiotic coatings for bone substitutes and implantable devices. Materialwissenschaft und Werkstofftechnik 36:814–819

von Eiff C, Jansen B, Kohnen W, Becker K (2005) Infections Associated with Medical Devices: Pathogenesis, Management and Prophylaxis. Drugs 65(2):179–214

Wafa H, Grimer RJ, Reddy K, Jeys L, Abudu A, Carter SR, Tillman RM (2015) Retrospective evaluation of the incidence of early periprosthetic infection with silver-treated endoprostheses in high-risk patients: case-control study. Bone Joint J. 97–B(2):252–257

Wahlig H, Buchholz HW (1972) Experimental and clinical studies on the release of gentamicin from bone cement. Chirurg 43:441–445

Warren DK, Quadir WW, Hollenbeak CS, Elward AM, Cox MJ, Fraser VJ (2006) Attributable cost of catheter-associated bloodstream infections among intensive care patients in a nonteaching hospital. Crit Care Med 34(8):2084–2089
Wilding CP, Cooper GA, Freeman AK, Parry MC, Jeys L (2016) Can a Silver-Coated Arthrodesis Implant Provide a Viable Alternative to Above Knee Amputation in the Unsalvageable, Infected Total Knee Arthroplasty? J Arthroplasty 31(11):2542–2547
Xue C, Jia S, Zhang J, Ma J (2010) Large-area fabrication of superhydrophobic surfaces for practical applications: an overview. Sci Tech Adv Mat 11(3):1–15
Yamamura K, Iwata H, Yotsuyanagi T (1992) Synthesis of antibiotic-loaded hydroxyapatite beads and in vitro drug release testing. J Biomed Mater Res 26(8):1053–1064
Yount NY, Yeaman MR (2012) Emerging themes and therapeutic prospects for anti-infective peptides. Annu Rev Pharmacol Toxicol 52:337–360
Zhang F, Zhang Z, Zhu X, Kang ET, Neoh KG (2008) Silk-functionalized titanium surfaces for enhancing osteoblast functions and reducing bacterial adhesion. Biomaterials 29:4751–4759
Zhao C, Li X, Li L, Cheng G, Gong X, Zheng J (2013) Dual functionality of antimicrobial and antifouling of poly(N-hydroxyethylacrylamide)/salicylate hydrogels. Langmuir 29(5):1517–1524
Zhou B, Li Y, Deng H, Hu Y, Li B (2014) Antibacterial multilayer films fabricated by layer-by-layer immobilizing lysozyme and gold nanoparticles on nanofibers. Colloids Surf B Biointerfaces 116:432–438
Zhu H, Guo Z, Liu W (2014) Adhesion behaviors on superhydrophobic surfaces. Chem Commun 50(30):3900–3913

Servicepart

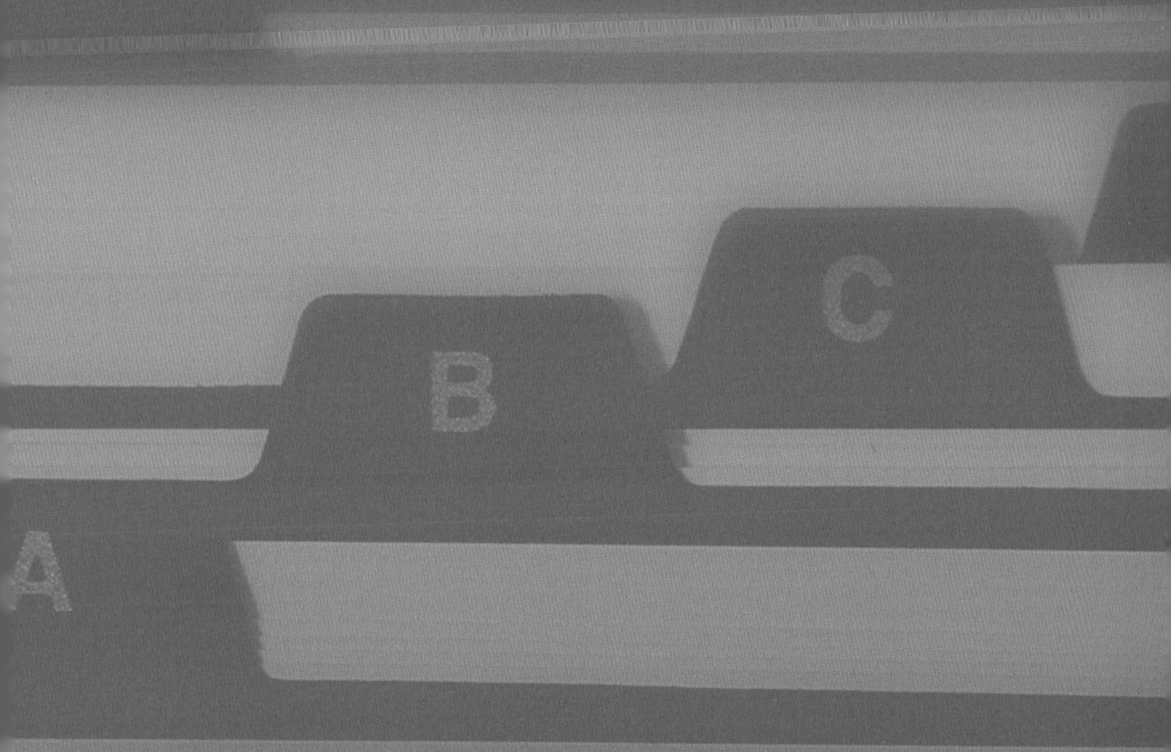

K.-D. Kühn (Ed.), *Management of Periprosthetic Joint Infection*
DOI 10.1007/978-3-662-54469-3

Subject Index

D

E

F

G

H

I

O

P

Q

R

S

T

U

V

W

X

Z